Celia Reed.

Drug Metabolism —
from Molecules to Man

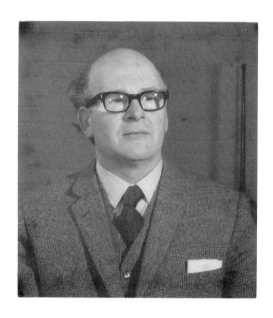

Dedicated to Professor Dennis Parke
in recognition of his extensive
contributions to the field of drug
metabolism

Drug Metabolism — from Molecules to Man

Edited by

D. J. Benford, J.W. Bridges and G.G. Gibson

University of Surrey, UK

Taylor & Francis
London, New York, Philadelphia
1987

UK Taylor & Francis Ltd, 4 John St, London WC1N 2ET

USA Taylor & Francis Inc., 242 Cherry St, Philadelphia,
PA 19106-1906

British Library Cataloguing in Publication Data

Drug metabolism from molecules to man.
   1. Drugs — Metabolism
   I. Benford, D.   II. Bridges, J.W.
   III. Gibson, G. Gordon
   615'.7   RM301.55

   ISBN 0-85066-373-3

**Library of Congress Cataloging-in-Publication Data
is available**

*Printed in Great Britain by WBC Print Ltd,
Bristol, Avon.*

CONTENTS LIST

PREFACE

The European Drug Metabolism Workshops began at the University of Surrey, Guildford, UK, in 1970. Since then Workshops have been held in Guildford (1971), Tubingen (1972), Mainz (1974), Stockholm (1976), Leiden (1978), Zurich (1980), Liege (1982), Nancy (1984). From the moment the concept of a workshop was proposed Professor Dennis Parke who was Head of the Biochemistry Department at Surrey, provided the strong encouragement and practical support which was crucial in getting it underway. It was therefore particularly appropriate that the Tenth European Drug Metabolism Workshop should be held at Guildford in honour of Professor Parke.

Professor Parke's contributions to the field of drug metabolism are immense. In addition to his many important research contributions (which number over 300 publications) and the key role he played in the Drug Metabolism Workshops he founded the first journal dedicated to drug metabolism, Xenobiotica, of which he remains the Editor. He also started the still thriving section of Pharmacological Biochemistry of the Biochemical Society (UK) and began the first taught postgraduate degree course in the world in Toxicology. This course lays strong emphasis on the molecular basis of toxicity and incorporates a major element of instruction on the principles of drug metabolism.

Professor Parke's career in drug metabolism began when he joined Professor R. T. Williams' Department at St Mary's Hospital Medical School in 1949 as a Research Assistant. He was one of the earliest workers to use radiolabelled substrates to study the metabolic fate of chemicals, in this case benzene and aniline. During the fifties and early sixties he was involved in establishing with others a firm scientific basis both in the technical and structure activity aspects of in vivo drug metabolism studies. As a natural outcome of his increasing interests in biochemistry during the sixties and early seventies the emphasis of his research shifted progressively to in vitro based investigations of drug metabolism pathways and particularly to the identification of the role of cytochrome P450 in chemical toxicity and the influences on factors which modify P450 activity. In the last few years he has initiated an entirely new phase of drug metabolism studies namely computer modelling of substrate enzyme interactions again using cytochrome P450 as the model. A consistent hallmark of Dennis Parke's work has been his outstanding ability to link fundamental discoveries to practical human medicine and to communicate to scientists and laymen alike the excitement of his subject.

He has been a true visionary for his subject, never afraid to challenge existing dogma or to adopt new techniques and approaches to investigate problems. Dennis Parkes' very positive approach, enormous span of knowledge and willingness to discuss research ideas and to help others has never faltered and has been an inspiration to all who have been involved with him. The large number of his PhD students who have gone on to hold senior positions in academia, industry and govenment departments all over the world is a continuing record of his great achievements as a teacher. He has dedicated much time to helping developing countries both in establishing research activities and in practical advice on chemical safety. Some measure of the respect in which his judgement is held is reflected in the very impressive list of major national and international committees on which he has served. These include:

Member of the Committee of Safety on Drugs, U.K., 1968-70; Committee on Safety of Medicines, U.K., 1970-83. Member of Committee on Medical Aspects of Chemicals in Food and the Environment, Department of Health and Social Security, U.K., 1972-. Member of the Biology committee, 1970-76, and Life Sciences Committee, Ministry of Defence, U.K., 1978-1984. Member of Food Additives and Contaminants Committee, Ministry of Agriculture, Fisheries and Food, 1972-78. Member of the Council and Medical and Scientific Committee, Marie Curie Memorial Foundation 1970-. WHO Expert Panel on Food Additives, 1975- ;Joint FAO/WHO Committee on Pesticide Residues, Geneva, 1975- ; WHO Scientific Group on Toxicity Evaluation of Chemicals, 1975-76; WHO Consultant on Industrial Toxicology, Poland, 1974, 1978, 1980, 1982; WHO Consultant on Environmental Health, Vienna, 1983; British Council Consultant on Toxicology DSIR, India, 1976; Member of Advisory Committee for Center of Toxicology, Ontario, Canada; U.K., 1977; Member of the British National Committee on Pharmacology 1976-81; Member of SGOMSEC (WHO and SCOPE), 1978- ; Member of the Expert Committee of Pathologists and Toxicologists, ILSI, Washington, 1978-1982.

Although Dennis Parke is stepping down from the Headship of the Biochemistry Department of the University of Surrey in 1987, no one should presume that this means a lessening of commitment to drug metabolism research. Although his research into computer modelling of the drug metabolising enzymes is still at an early stage his determination to open another new and exciting chapter in drug metabolism is as strong as ever.

We look forward to Dennis' continued involvement with drug metabolism for many years to come.

We hope that this volume will make a worthy and fitting tribute to Professor Dennis Parke. In addition to identifying recent advances in specific aspects of drug metabolism we believe that the book will be useful in providing an overview of the growing importance of the subject and give valuable pointers to likely future developments.

D. J. Benford	J. W. Bridges
M. D. Burke	G. M. Cohen
C. R. Elcombe	G. G. Gibson
J. D. Houston	M. J. Humphrey
L. J. King	B. G. Lake
C. R. Wolf	

ACKNOWLEDGEMENTS

The editors would like to thank the other members of the DMW '86 Organising Committee for their assistance in compiling the scientific programme which has resulted in a rather comprehensive analysis of the 'state of the art' from both theoretical and practical viewpoints.

In addition we would particularly like to express our sincere gratitude to the typists - Michele Brookes and Sally Coel - for their long hours spent producing the final copy for this volume and the great care they have taken with it.

D.J. Benford
J.W. Bridges
G.G. Gibson

1. Drug metabolizing enzymes at the molecular level.

SIMILARITIES AND DIFFERENCES IN PROPERTIES BETWEEN CONSTITUTIVE FORMS OF CYTOCHROME P-450

John B. Schenkman[1], Leonard V. Favreau[1], Ingela Jansson[1] and John E. Mole[2]

[1]Department of Pharmacology, University of Connecticut Health Center, Farmington, CT 06032, USA and [2]Department of Biochemistry, University of Massachusetts Medical School,Worcester,MA01605, USA.

INTRODUCTION

In interactions with the environment, the animal is continuously exposed to various chemicals and compounds of biological or man-made origin. Many of these compounds are hydrophobic in nature and thus require a means of modification to enhance their excretion from the body. A number of enzymes have evolved for this task (Table 1) and involve four basic reactions : the hydrolytic enzymes cleave esters and amides to release masked functional groups, reductive and oxidative enzymes alter and create new functional groups on compounds and conjugative enzymes couple compounds of endogenous origin, products of intermediary metabolism, to the chemicals and compounds to be eliminated.

Table 1. Enzymes of Drug Metabolism

Hydrolytic	Oxidative
Reductive	Conjugative

By and large these are the major routes utilized by the animal to remove unwanted chemicals from the body and constitute the pathways of drug metabolism. As the reader is no doubt aware, each of these major pathways has a number of enzymes catalyzing a number of reactions typical of that pathway. In the presentations to follow you will learn more about the enzymes of drug metabolism and in particular about enzymes of the oxidative and the conjugative pathways, two pathways of major importance in the body.

The oxidative pathway contains a number of enzymes responsible for drug metabolism, including a class of enzymes termed cytochrome P-450. A number of cytochrome P-450 enzymes are known, the majority observed to be elevated (induced) in the liver microsomal fraction by prior treatment of animals with one chemical or another. Our own interest has been in the constitutive forms of cytochrome P-450, those forms commonly present in the animal that has not been pretreated with xenobiotics. The rest of my presentation is concerned with these P-450 enzymes.

RESULTS AND DISCUSSION

Early attempts to isolate constitutive forms of cytochrome P-450 were slowed by the low levels of these forms in the microsomes. However success came with the isolation of RLM3 and RLM5 (Cheng and Schenkman, 1982) two forms with considerable homology in the N-terminal amino acid partial sequence (Table 2). Subsequently, RLM2, RLM4 and RML6 were isolated (Schenkman et al., 1982). Characteristics of RLM2 (Jansson et al., 1985a, 1985b) as well as RLM5a (Jansson et al., 1985b, Schenkman, et al., 1986) the latter previously isolated as PBRLM4 in phenobarbital-induced rats (Backes et al., 1985) are shown. FRLM4 was isolated from microsomes of female rats and studied (Schenkman et al., 1986). RML6 and RLM5b, new forms isolated by this laboratory, will be described elsewhere.

Table 2 shows a comparison of the characteristics of the different cytochrome P-450 enzymes. The constitutive forms RLM2, 2b, 3, 5, 5a, 5b, and possibly 6 are all found in the liver microsomes of the untreated male rat. In contrast, RLM2b, fRLM4, RLM5a, RLM5b, and possibly RLM6 are found in the untreated female. RLM5a of male and female rat have been compared and found to be the same enzyme as well as to be identical to PBRLM4. Whether its content is increased by phenobarbital has not been determined by this laboratory.

The NH_2-terminal partial amino acid sequence data for P-450 PCN was obtained from Gonzalez et al (1985) and that of P-452 was obtained from Hardwick et al (1986) at the Washington, D.C. ASBC meeting. These forms of cytochrome P-450 are induced respectively by the synthetic steroid pregnenolone 16α-carbonitrile (PCN) and the hypolipidaemic

Table 2. Physical characteristics of constitutive and some inducible forms of cytochrome P-450 from rat liver microsomes.

TABLE II

PHYSICAL CHARACTERISTICS OF CONSTITUTIVE AND SOME INDUCIBLE FORMS OF CYTOCHROME P-450 FROM RAT LIVER MICROSOMES

SUB-GROUP	ENZYME	PI	M$_R$	B5 STIM.	PEAK (FE^{2+} CO)
I	P-452	7.9	51.5	( )	452
	RLM2	7.3	49.0	(-)	449
	RLM2B	>8	49.0	(-)	452
II	RLM3	7.1	51.0	(-)	449
	FRLM4	7.6	51.3	(-)	449
	RLM5	7.4	52.0	(+)	451
III	RLM5B	>8	52.5	(-)	447.5
	RLM5A/PBRLM4	7.6	52.5	(+)	452
	P-450 PCN		51.0	( )	450
	RLM6	7.9	53.0	( )	451

NH$_2$-TERMINAL PARTIAL AMINO ACID SEQUENCES

P-452 DATA FROM HARDWICK, ET AL., 1986.
P-450 PCN DATA FROM GONZALEZ, ET AL., 1985.

drug clofibrate respectively. RLM6 is a form we recently
isolated from liver microsomes of streptozotocin diabetic
rats. As will be described elsewhere, this form appears to
increase during diabetes and to return to initial levels
upon administration of insulin to the rats.

It is at once apparent from Table 2 that all the
constitutive forms of cytochrome P-450 (2, 2b, 3, f4, 5,
5a, 5b) belong to the same gene family; they demonstrate an
extensive homology just in the amino terminal first 20
amino acid residues. All of these have a methionine
residue in position 1 and leucine in position 7.
Thereafter, homologies are still seen but three subgroups
are differentiated. Subgroup 1 seems to have split off
earliest and to embrace RLM2 and RLM2b (in our earliest
report RLM2 was called RLM2a, Schenkman et al., 1982, but
later was named RLM2, Jansson et al., 1985). RLM2 and
RLM2b have the same NH_2-terminal amino acid sequence,
differing only in residue 19 in the first 20 residues.
That residue in RLM2b resembles residue 19 of the Group II
cytochromes P-450, i.e. RLM3, fRLM4 and RLM5. Group II and
III cytochromes P-450 differ from Group I by having
aspartate as residue 2 instead of leucine and leucine as
residues 9, 14 and 16 instead of valine, serine and serine
respectively and leucine and tryptophan at positions 17 and
20 instead of valine and leucine respectively. Groups II
and III subdivide on the basis of amino acid sequence as
well. Thus, Group II has proline as residue 3 and leucine
as residue 15 instead of leucine and isoleucine
respectively. Group II also have valine for residue 6.
Thereafter, overlaps appear respectively for individual
members of the two groups. Thus Group III enzymes have
serine for residues 13 and 18 while only RLM5 also has
serine at these positions. Both fRLM4 and RLM5b have
serine at position 12, RML5b but not RLM5a have this
homology. Also, both RLM5a and RLM5b have threonine at
position 10, as does RLM5, but RLM3 and fRLM4 have serine.
Finally, except for fRLM4, all members of Group II and III
have valine at position 4; fRML4 has phenylalanine.

Attempts have been made to determine when certain of
the induced forms of cytochrome P-450 evolved from each
other (Kimura et al., 1984; Nebert and Gonzalez, 1985).
Based upon the above sequence overlaps, Groups II and III
may have evolved from each other much more recently than
did Group I enzymes.

More detailed nucleotide sequence data will be needed
to estimate structural similarities and differences between
the proteins. However, assuming the constitutive
cytochromes P-450 represent a single gene family, it is of

interest to determine relatedness of some of the inducible forms of cytochrome P-450 to these proteins on the sole basis of amino terminal amino acid sequence. On that basis, the 3-methylcholanthrene-inducible form of cytochrome P-450, P-450c, held no discernable relationship, perhaps in agreement with estimates of its evolving hundreds of million years ago from some ancestral gene (Nebert and Gonzalez, 1985). In contrast, the phenobarbital inducible forms of cytochrome P-450, PBRLM5, PBRLM6 and PBRLM7, all of which possess identical amino-terminal amino acid sequence for the first 40 residues (Backes et al., 1985) showed considerable homology with Group II of the constitutive cytochromes P-450. The sequence MEPSILLLLALLVGFLLLLV shows homology in 8 of the 20 initial residues (40%) of Group II enzymes, too many to merely be coincidental. Since there are 20 amino acids, if we assume a random arrangement we could expect about 20^{20} or 2×10^{21} possible arrangements of amino acids. That 40% of the N-terminal sequence of the phenobarbital inducible form exhibits homology in these first 20 residues indicates this is not coincidental. In contrast, the homology with enzymes of Groups I and III are 25% and 30% respectively. If the degree of homology is any indication, the phenobarbital inducible forms of P-450 evolved from the Group II subfamily before Group III split off, the latter having a 65% homology with Group II. Since there is only 15% homology between Group I and II (residues 1, 7 and 15) although partial overlap with residues 8 and 19 exist, the phenobarbital inducible form must have evolved much later from Group II-III before these latter evolved apart.

We can compare other inducible forms of cytochrome P-450 with these three constitutive subgroups. A form of cytochrome P-450, P-452 has been shown to be induced by pretreatment of rats with the hypolipidaemic agents clofibrate and ciprofibrate (Gibson et al., 1982; Tamburini et al., 1984). The NH_2-terminal partial amino acid sequence of this cytochrome P-450 enzyme (Hardwick et al., 1986) puts it in the Group I constitutive P-450 subfamily with a 25% homology with the group.

PCN, a synthetic steroid, induces a different cytochrome P-450 mono-oxygenase activity (Lu et al., 1972) which has been shown on purification to be due to a distinctly different form of P-450 from other inducible forms (Elshourbagy and Guzelian, 1980). The amino terminal partial amino acid sequence of this enzyme (Gonzalez et al., 1985) suggests (Table 2) that this form of P-450 evolved from the constitutive family of cytochrome P-450, probably Group III, but equally possibly Group II. A related, but different form of the PCN-induced enzyme, P-450p, has the NH_2-amino acid sequence MDLIFMLQTSSLA (Wrighton et al., 1985). While RLM5a and RLM5b share an 80% homology with each other at the NH_2-terminal end shown, P-450 PCN has a 35% homology with Group III. Its homology with Group II is also 35%. Members of Group II have greater than 65% homology within the Group II amino terminal sequence (Table 2) if partially variable regions are ignored. In contrast, P-450 PCN exhibits only a 15% homology with the sequence of the Group I subfamily.

The constitutive forms of cytochrome P-450 appear to be under homeostatic control. RLM6 responds to the hormone insulin; its presence is suppressed by insulin and it is elevated during diabetes (Favreau, Mallkoff, Mole and Schenkman, manuscript in preparation). In contrast, RLM2, 3 and 5 respond to male hormone. From its amino-terminal partial amino acid sequence it would appear that RLM6 evolved early from a constitutive form of cytochrome P-450 in Subgroup III, with which it exhibits a 20% homology; its homology with Subgroup II is only 15% and with Subgroup I is 0%. Of interest, RLM6 exhibits a 25% homology with the P-450 PCN NH_2-terminal sequence mainly in regions exhibiting variability between subfamilies. From the fairly low (20%) level of homology between Group III and RLM6, it is possible that this reflects an earlier evolution from Group III of this form of cytochrome P-450. Its homology with P-450 PCN at residues 12, 13 and 18 as well as 3 and 9 suggest both of these forms may fit in a separate inducible P-450 family, the characteristics of which remain to be elucidated. Like RLM6, P-450 PCN appears to be present in low levels in untreated rats.

At this point, it might be appropriate to consider the physical properties of these cytochromes P-450. As seen in Table 2, the different forms when reduced and complexed with carbon monoxide absorb maximally at wavelengths ranging from 447.5nm to 452nm. Nothing consistent with subfamily is seen in this characteristic. The minimal molecular weights as determined by SDS-PAGE likewise provide no predictive information about the forms of P-450. Some of the forms exhibit neutral isoelectric points and some are slightly basic proteins. Of these forms of cytochrome P-450, only RLM5 and RLM5a undergo appreciable spin shift of the ferric hemoprotein on addition of cytochrome b_5 (Jansson et al., 1985b) or a significant increase in reduction or turnover rates.

The individual forms of cytochrome P-450 described in Table 2 show considerable epitopic similarity when tested with polyclonal rabbit or goat antibodies. When viewed in

Ouchterlony double diffusion plates all of the antibodies showed white precipitin bands only to the inducing antigen except for anti RLM3 which also formed a precipitin band to RLM5b. On staining, with Coomassie Blue stain, other faint precipitin bands were seen. Using the more sensitive Western Blot procedure, the polyclonals, except for RLM6, were found to recognise all of the forms of P-450. In contrast, RLM6 antibody only showed recognition to RLM6. Table 3 shows the results of an ELISA of the immuno-relatedness of the constitutive forms of cytochrome P-450.

Table 3. Cross-Reactivity of Polyclonal Antibodies to Constitutive Cytochromes P-450 as Determined by an ELISA

	Relative Absorbance at 405nm				
Antigen	Anti-RLM3	Anti-RLM5	Anti-RLM5a	Anti-RLM5b	Anti-RLM6
RLM2	.48	.16	.02	.39	.06
RLM3	1.00	.63	.55	.87	.52
fRLM4	.76	.55	.39	.62	.43
RLM5	.72	1.00	.40	.71	.10
RLM5a	.73	.58	1.00	.75	.60
RLM5b	.66	.34	.38	1.00	.49
RLM6	.68	.16	.12	.59	1.00

All of the activities are relative to recognition of the antigen used to produce the individual antibodies. In each case the antibodies show considerable recognition of other forms of P-450. Thus, antibodies raised to RLM3 and RLM5b reacted strongly with all of the forms of P-450. RLM2 and RLM6 exhibited the least cross-reactivity with the different antibodies; RLM6 did not cross-react to any extent with antibodies raised to RLM5a, and similarly RLM2 did not cross-react with antibodies raised to RLM5, RLM5a, or RLM6 (Table 3).

As a further indication of antigenic similarity between the forms of cytochrome P-450, monoclonal antibodies to various induced forms of cytochrome P-450 generously provided by Dr. Harry Gelboin were tested against five of the constitutive forms of P-450 (Table 4).

Schenkman et al.

Table 4. Western Blot Staining for Antigen Recognition by Mono-Clonal Antibodies

Antibody	RLM2	RLM3	fRLM4	RLM5	RLM5a
Goat anti RLM5	+++	+++	++++	+++++	++++
RLM5 1-68-11	tr	tr	tr	+	tr
MC 1-31-2	0	0	0	0	0
MC 1- 7-1	0	0	0	0	+
PB 2- 8-1	0	0	tr	tr	tr
PB 4-29-5	0	0	0	0	0
PB 2-66-3	+	++	+++	tr	+++
PB4- 7-1	+	1/2 +	1/2 +	++	1/2tr
PCN 2- 3-2	0	0	tr	1/2 +	1/2 +
PCN 2-13-1	0	0	0	0	+

0   = No reaction
tr = barely discernable
+   = weak reaction
++ = good reaction
+++ = strong reaction

The monoclonal antibodies used were the generous gift of Dr. Harry Gelboin.

The data shows the results of semiquantitative Western Blot analysis and a comparison with goat polyclonal anti RLM5 IgG. An anti RLM5 IgM monoclonal antibody preparation showed slight recognition to all of the constitutive forms of P-450 and definite recognition of RLM5. Similarly, 3 or 4 monoclonals against phenobarbital induced P-450 showed some differential recognition of the constitutive forms of P-450. PB 2-66-3 recognised all of the enzymes, but reacted strongly with fRLM4 and RLM5a. In contrast, PB 4-7-1 showed strong reactivity with RLM5 and definite reactivity with RLM2. Two of the monoclonals raised against P-450 PCN showed recognition of the constitutive forms of P-450. PCN 2-13-1 showed definite recognition of RLM5a and the other antibody showed faint reactivities with fRLM4, RLM5 and RLM5a. In contrast, only one of the constitutive forms of P-450 reacted with a MC clone

antibody, albeit weakly; RLM5a showed some interaction with
MC 1-7-1. The results of these and the above studies
strongly indicate considerable homologies exist between
induced forms and the different constitutive forms of
cytochrome P-450.

At this point our interest turned to the function of
the individual constitutive forms of cytochrome P-450. All
of these forms examined metabolise drugs and other
chemicals, but at relative rates differing with the
individual mono-oxygenases and substrates. They differ,
however, with respect to their site specificity for
metabolism of endogenous substrates such as fatty acids,
prostenoids and steroids. In Figure 1 is shown the site
specificities of the different constitutive forms of
cytochrome P-450 toward testosterone.

**Figure 1. Sketch of isomeric sites of hydroxylation of
testosterone by different constitutive cytochrome P-450
enzymes.**

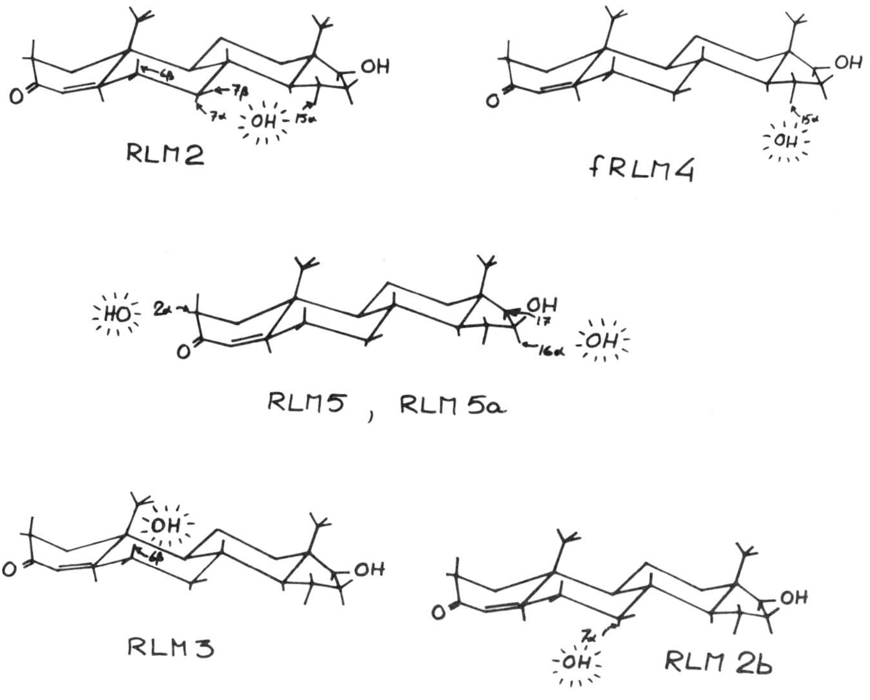

Form 6, which appears to be induced when insulin production and levels are diminished, shows a distinctive difference from the other P-450 enzymes; it is unable to metabolise testosterone at detectable rates.

Note the essential singularity of sites of attack of RLM3, fRML4 and RLM2b. These enzymes are highly specific for a single site of attack, suggesting a fair degree of rigidity in fitting of the substrate in the active site of the enzyme. Such a concept is consistent with crystal structure studies on cytochrome P-450 CAM (Poulos et al., 1985), which suggest substrate is held fairly tightly by hydrophobic as well as by hydrogen bonds in juxta-position to the heme.

If one assumes a similarity between the substrate binding sites of the RLM P-450 enzymes and P-450 CAM, how does one explain the multiplicity of isomeric metabolites produced by RLM2 and RLM5 and RLM5a? With the former enzyme a number of B- and D-ring isomeric sites are hydroxylated. With the latter two enzymes, sites on the A- and D-rings, at opposite ends of the molecule are hydroxylated. One can suggest a mechanism for these observations without evoking suggestions of multiple binding sites, a possibility not consistent with the dissociation constant data and K_m values for testosterone in assays of specific isomeric products with RLM2 (Jansson et al., 1985a) as well as with RLM5. As shown in Figure 2, one can, by the use of 3-dimensional imaging, arrive at an orientation of the steroid relative to a point source (the active oxygen in the figure), using an inverse relationship between distance and rate of hydroxylation of the individual isomeric sites. Such calculations suggest a fairly rigid orientation of the substrate, i.e. little wobble, a conclusion supported by the fairly rigid regiospecificity of the individual P-450 enzymes (Figure 1).

In summary, multiple forms of the cytochrome P-450 enzymes have evolved. These appear to fit in specific families. Thus, one speaks of a polycyclic hydrocarbon-induced gene family of rat P-450 which includes P-450c and P-450d (Nebert and Gonzalez, 1985) and a phenobarbital-inducible gene family, which includes a P-450b and P-450e (PBRLM5 and PBRLM6) and probably also PBRLM7 (Backes et al., 1985), and possibly also a steroid inducible gene family, of which P-450 PCN is a representative. Based upon sequence comparisons of the first 20 amino acids from the NH_2-terminal end, the constitutive family of cytochrome P-450 all have methionine as residue 1 and leucine as residue 7. After this they split into three subgroups, the members

Figure 2. Sketch of possible testosterone orientation in the active site of RLM2.

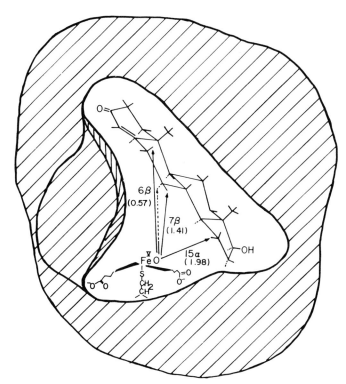

of which demonstrate greater than 65% homology in the first 20 residues within each group. A representative of the phenobarbital inducible family, P-450b, showed more than 40% homology with members of Subgroup II. Clofibrate, a hypolipidaemic drug, induces what may be a different gene-family of P-450. P452, the representative of this potentially new gene family, showed remarkable residue homology with members of Subgroup 1 (25%). By comparison, the representative of the steroid inducible gene family, P-450 PCN, showed about 35% NH_2-terminal sequence homology for the first 20 residues with Subgroup III.

While it is of interest to consider the evolutionary development of these forms of P-450 it must be recognised that such groupings of the P-450 enzymes into different gene families do not reveal anything about the functionality of the enzymes. Despite the similarities of enzymes in any of the designated subgroups their catalytic activities, substrate preferences and site specificities of hydroxylations show marked difference, attesting to major evolutionary alterations of amino acid sequences in locations where the count, i.e. in regions influencing properties of the enzymes, like substrate binding. Why so many constitutive forms of cytochrome P-450 have evolved is a question which must be asked. The answer remains to be found. Perhaps a fertile field to explore will be the biological activity of P-450 hydroxylated steroids and ω- and ω-1 hydroxy fatty acids.

ACKNOWLEDGEMENTS

Supported in part by a grant GM26114 from the US Public Health Service. Parts of this work were made possible by a Stauffer Chemical Company predoctoral fellowship to Leonard V. Favreau.

REFERENCES

Backes, W.L., Jansson, I., Mole, J.E., Gibson, G.G. and Schenkman, J.B. (1985). Pharmacology, 31, 155.
Cheng, K.-C. and Schenkman, J.B. (1982). J. Biol. Chem, 257, 2378.
Elshourbagy, N.A. and Guzelian, P.S. (1980). J. Biol. Chem, 255, 1279.
Gibson, G.G., Orton, T.C. and Tamburini, P.P. (1982). Biochem. J, 203, 161.
Gonzalez, F.J., Nebert, D.W., Hardwick, J.P. and Kasper, C.S. (1985). J. Biol. Chem, 260, 7435.
Hardwick, J.P., Song, B.-J. and Gonzalez, F.J. (1986). Federation Proc, 45, 1855.
Jansson, I., Mole, J.E. and Schenkman, J.B. (1985a). J. Biol. Chem, 260, 7084.
Jansson, I., Tamburini, P.P., Favreau, L.V. and Schenkman, J.B. (1985b). Drug Metab. Disp, 13, 453.
Kimura, S., Gonzalez, F.J. and Nebert, D.W. (1984). J. Biol. Chem, 259, 10705.
Lu, A.Y.H., Somogyi, A., West, S., Kuntzman, R. and Conney, A.H. (1972). Arch. Biochem. Biophys, 152, 457.
Nebert, D.W. and Gonzalez, F.J. (1985). TIPS, April 160.
Poulos, T.L., Finzel, B.C., Gunsalus, I.C., Wagner, G.C. and Kraut, J. (1985). J. Biol. Chem, 260, 16122.
Schenkman, J.B., Jansson, I., Backes, W.L., Cheng, K.-C. and Smith, C. (1982). Biochem. Biophys. Res. Comm, 107, 1517.
Schenkman, J.B., Favreau, L.V., Mole, J., Kreutzer, D.L. and Jansson, I. (1986). Arch. Tox, in press.

Tamburini, P.P., Masson, H.A., Bains, S.K., Makowski, R.J., Morris, B. and Gibson, G.G (1984). Eur. J. Biochem. 139, 235.

Wrighton, S.A., Maurel, P., Schuetz, E.G., Watkins, P.B., Young, B. and Guzelian, P.S. (1985). Biochemistry, 24, 2171.

MOLECULAR ASPECTS OF CYTOCHROME P-450 MONOOXYGENASES : CHARACTERISATION OF SOME CONSTITUTIVELY EXPRESSED FORMS.

C. Roland Wolf[1], Richard Meechan [1,2], M.Danny Burke[3], David J. Adams[1a], Franz Oesch[4], Thomas Friedberg[5a], Milton Adesnik[5] and Nicholas Hastie [2].

[1]Imperial Cancer Research Fund, Laboratory of Molecular Pharmacology, Department of Biochemistry, Edinburgh, UK. [2]MRC, Clinical and Population Cytogenetics Unit, Edinburgh, [3]Department of Pharmacology, University of Aberdeen, [4]Institute of Toxicology, University of Mainz, FRG, [5]Department of Cell Biology, New York University, USA

INTRODUCTION

Mammalian cytochrome P-450's are membrane bound proteins of molecular weight between 48 and 60kD. These enzymes are localised in either the endoplasmic reticulum, or the mitochondria, of almost all tissues but in a cell specific manner. With only one exception, P-450's catalyse monooxygenation reactions as outlined below :

$$RH + O_2 + NADPH + H^+ --------->ROH + NADP^+ + H_2O .....(1)$$

$$R=R' + O_2 + NADPH + H^+ ------->R-R' + NADP^+ + H_2O ...(2)$$

These monooxygenations are central to a wide variety of biological processes. In normal intermediary metabolism such reactions result in the synthesis of steroid hormones, glucocorticoids, dihydroxyvitamin D_3, bile acids and in the oxidation of fatty acids, prostaglandins, leukotrienes and steroid hormones. The other major function of this enzyme system is the metabolism of foreign compounds. As shown in equations 1 and 2 foreign compounds such as drugs and chemical carcinogens can be oxidised at carbon atoms to alcoholic or phenolic products which are in most cases then conjugated and excreted. On the other hand oxidations at carbon atoms can lead to the formation of epoxides, and at heteroatoms such as nitrogen and sulphur to N and S oxides,

[a]Present addresses of DJA and TF are Dept. Microbiology, University of Leeds, and University of Mainz, Institute of Toxicology respectively.

these products are usually more toxic than the parent compound. This metabolite step is an initial event in many chemical-induced toxic reactions and also in carcinogenesis (Wislocki et al., 1980; Wolf, 1982).

Cytochrome P-450's are a supergene family of proteins containing possibly fifty or more genes. These genes can be divided into subfamilies[b] based either on structural homology or chromosomal localisation (Adesnik and Atchison 1986; Wolf, 1986). The development of recombinant DNA techniques has brought tremendous advances in our understanding of cell biology. The application of thee techniques to the cytochrome P-450 area have also markedly increased our knowledge of this complex enzyme system. Some of the areas in which progress has been made are outlined below.

CYTOCHROME P-450 EVOLUTION

Cytochrome P-450 can be detected in all living organisms including bacteria and therefore appears to have developed at a very early time. It is tempting to speculate that this enzyme may have evolved as a mechanism for the conversion of inert hydrocarbons within the environment to products such as alcohols, which could then be usefully used by cells to produce energy. Indeed, certain yeasts which grow on hydrocarbons as the sole energy source do so because of P-450's which catalyse such reactions. An alternative role of the ancestral gene stems from the finding that cytochrome P-450 has peroxidase activity and can convert organic hydroperoxides to alcohols. The removal of toxic hydroperoxides by this mechanism may have been important for primitive organisms which used oxygen in cellular respiration.

The role of P-450's in the detoxification and elimination of foreign compounds is a less likely function of the ancestral gene. However, a large number of cytochrome P-450 isozymes have evolved which are active in foreign compound metabolism. The vast variety of structurally diverse molecules which this enzyme system needs to metabolise provides a reason why many P-450 isozymes have evolved, the generation of new P-450 forms with new substrate specificities being a basis for selective advantage.

[b]A cytochrome P-450 subfamily has been loosely defined here as proteins with either a high degree of structural homology or genes that map to the same chromosome.

Wolf et al.

The use of recombinant DNA techniques to determine the genomic structure and protein sequence of P-450 genes has given valuable information about how the multigene subfamilies evolved. In the rest of this article only the cytochrome P-450's which have been shown to be active against foreign compounds will be discussed.

Some cytochrome P-450 subfamilies are listed in Table 1.

Table 1. Some Cytochrome P-450 Subfamilies in Mouse and Human

| | Mouse | | Human | |
	Location	Number of Genes	Location	Number of Genes
PB_1	(19)	8-9	10	2-3
PB_2	?	?	?	?
PB_3	7	8-9	19	2-3
MC_1	9	2	15	2
PCN	6	6	?	?

PB = subfamilies contain members inducible with phenobarbital; MC = 3-methylcholanthrene-inducible; PCN = inducible with pregnenolone-16α-carbonitrile; ? = unknown.

The number of genes is probably the minimum number. The chromosomal assignments are reviwed (Adesnik and Atchison 1986) with the exception of the human assignment of PB_3 (Wainwright et al, 1985), MC_1 (Hildebrand et al, 1986) and PB_1 (unpublished).

On the basis of our findings and published literature we have divided proteins which contain members inducible by phenobarbital into three groups. The PB_1 subgroup which is marginally inducible by phenobarbital in the rat has approximately 50% structural homology to PB_3 (Adesnik and Atchison, 1986, Friedberg et al, 1986). PB_3 proteins are highly inducible (100-300 fold) and localised on a different chromosome to PB_1. The PB_1 and PB_2 show some structural homology and it is not clear if they represent different subfamilies[c] (Wolf et al., 1986).

However, some criteria which differentiate these groups of proteins are described later in this text. Other P-450's which may be part of different subfamilies which have not been adequately characterised to give an assignment are those inducible by ethanol and clofibric acid, as well as certain constitutively expressed forms. DNA sequences indicate that the PB subfamilies diverged from those induced by PCN and MC approximately 200 million years ago; the PB_1 and the PB_3 subfamilies appear to have diverged approximately 140 million years ago (Leighton et al., 1984). Within each of the P-450 subfamilies several gene products have been identified. Those relating to the PB groups are shown in Table 2.

To date only two gene products have been identified for the MC_1 group of proteins. There are significant similarities in the genomic arrangement, i.e. the organisation of the segments of the genes containing the coding sequences of these two genes. In the mouse both genes have seven exons and equivalent exons are of very similar size. These two proteins have approximately 70% sequence homology at the DNA level (Kimmura et al., 1984). It is very interesting that certain regions of the two genes are highly homologous and other regions had diverged to a greater extent (Adesnick and Atchison, 1986). Similar findings were made when the gene structure of the rat b and e genes were compared (Table 2 forms PB_{3a} and PB_{3b}). These two proteins also have very similar intron-exon structure and have 97% sequence homology, i.e. only 14 amino acid residues are different between the proteins (Suwa et al 1985), the major differences being exon 7 and exon 8. Only two amino acid substitutions were found within the first six exons and two in exon 9. These findings provide evidence that gene conversion, i.e. the non-reciprocal transfer of DNA from one gene to another with concomitant deletion of an equivalent section of the DNA from the recipient strand, is a mechanism involved in the evolution of cytochrome P-450 genes. Such a mechanism can either result in increasing the homology between genes or give rise to small areas of difference. A possible sequence of events for the evolution of this multigene family could therefore involve an amplication which would leave the new gene free to diverge, allowing a single or multiple

[c]In recent studies a human PB_{2c} c-DNA clone has been shown to give different restriction fragments to PB_1 clones indicating that at least some of the PB_2 proteins may belong to a separate subfamily to PB_1.

Table 2. Literature Nomenclatures of Proteins Associated With Rat Liver P-450 Subfamilies Containing Members Inducible with Phenobarbital.

NOMENCLATURES

M.Wt	Wolf	Levin	Guengerich	Waxman	Other
52700	PB_{1a}	-	-	-	-
52900	PB_{1b}	k	PB-C	PB_1	-
52900	(PB_{1c})	-	-	-	-
52900	PB_{2a}	h	UTA	2c	RLM5,P-450 male,16α
	-	i	UT1	2d	P-450 female,15α
	-	f	-	-	-
	-	g	-	-	-
52900	PB_{2b}	-	-	-	-
52900	(PB_{2c})	-	-	-	-
50800	PB_{2d}	-	-	-	-
53300	PB_{3a}	b	PB-B	PB_4	-
54700	PB_{3b}	c	PB-D	PB_5	-

Apparent molecular weights are based on electrophoretic mobility. PB_{1c} and PB_{2c} were isolated from a different rat strain and therefore may be the same as PB_{1b} and PB_{2b}.

mutations to occur. Unequal crossing over could then amplify the genes further and gene conversion would increase the homology of some genes while changing others (shown diagramatically in Figure 1). It is interesting that in spite of the high degree of sequence homology between the PB_{3a} and PB_{3b} genes there is up to 100 fold difference in enzymic activity, PB_{3a} being invariably more active than PB_{3b}. The amino acid substitutions have therefore significantly altered the properties of the enzymes. It is worthy of note that the variable sequences flank a structurally conserved region of the P-450 gene first described by Ozols et al (1981).

Many cytochrome P-450 subfamily members have 60% or greater sequence homology at the protein level. Within a particular mammalian species the sequence homology between subfamilies ranges between 30 to 50%. A comparison of

Figure 1. A Representative Sequence of Events Showing the
Manner in which Cytochrome P-450 Genes could have Evolved.

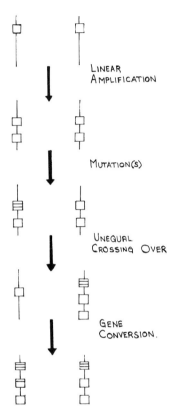

bacterial P-450 with the mammalian enzymes reveals an
extremely low degree of sequence homology. Indeed the
majority of the similiarities lie within short highly
conserved regions. Two regions have received most
attention. One of these lies towards the carboxyl end of
the protein and the other towards the amino terminus. As
these regions have been conserved through evolution it is
reasonable to assume that they are important for the
function of cytochrome P-450 as a monooxygenase. Both of
these sequences contain a cysteine atom which has been
implicated in heme binding. There is now considerable
evidence, however, including X-ray crystallographic data
(Poulos et al 1985), which indicates it is the cysteine at
the carboxyl end of the protein which is responsible for
heme binding.
      Between mammalian species there also seems to be a high
degree of sequence homology between genes, though it is

20 *Wolf et al.*

difficult to equate genes between species. PB_3 (and MC_1) gene subfamily for the mouse, rat, rabbit and human are 60-70% homologous.

CHARACTERISATION OF PB_1/PB_2 P-450 GENES AND THEIR EXPRESSION

In our studies we have concentrated on the characterisation of cytochrome P-450 genes and proteins within the PB_1/PB_2 gene subfamilies. In previous reports (Adams et al., 1985; Wolf et al, 1984; Buchmann et al., 1985) we have isolated two proteins from rat liver termed PB_1 (now PB_{1c}) and PB_2 (now PB_{2c}) and showed that both of these proteins were constitutively expressed and were marginally inducible by PB. PB_1 was diffusely localised in the centrilobular region of the liver whereas PB_2 was localised in a much more confined area of this region. Antibodies to both PB_1 and PB_2 reacted with microsomal proteins from a variety of animal species including human (Adams et al, 1985 and Figure 2). On the basis of this apparent structural conservation of PB1 and PB_2 proteins between species we have recently isolated human c-DNA clones for these genes from a human liver c-DNA library using either a rat c-DNA clone for a PB_1 gene (Friedberg et al, 1986) or by immunoscreening of human c-DNA libraries in the expression vector λ gt11.

Figure 2. **Western Blot of Liver Microsomal Samples from Various Species With an Antibody to PB_{2c}**

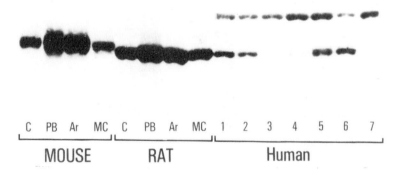

Animals were treated in the following manner C = control; PB = phenobarbital; Ar = Aroclor 1254; MC = 3-methylcholanthrene. The human samples 1-7 were from seven independent samples.

Southern blots of genomic DNA isolated from various species indicated the PB_1 gene family is highly conserved through species. Indeed the PB_1 c-DNA probe hydridized to drosphila DNA. These studies also showed that the PB_1 subfamily contains a large number of genes in rat and mouse and several genes in man (Table 1) (Meehan et al, unpublished).

Southern analysis cannot differentiate between genes which are expressed and pseudogenes. However, several laboratories have isolated gene products which appear to be part of the PB_1/PB_2 subfamily (Table 2). PB_{1a} and PB_{1b} have identical N-terminal amino acid sequences but have different molecular weights, absorption spectra and proteolytic fragments with papain (Wolf et al, 1986) PB_{1c} does exhibit some differences to the other members of this group. However this protein was isolated from a different strain of rat, using a different procedure, and therefore it is not possible to state conclusively that it is a different gene product to PB_{1a} or PB_{1b}. One of the most significant differences between these proteins is the differences in their activities towards substrates (Figure 3).

Figure 3. Specificity of Various Members of the PB_1 and PB_2 Subfamilies in the Metabolism of Mono-oxygenase Substrates.

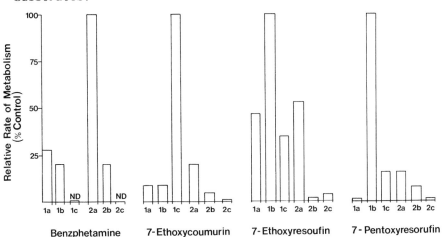

The 100% values were : Benzphetamine 15.9; 7-ethoxycoumarin 3.4; 7-ethoxyresorufin 0.87 and 7-pentoxyresorufin 0.25 nmol/nmol P-450/min. 1a and 1b etc are PB_{1a} PB_{1b} etc. N.D. = Not determined.

Wolf et al.

The classification of PB_1 and PB_2 proteins into separate subgroups is based on the peptide maps produced on digestion with papain and immunochemical cross-reactivity and more recently Southern blots of genomic DNA. The immunochemical cross-reactivity is shown in Figure 4. Polyclonal antibodies to members of the PB_1 family reacted strongly with other members of this group and also reacted with PB_{2a} and PB_{2d}. PB_{2a} reacted strongly with the PB_2 proteins and to a lesser extent with the PB_1 enzymes. PB_{2c} however only reacted significantly with the PB_2 proteins. The peptide maps for PB_1 and PB_2 proteins were clearly different. However, there were many similarities in the peptides produced within a group (Wolf et al., 1986).

Figure 4. Immunochemical Cross-reactivity of Members of the PB_1, PB_2 and PB_3 Subfamiles.

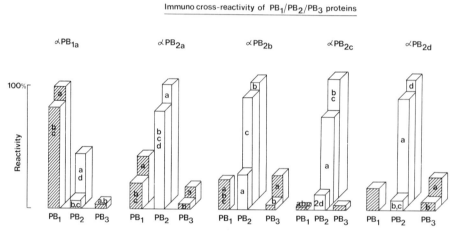

Immuno cross-reactivity of $PB_1/PB_2/PB_3$ proteins

100% reactivity was based on reactivity observed by dot blot analysis or on Western Blots.
α = antibody.

On the basis of absorption spectra, N-terminal sequence analysis substrate specificity, mobility in SDS gels, proteolytic fragments on digestion with papain and immunochemical reactivity, PB_{2a}, PB_{2b} and PB_{2d} appear different to each other. However, similar to PB_{1c}, PB_{2c} was isolated from a different source and by a different method (Wolf et al, 1984). PB_{2c} by all the above criteria however is very similar to PB_{2b}. The N-terminal sequence of PB_{2b} is novel and does not resemble other forms of cytochrome P-450 described so far. Table 2 shows other possible members of the PB_1/PB_2 subfamilies. A number of other forms have been described by Ryan et al (1984) which can be differentiated by their N-terminal sequences. The existence of these forms together with those described above indicates that at least eight proteins belonging to this group are expressed.

CHROMOSOMAL ORGANISATION AND MAPPING OF THE PB_1 SUBFAMILY

In our studies we have been using genetic models to study the organisation and function of cytochrome P-450 genes. One of these models involves the use of recombinant inbred mouse strains. Recombinant inbred strains result from the systematic inbreeding of the F_2 cross of progenitor mouse strains. Production of the F_2 generation essentially randomises genetic differences between the parent strains which are then stabilised by inbreeding. Each line (RI line) is then typed for chromosomal markers and the strain distribution pattern established for each marker. Unknown markers can be typed for their distribution pattern between the lines and compared to the known markers. Such an analysis allows close linkage between genes to be established. Examination of restriction fragment linked polymorphisms (RFLPs) in RI lines resulting from a C57 BL/6-DBA/2 cross (using three different restriction enzymes Sst 1, Hind III and Taq 1) showed that with one exception, of 26 lines either the C57 BL/6 or the DBA/2 restriction pattern was observed. In one sample using the restriction enzyme Sst 1, a DBA band was observed on a C57 BL/6 background indicating that one recombination event had occurred during the generation of the lines (Meehan et al, unpublished). The above data provides evidence that the PB_1 multigene subfamily in the mouse is a tightly linked cluster of genes located on the same chromosome. This data together with the Southern blot analysis indicates that this gene subfamily covers approximately 200kb and 70kb of genomic DNA in mouse and man respectively. Initial studies using either mouse/human or hamster/human somatic cell hybrids indicates that the PB_1 gene subfamily maps to chromosome 10 in human and possibly to chromosome 19 in the mouse. It is intriguing that almost all the cytochrome P-450 subfamilies mapped so far are localised on different chromosomes (Table 1). The chromosomal localisation of these gene clusters would therefore appear a good criterion for their classification into subfamilies.

REGULATION OF CYTOCHROME P-450 GENES

The regulation of cytochrome P-450 genes is clearly very complex and a large variety of factors determines the level of these proteins within cells. For convenience the regulation of the liver genes can be split into three categories: 1) Genes that are highly inducible by foreign compounds, e.g. PB_3 and MC_1 subgroups, and in some cases the PCN group. 2) Genes which are marginally inducible by foreign compounds, e.g. some members of the PB_1 and PB_2 subgroups, and 3) Genes which are regulated by endogenous molecules such as hormones and interferons etc. In rats, P-450's within the PB_1 subgroup of proteins, PB_{2a} form i in the PB_2 group as well as P-450's within the PCN group (Tables 1 and 2) show marked sex differences in their expression (Friedberg et al, 1986, Waxman et al, 1985, Wrighton et al, 1985). In certain cases this has been associated with steroid hormone levels (Waxman et al, 1985). Northern blots of hepatic male and female RNA from rat or mouse liver probed with a PB_1 clone are shown in Figure 5. In rats, females have a much higher PB_1 RNA content than males (Friedberg et al, 1986). This difference is not observed in the mouse RNA levels studied so far.

Figure 5. Northern Blot Analysis of Rat and Mouse Liver RNA with c-DNA to PB_1 from Untreated Animals.

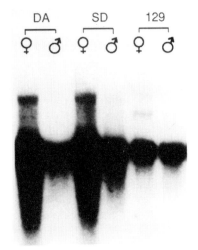

15μg of RNA was run per tract. DA and SD were samples from DA and Sprague Dawley rat liver. 129 are mouse liver samples.

Apart from the steroid hormones, the molecules which control the constitutive levels of P-450's within cells are poorly understood. Regulation by endogenous molecules may prove extremely important in determining the levels of specific isozymes within cells. This possibility is exemplified by the finding that factors released during inflammatory response or infection can modulate P-450 levels. The mechanism of modulation by molecules such as interferons is unclear but results from either altered transcription rates or possibly other mechanisms involving increased rates of P-450 degradation (Deloria et al, 1985). We have been using bacterial endotoxin, as well as recombinant interferon, to study the modulation of P-450 by endogenous factors. Endotoxin is often used as a model for the study of gene expression during 'acute phase' or inflammatory response and has been shown to induce the production of lymphokines such as interferons, tumour necrosis factor and interleukin 1. Treatment of mice with high levels of bacterial endotoxin (25µg) causes very marked changes in hepatic P-450 levels, overall cytochrome P-450 content being reduced to 40% of control values. Western blot analysis of the hepatic microsomes using antibodies to PB_{1a} and PB_{2c} show a very marked reduction in the expression of these proteins. When animals were treated concomitantly with endotoxin and the inducing agents PB or MC the synthesis of PB_1 and PB_2 proteins was still markedly suppressed. Northern blot analysis indicated that these changes do not appear to be paralled by changes in mRNA levels, which suggests that altered m-RNA production is not the only mechanism involved in these effects. The levels of the highly inducible proteins, PB_3 and MC_1, were affected to a lesser extent by high endotoxin. Interestingly when a lower dose of endotoxin was used in such experiments (7.5 µg per mouse) the microsomal metabolism of 7-ethoxyresorufin was actually enhanced indicating that endotoxin can cause both elevation or suppression of cellular P-450 activities and levels. This finding indicates that infection or inflammation may affect the rate of toxin metabolism or the activation of chemical carcinogens within cells.

It has been known for some time that interferons can suppress cytochrome P-450 levels (Renton and Singh 1984; Balkwill et al, 1984). Interestingly when recombinant interferon is dosed in combination with P-450 inducing agents such as MC similar to the effects observed with low doses of endotoxin, an enhancement (approx 2 fold) of the metabolism of 7-ethoxyresorufin was measured (unpublished). This indicates that interferons can also lead to increased as well as reduced levels of P-450's within cells.

Certain P-450 forms are marginally inducible with compounds such as PCN and PB, for example some proteins within the PB_1 and PB_2 subgroups. The synthesis of PB_{2a} on the other hand is suppressed by treatment with this compound (Waxman et al, 1985).

The mechanisms which regulate cytochrome P-450 levels in cells in almost all cases remain obscure. The greatest progress has been on the genes inducible by MC. The regulation of these genes involves the binding of the inducing agent to a receptor molecule which through an, as yet, unidentified mechanism, initiates transcription (Nebert and Jensen 1979). A positive regulatory element at the 5' end of one of the genes within this subfamily has recently been identified (Jones et al., 1986). However, genetic studies on this induction process indicate it to be complex involving several different genetic loci.

CYTOCHROME P-450 SUBSTRATE SPECIFICITY

A major problem resulting from the multiplicity of the cytochrome P-450 dependent mono-oxygenases is to associate specific microsomal or in vivo activities with particular P-450 subfamilies or with the expression of specific P-450 forms. It is now clear that analagous cytochrome P-450's between species have structural and functional homology although this is not absolute. There are several techniques which can be applied to relate activities with the expression of specific P-450 forms. The first is the isolation of the specific proteins and characterisation of their activities. This is a difficult approach and many proteins with important function may be missed if they are not present in the microsomal samples used in the purification. The second involves the isolation of full length c-DNA and their subsequent expression in cells. This approach has the advantage that all P-450 genes could be tested individually in this manner. Thirdly, antibodies raised against purified P-450's can be used as inhibitors of enzymic activities in microsomal samples. This powerful technique has been used by many groups and allows the association of enzyme activities with either P-450 subgroups and, if the antibodies are sufficiently specific, with specific proteins. A fourth approach is to use genetic differences in foreign compound metabolism, for example, using the recombinant inbred mouse strains, to associate the expression of a specific gene or subfamily of genes with an enzymic activity.

We are currently using these approaches to study the

polymorphic P-450 expression in relation to adverse drug-side effects and genetic susceptibility to drug or hormone induced disease (Idle and Ritchie, 1983). There have recently been several reports on the isolation and characterisation of P-450 proteins associated with polymorphic drug metabolism in humans. These include enzymes involved in the metabolism of nifedipine, mephenytoin and debrisoquine (see Meyer et al, this volume; Shimada, et al, 1986; Guengerich et al, 1986; Gut et al., 1986). As part of our interest in P-450's which are constitutively expressed we have been investigating the properties of the PB_1/PB_2 proteins in this regard. There is direct evidence from N-terminal sequence analysis which indicates that the human genes involved in mephenytoin metabolism (Shimada et al, 1986) are part of this subfamily(ies) as well as circumstantial evidence linking debrisoquine metabolism to these genes. Recombinant inbred mouse lines derived from AKR and C57L mice have a difference in their constitutive arylhydrocarbon hydroxylase activity. The segregation pattern of retriction fragments obtained with the PB_1 c-DNA clone co-segregates with constitutive arylhydrocarbon hydroxylase activities (Meehan, Hastie, Friedberg, Adesnick, Hutton, Taylor and Wolf, unpublished), indicating that a member (or members) of this subfamily is involved in this reaction. These data are supported by the finding that antibodies to PB_1 are highly efficient inhibitors of 7-ethoxyresorufin deethylase activity, an activity associated with arylhydrocarbon hydroxylase, in liver microsomal fractions from untreated rats (Burke and Wolf, unpublished). Similar antibody inhibition studies indicate that constitutive aromatic amine activation may be associated with this gene subfamily (Robertson et al, unpublished). Thus the expression of a constitutively expressed P-450 may be important in the activation of chemical carcinogens. At the present time the role of constitutively expressed cytochrome P-450 forms, relative to the highly inducible forms in drug metabolism in the epidemiology of foreign compound-induced disease is unclear. The fact that the polymorphic metabolism of drugs has been associated with many P-450 forms which are constitively expressed, emphasises the potential importance of these proteins in these reactions.

ACKNOWLEDGEMENTS

RM would like to express his thanks to ICI Corporate Bioscience laboratories for financial support and Professor

H.J. Evans for continued backing and laboratory support.

REFERENCES

Adams, D.J., Seilman, S., Amelizad, Z., Oesch, F. and Wolf,
    C.R. (1985). Biochem. J. 232, 869.
Adesnik, M. and Atchison, M. (1986). CRC Crit. Rev.
    Biochem. 19, 247.
Balkwill, F.R., Mowshowitz, S., Seilman, S., Moodie, E.M.,
    Griffin, D.B., Fantes, K.H. and Wolf, C.R. (1984).
    Cancer Res, 44, 5249.
Buchmann, A., Kuhlmann, W., Schwartz, W., Kunz, W., Wolf,
    C.R., Moll, E., Friedberg, T. and Oesch, F. (1985).
    Carcinogenesis, 6, 513.
Deloria, L., Abbott, V., Gooderham, N., Mannering, G.J.
    (1985). Biochem. Biophys. Res. Commun, 131, 109.
Distlerath, L.M., Reilly, P.E.B., Martin, M.V., Davis,
    G.G., Wilkinson, G.R. and Guengerich, F.P. (1985). J.
    Biol. Chem. 260, 9057.
Friedberg, T.F., Waxman, D.J., Atchison, M., Kumar, A.,
    Haarparanta, T., Raphael, C. and Adesnick, M. (1986).
    Biochemistry, 25, 7975.
Guengerich, F.P., Martin, M.V., Beaune, P.H., Kremers, P.,
    Wolff, T. and Waxman, D.J. (1986). J. Biol. Chem. 261,
    5051.
Gut, J., Catin, T., Dayer, P., Kronbach, T., Zanger, U.,
    Meyer, U.A. (1986). J. Biol. Chem, 261, in press.
Hildebrand, C.E., Gonzalez, F.J., McBride, O.W. and Nebert,
    D.W. (1986). Nucleic Acid Res, 13, 2009.
Idle, J.R. and Ritchie, J.C. (1983). In : "Human
    Carcinogenesis", Academic Press, p.857.
Jones, P.B.C., Durring, L.K., Galeazzi, D.R., Whitlock,
    J.P. (1986). Proc. Natl. Acad. Sci. USA, 83, 2802.
Kimmura, S., Gonzalez, F.J. and Nebert, D.W. (1984). J.
    Biol. Chem. 259, 10705.
Leighton, J.K., Debrunner-Vossbrinck, B.A. and Kemper, B.
    (1984). Biochemistry, 23, 204.
Nebert, D.W. and Jensen, N.M. (1979). CRC Crit. Rev.
    Biochem, 401.
Nebert, D.W. and Gonzalez, F.J. (1985). Trends in Pharm.
    Sci 6, 160.
Ozols, J., Heinmann, F.S. and Johnson, E.F. (1981). J.
    Biol. Chem, 256, 11405.
Poulos, T.L., Finzel, B.C., Gunsalus, I.C., Wagner, G.C.
    and Kraut J. (1985). J. Biol. Chem, 260, 16122.
Renton, K.W., Singh, G. (1984). Biochem. Pharmacol, 33,
    3899.
Ryan, D.E., Iida, S., Wood, A.W., Thomas, P.E., Lieber,

C.S. and Levin, W. (1984). J. Biol. Chem, 259, 1239.
Shimada, T., Misono, K.S. and Guengerich, F.P. (1986). J. Biol. Chem, 261, 909.
Suwa, Y., Mizukami, Y., Sogawa, K. and Fujii-Kuryama, Y. (1985). J. Biol. Chem, 260, 7980.
Wainright, B.J., Watson, E.K., Shepherd, E.A. and Phillips, I.R. (1985). Nucleic Acid Res, 13, 4610.
Waxman, D.J., Dannan, G.A. and Guengerich, F.P. (1985). Biochemistry, 24, 4409.
Wislocki, P.G., Miwa, G.T. and Lu, A.Y.H. (1980). In : "Enzymatic Basis of Detoxification" (Jakoby, W.B. ed). Academic Press Vol 1, p135.
Wolf, C.R. (1982). In : "Metabolic Basis of Detoxification" (Jakoby, W.B., Bend, J.R. and Caldwell, J. eds). Academic Press p5.
Wolf, C.R., Moll, E., Friedberg, T., Oesch, F., Buchmann, A., Kuhlmann, W.D. and Kunz, W.D. (1984). Carcinogenesis, 5, 993.
Wolf, C.R. (1986). Trends in Genetics, August 2, 209.
Wolf, C.R., Seilman, S., Oesch, F., Meyer, R.T. and Burke, M.D. (1986). Biochem. J, 240, 27.
Wrighton, S.A., Schvetz, E.G., Watkins, P.B., Maurel, P., Barwick, J., Bailey, B.S., Hartle, H.T., Young, B. and Guzelian, P. (1985). Molec. Pharmacol, 28, 312.

GLUTATHIONE TRANSFERASE

Bengt Mannervik

Department of Biochemistry, Arrhenious Laboratory,
University of Stockholm, S-106 91 Stockholm, Sweden.

INTRODUCTION

Glutathione transferase (EC 2.5.1.18) was originally identified as an enzyme involved in drug metabolism. Combes and Stakelum (1961) and Booth et al (1961) found that bromosulphothalein and other halogen-containing aromatic compounds were conjugated with glutathione in the presence of liver extracts. It is now known that an organism, or even a single tissue, may contain multiple forms of glutathione transferase (Jakoby, 1978; Mannervik, 1985a), and that electrophilic chemicals can serve as substrates for this group of enzymes (Chasseaud, 1979; Jakoby and Habig, 1980; Mannervik, 1985a). Glutathione transferases occur in high concentrations in certain tissues and have also been recognised as intracellular binding proteins under the name of ligandins (Litwack et al., 1971; Smith and Litwack, 1980). In their capacity as binding proteins, the glutathione transferases may serve important functions in the intracellular transport of drugs, carcinogens, and other xenobiotics (Ketterer and Tipping, 1978; Arias et al., 1980). Originally, investigations of glutathione transferases were focussed on their interaction with chemical substances foreign to the organism, but more recently attention to endogenous compounds and their metabolism has been increasing (cf. Mannervik et al., 1985a; Mannervik, 1985a).

MULTIPLE FORMS OF MAMMALIAN GLUTATHIONE TRANSFERASE

Two fundamentally different types of protein with glutathione transferase activity have been identified in mammalian tissues (cf. Mannervik, 1985a). One occurs in certain cellular membrane fractions and is generally referred to as "microsomal" glutathione transferase; another is predominantly recovered in the post-microsomal supernatant fraction and is called "cytosolic" glutathione transferase. The microsomal enzyme in rat liver has been purified and shown to be distinct from the cytosolic enzyme forms by various criteria, including reactions with specific antibodies (Morgenstern et al., 1982a). The relative molecular mass of its polypeptide chain is 17,237 daltons, as calculated from the primary structure (Morgenstern et al., 1985). A microsomal glutathione transferase in mouse liver with very similar molecular properties, and which reacts with antibodies raised against the rat enzyme, has recently been purified to homogeneity (M. Soderstrom; C. Andersson and B. Mannervik, unpublished work).

More than 10 different forms of cytosolic glutathione transferase have been isolated and characterised in the rat. Some of them have been shown to be bound to the microsome fraction of rat liver (Friedberg et al., 1979; Morgenstern et al., 1983), but the contribution of these proteins to the total concentration of glutathione transferase in microsomes is only about 10% as determined by quantitative immunochemical analysis (Morgenstern et al., 1983).

The primary structure of one of the cytosolic enzymes, rat glutathione transferase 4-4, has been determined by conventional techniques of protein chemistry (Alin et al., 1986). Its relative molecular mass is 25,457 daltons and the amino acid sequence shows no obvious similarity to that of the microsomal enzyme. Several additional primary structures of cytosolic rat glutathione transferases have been deduced from corresponding cDNA structures (for references, see Alin et al., 1986). Similarities between the cytosolic enzymes are clearly discerned, but none of the structures shows any sequence homology with the microsomal transferase. The only common feature of the microsomal and the cytosolic types so far noted is the catalytic activity and its requirement of glutathione as cofactor. The available partial amino acid sequences of glutathione transferases from mammalian species other than the rat indicate strongly that the distinction between the microsomal and the cytosolic enzyme types applies generally.

All the cytosolic glutathione transferases characterised are dimeric proteins composed of two subunits with a relative molecular mass of approximately 25,000 daltons. The subunits may be identical or nonidentical, and it has been proposed that the various isoenzymes should be named on the basis of their subunit composition (Mannervik and Jensson, 1982). This principle has been agreed upon by several investigators in the field and to date eight different subunits of rat glutathione transferase have been designated by Arabic numberals (cf. Jakoby et al., 1984; Jakoby, 1985). Thus, a homodimer of subunit 8 would be named rat glutathione transferase 8-8 and a heterodimer of subunits 3 and 4 would be named rat glutathione transferase 3-4. Recently, four cytosolic mouse glutathione transferases have been named according to the same principle (Warholm et al., 1986). However, it should be noted that the subunits are named in the order that they are sufficiently well characterised for clear identification. Therefore, a given number will not in general imply similarity between subunits of different animal species. At least seven forms of human glutathione transferase have been isolated (cf. Mannervik, 1985a), but the possible structural relationships among the dimeric structures are not entirely clear and the subunits of the human transferases have not yet been named by Arabic numerals.

The large number of glutathione transferases in a given species necessitates the use of a battery of tests for definitive identification of a given isozymes., For this purpose, properties such as physical parameters, substrate specificities, sensitivities to inhibitors, and reactions with specific antibodies have been determined for rat (Alin et al., 1985a), mouse (Warholm et al., 1986), and human glutathione transferase (Mannervik, 1985a). Since the properties of the transferases appear to reflect the subunit composition in a simple additive manner (Danielson and Mannervik, 1985; Tahir and Mannervik, 1986), the properties of a heterodimeric enzyme can be predicted quantitatively from those of the corresponsing homodimers.

CLASSIFICATION AND EVOLUTION OF GLUTATHIONE TRANSFERASES

When the multiple forms of glutathione transferase in different species were first discovered and characterised it was not obvious how they were related to one another. In the rat, it was clear that enzymes composed of subunits 1 and 2 were closely related and distinct from those containing subunits 3 and 4 (Mannervik and Jensson, 1982; in the reference cited these subunits are referred to as L,B,A and C, respectively). In human tissues, five gluta- thione transferases with basic isoelectric points named α, β,γ, δ and ε appeared closely related (Kamisaka et al., 1975), but distinct from the near-neutral transferase μ (Warholm et al., 1983) and the acidic transferase ρ or π (Marcus et al., 1978; Guthenberg and Mannervik, 1981).

The clues to understanding of the relationships among the glutathione transferases between different species came from comparisons of the enzymatic properties of three distinct mouse enzymes with the three major types of human enzymes (Mannervik et al., 1984a). One type of enzyme displayed high glutathione peroxidase activity with cumene hydroperoxide. Another type gave high activity in the conjugation of ethacrynic acid with glutathione and a third type was active with either bromosulphophthalein or trans-4-phenylbut-3-en-2-one as the electrophilic substrate. The three types of glutathione transferase have now been designated as classes Alpha, Pi and Mu, respectively (Mannervik et al., 1985b), and the classification has been rigorously supported by reactions with specific antibodies and, most importantly, by primary structure analysis. Figure 1 shows the composite N-terminal amino acid sequences of the structures analysed so far.

The known primary structures of rat glutathione transferases have made possible comparisons of predicted secondary structures and hydropathy profiles of members from different classes (Alin et al., 1986, B. Persson, H. Jornvall, P. Alin and B. Mannervik, unpublished work). The comparative analysis reinforces the picture of strong structural similarities within a class and weaker, but significant, relationships between members of different classes. It is also clear that the enzymes all have alternating α-helices and β-strands along the polypeptides chain (Alin et al., 1986). The glutathione transferases should therefore be referred to as α/β proteins (Chothia, 1984).

The structural comparison of the multiple forms of glutathione transferase suggests that the cytosolic forms have evolved from a common protein structure (Mannervik 1985a, 1986; Mannervik et al., 1985b). The segregation into three distinct classes of cytosolic transferases must have preceded the evolution of the various mammalian species, since the sequence homologies between members of a class irrespective of species are greater than homologies between tranferases of different classes from the same species.

The possible evolutionary relationship between the microsomal and the cytosolic glutathione transferases has support only from the common catalytic properties. It has been hypothesized that the two distinct types may both have originated from an ancestral glutathione-binding protein (Mannervik, 1985a, 1986).

SUBSTRATES FOR GLUTATHIONE TRANSFERASES

A wide variety of electrophilic compounds may serve as

Figure 1. Composite N-Terminal Amino Acid Sequences of
Different Classes of Glutathione Transferase[a]

Cytosolic

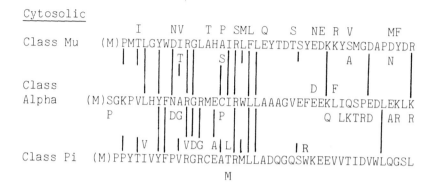

Class Mu

Class Alpha

Class Pi

Microsomal   ADLKQLMDNEVLMAFTSYATIILAKVMFLSSATAFQRLTNKV

a - The classes have been defined by Mannervik et al.,
(1985b). The sequences (in one-letter code) are composites
of available N-terminal primary structures from several
mammalian species, showing alternative amino acid residues
in the positions indicated (Mannervik, 1986). Inter-class
identities are marked with vertical bars. The N-terminal
methionine residues (M) deduced from complementary DNA
structures are not present in the peptides analysed. The
stucture of the microsomal transferase is from Morgenstern
et al (1985).

substrates for glutathione transferase. Most of the
substrates used are xenobiotics, including drugs,
pesticides and environmental pollutants. Three fundamental
types of chemical reaction are encountered: nucleophilic
displacements, additions and isomerisations. Many of the
substitution and isomerisation reactions give rise to
chemically stable glutathione conjugates that may serve as
vehicles for excretion, either directly or after
biotransformation. The possible excretion products include
the classical mercapturic acid derivatives, N-acetyl-S-
(substituent)-cysteine, formed by degradation of the
primary glutathione derivative. More recently it was found
that the conjugates can be degraded to the extent that only
the sulphur atom of glutathione remains bound to the group
originally linked to glutathione. Such a mercapto
derivative may be glucuronosylated with uridine
diphosphoglucuronate to give a thioglucuronide or
methylated with S-adenosylmethionine to give a thiomethyl

conjugate. These metabolites, as well as the oxidised methylsulphinyl and methylsulphonyl derivatives of the latter conjugate, have been recognised as important end products in the biotransformation of xenobiotics (for further references, see Mannervik, 1985a). Thus, the importance of the glutathione conjugations catalysed by glutathione transferases is well established.

Some substitution reactions involving glutathione yield labile conjugates of transient existence. The conjugates may react with a second molecule of glutathione to release the S-substituent and transform glutathione to its corresponding disulphide. The net effect is chemical reduction of the compound at the expense of reducing equivalents of the sulphydryl group of glutathione. Such reactions catalysed by glutathione transferases include organic nitrate esters, thiocyanates, hydroperoxides, and disulphides, in which the sulphur atom of glutathione attacks heteroatoms, such as nitrogen, sulphur or oxygen rather than carbon (Jakoby and Habig, 1980).

Glutathione transferases are also active in cis-trans or positional isomerisations of certain unsaturated organic compounds (Jakoby and Habig, 1980). The mechanism is believed to involve addition of glutathione to the double bond, sterical rearrangement, and subsequent elimination of free glutathione.

In spite of the established significance of glutathione transferase in drug metabolism, the products of pharmaceutical industries cannot have determined the molecular evolution of the various forms of the enzyme. Products of oxidative metabolism have been suggested as "natural" substrates that may have influenced the development of different classes of glutathione transferase (Mannervik, 1985a, 1985b; Mannervik et al., 1985a).

Thus, the members of class Alpha have high activity with organic hydroperoxides and can be identified with the non-selenium-dependent glutathione peroxidase (cf. Mannervik, 1985b). It has also been demonstrated that a member of this class (rat glutathione transferase 1-2, previously designated "B") catalyzes the conjugation of quinone derivatives of benzo(a)pyrene (Morgenstern et al., 1982b).

Transferases of class Mu have been found to have high activity with many epoxides. In particular the human enzyme, which appears to be present only in 60% of the population, has a pronounced activity with compounds such as styrene-7,8-oxide and benzo(a)pyrene-4,5-dihydro-4,5-oxide (Warholm et al., 1983). It should also be noted that the class Mu enzymes rat transferase 4-4 and human transferase μ display the highest activity of the enzymes tested with the epoxide leukotriene A$_4$ (Mannervik et al., 1984b; Soderstrom et al., 1985).

Class Pi transferases also have high catalytic activities with some epoxides. Particularly significant is the high activity with the ultimate carcinogenic metabolite of benzo(a)pyrene, 7β,8α-dihyroxy-9α,10α-oxy-7,8,9,10-tetrahydrobenzo(a)pyrene (Robertson et al., 1986a, b). Particularly noteworthy is the observation that whereas the human transferase μ is equally active with the (+)- and the (-)-enantiomer of the epoxide, the human transferase π is stereospecific for the most strongly carcinogenic (+)-enantiomer, which has R,S,S,R absolute stereochemical configuration (Robertson et al., 1986b).

Finally, the homologous series of 4-hydroxy-alk-2-enals, products of lipid peroxidation, have been shown to be excellent substrates for glutathione transferase (Alin et al., 1985b). However, these compounds are not generally superior for any of the classes of the cytosolic enzymes. Nevertheless, an enzyme, rat glutathione transferase 8-8 (not yet referred to any of the classes), has recently been found to have by far the highest catalytic activity of all the transferases with this group of substrates (Jensson et al., 1986).

The microsomal glutathione transferase has no significant activity with 4-hydroxyalk-2-enals, benzo(a)pyrene oxides, or leukotriene A$_4$ (M. Soderstrom, B. Jernstrom, S. Hammarstrom, and B. Mannervik, unpublished work) and its biological role is not yet understood.

INDUCTION OF GLUTATHIONE TRANSFERASES AND CARCINOGENESIS

In spite of the fact that the glutathione transferases are present in high intracellular concentrations in many tissues, it has been demonstrated that their concentrations can be elevated in experimental animals by administration of various chemicals or by alterations of the hormonal status (for references, see Jakoby and Habig, 1980; Mannervik, 1985a). In chemically induced preneoplastic rat liver nodules, the class Pi transferase 7-7, which is essentially undetectable in normal liver tissue is one of the major forms of glutathione transferase (Kitahara et al., 1984; Jensson et al., 1985). This form has also been identified in rat hepatomas (Meyer et al., 1985; M.K. Tahir, C. Guthenberg and B. Mannervik, unpublished work). It has been proposed as a suitable marker protein for hepatic tumor formation (Satoh et al., 1985; Soma et al., 1986). Particularly noteworthy are recent reports suggesting that overproduction of the class Pi transferase is linked to increased drug-resistance of cancer cells with respect to chemotherapeutic agents (Shea and Henner, 1986; Batist et al., 1986; Evans et al., 1986; Buller and Tew, 1986; Tulpule et al., 1986). Thus, the regulation of the cellular levels of glutathione transferases may have consequences for the survival of the cell as well as for the organism itself.

ACKNOWLEDGEMENTS

The work from the author's laboratory was supported from the Swedish Natural Research Council and the Swedish Council for Co-ordination and Planning of Research.

REFERENCES

Alin, P., Jensson, H., Guthenberg, C., Danielson, U.H., Tahir, M.K. and Mannervik, B. (1985a). Anal. Biochem, 146, 313.

Alin, P., Danielson, U.H. and Mannervik, B. (1985b). FEBS Lett, 179, 267.

Alin, P., Mannervik, B. and Jornvall, H. (1986). Eur. J. Biochem, 156, 343.

Arias, I.M., Ohmi, N., Bhargava, M. and Listowsky, I. (1980). Mol. Cell. Biochem, 29, 71.

Batist, G., de Muys, J.-M., Cowan, K.H. and Myers, C.E. (1986). Proc. Am. Assoc. Cancer Res, 27, 270.

Booth, J., Boyland, E. and Sims, P. (1961). Biochem. J. 79, 516.

Buller, A.L. and Tew, K.D. (1986). Proc. Am. Assoc. Cancer Res, 27, 263.

Chasseaud, L.F. (1979). Adv. Cancer Res, 29, 175.

Chothia, C. (1984). Annu. Rev. Biochem, 53, 537.

Combes, B. and Stakelum, G.S. (1961). J. Clin. Invest. 40, 981.

Danielson, U.H. and Mannervik, B. (1985). Biochem. J, 231, 263.

Evans, C.G., Bodell, W.J., Ross, D., Doane, P. and Smith, M.T (1986). Proc. Am. Assoc. Cancer Res, 27, 267.

Friegberg, T., Bentley, P., Stasiecki, P., Glatt, H.R., Raphael, D. and Oesch, F. (1979). J. Biol. Chem. 254, 12028.

Guthenberg, C. and Mannervik, B. (1981). Biochim. Biophys. Acta, 661, 255.

Jakoby, W.B. (1978). Adv. Enzymol, 46, 383.

Jakoby, W.B. (1985). Methods Enzymol, 113, 495.

Jakoby, W.B. and Habig, W.B. (1980). In : "Enzymatic Basis

for Detoxication" (Vol 2, (Ed. by Jakoby, W.B), Academic Press, New York, p.63.

Jakoby, W.B., Ketterer, B. and Mannervik, B. (1984). Biochem. Pharmacol, 33, 2539.

Jensson, H., Eriksson, L.C. and Mannervik, B. (1985). FEBS Lett. 187, 115.

Jensson, H., Guthenberg, C., Alin, P. and Mannervik, B. (1986). FEBS Lett, in press.

Kamisaka, K., Habig, W.H., Ketley, J.N., Arias, I.M. and Jakoby, W.B. (1975). Eur. J. Biochem, 60, 153.

Ketterer, B. and Tipping, E. (1978). "Conjugation Reactions in Drug Biotransformation" (Ed. by Aitio, A). Elsevier/North Holland Biomedical Press, Amsterdam, p.91.

Kitahara, A., Satoh, K., Nishimura, K., Ishikara, T., Ruike, K., Sato, K., Tsuda, H. and Ito, N. (1984). Cancer Res, 44, 2698.

Litwack, G., Ketterer, B. and Arias, I.M. (1971). Nature 234, 466.

Mannervik, B. (1985a). Adv. Enzymol, 57, 357.

Mannervik, B. (1985b). Meth. Enzymol, 113, 490.

Mannervik, B. (1986). Chemica Scripta, 26, in press.

Mannervik, B. and Jensson, H. (1982). J. Biol. Chem, 257, 9909.

Mannervik, B., Guthenberg, C., Jensson, H., Tahir, M.K., Warholm, M. and Alin, P. (1984a). In : Proceedings IUPHAR 9th Intern. Congr. Pharmacol, Vol 3, (ed. by Paton, W., Mitchell, J. and Turner, P). Macmillan Press, London, p.225.

Mannervik, B., Jensson, H., Alin P., Orning, L. and Hammarstrom, S. (1984b). FEBS Lett, 175, 289.

Mannervik, B., Alin, P., Guthenberg, C., Jensson, H. and Warholm, M. (1985a). In : "Microsomes and Drug Oxidations" (Ed. by Boobis, A.R., Caldwell, J., DeMatteis, F. and Elcombe, C.R). Taylor and Francis, London. p.221.

Mannervik, B., Alin P., Guthenberg, C., Jensson, H., Tahir, M.K., Warholm, M. and Jornvall, J. (1985b). Proc. Natl. Acad. Sci, USA, 82, 7202.

Marcus, C., Habig, W.H. and Jakoby, W.B. (1978). Arch. Biochem. Biophys, 188, 287.

Meyer, D.J., Beale, D., Tan, K.H., Coles, B. and Ketterer, B. (1985). FEBS Lett, 184, 139.

Morgenstern, R., Guthenberg, C. and DePierre, J.W. (1982a). Eur. J. Biochem, 128, 243.

Morganstern, R., Guthenberg, C., Mannervik, B., DePierre, J.W. and Ernster, L. (1982b). Cancer Res, 42, 4215.

Morganstern, R., Guthenberg, C., Mannervik, B. and

DePierre, J.W. (1983). FEBS Lett, 160, 264.

Morganstern, R., DePierre, J.W. and Jornvall, H. (1985). J. Biol. Chem. 260, 13976.

Robertson, I.G.C., Jensson, H., Mannervik, B. and Jernstrom, B. (1986a). Carcinogenesis, 7, 295.

Jernstrom, B. (1986b). Cancer Res 46, 2220.

Satoh, K., Kitahara, A., Soma, Y., Inaba, Y., Hatayama, I. and Sato, K. (1985). Proc. Natl. Acad. Sci. USA, 82, 3964.

Shea, T. and Henner, W.D. (1986). Proc. Am. Assoc. Cancer Res, 27, 5.

Smith, G.J. and Litwack, G. (1980). Rev. Biochem. Toxicol, 2, 1.

Soderstrom, M., Mannervik, B., Orning, L. and Hammerstrom, S. (1985). Biochem. Biophys. Res. Commun, 128, 265.

Soma, Y., Satoh, K. and Sato, K. (1986). Biochim. Biophys. Acta, 869, 247.

Tahir, M.K. and Mannervik, B. (1986). J. Biol. Chem, 261, 1048.

Tulpule, A., Batist, G., Sinha, B., Katki, A., Myers, C.E. (1986). Proc. Am. Assoc. Cancer Res, 27, 271.

Warholm, M., Guthenberg, C. and Mannervik, B. (1983). Biochemistry 22, 3610.

Warholm, M., Jensson, H., Tahir, M.K. and Mannervik, B. (1986). Biochemistry, 25, in press.

MOLECULAR CHARACTERISATION OF HEPATIC UDP-GLUCURONYL TRANSFERASES

Brian Burchell[1], Michael R. Jackson[1], Michael W.H. Coughtrie[1], David Harding[1], Stuart Wilson[1] and John R. Bend[2]

[1]Department of Biochemistry, The University, Dundee, DD1 4HN, Scotland and [2]Laboratory of Pharmacology, NIH/NIEHS, Research Triangle Park, N.C. 27709, USA.

INTRODUCTION

Glucuronide formation is a major pathway in the biotransformation and elimination of a wide variety of endogenous and xenobiotic compounds (Dutton, 1980). The glucuronidation reactions have been determined to be catalysed by a number of closely related UDP-glucuronyltransferases (GTs) (See Burchell 1981).

We are attempting to define the boundaries of specificity of individual GTs, to eventually predict whether effective glucuronidation will occur during perinatal development and disease.

Some studies of substrate specificity of rat enzymes have already been performed using transferases purified to apparent homogeneity (See Burchell et al., 1985), but this approach becomes even more difficult and laborious when several enzymes have been identified with some overlapping specificity. All of these transferases must be isolated and their properties directly compared. This problem becomes considerably greater when attempting to study human liver UDP-glucuronyltransferase, with limited tissue availability and more difficult purification work.

The question which is always raised - "does the individual UDP-glucuronyltransferase exhibit a 'true' substrate specificity when purified from a membrane microenvironment using detergents?", may not be satisfactorily answered. Therefore, our intention is to place individual rat or human liver GTs into the correct cellular microenvironment to study glucuronidation in the whole cell in vitro to obtain a 'true' assessment of the substrate specificity of each transferase. Further, the regulation of GTs by drugs and hormones can be studied in these modified cells. It is necessary to perform purification work, raise specific antibodies, and obtain cloned genes to achieve these aims.

Our current progress with the molecular characterisation of UDP-glucuronyltransferases will be described in this manuscript.

PURIFICATION OF UDP-GLUCURONYLTRANSFERASES

The purification of several UDP-glucuronyltransferases catalysing the glucuronidation of various endogenous substrates and numerous xenobiotic substrates is reviewed in Table 1. Six of the nine GTs identified have been purified to apparent homogeneity; three of the transferases to date do not glucuronidate the most known endogenous substrates. The newcomer to the list since its compilation in 1984 (See Burchell et al., 1985) is a phenol UDPGT present at high levels in foetal liver, but which is present at much lower levels in adult liver, as judged by immunoblot analysis (Burchell et al., 1986), although this transferase can be dramatically induced in liver by treatment of adult rats with β-naphthoflavone (M. Coughtrie et al., unpublished work).

Careful studies of GT purification and substrate specificity by Tom Tephly's group are helping to resolve minor controversies. Recently, morphine GT has been separated from a transferase catalysing the glucuronidation of 4-hydroxybiphenyl (Puig and Tephly, 1986) which updates previous work (Bock et al., 1979), suggesting the possible existence of another GT. The information reported by Tephly and Green (1986) indicates that N-glucuronidation of naphthylamines is catalysed to purified 17-β-hydroxy steroid GT, whereas N-glucuronidation of 4-aminobiphenyl is catalysed by 3α-hydroxysteroid GT.

The first extrahepatic GTs, a mixture of phenol GT, and bilirubin GT have been purified from rat kidney microsomes. The major transferases present in this tissue exhibit the same molecular weights as the equivalent liver enzymes, bilirubin GT (54 kDa) and the foetal phenol GT (53 kDa), (M. Coughtrie et al, submitted for publication).

Irshaid et al (1986) have recently reported the purification of a human liver (53 kDa) GT exhibiting broad substrate specificity and catalysing O-and N-glucuronidation.

Obviously, the difficult purification work must continue and substrate specificity studies performed simultaneously on several different purified GTs. The existence of an increasing number of GTs and the vast range

Table 1. Substrate Specificity of Purified Rat Hepatic UDP-Glucuronyltransferases (GTS)

ENZYMES	SUBSTRATES	SUBUNIT	SPECIFIC INDUCERS	REFERENCES
4-Nitrophenol-GT (GT-1)	4-nitrophenol 1-naphthol 2-aminophenol 4-methylumbelliferone 3-hydroxybenzo(a)pyrene	56	3-methyl-cholanthrene	Burchell, 1977 Bock et al, 1979 Falany & Tephly, 1983 Tephly & Green, 1986
Bilirubin GT	bilirubin	54	clofibrate	Burchell, 1980; Burchell & Blankaert, 1984
Phenol-GT (foetal)	phenol 1-naphthol 2-aminophenol 4-nitrophenol	53	β-naphthoflavone	Scragg et al, 1985
3α-hydroxy-steroid-GT	etiocholanolone androsterone lithocholic acid chenodeoxycholic acid 4-aminobiphenyl	52	phenobarbital	Kirkpatrick et al, 1984 Tephly & Green, 1986
17β-hydroxy-steroid-GT	testerone 4-nitrophenol 1-naphthol naphthylamine	50	phenobarbital	Matern et al, 1982 Falany & Tephly, 1983 Kirkpatrick et al, 1984 Tephly & Green, 1986

Table 1 (cont'd)

ENZYMES	SUBSTRATES	SUBUNIT	SPECIFIC INDUCERS	REFERENCES
Morphine GT	(-)morphine	56	phenobarbital	Puig & Tephly, 1986
GT-2	4-hydroxybiphenyl chloramphenicol	?	phenobarbital	Bock et al, 1979
GT-3	oestrone	?	aroclor 1254	Weatherill & Burchell, 1980; Lillienblum et al, 1982
GT-4	digitoxigenin-monodigitoxoside	?	spironolactone pregnenolone-16α-carbonitrile	Richards & Lage, 1977 Watkins et al, 1982 Von Meyerinck et al, 1985.

GTs 2,3 and 4 are possible different transferases which have not been completely purified.

of substrates presents a formidable challenge to the
protein chemist.

IMMUNOCHEMICAL ANALYSES WITH ANTI-GT ANTIBODIES

Many anti-GT antibodies have been raised in rabbits,
sheep, chickens and mice using various apparently
homogenous preparations of individual UDPGTs as antigens.
To date, a monospecific antibody preparation which will
recognise a single isoenzyme has not been obtained in this
laboratory or reported elsewhere. The extensive sequence
homology predicted from cDNA clones (see below) emphasises
the difficulties that will be encountered in raising
antibodies with an apparently homogeneous preparation of
antigen, due to the presence of common epitopes on
different GTs.

To overcome this problem we have used antigens purified
from different tissues or species, and attempted affinity
purification of antibody preparations. The use of purified
rat kidney bilirubin/phenol UDP-glucuronyltransferase has
proved to be the most successful method of obtaining a more
specific preparation of anti-GT antibodies. Polyclonal
anti-rat liver GT antibodies raised in sheep (Burchell et
al., 1984) specifically inhibited up to 85% of the
transferase activities towards bilirubin, testosterone,
androsterone, morphine, 1-naphthol and 4-methyl-
umbelliferone. Assay of these activities is believed to
represent at least five or six different isoenzymes based
on purification work (See Table 1). Indeed, immunoblot
analysis of rat liver microsomes revealed the existence of
at least five immunoreactive polypeptides, which exhibit
molecular weights of 50-56 kDa (Burchell et al., 1986).
Individual isoenzymes can be identified by immunoblot
analysis of microsomes from developing, genetically
deficient and xenobiotic pre-treated animals compared to
purified transferases (Scragg et al., 1985; Burchell et
al., 1986 and unpublished work).

This sheep anti-rat liver GT antibody preparation was
tested for its ability to interact with human liver
microsomal GTs. Transferase activities towards 1-naphthol,
bilirubin and testosterone were specifically inhibited up
to 85% by incubation with anti-rat liver UDPGT antibodies.
Further, the antibody recognises a similar spectrum of GT
isoenzymes (52-56 kDa) to those observed on immunoblot
analysis of rat hepatic microsomes (See Figure 1A). This
work illustrates for the first time the existence of
separable UDPGT isoenzymes in human liver, a feature well
documented for rat liver GTs (Burchell et al., 1985; Scragg

et al., 1985).
    Polyclonal anti-rat kidney GT antibodies raised in goats have been used to specifically identify bilirubin GT (Mr 54 kDa) in clofibrate-treated rat liver microsomes and a phenol GT (Mr 53 kDa) present in β-naphthoflavone-treated livers (Figure 1).

Figure 1.   Immunoblot analysis of human and rat liver microsomal proteins with anti-rat GT IgGs.

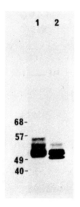 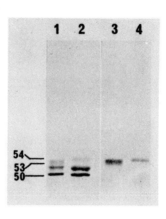

A. Microsomal proteins from the liver of an adult human (lane 1,20μg) or Wistar rat (lane 2,10μg) were analysed by electrophoresis on a 7% SDS-polyacrylamide gel.   Proteins were transferred to nitrocellulose and the blot incubated with anti-rat liver GT.
B. Microsomal proteins (10 μg) from β-naphthoflavone-treated Wistar rat livers (lanes 1 and 3) and clofibrate-treated rat livers (lanes 2 and 4) were analysed on a 7% SDS-polyacrylamide gel. Proteins were transferred to nitrocellulose and the blot incubated with anti-rat liver GT IgG (lanes 1 and 2) or anti-rat kidney GT IgG (lanes 3 and 4).   Chromogenic detection of specifically bound IgG was achieved using the immunoperoxidase system utilising 4-chloro-1-naphthol as substrate.

    The improved specificity of this preparation could be due to the presence of antibodies which recognise possible carbohydrate structures attached to the kidney proteins. In a different glycosylated protein, it was determined that antiserum raised against deglycosylated kidney γ glutamyl-transpeptidase failed to recognise the native form of the enzyme (Coloma and Pitot, 1986), indicating the role of carbohydrate structures in the specific immunodetection of glycoproteins.

ISOLATION OF RAT AND HUMAN LIVER GT cDNA CLONES

Our use of affinity-purified anti-GT antibodies to clone cDNAs coding for UDPGTs from rat liver cDNA libraries in the expression vector λ gt11 have already been described (Jackson et al., 1985; Jackson and Burchell, 1986). More recently, additional GT cDNA clones have been obtained by further screening of (i) a foetal rat liver cDNA library (S. Wilson et al, unpublished work) with cDNA probes or (ii) adult rat liver cDNA library using anti-kidney-GT antibodies (D. Harding et al., unpublished work). A comparison of the nucleotide sequences of 35 rat GT cDNAs allowed their categorisation into four classes of cDNA which presumably code for four different GT mRNAs (Jackson and Burchell, 1986; Jackson et al., 1986). The sequences of the different cDNAs are 85-96% homologous within the coding regions. Indeed, the close similarities of some class 3 cDNAs indicates the existence of microheterogeneities where 6 nucleotide changes are found over 1170 base pairs of sequence. Only one of these changes results in a significant non-conservative change of amino acid (unpublished work). Some of our cDNAs isolated more recently have more extensive 5'sequences, e.g. rlug38 (Class 3 GT cDNA), than those previously reported (Jackson and Burchell, 1986 and Figure 2).

A cDNA clone encoding a human liver GT has been isolated from a λ gt11 human liver cDNA library and exhibits extensive sequence homology to the rat liver GT cDNAs (Jackson et al., 1986).

COMPARISON OF THE AMINO ACID SEQUENCE DEDUCED FROM RAT AND HUMAN GT cDNAs

The nucleotide sequence of the junction between the lacZ gene and GT cDNAs in bacteriophage λ gt11 recombinants is obtained by nucleotide sequence analysis and allows identification of the translation reading frame of GT cDNAs (See Jackson and Burchell, 1986).

It is difficult to predict the 5'methionine codon at the start site of the cDNA clones without knowledge of the amino-terminal sequence analysis of individual proteins. This problem is heightened by the size of some cDNA clones (possibly not full length) and possibly post-translational processing of the GTs. The size of proteins predicted from nucleotide sequences compared with fusion proteins, mature purified GTs and the transferases synthesised in vitro (Jackson et al., 1985; Jackson and Burchell, 1986) can also lead to possible errors in identification of the

Figure 2. Comparison of the amino acid sequences (single letter code) deduced from rat and human liver cDNAs.

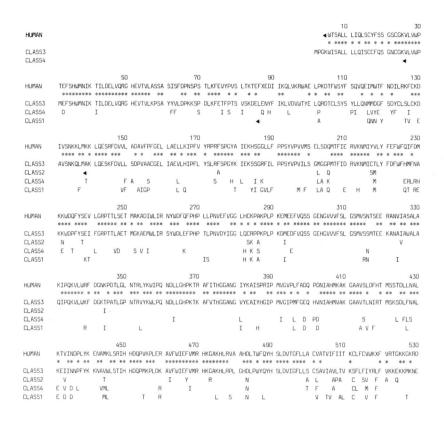

The amino acid sequences are deduced using the predicted start site of rlug38 (Class 3 cDNA). The limit of amino-terminal sequences of hlug24 and other rat cDNA is indicated by the arrows (←). The homology of hlug24 to rlug38 is indicated by the asterisks. Two additional residues observed in rlug38 at residues 87 and 519 are introduced into hlug24 to maximise the homology. The differences of class 2, 4 and 1 sequences from rlug38 are indicated by the replacement amino acids.

translation start site. The concensus start site sequence
described by Kozak (1985) for ribosomal proteins does not
appear to be generally useful, although the first ATG in an
mRNA is usually used (Kozak, 1984).

The deduced amino acid sequences translated from rat
and human GT cDNA clones are compared in Figure 2 using the
methionine codon (ATG) at nucleotide position 72-75 in
rlug38. The human cDNA clone (hlug24) which is very highly
homologous to the sequence of rlug38 over the 5'region
might then be considered too short to encode the complete
coding sequence. Amino acid composition analysis (Falany
et al., 1986) and preliminary amino terminal sequence
analysis (M. Green and T. Tephly, personal communication)
of androsterone GT confirm that rlug23 encodes this
transferase.

The predicted molecular weight of the unmodified rat
and human GTs, translated from this initiation codon, are
now calculated to be over 60 kDa whilst the GT synthesised
in reticulocyte lysates have been estimated to have
molecular weights of approximately 52 kDa (Jackson et al.,
1985). Anomalous migration of GT on SDS polyacrylamide gel
electrophoresis might explain some of this discrepancy.
Recently Mackenzie (1986) has reported the sequence of a
rat liver cDNA which is homologous (61-65%), but shows
differences from the sequences in Figure 2. The deduced
amino acid sequence from this cDNA clone predicts a
sequence of 529 amino acids, Mr 60.5 kDa, but in vitro
translation of this cloned mRNA released a protein of 52
kDa.

Inspection of the rat (rlug38) and human (hlug24)
sequences indicate at least 65% homology rising to 79% if
conservative amino acid changes are taken into
consideration. However, it should be noted that we may not
be comparing cloned cDNAs coding for the same transferases
in rat and human liver, and therefore the homologies of rat
and human GTs may be even greater than observed in this
comparison.

Differences between rat and human amino acid sequences
do not seem to occur at random in the proposed coding
region, perhaps implicating a functional role for highly
conserved regions, for example, a UDPglucuronic acid
binding site or maintenance of membrane topology. Atchison
and Adesnick (1986) have proposed that divergent residues
in very homologous cytochrome P450 b and e occur mainly in
two short segments, which in P450e are located in exon 7.

The presence of apparently constant and variable
regions might indicate that these different segments are
encoded by different exons, and that newly evolved GTs may

arise by gene duplication with gene conversion resulting in sequence homogenisation in constant regions.

Comparison of computer derived hydrophobicity plots by the method of Hopp and Woods (1981) also showed that predicted human and rat GT proteins have a very similar overall pattern of conserved hydrophobic segments.

Inspection of the amino terminal sequence of the predicted human and rat proteins translated shows a highly conserved sequence which might act as a signal sequence (See Figure 3) for co-translational insertion into the endoplasmic reticulum membrane (See Rapoport, 1985).

Figure 3. Possible cleavage site of pre-UDP glucuronyl-transferases.

```
←--CLEAVED SIGNAL SEQUENCE ? --->  ← MATURE UDP GLUCURONYLTRANSFERASE-

       -20    -15   -10    -5  -1 1    5     10     15    20

HUMAN    ? ? ? ? W T S A L L L I Q L S C Y F S S G S C G K V L V W P T E F S H W M N I K T I L -
RLUG38   M P G K W I S A L L L L Q I S C C F Q S G N C G K V L V W P M D F S H W M N I K T I L -
RLUG23                              ? ? ? L V W P M D F S H W M N I K T I L -
```

A comparison of three GT amino acid sequence is shown. The extension of the mature androsterone GT amino terminal sequence was deduced from rlug23 cDNA and amino terminal sequence analyses (M.D. Green and T. Tephly, personal communication). The possible cleavage site further identified from concensus sequence analysis (Von Heijne, 1983, 1984). The ?'s indicate the presence of unknown residues.

POST-TRANSLATIONAL MODIFICATION OF UDP-GLUCURONYLTRANS-FERASES

GTs may be post-translationally modified by proteolytic cleavage, glycosylation or fatty acid acylation which would occur in the lumen of the endoplasmic reticulum following insertion of the protein into the membrane (See Rapoport, 1985).

The evidence for post-translational cleavage of a signal sequence from GT is not particularly strong. Mackenzie and Owens (1984) have reported that a 2 kDa peptide is cleaved from some in vitro synthesised rat GTs by inclusion of dog pancreas microsomes in the reticulocyte lysate incubation mixture. These microsomes contain the components necessary for post-translational modification of proteins (Shields and Blobel, 1978; Hanover and Lennarz, 1981). Improved electrophoretic separation, which showed

at least three in vitro synthesised GTs with Mr of 5052 kDa
(Jackson, 1986) presents a more confused picture; the
reported processing of a 52 kDa GT to 50 kDa was not
obvious and a clearer analysis is required. Mackenzie
(1986) has cloned a GT cDNA into the expression vector
pSP64, which allows synthesis of GT mRNA in vitro by SP6
RNA polymerase. This mRNA translated in vitro in
reticulocyte lysates in the presence or absence of dog
pancreas microsomes indicated a partial cleavage of the
protein (Mackenzie, 1986).

The best evidence in support of a cleaved signal
sequence has been very recently indicated from preliminary
amino terminal sequence analysis of purified rat liver
androsterone GT (M.D. Green and T. Tephly, personal
communication). The work suggests that the mature
androsterone GT begins 3 residues upstream of the amino
acid sequence deduced from rlug23 cDNA (Jackson and
Burchell, 1986, see Figure 3). Thus, by analogy of GT
sequences deduced from rlug38 of hlug24 cDNAs starting from
the earlier initiation codon might be assumed to encode
pre-GT sequences (see Figure 3). Cleavage of the
hypothetical pre-GT at a position consistent with the amino
terminus of mature androsterone GT would indeed be
predicted based on the pattern of amino acids identified
near signal sequence cleavage sites (Von Heijne 1983, 1984;
Watson, 1984). The evidence presented here is by no means
conclusive, and it is possible that the amino terminal
residue determined by protein sequence analysis may be the
result of 'artefactual' proteolytic cleavage during
purification. Other microsomal proteins, cytochrome P450's
(see Coon et al, 1985) and epoxide hydrolase (Dubois et al,
1979) do retain their "signal" sequences. Further work is
required to unequivocally determine if GT is produced as a
pre-protein. The use of a coupled in vitro transcription-
translation system (Steuber et al, 1984) or SP6 (See
Mackenzie, 1986) with cloned GT cDNA and purified signal
peptidase (see Finidori et al, 1984) should help to resolve
this problem.

The size of some GTs present in vivo (50-56 kDa)
indicated by purification work and immunochemical analysis
(see previous sections) which are greater than the GTs
synthesised in vitro (52 kDa), suggests that post-
translational glycosylation might be responsible for the
differences. Most purified GTs have been reported to be
glycoproteins following periodic acid/Schiff reagent
staining (Roy Chowdhury et al, 1986). Glycosylation of a
rodent liver GT has been demonstrated by inclusion of dog
pancreas microsomes during in vitro synthesis of GTs

(Mackenzie et al, 1984; Mackenzie, 1986). The carbohydrate moiety could be subsequently removed by treatment of the proteins with endoglycosidase H.

Putative glycosylation sites in the GT amino acid sequences deduced from cDNA clones suggest that this form of post-translational modification could occur (Burchell and Jackson, 1986; Mackenzie, 1986; See Figure 2). Our preliminary experiments using endoglycosidase F to deglycosylate purified bilirubin GT indicates that this GT is post-translationally glycosylated (unpublished work).

An alternative explanation of the discrepancy in mobility of in vivo and in vitro synthesised GTs during SDS polyacrylamide gel electrophoresis might be due to N-terminal acylation (Towler and Glaser, 1986). The deduced amino terminal amino acid at putative cleavage sites in rlug38 and hlug24 is glycine (See Figure 3). At least one microsomal protein, NADH cytochrome b_5 reductase, is myristoylated at the N-terminal glycine (Ozols et al, 1984) it is possible that some GTs could be myristoylated to 'cement' the membrane orientation.

MEMBRANE TOPOLOGY OF UDP-GLUCURONYLTRANSFERASE

The characteristics of GT described above would suggest that GT might be anchored into the endoplasmic reticulum membrane by the carboxy-terminal transmembrane domain, with the majority of the protein including the amino-terminus being located on the lumenal side. The highly hydrophobic sequence followed by the short and very highly charged carboxy-terminal tail protruding from the membrane into the cytoplasm could act as a stop transfer signal, and might help to maintain the membrane orientation of the protein (Rapoport, 1985). A putative glycosylation site (Hanover and Lennarz, 1981) is found in the predicted human and rat class 1 and 4 GT sequence at residue 316, and also at residue 442 in rat class 2, consistent with the above model. The proposed topology suggests the active site of the enzyme has a lumenal location, and this would certainly help to explain the trypsin insensitivity of GT in intact microsomes (Wilkinson and Hallinan, 1977) and influence theories concerning the known latency of this enzyme (Dutton, 1980).

CONCLUDING REMARKS

Whilst considerable advances have been achieved over the last two years in molecular characterisation of rat and human GTs, more work is required to identify more members

of this family of enzymes. In particular, various human
and rat liver cDNAs need to be identified with particular
GT activities and this should be achieved by further amino
acid sequencing and expression of full length cDNAs in
yeast or cell cultures. In this way we should rapidly
obtain an understanding of the molecular heterogeneity of
this family of proteins, which play such a key role in the
metabolism of drugs and detoxification of foreign
compounds. The future advantages of cloning of human GT
cDNAs should be that the metabolic activities of these
enzymes can be studied following their expression in
various cell culture lines. Stable integration of GT
cDNAs in cell cultures using retroviral vectors (see Ledley
et al, 1986) should facilitate the determination of the
substrate specificity and drug glucuronidation by the
expressed transferases.

ACKNOWLEDGEMENTS

We are especially grateful to Richard Hynes and Savio
Woo for supplying their liver cDNA libraries, to Roland
Wolf for making available human liver samples and to
Mitchell Green and Tom Tephly for communicating preliminary
amino terminal sequence analysis of purified rat liver
androsterone UDPGT prior to publication. We also thank the
Medical Research Council and the Wellcome Trust for grants
supporting this work. MWHC and SW hold SERC studentships.
BB is a Wellcome Trust Senior Lecturer.

REFERENCES

Atchison, M. and Adesnik, M. (1986). Proc. Natl. Acad. Sci
     (USA), 83, 2300.
Bock, K.W., Josting, D., Lillienblum, W. and Pfeil, H.
     (1979). Eur. J. Biochem, 98, 19.
Burchell, B. (1977). FEBS Lett, 78, 101.
Burchell, B. (1980). FEBS Lett, 111, 131.
Burchell, B. (1981). Rev. Biochem. Toxicol, 3, 1.
Burchell, B. and Blankaert, B. (1984). Biochem. J. 223,
     461.
Burchell, B., Kennedy, S.M.E., Jackson, M.R. and McCarthy,
     L. (1984). Biochem. Soc. Trans, 12, 50.
Burchell, B., Jackson, M.R., Kennedy, S.M.E., McCarthy,
     L.R. and Barr, G.C. (1985). In "Microsomes and Drug
     Oxidations" (Ed. Boobis, A.R., Caldwell, K., De
     Matteis, F. and Elcombe, C.R.) Taylor and Francis,
     LondonandPhiladelphia, p.212.
Burchell, B., Coughtrie, M.W.H., Shepherd, S.R.P., Scragg,

I., Leakey, J.E.A., Hume, R. and Bend, J.R. (1986). Zbl. Pharm. in press.

Coloma, J. and Pitot, H.C (1986). Biochem. Biophys. Res. Commun, 135, 304.

Coon, M.J., Black, S.D., Fujita, V.S., Koop, D.R. and Tarr, G.E. (1985). In "Microsomes and Drug Oxidations" (Ed by Boobis, A.R., Caldwell, J., De Matteis, F. and Elcombe, C.R.) Taylor and Francis, London and Philadelphis, p.42.

Dubois, G.C., Appella, E., Armstrong, R., Levin, W., Lu, A.Y.H and Jerina, D.M. (1979). J. Biol. Chem, 254, 6240.

Dutton, G.J. (1980). "Glucuronidation of Drugs and other compounds", CRC Press, Boca Raton, Florida, USA.

Falany, C.M. and Tephly, T.R. (1983). Arch. Biochem. Biophys, 227, 248.

Finidori, J., LaPerche, Y., Haguenauer-Tsapsis, R., Barouki, R., Guellaen, G. and Hanoune, J. (1984). J. Biol. Chem, 259, 4687.

Hanover, J.A. and Lennarz, W.J. (1981). Arch. Biochem. Biophys, 211, 1.

Hopp, T.P. and Woods, K.R. (1981). Proc. Natl. Acad. Sci, (USA), 78, 3824.

Irshaid, Y., Nghiem, D.D. and Tephly, T.R. (1986). Fed. Proc, 45, 933.

Jackson, M.R. (1986). PhD Thesis, University of Dundee.

Jackson, M.R., McCarthy, L.R., Corser, R.B., Barr, G.C. and Burchell, B. (1985). Gene 34, 147.

Jackson, M.R. and Burchell, B. (1986). Nuc. Acid. Res, 14, 799.

Jackson, M.R., McCarthy, L.R., Harding, D., Wilson, S., Coughtrie, M.W.H. and Burchell, B. (1987). Biochem, J, 242, 581.

Kirkpatrick, R.B., Falany, C.N. and Tephly, T.R. (1984). J. Biol. Chem, 259, 6176.

Kozak, M. (1984). Nuc. Acids. Res, 12, 857.

Kozak, M. (1986). Cell, 44, 283.

Ledley, F.D., Grennett, H.E., McGinnis-Shelnutt, M. and Woo, S.L.C. (1986). Proc. Natl. Acad. Sci (USA), 83, 409.

Lillienblum, W., Walli, A.K. and Bock, K.W. (1982). Biochem. Pharmacol, 31, 907.

Mackenzie, P.I. (1986). J. Biol. Chem, 261, 6119.

Mackenzie, P.I. and Owens, I.S. (1984). Biochem. Biophys. Res. Commun, 122, 1441.

Mackenzie, P.I., Gonzalez, F.J. and Owens, I.S. (1984). Arch. Biochem. Biophys, 230, 676.

Matern, H., Matern, S. and Gerok, W. (1982). J. Biol.

Chem, 257, 7422.

Ozols, J., Carr, S.A. and Strittmatter, P. (1984). J. Biol. Chem, 259, 13349.

Puig, J.F. and Tephly, T.R. (1986). Fed. Proc, 45, 933.

Rapoport, T.A. (1985). FEBS Lett, 187, 1.

Richards, L.G. and Lage, G.L. (1977). Toxicol. App. Pharmacol, 42, 309.

Roy Chowdhury, J., Roy Chowdhury, N., Falany, C.N. and Tephly, T.R. (1986). Biochem. J. 233, 827.

Scragg, I., Celier, C. and Burchell, B. (1985). FEBS Lett, 183, 37.

Sheilds, D. and Blobel, G. (1978). J. Biol. Chem, 253, 3753.

Steuber, D., Ibrahimi, I., Cutler, D., Dobberstein, B. and Bujard, H. (1984). EMBO. J. 3, 3143.

Tephly, T.R. and Green, M.D. (1986). Fed. Proc, 45, 934.

Towler, D. and Glaser, L. (1986). Proc. Natl. Acad. Sci (USA), 83, 2812.

Von Heijne, G. (1983). Eur. J. Biochem, 133.

Von Heijne, G. (1984). EMBO J. 3, 2315.

Von Myerinck, L., Loffmann, B.L., Green, M.D., Kirkpatrick, R.B., Schmoldt, A. and Tephly, T.R. (1985). Drug Metab. Disp, 13, 700.

Watson, M.E.E. (1984). Nuc. Acids. Res, 12, 5145.

Watkins, J.B., Gregus, Z., Thompson, J.N. and Klaassen, C.D. (1982). Toxicol. App. Pharmacol, 64, 439.

Weatherill, P.J. and Burchell, B. (1980). Biochem. J, 189, 377.

Wilkinson, J. and Hallinan, T. (1977). FEBS Lett, 75, 138.

THE REGULATION OF RAT LIVER EPOXIDE HYDROLASES IN RELATION TO THAT OF OTHER DRUG-METABOLIZING ENZYMES

Christopher Timms, Ludwig Schladt, Larry Robertson, Petra Rauch, Helga Schramm and Franz Oesch.

Institute of Toxicology, University of Mainz, Obere Zahlbacher Strasse 67, Mainz, FRG.

INTRODUCTION

Since 1950, when Boyland first proposed that the hydrolysis of polycyclic aromatic hydrocarbon epoxides proceeds enzymically, a wealth of information has been obtained regarding the enzyme system, epoxide hydrolase (E.C.3.3.2.3).

Indeed, recent work has concentrated on identifying and characterising the following multiple forms of this enzyme all of which, with the possible exception of cEH and mEH_t (as defined below), differ in substrate-specificity, molecular weight, immunological and activity-modulation characteristics :

1. mEH_b : microsomal, metabolizing both exogenous, e.g. polycyclic aromatic hydrocarbon epoxides (Bentley et al, 1976), alkene epoxides (Brooks et al, 1970; Dansette et al, 1978), and endogenous compounds, e.g. oestrogen and androgen epoxides (Oesch et al, 1981). Present in all species investigated.
Standard substrate : Benzo(a)pyrene 4,5-oxide.

2. mEH_{ch} : microsomal, metabolizing exclusively steroids, particularly certain epoxides of cholesterol and pregnenolone (Watabe et al, 1981; Levin et al., 1983; Oesch et al, 1984). Present in all species investigated.
Standard substrate : Cholesterol 5,6-oxide.

3. mEH_t : microsomal, and probably specifically peroxisomal (see later), with substrate specificity similar to cEH (Guenthner, 1986). Present in species investigated, i.e. mouse and human (Guenthner and Karnezis, 1986).
Standard substrates : trans-stilbene oxide and trans-ethylstyrene oxide.

4.   cEH : cytosolic, with complementary substrate
specificity to mEH_b (Oesch and Golan, 1980), but also
metabolising exogenous e.g. certain alkene epoxides
(Hammock and Hasegawa, 1983), and endogenous compounds,
e.g. fatty acid epoxides (Gill and Hammock, 1979; Chacos et
al, 1983). A soluble enzyme in human leukocytes has been
reported to catalyse the hydrolysis of leukotriene A_4 to
the dihydroxy acid leukotriene B_4, but this is probably a
different enzyme (Radmark et al 1984); however, a purified
mouse liver cEH has been reported to catalyze the formation
of a 5,6-dihydroxyeicosatetraenoic acid from leukotriene A_4
(Haeggstrom et al., 1986).   Present in all species
investigated.
Standard substrates : trans-stilbene oxide and trans-
ethylstyrene oxide.

    For the purpose of this review, we would like to
concentrate on the two forms, mEH_b and cEH, with a minor
section concerning mEH_t. Although recent studies have
investigated the substrate-specificity and the inhibition
of mEH_{ch}, (Sevanian and McLeod, 1986; Nashed et al, 1986),
an inducer for this enzyme has not been described.

1. mEH_b INDUCTION

    In analogy to several other drug-metabolizing enzymes,
microsomal epoxide hydrolase, mEH_b (Timms et al., 1984) is
inducible by a wide range of xenobiotics. These include
epoxides, halogenated industrial compounds, phenolic
antioxidants, polycyclic aromatic hydrocarbons as well as
various drugs and pharmaceuticals (for a comprehensive
review, see Parkki, 1982).
    The list of potent inducers of mEH_b can be further
divided into those compounds which are good substrates for
the enzyme, e.g. cis-stilbene oxide (CSO) (Watabe et al.,
1971) and those which are not, e.g. trans-stilbene oxide
(TSO) (Oesch and Schmassmann, 1979) and the phenolic
antioxidants, 2(3)-tert-butyl-4-hydroxyanisole (BHA), and
3,5-di-tert-butyl-4-hydroxy-toluene (BHT), (Seidegard and
De Pierre, 1983).
    Although the broad inducibility of mEH_b is comparable
with that of other drug-metabolizing enzymes, certain
differences exist. Historically, xenobiotics have been
classified as inducers on the basis of the cytochrome P-450
isozymes affected. Many compounds in addition to
phenobarbital (PB), cause increases in cytochromes $P-450_b$
and $P-450_e$ (Thomas et al., 1983) while other xenobiotics
like the polycyclic aromatic hydrocarbon 3-

methylcholanthrene (MC) increase the isozymes cytochrome P-450_c and P-450_d. Indeed, many xenobiotics have been classified as inducers of drug-metabolizing enzymes on the basis of comparison to these 'classical' inducers. The description of the inductive effects of TSO (Schmassmann and Oesch, 1978) however, made it clear that this classification may not be universally applied. Although TSO induces the same cytochrome P-450 isozymes as PB (Meijer et al., 1982; Thomas et al., 1983), TSO is somewhat weaker than PB as a cytochrome P-450 inducer whilst being much more potent than PB as an inducer of mEH_b and several conjugating (phase II) enzymes (De Pierre et al., 1984; Kuo et al., 1984). Compounds like TSO and CSO (Seidegard et al, 1981) are of particular interest to the toxicologist since they are able to shift the spectrum of xenobiotic-metabolizing enzyme activities in that conjugating, and other potentially detoxifying, activities are enhanced. Administration of TSO, for example, leads to a profound shift in the metabolism of benzo(a)pyrene which is accompanied by a marked lowering of mutagenic metabolites (Bucker et al, 1979).

Inspection of Table 1 reveals that despite quantitative differences, compounds like PB which lead to an increase in cytochromes P-450_b and P-450_e, shown here as increases in the specific activity of aminopyrine N-demethylase, also lead to increases in mEH_b activity. Other examples of this inducer type include racemic TSO as well as the TSO enantiomers, and the TSO analogue trans-1,2-diphenyl-aziridine (TSI). In direct contrast to mEH_b activity, cEH activity was not increased by any of the xenobiotics whilst the activity of glutathione transferase, towards the broad spectrum substrate 1-chloro-2,4-dinitrobenzene (CDNB) was increased in all treatment groups.

The attractive possibility that cytochrome P-450_b + P-450_e and mEH_b are coordinately regulated prompted the immunoquantitation of these enzymes, following administration of a homologous series of polyhalogenated biphenyls. Although each PCB or polybrominated biphenyl (PBB) which led to an increase in cytochromes P-450_b and P-450_e also increased the level of mEH_b, statistical analysis demonstrated a poor correlation (Parkinson et al., 1983a; Dannan et al., 1983). Differential turnover rates may partly explain this poor correlation and indeed Parkinson et al (1983b) have provided evidence that in the livers of Aroclor 1254-treated rats, cytochromes P-450_b + P-450_e have half-lives of 37 and 28 h for the apoprotein and heme moieties respectively, whilst mEH_b has a much longer half-life of 132 h. Perhaps it is also of relevance to note

Table 1. Effects of various xenobiotics on hepatic microsomal and cytosolic enzyme activities in young male Sprague-Dawley rats[1]

	Cytochrome P-450 content (nmol/mg protein)	Aminopyrine N-demethylase (nmol/mg/min)	Microsomal EH[2] (nmol/mg/min)	Cytosolic EH[3] (pmol/mg/min)	Glutathione transferase[4] (nmol/mg/min)
Control n=7	0.41	4.0	5.8	21	576
PB n=7	1.30**	12.0**	9.8***	15	1520**
MC n=7	0.99**	5.2	6.3	21	1330**
(+)-TSO n=4	1.00**	9.1**	15.5**	23	1340**
(+)-TSO n=4	1.10**	9.8***	17.8***	15	1520**
(-)-TSO n=4	0.74**	6.3**	16.7**	11	1400**
(+)-TSI n=3	0.61	7.1	9.7	18	1380**

1-one-month old rats were treated for 3 consecutive days and killed on the fourth day
2-measured using benzo(a)pyrene 4,5-oxide. 3-measured using trans-stilbene oxide.
4-measured using CDNB.
All rats were fasted 24 hours prior to sacrifice.
*,** significantly different from the control mean at $p < 0.05$ or $p < 0.01$, respectively.

here, that Guengerich and Davidson (1982) have observed coupling of mEH$_b$ to the two cytochrome forms induced by PB and β-napthoflavone, with a tighter binding of mEH$_b$ to the latter. However, the consequences of this observation for corregulation of the two enzyme systems are unclear.

Interestingly, we have recently discovered a compound which increases both mEH$_b$ and cEH activities. Perfluorodecanoic acid (PFDA) has unexpectedly long lasting effects after a single i.p. application (up to 21 days) (Table 2). The concurrent induction of mEH$_b$ and cEH was quite unexpected, since compounds which potently induce cytochrome P-450 and mEH$_b$ do not alter cEH activity (Table 1) and conversely, the potent inducers of cEH, notably the peroxisome proliferators (see discussion below), do not increase mEH$_b$ in the rat. In contrast to cEH however, another cytosolic enzyme, namely glutathione transferase, exhibited slightly reduced activity after PFDA treatment. Unfortunately, PFDA is not suitable as an experimental probe for investigating the interrelationship between cytochromes P-450$_b$ + P-450$_e$ and mEH$_b$ since this compound selectively destroys these PB-inducible cytochrome P-450 isozymes (Rauch, Oesch and Robertson, unpublished data.

2. cEH INDUCTION

As indicated in the introduction, the induction of mEH$_b$ and cEH in rats is almost mutually exclusive, i.e. compounds which induce mEH$_b$ have little effect on cEH and vice versa. In fact, only hypolipidaemic agents and plasticisers are known to be inducers of cEH activity.

The discovery that hypolipidaemic agents induce peroxisome proliferation and hepatomegaly (hypertrophy) was made in the 1960's (Paget, 1963; Hess et al, 1965) and later work showed peroxisome proliferation to be frequently associated with hypotriglyceridemic compounds but not with hypocholesteremic agents, such as probucol (Cohen and Grasso, 1981). Also, the corresponding induction of the various peroxisomal enzymes, e.g. catalase, carnitine acyl transferase, and the peroxisomal fatty acid β-oxidation system has also been thoroughly investigated (for review see Reddy and Lalwani, 1983). In contrast, characterisation of the phthalate ester plasticisers has only been carried out more recently, using the two common plasticisers involved in the manufacture of polyvinylchloride plastics, di-(2-ethylhexyl)-phthalate (DEHP) and di-(2-ethylhexyl) adipate (DEHA). The main sources of exposure to man of such compounds are supermarket meat wraps, disposable medical devices, e.g.

Table 2. Effects of perfluorodecanoic acid (PFDA)-administration on various hepatic microsomal and cytosolic enzyme activities in young male Sprague-Dawley Rats[1]

	n	Cytochrome P-450 content (nmol/mg protein)	Aminopyrine N-demethylase (nmol/mg/min)	Microsomal EH[2] (nmol/mg/min)	Cytosolic EH[3] (pmol/mg/min)	Glutathione transferase[4] (nmol/mg/min)
Control	5	0.64	4.4	6.5	32	1170
PFDA day 3	3	0.70	2.7**	11.9**	140**	1020
PFDA day 6	3	0.78**	1.8***	13.6***	250***	850*
PFDA day 9	3	0.89*	2.1***	10.1***	200***	742**
PFDA day 12	3	0.96***	2.6***	9.5***	280***	717***
PFDA day 15	3	0.72	2.0***	11.0***	310***	570**
PFDA day 18	3	0.94**	2.9***	13.0***	220***	662**
PFDA day 21	3	0.89	5.2*	11.7	210	868**

1. A single i.p. injection of 70 mg PFDA/kg body weight was administered at various times and all rats were killed on the same day. Rats were 2 months old at the time of sacrifice and had been fasted for 24 hours.

2 Measured using benzo(a)pyrene 4,5-oxide.

3 Measured using trans-stilbene oxide

4 Measured using CDNB.

* ** significantly different from the control mean at $p < 0.05$ or $p < 0.01$, respectively.

polyvinylchloride plastic haemodialysis tubing, and environmental contamination, e.g. in estuarine and marine sediment (Reddy and Lalwani, 1983). These compounds have also been found to induce peroxisome proliferation and hepatomegaly in rats and mice in addition to their hypolipidaemic activity. However, the significance of peroxisome proliferators with respect to the various drug metabolizing enzyme system has largely been ignored until recently.

In 1983, Hammock and Ota showed that di-(2-ethylhexyl) phthalate, 2-ethyl-1-hexanol, and clofibrate are potent inducers of cEH in male Swiss-Webster mice, and that the induction of cEH and mEH_b in mice is not mutually exclusive. For example, whilst cEH was induced by these compounds, mEH_b was induced in parallel (2-fold). These authors also observed the aforementioned distinction between various types of hypolipidaemic agents : clofibrate which lowers the serum triglyceride and cholesterol concentration induces cEH and mEH_b to a similar extent whilst probucol, which specifically lowers the cholesterol level, has no significant effect on either of the two enzymes. Furthermore, although the evidence is very limited, it was also observed that whilst the two plasticisers investigated, DEHP and 2-ethyl-1-hexanol, induced the cytosolic glutathione transferase (using, 1,2-dichloro-4-nitrobenzene as substrate) approximately 2-fold, clofibrate exerted a weak inhibitory effect. Waechter et al (1984) have also reported the induction of both mouse liver cEH and mEH_b, but no change in glutathione transferase activity (using CDNB), with nafenopin. Recently, Loury et al (1985) investigated the organ specificity in male Swiss-Webster mice, showing that cEH was significantly induced in liver and kidney by clofibrate, whilst mEH_b induction showed substrate differentiation : although hydration of CSO was induced in liver and kidney, activity towards benzo(a)pyrene 4,5-oxide was induced only in liver. The authors used these and other data as evidence for the possible existence of novel forms of epoxide hydrolase. Also, in contrast to previous results, an induction by clofibrate of glutathione transferase in the liver was reported, using CSO as substrate.

Recently, work in our laboratories has been concentrated on the rat, and initial results, using Sprague-Dawley rats, showed significant induction of cEH with clofibrate in liver and kidney but in no other organs, with no significant effect on mEH_b. However, the large interindividual variation of cEH observed using this

outbred rat strain made it very difficult to obtain
statistically significant data, as can be observed in Table
3, using both controls and animals treated with
dibenz(a,h)anthracene (no induction) and clofibrate
(induction). Therefore in an effort to reduce the inter-
individual variation, it was decided to use an inbred
strain for further work, and Fischer 344 rats were used
thereafter.

   In an extended study, both triglyceride- and
cholesterol- lowering agents were investigated, as well as
various other compounds. Figure 1 presents the effects of
Aroclor 1254 and six hypolipidaemic compounds on the
relative activities of peroxisomal β-oxidation, palmitoyl
CoA hydrolase and the two epoxide hydrolase activities. In
contrast to Aroclor 1254, which only induces mEH_b, the
cholesterol-lowering agent probucol induces both palmitoyl
CoA hydrolase and mEH_b, although the latter is only weakly
induced (1.5-fold). In fact, the largest induction of mEH_b
(4.5-fold) was caused by benzylimidazole, with a
correspondingly weak induction of peroxisomal β-oxidation
and cEH (1.5-fold). In contrast, a weak triglyceride
agent, acetylsalicylic acid, induced all enzymes except
mEH_b, the extent of induction being dependent on the dose
administered : for example, a maximal induction of 5-fold
was observed for peroxisomal β-oxidation and cEH.
Furthermore, a similar, but exaggerated dose-dependent
response was obtained when potent triglyceride and
cholesterol-lowering agents, like clofibrate or
fenofibrate, were used. For example, 0.25% fenofibrate
(w/w) in the diet, induced peroxisomal β-oxidation
approximately 20-fold whilst cEH and palmitoyl CoA
hydrolase activities were both induced about 15-fold. In
addition, the typical hepatomegaly and peroxisome
proliferation were observed with all hypolipidaemic agents
except probucol as already reported (Cohen and Grasso,
1981). cEH induction was also observed in kidney, although
the effect was always weaker than in liver (the largest
increase seen was approximately 2-fold).

   However, it was important to discover if the increases
in enzyme activities can truly be classified as induction.
When the test compounds were added to an in vitro
incubation, cEH activity was weakly inhibited, whereas mEH_b
activity remained unchanged except in the presence of
benzylimidazole which caused an activation (2.6-fold).
Therefore, these results confirmed that the measured
increases in cEH activity are a result of induction,
whereas it cannot be ruled out that activation

Table 3. Response of rat liver and kidney cytosolic epoxide hydrolase following treatment with dibenz (a,h)anthracene (DBA) and clofibrate.

Tissue	Individual	Control	DBA	Clofibrate
			Specific activity of cEH (pmol TSO/mg protein/min)	
LIVER	1	47.1	16.9	47.7
	2	30.0	19.8	110.3
	3	43.9	44.6	105.5
	4	7.0	39.2	261.2
	5	24.4	40.7	197.5
	6	46.3	38.8	188.8
	$\bar{x}$	33.1	33.3	151.8**
KIDNEY	1	90.3	47.5	68.4
	2	84.8	37.8	163.7
	3	87.5	77.7	121.5
	4	2.8	91.4	117.4
	5	36.3	100.1	121.3
	6	100.9	91.1	106.3
	$\bar{x}$	60.3	74.3	109.8*

Animals were treated by i.p. injection of 25 mg/kg DBA or 200 mg/kg clofibrate on three consecutive days. After fasting overnight, animals were sacrificed on the fourth day.

* ** significantly different from control animals (*α= 0.05 and, ** α = 0.01) according to the u-test of Wilcoxon, Mann and Whitney.

Figure 1. Inducibility of peroxisome β-oxidation, cytosolic epoxide hydrolase, microsomal epoxide hydrolase and palmitoyl-CoA hydrolase activities.

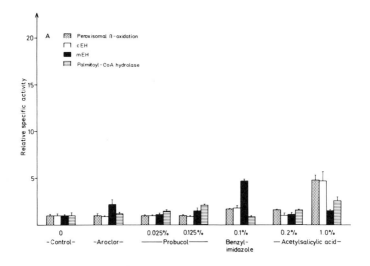

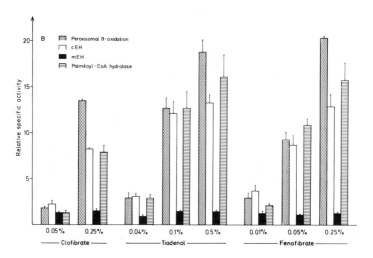

The drugs were given in the diet for one week. The concentration of the drugs in the diet (% w/w) is given. Animals were treated with Aroclor 1254 by two i.p. injections of 500 mg/kg seven, and four days before killing.

significantly contributes to the increased mEH_b activity observed with benzylimidazole.

Furthermore, as can be observed in Table 4, the induction of cEH and peroxisomal β-oxidation is species-specific, with the rat and mouse being positive and the guinea-pig negative in this respect, the specific activities remaining unchanged after treatment with the test substances. The significance of this result for toxicological risk estimation for man remains however, to be fully elucidated.

3. INDUCTION OF mEH_t

After the initial discovery of this enzyme in mouse liver (Guenthner et al, 1981), further characterization has shown many similarities between mEH_t and cEH, particularly in substrate-specificity, inhibition and induction characteristics (Guenthner, 1986).

Apart from these studies there is a relative lack of information in the literature characterising this form, which may be due to the relatively low amounts of this enzyme present. However, recently, using sucrose gradients in isopycnic centrifugation in a zonal rotor, we have observed the presence of this enzyme in the peroxisomal fraction of the rat liver, which agrees with similar evidence presented for mouse liver activity (Waechter et al, 1983; Patel et al, 1986). Also after administration of 0.1% fenofibrate (w/w) in the diet to the rats for 10 days, a significant increase of the activity was observed in the purified peroxisomes, paralleling the situation described for cEH, and thereby providing more evidence of the similarities of these two enzyme forms.

CONCLUSIONS

1. mEH_b is inducible by a wide range of xenobiotics which also induce cytochrome P-450, although convincing evidence for coregulation with specific forms of cytochrome P-450 has not yet been presented.

2. mEH_b and cEH inducers are mutually exclusive in the rat, with the exceptions of perfluorodecanoic acid and 1-benzylimidazole which significantly induce both enzymes.

3. cEH is induced in parallel with peroxisomal β-oxidation but with neither mEH_b nor other drug-metabolizing enzymes such as the cytosolic glutathione transferase.

Table 4. Species differentiation of peroxisomal proliferation and epoxide hydrolase induction in response to clofibrate.

SUBSTRATE	MOUSE		RAT			GUINEA-PIG		
	mEH_b(BPO)[1]	cEH(TSO)	MEH_b[2](STO)	cEH(TSO)*	Peroxisomal β-Oxidation[3]	mEH_b(STO)	cEH(TSO)*	Peroxisomal β-Oxidation
Control	3.45 ±0.55	68.1 ±18.8	4.0 ±0.5	38.0 ±8.0	5.2 ±0.3	31.02 ±2.05	294.1 ±7.4	2.26 ±0.38
Clofibrate-treated	7.66 ±0.51	174 ±6.0	5.8 ±0.6	312 ±7.0	70.0 ±3.89	29.64 ±3.89	296.5 ±18.5	1.89 ±0.10
	0.5% clofibrate (w/w) for 10 days		0.25% clofibrate (w/w) for 7 days			0.25% clofibrate (w/w) for 28 days		

1 Benzo(a)pyrene 4,5-oxide as substrate
2 Styrene 7,8-oxide as substrate
3 Measured according to Bieri et al (1984)

All values expressed as nmol/min/mg protein except, * which are pmol/min/mg protein
All mouse data taken from Hammock and Ota (1983)

4. mEH$_t$ is probably of peroxisomal origin, and resembles cEH very closely in substrate-specificity and induction characteristics. We are now characterising this former activity and investigating possible interrelationships with cEH, and it cannot be excluded that the two forms are identical.

5. Species differences in enzyme induction are becoming apparent, e.g. absence of peroxisome proliferation in guinea-pigs and the consequences of these dissimilarities for the control of drug-metabolising enzymes have yet to be elucidated.

ACKNOWLEDGEMENTS

Trans-2,3-Diphenylaziridine and the trans-stilbene oxide enantiomers were provided by Professor E.P. Muller, Innsbruck and Professor Y. Okamoto, Osaka, respectively. This work was supported by the Deutsche Forschungsgemeinschaft (SFB 302) and the "Pole de Toxicologie de Bourgogne". Some of the work presented in this study represents a part of the PhD Thesis of H.S and P.R.

REFERENCES

Bentley, P., Schmassmann, H., Sims, P. and Oesch, F. (1976). Eur. J. Biochem, 69, 97.
Bieri, F., Bentley, P., Waechter, F. and Staubli, W. (1984). Carcinogenesis, 5, 1033.
Boyland, E. (1950). Biochem. Soc. Symp, 5. 40.
Brooks, G.T., Harrison, A. and Lewis, S.E (1970). Biochem. Pharmacol, 19, 255.
Bucker, M., Golan, M., Schmassmann, H.U., Glatt, H.R., Stasiecki, P. and Oesch, F. (1979). Mol. Pharmacol, 16, 656.
Chacos, N., Capdevilla, J., Falck, J.R., Manna, S., Martin-Wixtrom, C., Gill, S.S., Hammock, B.D. and Estabrook, R.W. (1983). Arch. Biochem. Biophys, 233, 639.
Cohen, A.J. and Grasso, P. (1981). Fd. Cosmet. Toxicol, 19, 585.
Dannan, G.A., Guengerich, F.P., Kaminsky, L.S. and Aust, S.D. (1983). J. Biol. Chem, 258, 1282.
Dansette, P.M., Makedonska, V.B. and Jerina, O.M. (1978). Arch. Biochem. Biophys, 187, 290.
De Pierre, J.W., Seidegard, J., Morganstern, R., Balk, L., Meijer, J., Astrom, A., Norelius, I. and Ernster, L. (1984). Xenobiotica, 14, 295.

Gill, S.S. and Hammock, B.D. (1979). Biochem. Biophys. Res. Commun, 89, 965.

Guengerich, F.P. and Davidson, N.K. (1982). Arch. Biochem. Biophys, 215, 462.

Guenthner, T.M. (1986). Biochem. Pharmacol, 35, 839.

Guenthner, T.M. and Karnezis, T.A. (1986). Drug. Metab. Disp. 14, 208.

Guenthner, T.M., Hammock, B.D., Vogel, U. and Oesch, F. (1981). J. Biol. Chem, 256, 3163.

Haeggstrom, J., Meijer, J. and Radmark, O. (1986). J. Biol. Chem, 261 : 6332.

Hammock, B.D. and Hasegawa, L.S. (1983). Biochem. Pharmacol, 32, 1155.

Hammock, B.D. and Ota, K. (1983). Toxicol. Appl. Pharmacol, 71, 254.

Hess, R., Staubli, W. and Riess, W. (1965). Nature, 208, 856.

Kuo, C-H., Maita, K., Rush, G.F., Sleight, S. and Hoo, J.B. (1984). Toxicol. Lett, 20, 13.

Levin, W., Michaud, D.P., Thomas, P.E. and Jerina, D.M. (1983). Arch. Biochem. Biophys, 220, 485.

Loury, D.N., Moody, D.N., Kim, B.W. and Hammock, B.D. (1985). Biochem. Pharmacol, 34, 1827.

Meijer, J., Astrom, A., De Pierre, J.W., Guengerich, F.P. and Ernster, L. (1982). Biochem. Pharmacol. 31, 3907.

Nashed, N.T., Michaud, D.P., Levin, W. and Jerina, D.M. (1986). J. Biol. Chem, 261, 2510.

Oesch, F., Beermann, D., Sparrow, A.J., Bentley, P. and Vogel-Bendel, U. (1981). Anal. Biochem, 117, 223.

Oesch, F. and Golan, M. (1980). Cancer Lett, 9, 169.

Oesch, F. and Schmassmann, H. (1979). Biochem. Pharmacol, 28, 171.

Oesch, F., Timms, C.W., Walker, C.H., Guenthner, T.M., Sparrow, A., Watabe, T. and Wolf, C.R. (1984). Carcinogenesis, 5, 7.

Paget, J.E. (1963). J. Atheroscler, Res 3, 729.

Parkki, M.G. (1982). Academic Dissertation, University of Turku, Finland.

Parkinson, A., Safe, S.H., Robertson, L.W., Thomas, P.E., Ryan, D.E., Reik, L.M. and Levin, W. (1983a). J. Biol. Chem, 258, 5967.

Parkinson, A., Thomas, P.E., Ryan, D.E. and Levin, W. (1983b). Arch. Biochem. Biophys, 225, 216.

Patel, B.N., Mackness, M.I., Nwosu, U. and Connock, M.J. (1986). Biochem. Pharmacol, 35, 231.

Radmark, O., Shimizu, T., Jornwall, H. and Samuelsson, B. (1984). J. Biol. Chem, 259, 12339.

Reddy, J.K. and Lalwani, N.D. (1983). CRC Critical Reviews

in Toxicology, 12, 1.
Schmassmann, H.U. and Oesch, F. (1978). Mol. Pharmacol, 14, 834.
Seidegard, J. and De Pierre, J.W. (1983). Biochim. Biophys. Acta, 695, 251.
Seidegard, J., De Pierre, J.W., Morgenstern, R., Pilotti, A. and Ernster, L. (1981). Biochim. Biophys. Acta, 672, 65.
Sevanian, A. and McLeod, L.L. (1986). J. Biol. Chem, 261, 54.
Thomas, P.E., Reik, L.M., Ryan, D.E. and Levin, W. (1983). J. Biol. Chem, 258, 4590.
Timms, C., Oesch, F., Schladt, L. and Worner, W. (1984). In Proceedings of the 9th International Union of Pharmacology Congress (Eds. Mitchell, J.F., Paton, W. and Turner, P). Macmillan Press, London, 231.
Waechter, F., Bentley, P., Bieri, F., Staubli, W., Volkl, A. and Fahimi, H.O. (1983). FEBS Lett, 158, 225.
Waechter, F., Bieri, F., Staubli, W. and Bentley, P. (1984). Biochem. Pharmacol, 33, 31.
Watabe, T., Akamatsu, K. and Kiyonaga, K. (1971). Biochem. Biophys. Res. Commun, 44, 199.
Watabe, T., Kanai, M., Isobe, M. and Ozawa, W. (1981). J. Biol. Chem, 256, 2900.

2. Human drug metabolizing enzymes.

HUMAN P-450 ENZYMES

Pierre Kremers[1] and Philippe Beaune[2]

[1]Laboratoire de Chimie Medicale, Institut de Pathologie
(B23), Universite de Liege, B - 4000, Sart Tilman par Liege
1, BELGIUM. [2]Inserm U 75, Laboratoire de Biochimie-CHU
Necker, Rue de Vaugirard, 156, F-75730 Paris-Cedex 15,
FRANCE.

INTRODUCTION

Cytochrome P-450, the catalytic moiety of the mixed
function mono-oxygenase, occurs as a large family of as yet
an unknown number of isozymes and catalyses the conversion
of multiple substrates into a variety of possible products
including detoxified metabolites as well as toxic and
carcinogenic compounds.

Human liver mono-oxygenases and cytochrome P-450 have
been extensively studied since 1975 (Boobis and Davies,
1984) and in recent years, human liver banks have been
established by several laboratories (Von Bahr et al, 1980;
Meier et al, 1983) and large liver samples have been
obtained from renal transplant donors in optimal conditions
(Kremers et al, 1981) enabling the determination of a wide
variety of enzymatic and biochemical characteristics of the
human mono-oxygenase system. Moreover, several
laboratories have undertaken the purification of the
different cytochrome P-450 isozymes from human liver (Wang
et al, 1983). A recent review article provides an overview
of the studies concerning human liver cytochrome P-450
(Boobis and Davies, 1984). The present paper summarises
some of the recent progress made in this field during the
last few years.

METHODS OF INVESTIGATION

Different methodological approaches have been used to
study human P-450, including "in vivo" studies, "in vitro"
studies on liver microsomes and experiments on purified
enzymes. These three aspects are fundamentally different
but complementary to each other and all present their
specific advantages and limitations.

"In vivo" Studies

Pharmacological studies were the first experimental insight into the field of drug metabolism and cytochrome P-450 dependent enzymes. This aspect is usually well documented in the numerous text-books dealing with pharmacology.

The principal limitation of these experiments is linked to the difficulty to interpret the data obtained since they result from the influence of various parameters like absorption, distribution, diffusion into membranes, and interaction with several components of the living organism. Nevertheless, the existence of a genetic polymorphism in drug odixation has been revealed by pharmacological studies. For example, the well-documented debrisoquine type polymorphism was discovered by pharmacokinetic and frequency distribution studies (Eichelbaum, 1984). In addition, pharmacokinetic studies have also established some induction effects (Remmer et al, 1979).

Use of Liver Microsomes

The availability of human liver tissue has considerably increased the number of publications using human liver microsomes. These studies include numerous measures of enzymatic activities (McManus et al, 1984; Boobis et al, 1985), electrophoretic profiles (Von Bahr et al, 1985), kinetic studies (McManus 1983; Inaba et al, 1985), correlation studies (Beaune et al, 1986; Meier et al, 1983) and inter-species comparison of activities (Kremers et al, 1981).

Since the discovery of genetic defects in drug oxidation, numerous studies were devoted to a large scale screening of drugs and substrates in order to identify the molecules whose metabolism was supported by the same P-450 isozyme (Meier et al, 1983; Wolff et al, 1985). At least 12 different drugs were metabolized by the P-450 responsible for debrisoquine hydroxylation as confirmed by immunochemical inhibition studies (Wolff, 1985).

Isozyme Purification

Since the purification by Guengerich and coworkers of six cytochrome P-450 isozymes from human liver (Wang et al, 1983), several attempts have been made to purify other P-450 isozymes (Beaune et al, 1985a). Particular attention has been devoted to the P-450's involved in drug polymorphism. An isozyme with high activity for bufuralol hydroxylation (Gut et al, 1984) has been purified. Guengerich's laboratory has purified the isozymes responsible for debrisoquine 4-hydroxylation, phenacetin-0-

deethylation and Nifedipine oxidation respectively (Distelrath et al, 1985; Guengerich et al, 1986). Others were prompted to look toward inducible P-450 forms in the human and a form inducible by glucocorticoids and macrolide antibodies has been identified and characterised (Watkins et al, 1985).

Use of Antibodies

Using purified and partially purified human liver P-450's, polyclonal as well as monoclonal antibodies have been prepared (Beaune et al, 1985b). These antibodies have been largely used for different purposes including quantification of individual isozymes in microsomal preparations (Cresteil et al, 1985), identification of P-450 isozymes (Thomas et al, 1984), immunopurification (Friedman et al, 1985) and interspecies comparisons (Adams et al, 1985). These antibodies and more particularly the specific monoclonal antibodies will be most helpful for studies in molecular biology.

CHARACTERISATION OF HUMAN LIVER P-450's

Correlated Monoxygenase Activities

A large characterization study has recently been undertaken in our laboratory (Beaune et al, 1986). 25 liver samples were screened for monooxygenase activity and P-450 content. P-450 isozymes were measured by an Elisa technique and by a Western blot procedure, using specific polyclonal and monoclonal antibodies (Table 1).

About 10 different substrates were used for the determination of more than 20 monooxygenase activities. The results obtained, partially depicted in Table 2, were analysed in a correlation study in order to determine the activities that are supported by one P-450 isozyme. This allowed us to classify the different monooxygenase activities into 5 groups (Table 3).
1. Cytochrome P-450-8 content was correlated with AHH and nitroanisole demethylase, both enzymatic activities are correlated with each other (Figure 1). 7-hydroxylation of S warfarin is also included in this group : it correlates with the content of isozyme 8 but not with AHH activity and nitroanisole demethylase. In a reconstituted system, the 7-hydroxylation of S-warfarin is the major activity supported by this isozyme (Wang et al, 1983). These conclusions are strengthened by the observation (Cresteil et al, 1985) that cytochrome P-450-8 is absent in human fetal liver microsomes where AHH and nitroanisole demethylase activity are very low.

Table 1. Cytochrome P-450 Content of Human Liver Microsomes

LIVER SAMPLE	CYTOCHROME P-450 spectrally determined (nmol.mg^{-1} protein)	P-450-5 immunochemically determined (nmol.mg^{-1} protein)	P-450-8	P-450-9
38	0.49	0.62	0.17	0.08
39	0.24	ND	0.13	ND
41	0.75	0.73	0.21	0.01
47	0.53	0.67	0.19	0.16
50	0.41	0.22	0.24	0.09
51	0.78	0.96	0.75	0.07
55	0.36	0.45	0.30	0.09
58	0.50	0.41	0.17	0.14
61	0.36	ND	ND	ND
62	0.23	0.38	1.06	0.22
66	0.32	0.33	0.66	0.11
69	0.51	0.33	0.67	0.09
70	0.61	ND	1.33	ND
72	0.52	0.51	1.2	0.05
73	0.39	ND	0.87	ND
75	0.67	ND	1.11	ND
76	0.40	ND	ND	0.06
77	0.68	0.24	0.16	ND
80	0.57	ND	ND	ND
81	0.64	ND	0.78	ND
83	0.55	0.54	1.0	0.03
84	0.48	0.13	1.25	0.04
85	0.53	0.28	ND	0.19
86	0.38	ND	ND	0.03
90	ND	0.56	0.90	0.02
Mean	0.49	0.44	0.66	0.09
S.D	0.14	0.21	0.41	0.07
n	24	16	20	17

ND = Not Determined
S.D. = standard deviation
n = number of samples measured

Table 2. Monooxygenase Activities in Human Liver Microsomes

ENZYMATIC ACTIVITIES (nmol product. min^{-1}. mg protein^{-1})	n	MEAN	S.D.
Aldrin epoxidase	19	0.34	0.15
Benzphetamine demethylase	23	1.5	0.6
4-nitroanisole-0-demethylase	23	2.5	1.0
Aryl hydrocarbon hydroxylase	24	0.18	0.06
Aniline hydroxylase	22	0.49	0.15
7-ethoxycoumarin-0-deethylase	22	0.17	0.13
Testosterone 6β-hydroxylase	23	1.2	0.6
DHEA 16α-hydroxylase	13	0.168	0.107
Pregnenolone 16α-hydroxylase	14	0.038	0.018

Figure 1. Human Liver Microsomes : AHH/isozyme 8

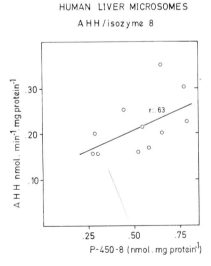

HUMAN LIVER MICROSOMES

AHH/isozyme 8

2. A second group involves P-450-5, benzphetamine-N-demethylase, aldrin epoxides and S warfarin 4'-hydroxylase which cross-react perfectly (Figure 2).

Figure 2. Human Liver Microsomes : benzphetamine N-demethylase/isozyme 5

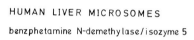

HUMAN LIVER MICROSOMES

benzphetamine N-demethylase/isozyme 5

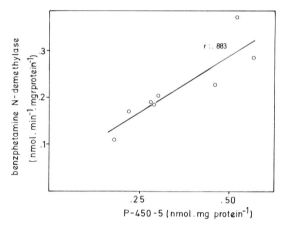

P-450-5 (nmol.mg protein^{-1})

Several other activities are associated to this group although they do not correlate with all the above activities (Table 3); it is the case for testosterone 6β-hydroxylase, cortisol 6β-hydroxylase, 10-hydroxylation of warfarin, formation of R-and S-dehydrowarfarin and the inhibition of 7-ethoxycoumarin-O-deethylase by metyrapone.

It is interesting to observe that these activities are supported in rat liver microsomes by forms induced by phenobarbital and/or pregnenolone-16α-carbonitrile. Moreover, the monoclonal antibody (KO3 13-7-10) developed against P-450-5 cross-reacts with P-450 PCN-E from rat liver.

The cytochrome P-450 induced in human liver by glucocorticoids or macrolide antibiotics shares some common properties with the present group in that it is recognised by the same antibody (KO3 13-7-10) (Watkins et al, 1985). The P450-NF isozyme recently purified (Guengerich, 1986) also supports most of these enzymatic activities.

3. The third group includes two enzymatic activities which correlate with total cytochrome P-450 level, but with none of the individual isozymes measured, namely 7-ethoxycoumarin-O-deethylase and dehydroepiandrosterone-16α-hydroxylase. These activities are both correlated to aniline-4-hydroxylase. One possible explanation is that an

Table 3. Human Liver Microsomes : Groups of Correlated Monooxygenase Activities.

Group 1 :   P-450-8

- Aryl Hydrocarbon Hydroxylase   - MAb : KO7
- 4-nitro-anisole-0-demethylase

also associated : S-Warfarin-7-hydroxylation

Group 2 :   P-450-5

- Aldrin epoxidase
- Benzphetamine N-demethylase   - MAb : KO3
- S-Warfarin-4-hydroxylase

also associated : Testosterone 6β-hydroxylase, inhibition by metyrapone, production of R- and S-dehydrowarfarin and of R and S-10-hydroxywarfarin, cortisol-6β-hydroxylase. P-450-NF, P-450-HLp

---

Group 3 :

- Dehydroepiandrosterone-16α-hydroxylase
- 7-ethoxycoumarin-0-deethylase

correlated to total cytochrome P-450

Group 4 :

- R-Warfarin-4-hydroxylation
- R-Warfarin-6-hydroxylation
- R-Warfarin-7-hydroxylation
- R-Warfarin-8-hydroxylation

associated to none of the measured P-450 isozyme

Group 5 :   P-450-9   - MAb : KO5

associated enzymatic activity : ?

---

undefined number of different P-450's all catalyse these
reactions.

4. A fourth group is represented by R warfarin-4,6,7 and 8
hydroxylations that are all cross-related. These enzymatic
activities are not correlated with the metabolism of other
xenobiotics and not correlated with the measured P-450
isozymes. They seem thus to be supported by a different
isozyme.

5. From a quantitative point of view, P-450-9 is a minor
form (Table 1) and correlates with none of the measured
enzymatic activities.

6. Debrisoquine hydroxylase activity does not correlate
with total cytochrome P-450 content or with the activities
of aldrin epoxidase, ethoxycoumarin-0-deethylase, arylhydrocarbon hydroxylase (Meier, 1983), but correlates with
most of the activities supporting the metabolism of drugs
associated to the same genetic defect.

Induction of P-450

There is abundant, albeit indirect, evidence that human
liver, like rodent liver, contains inducible cytochromes P-
450 (Remmer et al, 1979). Exposure of humans to inducers
of the animal P-450 system, like barbiturates, pesticides,
rifampicine, macrolide antibiotics and glucocorticoids
accelerates the metabolism and increases the blood
clearance of several drugs (Boobis and Davies, 1984).

Cytochrome P-450 analogous to forms induced in rat by
phenobarbital and methylcholanthrene have been identified
by immunochemical techniques in human liver (Adams et al,
1985). In a comparative study conducted on 6 human liver
samples it was demonstrated that administration of a
tricyclic antidepressant had an inductive effect on some
enzymatic activities (Cresteil et al, 1983).

From a study on human liver needle biopsy samples from
smokers and non smokers it appeared that cigarette smoking
induced ethoxyresorufin-0-deethylase and a P-450 isozyme
recognised by a monoclonal antibody directed against 3-
methycholanthrene induced P-450 from rat liver. Within the
same patients, smokers had a significantly higher
antipyrine clearance rate (Pelkonen, personnel
communication). P-450 HLp was induced by glucocorticoids
and was immunochemically related to the rat liver P-450p
(Watkins et al, 1985).

Comparison of Purified P-450's

The analytical data and criteria concerning purified P-450's vary from one laboratory to another so that it remains very difficult, if not impossible, to compare the different isozymes already purified. For instance, cytochrome P-450-5 (Wang et al, 1983), P-450-NF (Guengerich et al, 1986), P-450-HLp (Watkins) obviously share some common properties namely substrate specificity and reaction with the same monoclonal antibody (KO3-13-7-10). Whether or not these very similar proteins are derived from the same gene or gene family remains to be established. Monoclonal antibodies may be prepared in large amounts of reproducible material. Taking advantage of this opportunity it would be suitable to exchange antibodies between laboratories in order to systematise the characterisation of the isolated P-450's and to progress toward more homogeneity in the nomenclature of the various P-450 forms.

PERSPECTIVES

The amount of information concerning human P-450 has grown tremendously in recent years, and more recently, the molecular biology of the cytochrome P-450 family of isozymes is actively being investigated in several laboratories (Iversen, 1986; Molowa et al, 1986). On the other hand, experimental models using cultured hepatocytes (Hsu et al, 1985; Guillouzo et al, 1985) or established cell lines (Friedman et al, 1985) are in development. It is hoped that the information derived from all of these studies and a better knowledge of P-450 regulation will have broad implications in fields as diverse as drug design and risk of cancer assessment.

REFERENCES

Adams, D.J., Seilman, S., Amelizad, S., Oesch, F., Wolf, C.R. (1985). Biochem. J., 232, 869.
Beaune, Ph., Flinnois, J.P., Kiffel, L., Kremers, P., Leroux, J.P. (1985). Biochem. Bioph. Acta, 840, 364.
Beaune, Ph., Kremers, P., Letawe-Goujon, F.R., Gielen, J. (1985). Biochem. Pharmacol, 34, 3547.
Beaune, Ph., Kremers, P., Kaminsky, L.S., De Graeve, J., Albert, A., Guengerich, F.P. (1986). Drug Metab. Disp, in press.
Breimer, D.D. (1983). Clin. Pharmacokinetics, 8, 371.
Boobis, A.R., Davies, D.S. (1984). Xenobiotica, 14, 151.

Boobis, A.R., Murray, S., Hampden, C.E., Davies, D.S. (1985). Biochem. Pharmacol, 34, 65.

Cresteil, T., Celier, C., Kremers, P., Beaune, Ph., Leroux, J.P. (1983). Br. J. Pharmac, 16, 651.

Cresteil, T., Beaune, Ph., Kremers, P., Celier, C., Guengerich, F.P., Leroux, J.P. (1985). Eur. J. Biochem, 151, 345.

Distlerath, L.M., Reilly, P.E.B., Martin, M.V., Davis, G.G., Wilkinson, G.R., Guengerich, F.P. (1985). J. Biol. Chem, 260, 9057.

Ekstrom, G., Von Bahr, C., Glaumann, H., Ingelman-Sundberg, M. (1982). Acta. Pharmacol. Toxicol, 50, 251.

Eichelbaum, M. (1984). Fed. Proc, 43, 2298.

Friedman, F.K., Pastewka, J.V., Robinson, R.C., Park, S.S., Marletta, M.A., Gelboin, H.V. (1985) FEBS Lett, 185, 67.

Guengerich, F.P., Martin, M.V., Beaune, P.L., Kremers, P., Wolff, T., Waxman, D.J. (1986). J. Biol. Chem, 261, 5051.

Guillouzo, A., Begue, J.M., Campion, J.P., Gascoin, M.N., Guguen-Guillouzo, A. (1985). Xenobiotica, 15, 635.

Gut, J., Gasser, R., Dayer, P., Kronbach, T., Catin, T., Meyer, U.A. (1984). FEBS Lett, 173, 287.

Hsu, I.C., Lipsky, M.M., Cole, K.E., Su, C.H., Trump, B.F. (1985). In vitro C, 21, 154.

Inaba, T., Jurima, M., Mahon, W.A., Kalow, W. (1985). Drug Metab D, 13, 443.

Iversen, P.L., Hines, R.N., Bresnick, E. (1986). Bioessays, 4, 15.

Kremers, P., Beaune, Ph., Cresteil, T., De Graeve, J., Columelli, S., Leroux, J.P., Gielen, J. (1981). Eur. J. Biochem, 118, 599.

McManus, M.E., Boobis, A.R., Minchin, R.F., Schwartz, D.M., Murray, S., Davies, D.S., Thorgeirsson, S.S. (1984). Cancer Res, 44, 5692.

Meier, P.J., Mueller, H.K., Dick, B., Meyer, U.A. (1983). Gastroenterology, 85, 682.

Molowa, D.T., Schuetz, E.G., Wrighton, S.A., Watkins, P.B., Kremers, P., Mendez-Picon, G., Parker, G.A., Guzelian, P.S. (1986). Proc. Nat. Acad. Sci, in press.

Remmer, H., Fleischmann, R., Kunz, W. (1979). In "The induction of drug metabolism" (Ed. by Estabrook, R.W., Lindenlaub, E). Schattauer Verlag, Stuttgart, p.555.

Thomas, P.E., Reik, L.M., Ryan, D.E., Levin, W. (1984). J. Biol. Chem, 259, 3890.

Von Bahr, C., Spina, E., Birgersson, C., Ericsson, O., Goransson, M., Henthorn, T., Sjoqvist, F. (1985). Biochem. Pharmacol, 34, 2501.

Von Bahr, C., Groth, C.G., Janssen, H., Lundgren, G., Lind, M., Glaumann, H., (1980). Clin. Pharmacol. Ther, 27, 711.

Wang, P.H., Beaune, Ph., Kaminsky, L.S., Dannan, G.A., Kadlubar, F.F., Larrey, P., Guengerich, F.P. (1983). Biochemistry, 22, 5375.

Watkins, P.B., Wrighton, S.A., Maurel, P., Schuetz, E.G., Mendez-Picon, G., Parker, G.A., Guzelian, P.S (1985). Proc. Nat. Acad. Aci, 82, 6310.

Wolff, T., Distlerath, L.M., Worthington, M.T., Groopman, J.D., Hammons, G.J., Kadlubar, F.F., Prough, R.A., Martin, M.V., Guengerich, F.P. (1985). Cancer Res, 45, 2116.

HUMAN GLUTATHIONE S-TRANSFERASES

John D. Hayes, Lesley I. McLellan, Paul K. Stockman, John Chalmers, A Forbes Howie, Amanda J. Hussey and Geoffrey J. Beckett.

Department of Clinical Chemistry, University of Edinburgh, The Royal Infirmary, Edinburgh, EH3 9YW. Scotland, UK.

INTRODUCTION

The glutathione S-transferases (GST) play a pivotal role in drug metabolism. These enzymes catalyse the formation of a thioether bond between reduced glutathione (GSH) and a large number of lipophilic compounds that possess an electrophilic centre; this conjugation reaction is the first step in the synthesis of mercapturic acids (Jakoby, 1978; Chasseaud, 1979). Some of the compounds that serve as the second substrate for GST, such as halogenated hydrocarbons, may already possess an electrophilic centre and therefore require no modification prior to conjugation with GSH. Other potential substrates may require activation by the cytochrome P-450 dependent monooxygenases before they can be metabolised by GST. Although primarily thought to provide protection against xenobiotics (Smith et al, 1977; Sparnins et al., 1982; Glatt et al., 1983), it should be noted that the conjugation of GSH by GST to certain foreign compounds may markedly increase their toxicity (Rannug et al, 1978; Wolf et al, 1984).

GST are widely distributed in the animal kingdom and the cytosolic forms that have been isolated from mammalian sources are encoded by three multi-gene families (Mannervik et al., 1985; Hayes and Mantle, 1986a). The cytosolic GST each comprise two subunits of 24.0 - 27.5 kDa. Both homodimers and heterodimers exist but only subunits that are members of the same family can hybridise (Hayes, 1984, 1986; Stockman et al., 1985). An additional unique GST, composed of 14.0 kDa subunits, the activity of which is induced by N-ethylmaleimide, has been described in rodents, but not in man (Morgenstern et al., 1982, 1984). Each GST is active towards a distinct spectrum of electrophiles and the individual isozymes appear to serve different detoxification roles (Glatt et al., 1983; Coles et al., 1985; Jernstrom et al., 1985).

Recent work has focussed on the catalytic and molecular differences between the various rat GST forms but must less is known about the enzymes in man. Human cytosolic GST have been divided into three groups - 'basic', 'neutral' and 'acidic' (Mannervik, 1985). However, the structural and immunochemical properties of the GST in these groups is confused (cf Awasthi et al., 1980; Mannervik et al., 1985; Singh et al., 1985; Vander Jagt et al., 1985). Furthermore, variations in the GST content of individual human livers have been reported, but the polypeptide basis of these differences is poorly understood (Warholm et al., 1980; Board, 1981).

During the present study the polymorphism associated with human GST has been investigated and the properties of the purified enzymes are described. The relationship has been explored between human GST, rat microsomal GST and rat cytosolic Ya (25.5 kDa), Yb_1 (26.3 kDa), Yb_2 (26.3 kDa), Yc (27.5 kDa) and Yf (24.8 kDa) GST subunits (Hayes and Mantle, 1986b).

METHODS

Enzyme Assays
These were performed as described by Habig and Jakoby (1981).

Tissue and Preparation of Extracts
Human livers were obtained within 2h of death and were stored at -85°C until use. Human lung, that had no macroscopic evidence of disease, was obtained from a non-smoker 14h after death and was also stored at -85°C. Portions (20g or 300g) of frozen human liver were allowed to thaw at room temperature (20°C) and the resulting material was blended with 3 vols of ice-cold 50mM-Tris/HCl buffer pH 7.5. A portion of thawed human lung (approx. 500g) was blended in 2 vols of ice-cold 10mM-sodium phosphate buffer, pH 6.5. The cytosol and microsomal fractions were prepared by centrifugation using standard techniques.

Enzyme Purification
(a) Human GST - The hepatic cytosolic GST were purified using, sequentially, DEAE-cellulose (at pH 8.0), S-hexylglutathione affinity chromatography (by the method of Mannervik and Guthenberg, 1981), chromatofucusing and hydroxyapatite chromatography (Stockman et al., 1985). The

pulmonary GST was isolated using, sequentially, SP-Sephadex (at pH 6.5), S-hexylglutathione affinity chromatography and chromatofucusing (pH 6.0-4.0).

(b)   Rat GST - Rat GST were isolated to allow the preparation of antisera. The microsomal GST was purified by the method of Morganstern et al (1982), and the preparation of the cytosolic forms has been described previously (Hayes, 1983, 1984, 1986).

Immunoblotting
     This was performed using essentially the method devised by Towbin et al (1979) and is described elsewhere (Hayes and Mantle, 1986a). The antisera used were obtained by standard techniques and their specificities have been described (Hayes and Mantle, 1986a).

RESULTS

Polymorphism of Hepatic GST
     Differences in the microsomal and cytosolic GST content of several livers were studied. Unlike the cytosolic GST, the microsomal form is not retained by S-hexylglutathione-Sepharose. Human microsomes were therefore studied directly, whereas the cytosolic GST were purified by affinity chromatography before examination.
     The concentration of GST in microsomes prepared from five different human livers was examined by immunoblotting. Figure 1 shows a nitrocellulose blot of microsomes that had been subjected to SDS-PAGE. This demonstrated the presence of a 14 kDa poly-peptide in all human specimens examined; this co-migrated during electrophoresis with the rat microsomal GST and possessed similar immunochemical properties.
     Cytosolic GST represent a complex mixture of enzymes. The forms present in six different livers were examined by isoelectric focusing following S-hexylglutathione-Sepharose chromatography. Each purified GST pool produced a different electrophoretic pattern (Figure 2); the position of purified marker GST is indicated. Proteins at the cathodal, or basic, end of the gel were observed in all samples. Protein that migrated with GST ε (B_1B_1, pI 8.9) was represented strongly in livers B,C,D and E, whereas livers A and F contained predominantly GST γ (B_2B_2, pI 8.4); all livers possessed GST δ (B_1B_2, pI 8.75). Although the 'basic' GST were present in all liver samples, 'neutral' and 'acidic' GST were only detected in certain livers; GST μ was found in livers A,B and D, GST ψ was only

Figure 1. Identification of human microsomal GST by 'Western Blotting'

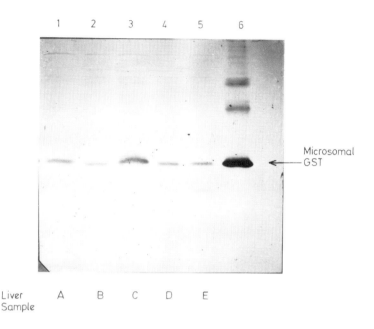

Human microsomes that were obtained by centrifugation at 100,000g from five separate livers were washed twice by repetitive ultracentrifugation. The pellets from the third centrifugation were re-suspended in 50mM-Tris/HCl buffer pH 7.5 and subjected to SDS/PAGE. Tracks 1-5 contain 100µg portions from livers A-E and track 6 contains 5 µg of purified rat microsomal GST. The polypeptides were transferred to nitro-cellulose paper which was probed with antisera raised against the rat microsomal GST (subunit 14.0 kDa). The immunoreactive protein was visualised with a peroxidase-labelled second antibody and 4-chloro-1-naphthol as substrate.

found in liver C and GST λ was faintly observed in liver C. Immunoblotting of cytosolic GST resolved by SDS/PAGE, showed that all livers contained GST subunits of 26.0 kDa that cross-reacted with anti-rat Ya-IgG. Livers A,B,C and D contained GST subunits of 26.7 kDa that cross-reacted with anti-rat Yb_1-IgG. Liver C showed very faint cross-reactivity with anti-rat Yf-IgG.

FIGURE 2.   Isoelectric focusing of purified cytosolic GST

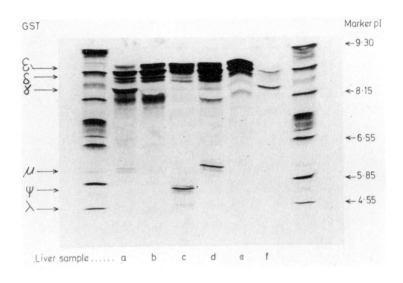

The cytosolic GST in six different liver specimens were separately purified by affinity chromatography on S-hexylglutathione-Sepharose that was developed by elution with 5mM S-hexylglutathione. IEF was performed using a broad range gel (pH 3.5-9.5) in thin-layer 5% (w/v) polyacrylamide. The liver samples applied (A-F) are indicated. The tracks on the extreme left and right contain the pI calibration proteins.

Purification of Human GST

(a) Hepatic Enzymes
   For preparative purposes, cytosol (normally from about 300g of liver) was dialysed against 10 litres of 20mM-Tris/HCl buffer pH 8.0 and applied to 4.4cm x 80.0cm columns of DEAE-cellulose that were equilibrated with the same buffer. The exchanger was developed with a 0-150mM NaCl gradient. Figure 3 shows the profile obtained from liver D; the initial peak of activity, the "flow through" fractions, contains both GST ϵ (B_1B_1) and GST δ (B_1B_2), the second peak of activity contains GST γ (B_2B_2) and the third peak of activity contains GST μ. GST ψ was isolated from liver C and it, like GST μ, was eluted by the salt gradient in peak 3. Although GST ϵ (B_1B_1) and GST δ (B_1B_2) were both recovered from DEAE-cellulose in peak 1 they were resolved

at a later stage in the purification scheme by chromatofocusing. Thus, the five major hepatic GST were each isolated using, sequentially DEAE-cellulose, S-hexylglutathione-Sepharose, chromatofocusing and hydroxyapatite. Table 1 summarises their chromatographic properties.

Figure 3. Resolution of Cytosolic GST in Human Liver by DEAE-Cellulose Chromatography

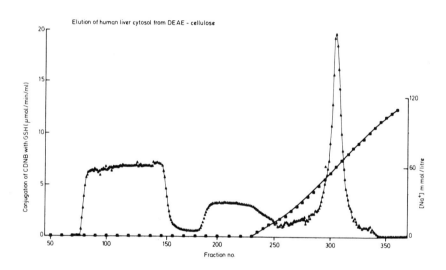

Elution of human liver cytosol from DEAE - cellulose

Hepatic cytosol from 300g of tissue was dialysed against 10 litres of 20mM Tris/HCl buffer pH 8.0. The resulting material (about 500ml) was applied to 4.4cm x 80.0cm columns of DEAE-cellulose. Fractions of 8.5ml were collected and the activity with 1-chloro-2,4-dinitrobenzene (CDNB, ▲) determined. The Na^+ concentration (■) was also measured.

(b) Pulmonary GST

GST λ was isolated from 500g of human lung. The cytosol, obtained following centrifugation at 100,000g, was dialysed against 15 litres of 10mM sodium phosphate buffer pH 6.5 and applied to SP-Sephadex (4.4cm x 80cm) equilibrated with the same buffer. The activity that was not retained by this exchanger was purified by affinity

Table 1.   Chromatographic Properties of Cytosolic GST Isoenzymes

GST	ORGAN	SUBUNIT SIZE (kDa)	DEAE-CELLULOSE	SP-SEPHADEX	CHROMATO-FOCUSING (pH eluted)	HYDROXY-APATITE ($[Na^+]$ mmol/1)
ψ	liver	26.7	peak 3	N.D.	7.1	85
μ	liver	26.7	peak 3	N.D.	7.8	100
γ	liver	26.0	peak 2	N.D.	N.D.	185
δ	liver	26.0	peak 1	N.D.	8.3	185
ε	liver	26.0	peak 1	N.D.	9.0	185
λ	lung	24.8	N.D.	Not retained	4.8	Not retained

DEAE-cellulose and SP-Sephadex chromatography were both performed in 4.4cm x 80.0cm columns at pH 8.0 and pH 6.5 respectively. Chromatofocusing was carried out using 1.6cm x 35.0cm columns of PBE 94. Hydroxyapatite columns (1.6cm x 19.0cm) were developed with 10-250 mM sodium phosphate gradients at pH 6.7. Abbreviation; N.D. - not determined.

chromatography and was finally eluted from the PBE 94
chromatofocusing gel at pH 4.8. The chromatographic
properties of GST are included in Table 1.

Distinguishing Features of Cytosolic GST

SDS/PAGE of the purified human GST showed that they
contain three subunit types of 24.8 kDa, 26.0 kDa and 26.7
kDa (Figure 4).

Figure 4. SDS/PAGE of Cytosolic GST

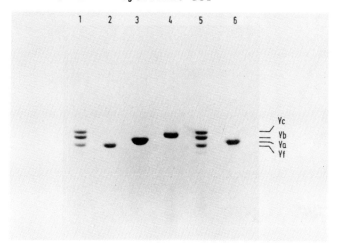

SDS/polyacrylamide-gel electrophoresis was performed in 12%
gels (w/v). Tracks 1 and 5 contain total rat lung GST.
Tracks 2, 3 and 4 contain GST ('acidic'), GST ('neutral')
and GST ('basic'). Track 6 contains rat liver GST (YaYa
protein). The position of the rat Yf (24.8 kDa), Ya (25.5
kDa), Yb (26.3 kDa) and Yc (27.5 kDa) is shown.

All the enzymes were found to comprise two subunits of
closely similar molecular mass. The 24.8 kDa polypeptide
(GST λ) cross-reacted with antisera raised against the rat
Yf GST subunit, the 26.0 kDa polypeptides (GST γ, δ and ϵ)
cross-reacted with antisera raised against the rat Ya GST
subunit and the 26.7 kDa polypeptides (GST μ and ψ) cross-
reacted with antisera raised against rat Yb_1 subunits
(Table 2).

All the GST purified catalyse the conjugation of 1-
chloro-2,4-dinitrobenzene with GSH but the subunit types
can be identified catalytically using other substrates,
such as ethacrynic acid, cumene hydroperoxide and p-
nitrobenzyl chloride. Thus, the GST that comprises 24.8
kDa subunits (λ) has a high activity with ethacrynic acid
as substrate. The GST that are composed of 26.0 kDa
subunits (γ, δ and ϵ) possess glutathione peroxidase

activity and are active with cumene hydroperoxide. The GST
that contain 26.7 kDa subunits (μ and ψ) have a high
activity towards p-nitrobenzyl chloride (Table 3).

Table 2. Immunochemical properties of GST

			INTENSITY OF CROSS-REACTIVITY WITH ANTISERUM AGAINST RAT SUBUNITS			
GST	Subunit Size (kDa)	pI	Anti-Yb$_1$	Anti-Ya	Anti-Yf	Anti-Yc
ψ	26.7	5.5	+++	-	-	-
μ	26.7	6.1	+++	-	-	-
γ	26.0	8.4	-	+	-	-
δ	26.0	8.75	-	+	-	-
ϵ	26.0	8.9	-	+	-	-
λ	24.8	4.8	-	-	+++	-

Antisera that were specific to the rat Ya (25.5 kDa), Yb$_1$
(26.3 kDa), Yc (27.5 kDa) and Yf (24.8 kDa) GST subunits
were obtained in female New Zealand White rabbits and their
crossreactivity with human GST was assayed by °Western
blotting' using a peroxidase labelled second antibody to
visualise the immunoreactive subunits.

DISCUSSION

     Human liver expresses both microsomal GST and cytosolic
GST. The microsomal enzyme appears to comprise subunits of
14.0 kDa that are immunochemically-related to the rat
microsomal form described by Morgenstern et al (1982;
1984). The cytosolic enzymes are composed of subunits of
either 24.8, 26.0 or 26.7 kDa that are respectively
immunochemically-related to the rat Yf, Ya and Yb GST
subunits. The cytosolic GST are dimeric and all the forms

identified were found to contain two subunits of equal size. The cytosolic enzymes in man have been grouped into the 'basic', 'neutral' and 'acidic' GST but the pI ranges used to identify the three families are not clear cut. The

Table 3. Discrimination between human GST using diagnostic substrates

GST	SUBUNIT SIZE (kDa)	pI	RELATIVE ACTIVITIES WITH				
			CDNB	pNBC	tPBO	CH	EA
ψ	26.7	5.5	+++++	+++	+++	−	+
μ	26.7	6.1	+++++	+++	+++	−	+
γ	26.0	8.4	++	−	−	+++	+
δ	26.0	8.75	++	−	−	++	+
ε	26.0	8.9	++	−	−	+	+
λ	24.8	4.8	++++	−	−	−	+++

Abbreviations -

CDNB, 1-chloro-2,4-dinitrobenzene; pNBC, p-nitrobenzyl chloride; tPBO, trans-4-phenyl-3-buten-2-one; CH, cumene hydroperoxide; EA, ethacrynic acid.

observation that the 'basic' GST comprise 26.0 kDa (Ya) subunits, the 'neutral' GST comprise 26.7 kDa (Yb) subunits and the 'acidic' GST comprise 24.8 (Yf) subunits suggests these enzymes might be more reliably classified, like the rat GST, according to their mobility during SDS/PAGE. A comparison between the equivalent rat and human GST revealed that the microsomal forms have a closely similar size as do the rat and human Yf subunits. However, differences in the electrophoretic mobilities of the rat Ya (25.5 kDa) and the human Ya (26.0 kDa) subunits as well as the rat Yb (26.3 kDa) and the human Yb (26.7 kDa) subunits are evident in Figure 4.

Significant differences in the cytosolic GST content of the six livers examined were revealed by isoelectric focusing; variations were observed in both the 'basic' (pI 8.0-8.9) and the 'neutral' (pI 5.5-6.1) regions of the IEF gel. Differences in the 'basic' GST expressed in individual livers have been shown to be due to the existence of two different Ya-type subunits, previously referred to as B_1 and B_2 (Stockman et al., 1985). During this study a marked difference was noted in the neutral' GST; the absence has been noted in certain livers of GST with either pI 6.1, or pI 5.5 or both. Subsequent purification of these enzymes showed the proteins of pI 6.1 and 5.5 both contained subunits of approximately 26.7 kDa, suggesting the existence of two Yb-type subunits in man.

Board (1981) used zymogram starch-gel analysis to investigate the variations in GST expressed in man and was the first to suggest that cytosolic forms could be ascribed to the existence of three loci; locus 1 is equivalent to the 'neutral' or Yb-containing forms, locus 2 is equivalent to the 'basic' or Ya-containing forms and locus 3 is equivalent to the acidic' or Yf-containing forms. The GST in human liver are primarily the products of locus 1 and 2. From his studies of the patterns of hepatic GST activity (towards 1-chloro-2,4-dinitrobenzene as electrophile) Board proposed that three autosomal alleles exist at locus 1 (one of which is null) and two autosomal alleles exist at locus 2. Our data are in broad agreement with that of Board but provide information about the polypeptide and catalytic differences between the GST in man.

The acidic' or Yf-containing GST are present in very low levels in normal human liver. This enzyme can be isolated from human lung; the Yf subunit is also present in rat lung (See Figure 4). Similarly, in rat liver the Yf sub-unit is normally only present in very low levels. However, the Yf subunit, in both rat and human livers, is specifically induced in experimentally produced preneoplastic nodules and hepatomas (Faber, 1984; Satoh et al., 1985; Soma et al., 1985; Meyer et al., 1985; Jensson et al., 1985).

The genetic variation associated with the Ya- and Yb-containing GST may affect the susceptibility of different individuals to toxic insult by carcinogens and other environmental pollutants.

ACKNOWLEDGEMENTS

This work was funded by grants from the Medical

Research Council (G8126392 SB) and the Scottish Home and Health Department (K/MRS/50/C570). We thank Mrs E. Ward for typing this script.

REFERENCES

Awasthi, Y.C., Dao, D.D. and Saneto, R.P. (1980). Biochem. J. 191, 1-10.
Board, P.G. (1981). Am. J. Hum. Genet, 33, 36-43.
Chasseaud, L.F. (1979). Adv. Cancer. Res, 29, 175-274.
Coles, B., Meyer, D.J., Ketterer, B., Stanton, C.A. and Garner, C. (1985). Carcinogenesis, 6, 693-697.
Farber, E. (1984). Biochim. Biophys. Acta, 738, 171-180.
Glatt, H., Friedberg, T., Grover, P.l., Sims, P. and Oesch, F. (1983). Cancer Res, 43, 5713-5717.
Habig, W.H. and Jakoby, W.B. (1981). Meth. Enzymol, 77, 398-405.
Hayes, J.D. (1983). Biochem. J. 213, 625-633.
Hayes, J.D. (1984). Biochem. J. 224, 839-852.
Hayes, J.D. (1986). Biochem. J. 223, 789-798.
Hayes, J.D. and Mantle, T.J. (1986a). Biochem. J. 233, 779-788.
Hayes, J.D. and Mantle, T.J. (1986b). Biochem. J. in press.
Jakoby, W.B. (1978). Adv. Enzymol. Relat. Areas Mol. Biol. 46. 383-414.
Jensson, H., Eriksson, L.C. and Mannervik, B. (1985). FEBS Lett, 187, 115-120.
Jernstrom, B., Martinez, M., Meyer, D.J. and Ketterer, B. (1985). Carcinogenesis 6, 85-89.
Mannervik, B. (1985). Adv. Enzymol, 57, 357-417.
Mannervik, B. and Guthenberg, C. (1981). Meth. Enzymol, 77, 231-235.
Mannervik, B., Alin, P., Guthenberg, C., Jensson, H., Tahir, M.K., Warholm, M. and Jornvall, H. (1985). Proc. Natl. Acad. Sci, USA, 82, 7202-7206.
Meyer, D.J., Beale, D., Tan, K.H., Coles, B. and Ketterer, B. (1975). FEBS Lett 184, 139-143.
Morgenstern, R., Guthenberg, C. and De Pierre, J.W. (1982). Eur. J. Biochem, 128, 243-248.
Morgenstern, R., Lundqvist, F., Andersson, G., Balk, L. and De Pierre, J.W. (1984). Biochem. Pharm, 33, 3609-3614.
Rannug, U., Sundvall, A. and Ramel, C. (1978). Chem-Biol. Interactions, 20, 1-16.
Satoh, K., Kitahara, A., Soma, Y., Inaba, Y., Hatayama, I. and Sato, K. (1985). Proc. Natl. Acad. Sci. USA, 82 3964-3968.
Singh, S.V., Dao, D.D., Partridge, C.A., Theodore, C.,

Srivastava, S.K. and Awasthi, Y.C. (1985). Biochem. J. 232, 781-790.

Smith, G.J., Ohl, V.S. and Litwack, G. (1977). Cancer Res, 37, 8-14.

Soma, Y., Satoh, K. and Sato, K. (1986). Biochim. Biophys. Acta, 869, 247-258.

Sparnins, V.L., Venegas, P.L. and Wattenberg, L.W. (1982). J. Natl. Cancer Inst, 68, 493-496.

Stockman, P.K., Beckett, G.J. and Hayes, J.D. (1985). Biochem. J. 227, 457-465.

Towbin, H., Staehlin, T. and Gordon, J. (1979). Proc. Natl. Acad. Sci, USA, 76, 4350-4354.

Vander Jagt, D.L., Hunsaker, L.A., Garcia, K.B. and Roger, R.E. (1985). J. Biol. Chem. 260, 11603-11610.

Warholm, M., Guthenberg, C., Mannervik, B., Von Bahr, C. and Glaumann, H. (1980)ˋ Acta. Chem. Scand, B34, 607-610.

Wolf, C.R., Berry, P.N., Nash, J.A., Green, T. and Lock, E.A. (1984). J. Pharmacol. Exp. Ther, 228, 202-208.

POLYMORPHISMS OF HUMAN DRUG METABOLISING ENZYMES

Urs A. Meyer,

Department of Pharmacology, Biocenter of the University,
CH-4056 Basel, Switzerland.

INTRODUCTION

Genetic polymorphisms of drug metabolising enzymes give rise to distinct subgroups in the population which differ in their ability to perform a certain drug biotransformation reaction. Genetic polymorphisms thus contribute considerably to interindividual variation in drug response. A well-known classical example of such a genetic polymorphism is the deficiency of liver N-acetyltransferase which affects the metabolism of caffeine, clonazepam, dapsone, hydralazine, isoniazid, nitrazepam, phenelzine, procainamide, sulphamethazine and sulphapyridine (for review, see Weber and Hein, 1985). In recent years a number of genetic polymorphisms of drug oxidation by hepatic microsomal monooxygenases (cytochrome P450) have been discovered (for review, see Franklin and Parke, 1986). Thus, independently occuring polymorphic drug oxidations with monogenic inheritance have been described for the metabolism of antipyrine (Penno and Vesell, 1983), debrisoquine (debrisoquine/sparteine-type polymorphism, see below), tolbutamide (Scott and Poffenbarger, 1979), mephenytoin (Kupfer and Preisig, 1984), carbocysteine (Mitchell et al, 1984) and nifedipine (Kleinbloessem et al, 1984). This review will concentrate on the debrisoquine/sparteine-type polymorphism and the mephenytoin-type polymorphism, because our laboratory has studied the mechanisms of these two deficiencies of drug-metabolising enzymes in liver tissue of extensive (EM)- and poor metabolizer (PM)-subjects (for review, see Meyer et al, 1986).

GENERAL CONSIDERATIONS IN REGARD TO THE MOLECULAR MECHANISMS RESPONSIBLE FOR GENETIC VARIATIONS IN CYTOCHROME P-450 ISOZYMES IN HUMAN BEINGS.

The principle mechanisms causing quantitative or

functional deficiencies in cytochrome P-450 isozymes in
human liver are summarised in Table 1. It is evident from
these considerations that the elucidation of the molecular
basis of these polymorphisms requires access to large
quantities of human liver tissue for isolation and
purification of proteins and RNA, but also access to tissue
(liver, DNA) from subjects of families phenotyped in vivo
to establish the causal relationship between in vitro and
in vivo findings. Moreover, sensitive assays for the
involved metabolic reactions are necessary to monitor the
purification of P-450 isozymes with affinity for the
substrates in question.

**Table 1. Possible mechanisms responsible for a deficiency
of cytochrome P450 isozymes in human.**

---

1.   Abnormal function of enzyme
     a. Decreased affinity for substrates (Km)
     b. Decreased maximal velocity (Vmax)
     c. Combination of a. and b.
     d. Change in the stereoselectivity of the reaction

2.   Decreased intracellular concentration or absence of
     enzyme protein
     a. Diminished rate of synthesis
     b. Accelerated degradation of labile enzyme variant

3.   At DNA/RNA level
     a. Deletion, insertion of rearrangement of gene
     b. Defect in transcription, RNA processing or RNA
         stability

ESTABLISHMENT OF A BANK OF HUMAN LIVER TISSUE

In order to investigate these polymorphisms we have
established a bank of human liver tissue. This bank
presently contains 28 human livers collected immediately
after circulatory arrest from kidney transplant donors.
Tissue from these livers was used to adapt and optimise
fractionation procedures, storage conditions and enzyme
assays. In addition, over 100 wedge biopsies of 0.5 to 2g
wet-weight were obtained from the livers of patients during
either diagnostic or therapeutic laparotomy and these
patients could (or can still) tested for one of these
polymorphisms. A large number of methods and techniques

have been developed for the fractionation, storage and enzymatic characterisation of human liver tissue and for the study of cytochrome P-450 dependent monooxygenase reactions (Meier et al, 1983).

THE DEBRISOQUINE/SPARTEINE-TYPE POLYMORPHISM OF DRUG OXI-DATION.

The best studied example of a genetically controlled polymorphism of hepatic cytochrome P-450 function is the debrisoquine/sparteine-type polymorphism. In 1977, at St. Mary's Hospital Medical School in London, it was discovered that some individuals were not able to oxidise the anti-hypertensive drug debrisoquine to 4-OH-debrisoquine (Mahgoub et al, 1977; Price-Evans et al, 1980). At about the same time, in Bonn (FRG), it was independently observed that a genetic deficiency of sparteine oxidative metabolism was a frequent cause of side-effects of this anti-arrhythmic and oxytocic drug (Dengler and Eichelbaum, 1977; Eichelbaum et al, 1979). It soon became clear that the impaired metabolism of both sparteine and debrisoquine was caused by the same genetic mechanism (Bertilsson et al, 1980a; Inaba et al, 1980). Subsequent studies have shown that the metabolism of debrisoquine and sparteine is impaired in 7 to 9% of the white population in Europe and North America (Price-Evans et al, 1980, Wedlund et al, 1984) and family studies have indicated that "poor metabolisers" of debrisoquine and sparteine are homozygous for an autosomal recessive gene (Price-Evans et al, 1980). Most importantly, these subjects also exhibit an impaired oxidation of numerous other drugs including antiarrhythmic agents (Woosley et al, 1985; Shah et al, 1982; Zekorn et al, 1983), beta-adrenoceptor blocking drugs (Alvan et al, 1982; Dayer et al, 1982a; Dayer et al, 1982b; Lennard et al, 1982; McNay et al, 1983; Lennard et al, 1984; Raghuram et al, 1984; Lewis et al, 1985; McGourty et al, 1985; Dayer et al, 1985) antidepressants (Bertilsson et al, 1980b; Balant-Gorgia et al, 1982; Bertilsson and Aberg-Wistedt, 1983; Alvan et al, 1984) and other clinical drugs (Sloan et al, 1978; Kitchen et al, 1979; Oates et al, 1982; Roy et al, 1985; Schmid et al, 1985; see Table 2).

Clinical studies have provided convincing evidence that poor metabolisers of the debrisoquine/sparteine-type poly-morphism represent a singular subgroup of the population with a propensity to develop exaggerated drug responses, untoward drug effects or therapeutic failure (Eichelbaum, 1982; Idle and Smith, 1984). Recent studies also have indicated that a link might exist between the

Table 2. Examples of drugs whose metabolism is known to be under the same or linked monogenic control as the debrisoquine/sparteine-type polymorphism.

Drug	Drug
Antiarrhythmic agents	Beta-adrenoceptor blocking drugs
Encainide	Alprenolol
Perhexiline	Bopindolol
Propylajmaline	Bufuralol
Sparteine	Metoprolol
	Penbutolol
	Propranolol
	Timolol
Antidepressants	Others
(+)-Amiflamine	Debrisoquine
Amitriptyline	Dextromethorphan
Clomipramine	Guanoxan
Desipramine	4-Methoxyamphetamine
Nortriptyline	Methoxyphenamine
	* Phenacetin
	Phenformin

*Oxidation probably mediated by other cytochrome P-450 isozyme(s) with linked genetic control (Distlerath et al, 1985).

debrisoquine/sparteine-type polymorphism and some forms of cancer (Ayesh et al, 1984) or with Parkinson's disease (Barbeau et al, 1985) presumbably related to environmental chemicals.

In vivo/in vitro correlation of the metabolism of debrisoquine, bufuralol and dextrometorphan.

In liver microsomes of 2 individuals identified as poor metabolisers by in vivo tests (debrisoquine urinary metabolic ratio) we found a markedly reduced hydroxylation rate of debrisoquine (Meier et al, 1983) confirming and extending previous studies by Davies et al (1981) who had observed a lack of 4-OH debrisoquine formation in the liver biopsy of one poor metaboliser.

This indicated that the deficient metabolism of debrisoquine in poor metabolisers is caused by a deficiency of a monooxygenase reaction in the liver. Moreover, our data demonstrated that defective hydroxylation of debrisoquine is not related to a general impairment of microsomal oxidation reactions.

In vitro/in vivo correlation of the metabolism of bufuralol.
   Bufuralol (Figure 1) is a beta-adrenergic receptor blocking drug which is under clinical investigation. One of the major pathways of bufuralol metabolism is its oxidation to 1'-OH-bufuralol (or carbinol).

**Figure 1.   Structures of bufuralol and its major metabolite
          1'-OH-bufuralol.**

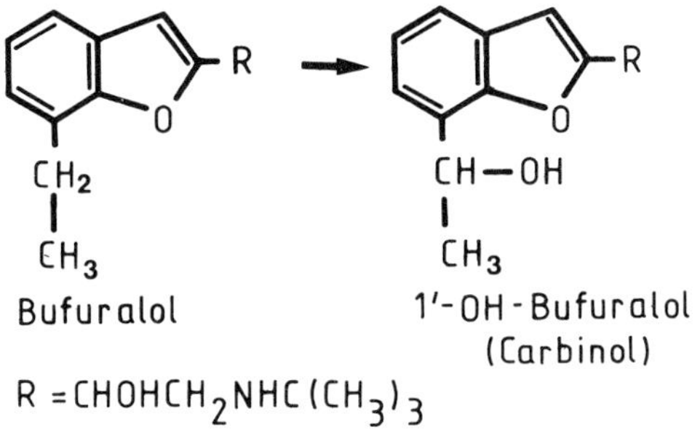

$$R = CHOHCH_2NHC(CH_3)_3$$

This reaction is under the same or linked genetic control as the metabolism of debrisoquine (Dayer et al, 1982b). We have developed a highly sensitive HPLC-assay for measurement of carbinol formation in small liver samples and in reconstituted cytochrome P-450 (Minder et al, 1984; Dayer et al, 1984a; Kronbach et al, 1986, submitted). The metabolism of bufuralol to carbinol showed substrate selectivity, preferring the (+)-isomer of bufuralol and exhibited saturation kinetics. The activity was competitively inhibited by other substrates sharing the same oxidation polymorphism in vivo. To rule out that the defect is related to a soluble modifier of enzyme activity, we mixed microsomes of a poor metaboliser with those of an extensive metaboliser. The rate of carbinol production of the mixture was equal to the sum of the rates in EM and PM microsomes measured separately (Minder et al, 1984). This excluded a transferable inhibitor as the cause of the lowered enzyme activity. These indirect studies in microsomes thus strongly supported the concept that a genetically variant cytochrome P-450 isozyme with high affinity for these substrates is defective in subjects of the poor metaboliser phenotype. They also supported the conclusions drawn from cross-over population studies that the metabolism of drugs involved in this polymorphism probably is coincidentally regulated by the same or a linked gene locus. These investigations however did not answer the question as to the nature of the oxidation impairment at the molecular level in poor metabolisers.

Michaelis constant (Km) and stereoselectivity of bufuralol 1'-hydroxylation in microsomes of poor metabolisers.

During the initial investigation of the kinetics of bufuralol-1'-hydroxylation in human liver microsomes (Minder et al, 1984) we observed that in extensive metabolisers the oxidation of bufuralol to carbinol is stereoselective, preferring the (+)-isomer, in agreement with in vivo studies (Dayer et al, 1984b). However, in microsomes of a total of 5 poor metabolisers, this stereoselectivity was virtually lost, suggesting that an isozyme stereoselective for (+)-bufuralol is deficient (Minder et al, 1984; Dayer et al, 1984a; Dayer et al, 1986, submitted). Moreover, the markedly decreased Vmax for (+)-bufuralol was associated with a 4 to 5-fold increase in the Km. This increase in Km was recently confirmed for several other substrates involved in this polymorphism, including sparteine (Osikowska-Evers et al, 1986, submitted).

Purification, functional and immunochemical characterisation of P-450 isozymes with high activity for bufuralol-1'-hydroxylation.

By using the specific enzymatic activity of bufuralol-1'-hydroxylation in a reconstituted system to optimise hydrophobic and ion-exchange chromatography, we have purified to electrophoretic homogeneity two cytochrome P-450 isozymes with high activity for bufuralol hydroxylation, namely "P450 buf I" and "P450 buf II" (Gut et al, 1984; Gut et al, 1986). Both isozymes had MW of ∿50000. However, P-450 buf I metabolised bufuralol in a highly stereoselective fashion, (-/+ ratio: 0.15) as compared to P-450 buf II (ratio: 1.03) and had a markedly lower Km for (+)- and (-)-bufuralol. Moreover, bufuralol 1'-hydroxylation by P-450 buf I was uniquely characterised by its extreme sensitivity to inhibition by quinidine. Rabbit antibodies against P-450 buf I and P450 buf II inhibited bufuralol metabolism in microsomes and with the reconstituted enzymes. Immunochemical studies with microsomes and in vitro translations of RNA from livers of extensive and poor metabolisers are not conclusive to date. Because the antibodies do not discriminate between P450 buf I and P450 buf II both a decreased content of P450 buf I or its functional alteration (to P450 buf II?) could explain the polymorphic metabolism in microsomes. However, a recently prepared polyclonal antiserum against a rat cytochrome P450 with high debrisoquine-4-hydroxylase activity crossreacted with microsomes of human liver. Immunoblots showed a markedly decreased or absent immunoreaction of a band of 50 Kd in PM-microsomes and this of course favours the hypothesis of a quantitatively decreased or absent enzyme protein as the mechanism of the debrisoquine/sparteine-type polymorphism. With this anti-body cDNA's in a λgt II expression library were identified by reaction with the corresponding lac Z fusion proteins and these clones are presently being analysed in order to study the mutation at the DNA level. A cytochrome P-450 isozyme named P-450 DB with a high catalytic activity towards debrisoquine has also been purified from human liver by Distlerath et al (1985).

THE MEPHENYTOIN-TYPE POLYMORPHISM OF DRUG OXIDATION

A genetic polymorphism of deficient metabolism of mephenytoin is observed in 2-5% of Causasian and over 20% of Japanese subjects (Kupfer and Preisig, 1984). This deficiency occurs independently of the debrisoquine/sparteine polymorphism. It also is inherited as a autosomal recessive trait and affects one of the two major pathways of mephenytoin metabolism, namely stereoselective aromatic 4-hydroxylation of S-mephenytoin. The other major pathway of mephenytoin metabolism, N-demethylation, remains unaffected (Kupfer and Preisig, 1984). To characterise this enzymatic deficiency, the rate of 4-hydroxylation and of N-demethylation of S- and R-mephenytoin was determined in liver microsomes of 13 extensive and 2 poor metabolisers of mephenytoin phenotyped in vivo (Meier et al, 1985a; Meier et al, 1985b). Detailed kinetic studies revealed that microsomes of PM are characterised by a high Km and a low Vmax for S-mephenytoin hydroxylation and a loss of stereoselectivity for the hydroxylation of S-mephenytoin versus R-mephenytoin. The microsomal formation of 4-OH-mephenytoin from R-mephenytoin and the rate of mephenytoin demethylation remains unaffected by the polymorphism. We have purified a P-450 isozyme from human liver with a high activity for mephenytoin 4-hydroxylation (P-450 meph, Gut

et al, submitted for publication). Rabbit antibodies
raised against this isozyme inhibited microsomal
mephenytoin hydroxylation by over 80%. On Western blots
there was no correlation between the in vivo hydroxylation
index, the microsomal activity of mephenytoin hydroxylation
and the extent of the immunochemical reaction. These
findings are very similar to those characteristic for the
enzymatic deficiency in livers of subjects with the
bufuralol-type polymorphism, namely increased Km and loss
of stereospecificity of the reaction. If the antiserum
specifically recognises P450 meph, they suggest the
presence of a functionally altered enzyme rather than a
quantitative decrease in enzyme protein as the cause of the
mephenytoin polymorphism. Two different but very similar
forms of cytochrome P-450 isozymes involved in S-
mephenytoin 4-hydroxylation were recently purified by
Shimada et al (1986). The role of these 2 isozymes in the
mephenytoin polymorphism is unclear as there was no
correlation between S-mephenytoin 4-hydroxylation and the
immunochemically determined concentration of the two P450
proteins.

CONCLUSIONS

·The presented data on two common genetic polymorphisms
of drug oxidation, using the stereospecific metabolism of
bufuralol and of mephenytoin as model reactions in
microsomes, and P450 isozymes purified from human liver,
suggest that a decreased content of a specific P-450
isozyme (P-450 buf I) may cause the observed functional
changes in microsomes of poor metabolisers of debrisoquine,
whereas the present data are more consistent with a
structural alteration of a cytochrome P-450 (P450 meph) as
the cause of the mephenytoin polymorphism. We believe that
because of their frequency of occurrence and clinical
significance, the elucidation of these and other genetic
polymorphisms of human P450 function deserves a major
effort. Similar polymorphisms may explain inter-individual
differences in the metabolism of endogenous substrates of
P-450 isozymes. An understanding of these mechanisms of
variation may ultimately explain the extreme multiplicity
of P450 isozymes.

ACKNOWLEDGEMENTS

This research was supported by grant 3.806.84 from the
Swiss National Science Foundation.

REFERENCES

Alvan, G., Von Bahr, C., Seideman, P. and Sjoqvist, F. (1982). Lancet 1, 333.

Alvan, G., Grind, M., Graffner, C. and Sjoqvist, F. (1984). Clin. Pharmacol. Ther, 36, 515.

Ayesh, R., Idle, J.R., Ritchie, J.C., Grothers, M.J. and Hetzel, M. (1984). Nature 312, 169.

Balant-Gorgia, A.R., Schulz, P., Dayer, P., Balant, L., Kubli, A., Gertsch, C. and Garrone, C. (1982). Arch. Psychiatr. Nervenkr, 232, 215.

Barbeau, A., Cloutier, T., Roy, M., Plasse, L., Paris, S.J. and Poirier, J. (1985). Lancet 2, 1213.

Bertilsson, L., Dengler, H.J., Eichelbaum, M., Schulz, H.-V. (1980a). Eur. J. Clin. Pharmacol, 17, 153.

Bertilsson, L., Eichelbaum, M., Mellstrom, B., Sawe, J., Schulz, H.-V and Sjoqvist, F. (1980b) Life Sci, 27, 1673.

Bertilsson, L. and Aberg-Wistedt, A. (1983). Br. J. Clin. Pharmac, 15, 388.

Davies, D.S., Kahn, G.C., Murray, S., Brodie, M.J., Boobis, A.R. (1981). Br. J. Clin. Pharmac, 11, 89.

Dayer, P., Courvoisier, F., Balant, L. and Fabre, J. (1982a). Lancet 1, 509.

Dayer, P., Kubli, A., Kupfer, A., Courvoisier, F., Balant, L. and Fabre, J. (1982b) Br. J. Clin. Pharmac, 13, 750.

Dayer, P., Leemann, T., Marmy, A. and Rosenthaler, J. (1985). Eur. J. Clin. Pharmacol, 28, 149.

Dayer, P., Gasser, R., Gut, J., Kronbach, T., Robertz, G.M., Eichelbaum, M. and Meyer, U.A. (1984a). Biochem. Biophys. Res. Comm, 125, 374.

Dayer, P., Leeman, T., Gut, J., Kronbach, T., Kupfer, A., Francis, R. and Meyer, U.A. (1984b). Biochem. Pharmacol, 34, 399.

Dengler, H.J. and Eichelbaum, M. (1977). Arznei-Forsch/Drug Res, 27, 1836.

Distlerath, L.M., Reilly, P.E.B., Martin, M.W., David, G.G., Wilkinson, G.R. and Guengerich, F.P. (1985). J. Biol. Chem, 260, 9057.

Eichelbaum, M., Spannbrucker, N., Steinke, B. and Dengler, H.J. (1979). Eur. J. Clin. Pharmacol, 16, 183.

Eichelbaum, M. (1982). Clin. Pharmacokinet, 7, 1.

Franklin, R.A. and Parke, D.V. (eds), (1986). Xenobiotica 16, No. 5, Special Issue on "Human Genetic Variations in Oxidative Drug Metabolism.

Gut, J., Gasser, R., Dayer, P., Kronbach, T., Catin, T. and Meyer, U.A. (1984). FEBS Letters, 173, 287.

Gut, J., Catin, T., Dayer, P., Kronbach, T., Zanger, U. and
    Meyer, U.A. (1986). J. Biol. Chem (in press).
Idle, J.R. and Smith, R.L. (1984). In "Proceedings of the
    Second World Conference on Clinical Pharmacology and
    Therapeutics". (Ed. by Lemberger, L. and Reidenberg,
    M). Am. Soc. Pharm. Exp. Ther, Bethesda, 148-164.
Inaba, T., Otton, S.V. and Kalow, W. (1980). Clin.
    Pharmacol. Ther, 27, 547.
Kitchen, J., Tremblay, J., Andre, J., Dring, L.G., Idle,
    J.R., Smith, R.L. and Williams, R.T. (1979).
    Xenobiotica 9, 397.
Kleinbloessem, C.H., van Brummelen, P., Faber, H., Danhof,
    M., Vermeulen, N.P.E. and Breimer, D.D. (1984).
    Biochem. Pharmacol, 33, 3721.
Kupfer, A. and Preisig, R. (1984). Eur. J. Clin.
    Pharmacol, 26, 753.
Lennard, M.S., Silas, J.H., Freestone, S. and Trevethick,
    J. (1982). Br. J. Clin. Pharmac, 14, 301.
Lennard, M.S., Jackson, P.R., Freestone, S., Tucker, G.T.,
    Ramsay, L.E. and Woods, H.F. (1984). Br. J. Clin.
    Pharmac, 17, 679.
Lewis, R.V., Lennard, M.S., Jackson, P.R., Tucker, G.T.
    Ramsay, L.E. and Woods, H.F. (1985). Br. J. Clin.
    Pharmac, 19, 329.
Mahgoub, A., Idle, J.R., Dring, L.G., Lancaster, R. and
    Smith, R.L. (1977). Lancet 2, 584.
McGourty, J.C., Silas, J.H., Fleming, J., McBurney, A. and
    Ward, J.W. (1985). Clin. Pharmacol. Ther, 38, 409.
McNay, J.L., Bechtol, L.D., Miner, D.J. and Bergstrom, R.F.
    (1983). In "Proceedings of the Second World Conference
    on Clinical Pharmacology and Therapeutics". (eds,
    Lemberger, L. and Reidenberg, M). Am. Soc. Pharm. Expt.
    Thera, Washington, p.14 (abstract).
Meier, P.J., Muller, H.K., Dick, B., Meyer, U.A. (1984).
    Gastroenterology, 85, 683.
Meier, U.T., Dayer, P., Male, P.J., Kronbach, T. and Meyer,
    U.A. (1985a). Clin. Pharmacol. Ther, 38, 488.
Meier, U.T., Kronbach, T. and Meyer, U.A. (1985b). Anal.
    Biochem, 151, 286.
Meyer, U.A., Gut, J., Kronbach, T., Skoda, C., Meier, U.T.
    and Catin, T. (1986). Xenobiotica 16, 449.
Minder, E., Meier, P.J., Muller, H.K., Meyer, U.A. (1984).
    Europ. J. Clin. Invest, 14, 184.
Mitchell, S.C., Waring, R.H., Haley, C.S., Idle, J.R. and
    Smith, R.L. (1984). Br. J. Clin. Pharmac, 18, 507.
Oates, N.S., Shah, R.R., Idle, J.R. and Smith, R.L. (1982).
    Clin. Pharmacol. Ther, 32, 81.

Penno, M.B. and Vesell, E.S. (1983). J. Clin. Invest. 71, 1698.
Price-Evans, D.A., Mahgoub, A., Sloan, T.P., Idle, J.R. and Smith, R.L. (1980). J. Med. Genet, 17, 102.
Raghuram, T.C., Koshakji, R.P., Wilkinson, G.R. and Wood, A.J.J. (1984). Clin. Pharmacol. Ther, 36, 51.
Roy, S.D., Hawes, E.M., McKay, G., Korchinski, E.D. and Midha, K.K. (1985). Clin. Pharmacol. Ther, 38, 128.
Schmid, B., Bircher, J., Preisig, R. and Kupfer, A. (1985). Clin. Pharmacol. Ther, 38, 618.
Scott, J. and Poffenbarger, P.L. (1979). Diabetes 28, 41.
Shah, R.R., Oates, N.S., Idle, J.R., Smith, R.L. and Lockhart, J.D.F. (1982). Br. Med. J. 284, 295.
Shimada, T., Misono, K.S. and Guengerich, F.P. (1985). J. Biol. Chem, 261, 909.
Sloan, T.P., Mahgoub, A., Lancaster, R., Idle, J.R. and Smith, R.L. (1978). Br. Med. J. 2, 655.
Weber, W.W. and Hein, D.W. (1985). Pharmacol. Rev. 37, 25.
Wedlund, P.J., Aslanian, W.S., McAllister, C.B., Wilkinson, G.R. and Branch, R.A. (1984). Clin. Pharmacol. Ther, 36, 773.
Woosley, R.L., Roden, D.M., Dai, G., Wang, T., Altenbern, D., Oates, J. and Wilkinson, G.R. (1985). Clin. Pharmacol. Ther. 39, 282.
Zekorn, C., Hausleiter, H.J., Achtert, G. and Eichelbaum, M. (1983). In "IUPHAR 9th International Congress of Pharmacology. Macmillan Press Ltd, London. p.108 (abstract).

A HUMAN ISOZYME OF GLUTATHIONE TRANSFERASE ACTIVITY IN DIFFERENT ORGANS AND ITS RELATION TO LUNG CANCER

Janeric Seidegard[1], Ronald W. Pero[1], Goran G. Jonsson[1], Sven-Ake Olsson[2], Lars Stavenow[3] and Karl-Fredrick Aronsen[4].

[1]Molecular Ecogenetics, The Wallenberg Laboratory, University of Lund, Box 7031, S-220 07, Lund, Sweden. [2]University Hospital, Lund, Sweden. [3]Department of Medicine, and [4]Department of Surgery, Malmo General Hospital, Malmo, Sweden.

INTRODUCTION

The glutathione transferases are a group of multifunctional proteins which play an important role in the biotransformation and detoxication of many different endogenous and exogenous compounds (Jakoby and Habig, 1980). It has been concluded that at least three distinct groups of human glutathione transferases exist based on their isoelectric points (Awasthi et al, 1980) : basic (α-ε), near-neutral (μ), and acidic (π). Thus, there are many different isozymes of glutathione transferase in human tissues. Recently, we discovered an isozyme of glutathione transferase having high activity towards the substrate trans-stilbene oxide (tSBO) in human mononuclear leukocytes (Seidegard et al, 1985). The interindividual differences of this activity showed a 100- to 200-fold variation and this property is inherited in an autosomal dominant fashion (Seidegard and Pero, 1985). Here we present the activity of this isozyme (GT-tSBO) in different human tissues.

MATERIALS AND METHODS

Various normal organs were taken from different individuals (n=85) at the time of a scheduled surgery and then either analysed directly or frozen in liquid nitrogen. The organ was homogenised in 0.25M sucrose and centrifuged at 10,000g for 15 min. The supernatant was further centrifuged at 105,000g for 1h. The 105,000g supernatant was then used for assaying different glutathione transferase activities.

The assay procedure for GT-tSBP has been reported in detail elsewhere (Seidegard et al, 1985). Glutathione transferase activity towards 1-chloro-2,4-dinitrobenzene (GT-CDNB) was carried out using the published procedure of Habig et al, 1974. In order to study the distribution of GT-tSBO phenotypes in various human populations, lung cancer patients (n=66) and control subjects (n=78) were recruited from an ongoing study of smokers which had been earlier designed to evaluate methods for early lung cancer detection at the PMI-Strang Clinic (National Lung Program, see Melamed et al, 1977). The lung cancer patients and control smokers were similar in age, sex and smoking histories (Seidegard et al, 1986).

RESULTS AND DISCUSSION

A recent characterisation of glutathione transferase activity towards trans-stilbene oxide (GT-tSBO) in peripheral resting mononuclear leukocytes showed very large inter-individual differences which were not paralleled by equal variation in GT-CDNB activity (Seidegard et al, 1985). Furthermore, GT-tSBO seemed to be lacking in about 50% of the general population (Seidegard and Pero, 1985).

The activities of GT-tSBO and GT-CDNB in different human organs is presented in Table 1. The GT-tSBO phenotypes determined in blood cells corresponds to the homo (++)- and hetero(+)-zygotes for the described GT-tSBO while the (-) phenotype reflects the lack of the same isozyme. As can be seen in Table 1 the activity in blood corresponds very well to the activity found in each specific organ investigated here. The highest activity was found in the liver and adrenal gland, but a relatively high activity was also found in other organs. The GT-CDNB activity was also high in liver and adrenal gland, but not significantly higher than was seen in those individuals that expressed the GT-tSBO activity. This information again demonstrates that GT-tSBO is very specific in the conjugation of the substrate trans-stilbene oxide.

The physiological consequences of having GT-tSBO may be of great importance, since the isozyme(s) involved probably can conjugate a large number of xenobiotics, especially when considering the broad substrate specificity of all the glutathione transferases characterised to date. This should be true at least for the liver and adrenal gland, since these organs have such high activity. The distributions of GT-tSBO phenotypes in lung cancer patients and control smokers are compared in Table 2. A greater proportion of the control smokers have GT-tSBO

Siedegard et al.

Table 1. Activities of glutathione transferase towards tSBO and CDNB in various human organs.

Organ	n	GT-tSBO[a]	GT-CDNB[b]	Blood[c]	Phenotype[d]
Liver	3	53.8-71.0	387-611	177-398	-
	6	36,500-45,000	526-837	787-1200	+
	2	51,900-62,800	757-767	1775-2301	++
Adrenal	2	45.1-60.7	727-1381	225-425	-
gland	1	27,000	1592	1305	+
Kidney	1	1770	325	975	+
Colon	11	9.0-30.5	91-122	177-435	-
	3	1036-1780	79-128	988-1235	+
	2	2710-3610	139-142	2112-2351	++
Small	7	17.2-35.6	74-252	277-325	-
intestine	1	1118	139	977	+
	3	2189-2650	121-272	1888-2112	++
Vein	12	30-119	35-161	252-364	-
	16	675-1740	56-112	624-1472	+
	4	1495-3421	90-225	1804-2666	++
Skin	6	3.5-36.0	36-211	326-367	-
	1	1250	45	976	+
Muscle	4	1.5-10.8	86-309	285	-

a GT-tSBO; specific activity in pmol/min/mg protein
b GT-CNDB; specific activity in nmol/min/mg protein
c Blood; GT-tSBO expressed in cpm of conjugates formed/15min/25µl whole blood
d The phenotypes (++), and (+) correspond to homo- and hetero-zygotes for the expression of GT-tSBO, while (-) represents the lack of this isozyme.

(59.0%), while the reverse occurs for those patients having lung cancer (34.8%). The distribution pattern of individuals having and lacking GT-tSBO between these two groups with and without lung cancer are significantly different (P<0.01, X^2-test).

Table 2. Proportion of GT-tSBO in individuals with and without lung cancer[a].

	Lung Cancer	No Lung Cancer	x^2-Test[c]
All smokers	23/66 (34.8%)	46/78 (59.0%)	P<0.01
Heavy smokers[b]	14/46 (30.4%)	38/65 (58.5%)	P<0.01
Light smokers[b]	9/20 (45.0%)	8/13 (61.5%)	P<0.70

a Data from Seidegard et al, 1986.

b Heavy smokers are arbitrarily defined as those who have been smoking >30 pack-yr and light smokers as those who have smoked between 10 and 30 pack-yr.

c x^2-test has been done by comparing individuals with and without lung cancer for the presence of GT-tSBO.

In addition, if control smokers and lung cancer patients are allocated into two separate groups according to the extent of their smoking, then controls and lung cancer patients smoking <30 pack-yr did not show any statistically significant difference in the proportion of GT-tSBO. On the other hand, among the heavy smokers (i.e. > 30 pack-yr) the proportion of individuals lacking GT-tSBO is significantly increased in patients with lung cancer when compared with control smokers. These data are at least consistent with the reasoning that there are health risks leading to an increased lung cancer incidence, for those individuals who smoke and lack GT-tSBO.

ACKNOWLEDGEMENTS

This study was supported by PMI-Strang Clinic in New York, and by Svenska Tobaks AB grant No. 8517.

REFERENCES

Awasthi, Y.C., Dao, D.D. and Saneto, R.P. (1980). Biochem, J. 191, 1.
Habig, W.H., Pabst, M.J. and Jakoby, W.B.J. (1974). J. Biol. Chem, 249, 7130.
Jakoby, W.B. and Habig, W.H. (1980). in "Enzymatic basis

of detoxification". (Ed. Jakoby, W.B).   Academic
Press, New York, vol 2, 63.

Melamed, M.R., Flehninger, B.J., Miller, D., Osbourne, R.,
Zaman, M.B., McGinnis, C. and Martini, N. (1977).
Cancer, 39, 369.

Seidegard, J. and Pero, R.W. (1985). Hum. Genet, 69, 66.

Seidegard, J., DePierre, J.W. and Pero, R.W. (1985).
Carcinogenesis, 6, 1211.

Seidegard, J., Pero, R.W., Miller, D. and Beattie, E.J.
(1986). Carcinogenesis, 7, 751.

STUDIES WITH MONOCLONAL ANTIBODIES AGAINST A HIGHLY PURIFIED ANTICONVULSANT-INDUCED HUMAN LIVER CYTOCHROME P-450.

Tristan S. Barnes , Peter M. Shaw[1] , Margaret D. Lobban , William T. Melvin and M. Danny Burke[1].

Departments of Biochemistry and [1]Pharmacology, University of Aberdeen, Marischal College, Aberdeen. AB9 1AS.

INTRODUCTION

Cytochrome P-450 is responsible for the metabolism of a wide variety of endogenous and exogenous compounds including steroids, prostaglandins, drugs, mutagens and carcinogens. The broad spectrum of reactions catalysed by P-450 is brought about by its extensive multiplicity of forms with characteristic but overlapping substrate specificities. Whilst P-450-mediated metabolism of compounds usually leads to their deactivation /detoxification and subsequent excretion, such metabolism can result in active, mutagenic or carcinogenic intermediates. The final metabolic outcome is often determined by the qualitative and quantitative distribution (or phenotype) of the P-450s within the individual. Hence the accurate 'P-450-phenotyping' of human individuals is of major value in the studies of carcinogenesis, pharmacology and toxicology. The unique specificity of monoclonal antibodies (Kohler and Milstein, 1975) make them particularly well suited for the phenotype analysis of a system as complex as the cytochromes P-450.

RESULTS

Murine monoclonal antibodies (MAbs) have been prepared against a human cytochrome P-450 by established immunological techniques (Kohler and Milstein, 1975) and using liver microsomes as immunogen. Four of the MAbs (HL3, HL4, HL5 and HP3), generated from two independent fusions, have been characterised in detail.
When immunoblotted against the human microsomes used for immunisation, all four MAbs recognised a single band of

protein corresponding to a molecular mass of 53kDa.
Moreover, the MAbs all bound to a highly purified form of
human cytochrome P-450 (15.5nmol/mg protein), also of
53kDa (Figure 1).

The MAbs exhibited different patterns when
immunoblotted against a series of differentially induced
rat liver microsomes. MAbs HL4 and HL5 each recognised a
single protein band corresponding to a molecular mass of
52kDa.

**Figure 1. Cross-reactivity of MAb HL5 with the proteins of
differentially induced rat liver microsomes.**

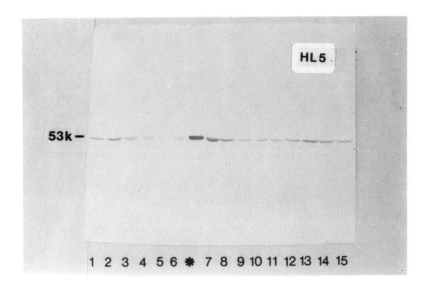

Rat liver microsomes submitted to SDS polyacrylamide gel
electrophoresis (Laemmli, 1970) and electroblotted on to
nitrocellulose were: untreated control (lane 1 & 9); PB-
induced (lane 2); PCN vehicle control (lane 3); PCN-induced
(lane 4); 3MC/IS/ARO vehicle control (lane 5); 3MC-induced
(lane 6); ISF-induced (lane 7); ARO-induced (lane 8); CL-
induced (lane 10) and IM-induced (lane 11). The
nitrocellulose sheet was immunochemically stained with MAb
HL5 as described for Figure 2.

This band was present in the microsomes of untreated
rats, was induced by pregnenolone-16α-carbonitrile (PCN),
was suppressed by 3-methylcholanthrene (3MC) or Aroclor

1254 (ARO) and was essentially unaffected by phenobarbitone (PB), isosafrole (IS), clofibrate (CL) or imidazole (IM) treatment. When immunoblotted against the same series of rat microsomes, MAb HL3 recognised two bands, one corresponding to the 52kDa band visualised by HL4/HL5 and a second, of molecular mass 54kDa, which was present in control microsomes, was extensively induced by PB, PCN, ISO and ARO, was induced less by CL and IM and was unaffected by 3MC. The fourth MAb, HP3, did not cross-react with any proteins present in the rat microsomes described.

Having partially characterised the MAbs against rat induced P-450s, MAb HL4 was used to investigate interindividual variation in the level of the 53kDa P-450 expressed in the human population. In immunoblots of liver microsomes from 15 adult individuals, the level of the antigenic P-450 varied 2- to 3-fold.

Figure 2. Interindividual differences in the level of cytochrome P-450$_{7:3}$ expressed in adult human livers.

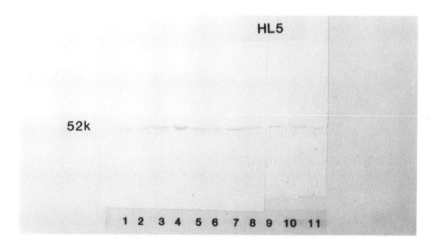

The microsomal fractions of 15 adult human livers (lanes 1-15, 25µg protein/lane) and a sample of pure cytochrome P-450$_{7:3}$ (lane '*', 1.5µg protein) were submitted to SDS polyacrylamide gel electrophoresis and electroblotted on to nitrocellulose paper. The nitrocellulose was immuno-chemically stained by incubating with solutions of: MAb HL5; anti-mouse IgG, horseradish peroxidase conjugate and diaminobenzidine/H_2O_2. The microsomes used for immunisation are present in lane 1 while lane 7 contains those of an epileptic chronically treated with phenobarbitone and phenytoin.

The level was approximately 10-fold higher in the liver microsomes obtained from an epileptic chronically treated with the anticonvulsants phenobarbitone and phenytoin and was, on average, 3-fold more abundant in human foetal liver microsomes (results not shown).

In 2-dimensional immunoblots of microsomes from the epileptic, MAb HL3 recognised two proteins of virtually identical molecular mass (53kDa) but of dissimilar isoelectric points (7.4 and 7.9). Only the 7.9 pI protein was found to be present in the liver microsomes of an individual who had not been receiving drug treatment (results not shown).

SUMMARY

MAbs HL4 and HL5, generated against human liver microsomes, recognised a major form of P-450 in human liver inducible by the anti-convulsant PB and phenytoin. An orthologous P-450 is also detected in rats and is inducible by the synthetic steroid PCN. The situation for MAb HL3 is more complex since it recognised at least two different proteins in both rats and humans. One of the proteins recognised by HL3 correlated with the P-450 bound by HL4 and HL5.

ACKNOWLEDGEMENTS

This work was supported by the S.E.R.C. Syntex Pharmaceuticals Ltd and the Aberdeen University Advisory Committee for Research. We acknowledge the essential assistance of Mr. J. Engeset (Department of Surgery) and Professor J.C. Petrie (Department of Medicine and Therapeutics) in providing human livers and patient histories.

REFERENCES

Kohler, G. and Milstein, C. (1975). Nature (London), 256, 495.
Laemmli, U.K. (1970). Nature (London), 227, 680.

OXIDATION OF QUINIDINE BY HUMAN LIVER CYTOCHROME P-450

Dieter Muller-Enoch[1] and F. Peter Guengerich[2]

[1]Abteilung Physiologische Chemie, Universitat, ULM, FRG and
[2]Department of Biochemistry and Center in Molecular
Toxicology, Vanderbilt University School of Medicine,
Nashville, TN, USA.

INTRODUCTION

Evidence exists that humans contain several different forms of cytochrome P-450 and that these forms play a role in polymorphisms of drug oxidation (Idle and Smith, 1979; Kupfer and Preisig, 1983). The first of these to be recognised involved the 4-hydroxylation of debrisoquine (P-450_{DB}) (Mahgoub et al., 1977). Recently quinidine has been reported to be a competitive inhibitor of sparteine oxidation and bufuralol hydroxylation, two activities of P-450_{DB} (Otton et al., 1984; Meyer et al., 1985). We report here that quinidine is not a substrate of P-450_{DB} or its rat orthologue, P-450_{UT-A}; instead another P-450 (P-450_{NF}) oxidizes quinidine.

MATERIALS AND METHODS

Chemicals : Quinidine was purchased from Aldrich Chemical Co. (Milwaukee, WI). (+) Bufuralol and 1'-hydroxybufuralol were gifts of the Hoffman-La Roche Co. (Nutley, NJ). Quinidine N-oxide was synthesised by peracid oxidation. 3-Hydroxy-quinidine was prepared by a modification of the method of Carroll et al., 1976.

Enzyme preparations : Sprague-Dawley rats were purchased from Harlan (Indianapolis, JN). Livers from DA strain rats were shipped from Dr. A. Kupfer, University of Bern, Switzerland. Human liver samples were obtained from organ donors through the Nashville Regional Organ Procurement Agency, Nashville, TN. Rat liver P-450_{UT-H} (Larrey et al., 1984) and human liver P-450_{DB} (Distlerath et al., 1985), P-450_{MP} (Shimada et al., 1986), and P-450_{NF} (Guengerich et al., 1986) were isolated as described previously and reconstituted with rabbit NADPH-P-450 reductase and L-α-dilauroyl-sn-glycero-3-phosphocholine as described in those references.

Assays : Microsomal enzyme incubations (generally equivalent to about 50 pmol P-450) were carried out in amber vials for 10-15 min at 37° with the substrate and 0.1M potassium phosphate buffer (pH 7.7) in the presence of an NADPH-generating system in a total volume of 0.50ml. For the analysis of 3-hydroxyquinidine and quinidine N-oxide an Altex cyanopropyl and an Altex octadecylsilyl (C_{18}) column were used, respectively. Bufuralol 1'-hydroxylation was measured as described previously (Distlerath et al., 1985; Hafelfinger, 1980), or using the cyanopropyl HPLC system.

RESULTS AND DISCUSSION

During the course of human liver microsomal bufuralol 1'-hydroxylase inhibition studies, the appearance of a new fluorescent peak in the HPLC profiles was noted (Figure 1).

Figure 1. Formation of a quinidine metabolite during the inhibition of the bufuralol 1'-hydroxylation.

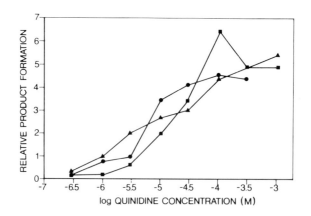

Microsomal protein from liver samples HL24 (■), HL39 (▲), or HL96 (●) equivalent to 500 pmol of P-450 was incubated under the standard conditions for 15 min with 0.5mM ($+$) bufuralol and varying concentrations of quinidine. The relative fluorescence of the new peak is plotted as a function of the quinidine concentration.

The area of the peak increased as a function of the quinidine concentration (apparent K_m 7-20μM). Two different HPLC systems were used to separate and quantify the quinidine metabolites, which were identified by comparison to authentic standards. At a quinidine concentration of 20µM, the major product is 3-hydroxy-quinidine and the only other prominent product is quinidine N-oxide, no significant amounts of 2-oxoquinidinone or O-desmethyl quinidine were found. The K_m values estimated for the formation of 3-hydroxyquinidine and quinidine N-oxide were about 4µM and 33µM respectively.

Table 1 indicates that microsomes prepared from DA strain females showed decreased catalytic activity for quinidine 3-hydroxylation when compared to preparations derived from DA strain males. However, the sex difference in quinidine 3-hydroxylation was apparent in Sprague-Dawley as well as DA strain rats. As indicated in Table 1, P-450_{DB} and its rat orthologue P-450_{UT-H} had little catalytic activity towards quinidine. Purified P-450_{MP} did not catalyse quinidine 3-hydroxylation either. Purified P-450_{NF} catalysed quinidine 3-hydroxylation and N-oxygenation, although the rates were low (< 0.2 nmol product/min/nmol P-450).

Table 1. Comparison of quinidine 3-hydroxylase and bufuralol 1'-hydroxylase activities in rat liver microsomes and purified enzymes.

Preparation	P-450	Bufuralol 1'-hydroxylase	Quinidine 3-hydroxylase
	nmol/mg microsomal protein	nmol/min/nmol P-450	nmol/min/nmol P-450
Female DA rat microsomes	0.92 ± 0.14	0.29 ± 0.08	0.11 ± 0.03
Male DA rat microsomes	1.07 ± 0.21	0.86 ± 0.06	0.82 ± 0.14
Female SD rat microsomes	1.06 ± 0.10	2.37 ± 0.15	0.64 ± 0.13
Male SD rat microsomes	0.90 ± 0.05	1.91 ± 0.16	1.42 ± 0.16
Rat P-450_{UT-H}	–	2.70 ± 0.51	0.23 ± 0.24
Human P-450_{DB}	–	0.98 ± 0.12	< 0.02

In order to circumvent problems in the interpretation of the relative rates of microsomal and purified P-450 forms, we utilised inhibitory antibodies to elucidate the contributions of individual P-450's. Anti P-450$_{UT-H}$ which extensively inhibits bufuralol 1'-hydroxylation in human liver microsomes, did not affect quinidine 3-hydroxylation or N-oxygenation in human liver microsomes (Figure 2).

Figure 2. Effects of antibodies on microsomal bufuralol and quinidine oxidation.

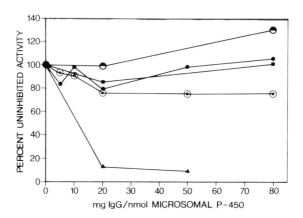

Liver microsomal sample HL96 and goat anti-P-450$_{UT-H}$ were used in the particular study shown; uninhibited rates of bufuralol 1'-hydroxylation (▲), quinidine 3-hydroxylation (●), and quinidine N-oxygenation (⊙) were 0.26, 0.82 and 0.19 nmol product formed/min/nmol P-450 respectively. Also shown are the effects of a pre-immune IgG preparation on quinidine 3-hydroxylation (■) and N-oxygenation (◓).

The addition of rabbit anti P-450$_{MP}$ preparation which completely inhibits human liver microsomal S-mephenytoin 4-hydroxylation when added at a ratio of 5mg IgG/nmol P-450 (Shimada et al., 1986) decreased the quinidine 3-hydroxylase activity of this microsomal preparation by <25%. However, the addition of rabbit anti-P-450$_{NF}$ to human liver microsomal preparations decreased both the quinidine 3-hydroxylation >95% (Figure 3A) and the N-oxygenation of quinidine >85% (Figure 3B). Thus, quinidine oxidation appears to be catalysed primarily by P-450$_{NF}$ and not by P-450$_{DB}$.

Figure 3. Effect of anti-P-450$_{NF}$ on microsomal quinidine 3-hydroxylation and N-oxygenation.

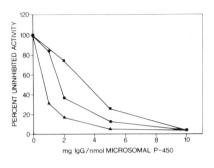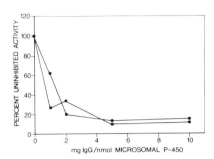

A. Effects of anti-P-450$_{NF}$ on quinidine 3-hydroxylation in liver samples HL94 (▲), HL39 (●), and HL95 (■); the respective uninhibited activities were 1.17, 1.24 and 0.38 nmol product formed.min^{-1}.nmol P-450^{-1}.
B. Effects of anti-P-450NF on quinidine N-oxygenation in liver samples HL39 (●) and HL95 (■); the uninhibited activity was 0.23 pmol product formed.min-1.nmol P-450-1 in both cases.

REFERENCES

Carroll, F.I., Philip, A. and Coleman, M.C. (1976). *Tetrahedron Letters*, 1757.
Distlerath, L.M., Reilly, P.E.B., Martin, M.V., Davis, G.G., Wilkinson, G.R. and Guengerich, F.P. (1985). *J. Biol. Chem*, 260, 9057.
Guengerich, F.P., Martin, M.V., Beaune, P.H., Kremers, P., Wolff, T. and Waxman, D.J. (1986). *J. Biol. Chem*, 261, 5051.
Haefelfinger, P. (1980). *J. Chromatog*, 221, 327.
Idle, J.R. and Smith, R.L. (1979). *Drug. Metab. Rev*, 9, 301.
Kupfer, A. and Preisig, R. (1983). *Sem. Liver Disease*, 3, 341.
Larrey, D., Distlerath, L.M., Dannan, G.A., Wilkinson, G.R. and Guengerich, F.P. (1984). *Biochemistry*, 23, 2787.
Mahgoub, A., Idle, J.R., Dring, L.G., Lancaster, R. and Smith, R.L. (1977). *Lancet* 2, 584.
Meyer, U.A., Gut, J., Dayer, P., Kronback, T., Meier, U.T., and Skoda, R. (1985). Abstracts, "Fourth International Symposium on Comparative Biochemistry", Janssen Research Foundation, Beerse, Belgium, p.63.

Otton, S.V., Inaba, T. and Kalow, W. (1984)   Life Sci, 34,
    73.
Shimada, T., Misono, K. and Guengerich, F.P. (1986).   J.
    Biol. Chem, 261, 909.

3. Conjugating enzymes.

THE INTERRELATIONSHIP BETWEEN DIFFERENT CONJUGATING ENZYMES IN VIVO

Gerard J. Mulder

Division of Toxicology, Center for Bio-Pharmaceutical Sciences, University of Leiden, Leiden, The Netherlands.

INTRODUCTION

Exposure of animals to xenobiotics usually gives rise to a wide variety of metabolites of these compounds, that are excreted in urine or faeces. Dependent on the chemical structure of the substance, various phase 1 and phase 2 reactions may occur in different regions of the molecule; therefore, often competition occurs for metabolism at the same or different sites. In this chapter only the conjugations, phase 2 reactions, will be discussed. Obviously, in many cases there is also competition between phase 1 and phase 2 reactions. For instance, phenol can be conjugated, but can also be further oxidised by cytochrome P-450-mediated activity (Mulder, 1982). Many of the more general statements discussed below will also apply to the competition between phase 1 and phase 2 reactions. One major difference, however, is that phase 1 reactions do not require a group-donating co-substrate. On the other hand, NADPH may be necessary in the reaction as electron donor, and somewhat similar problems with the availability of this co-factor may occur as will be discussed below for the co-substrates for conjugation.

Dependent on the available groups in the structure of a potential substrate for conjugation, one or more transferases may convert it to a conjugate. This is illustrated in Figure 1 for 1-hydroxy-4-aminobenzoic acid ("aminosalicylic acid"): in this simple structure three groups are available for conjugation, and at each several conjugations are possible. Moreover, the first conjugation may make another conjugation at other sites impossible. For instance, glucuronidation at one group most likely prevents further metabolism of most small compounds, presumably because the glucuronide is rapidly excreted, or because the changed physico-chemical properties of the glucuronide prevent conversion by other enzymes; yet, double conjugates (di-glucuronides or mixed glucuronide-

Figure 1. Metabolic pathways of p-aminosalicylic acid.

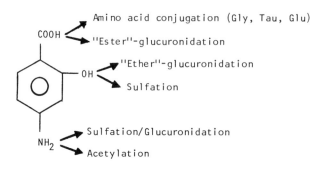

sulphate conjugates) do occur occasionally. Certainly N-acetylation of aromatic amines does not prevent conjugation at other sites; for instance, p-aminophenol and N-acetyl-p-aminophenol can be converted to their sulphate and glucuronide conjugates with equal efficiency. It is possible, however, that subsequent conjugation specificity is determined by the presence of the N-acetyl moiety on the amino group. Interestingly, the sulphate or glucuronide conjugate of p-aminophenol (or any aromatic amine), have never been reported (or tested?) to be substrates for N-acetylation.

The same group may be conjugated by very many different transferases; other groups in the structure will determine what the ratio between the different conjugations at that particular site or others in the structure will be. Table 1 lists a number of competing pathways for the metabolism of some of the major groups that can become conjugated.

A number of factors will determine the outcome of the simultaneous action of several of these enzymes on a dose of the xenobiotic. The major ones will be discussed, such as substrate specificity of the transferases involved, pharmacokinetics of distribution and elimination of the substrate, and availability of the co-substrates.

SPECIFICITY OF THE TRANSFERASES AND STRUCTURE OF THE SUBSTRATES

Obviously the substrate specificity of the transferases involved in conjugation is of decisive importance in the determination of the final outcome of competition for the same substrate. Most conjugating enzymes are complex mixtures of isoenzymes or enzymes with overlapping substrate specificity (Jacoby, 1980); therefore, when a

Table 1. Competitive pathways for biotransformation at certain groups of a xenobiotic.

Phenolic hydroxyl group	: Sulphation/Glucuronidation/Phosphorylation/O-Acetylation/Glycosylation.
Alcoholic hydroxyl group	: Glucuronidation/Sulphation/Oxidation.
N-Hydroxy group in substituted hydroxamic acids	: Sulphation/Glucuronidation/Deacylation/O-Acetylation.
Carboxylic acid group	: Glucuronidation/Amino acid conjugation (Taurine, glycine, glutamate, ornithine)/Incorporation in lipids/Conjugation to hydroxyl group of bile salts
Epoxides	: Glutathione conjugation/Epoxide hydrolase activity.
Aromaticaminogroup	: N-Acetylation/Sulphamate formation/N-Oxidation/N-Glucuronidation.

conjugation is characterised in vitro in an impure enzyme preparation by the K_m and V_{max} of the transferase, these kinetic parameters have been derived for the mixture of the enzyme forms present in that particular preparation (microsomes, cytosol etc), unless the various forms have been separated. When more than one transferase can convert the substrate, the relative K_m and V_{max} values of the transferases involved will determine the outcome of the competition, in relation to the substrate concentration. This may lead to changing product ratio's if the substrate concentration increases while competitive conjugation takes place, and one of the transferases becomes saturated (Figure 2). An evaluation of the relationship between K_m and V_{max} values of competing pathways in vivo can best be done with infusions of the substrate to steady state at various infusion rates.

The specificity of the enzyme determines whether a certain chemical structure fits in the active site and can be converted to the conjugate. For a series of arylacetic acids and benzoic acid derivatives this has been extensively investigated, mainly in vivo (Caldwell 1978; 1982). In this case the competition is between the UDP-

Figure 2. Change of conjugation ratio's of a substrate for two competing transferases as a function of substrate concentration.

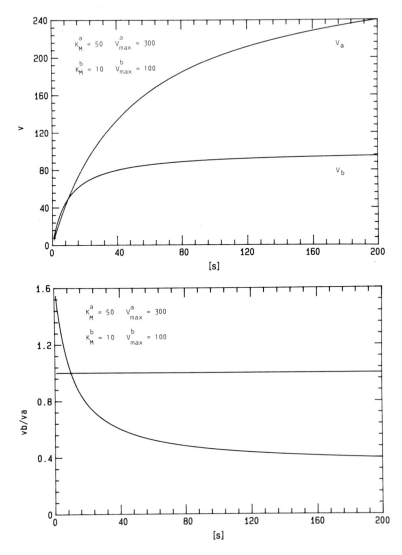

Transferase A (K_m=50, V_{max}=300) and B (K_m=10, V_{max}=100) compete for the same substrate. The conjugation rates as a function of substrate concentration (S) are given in Figure 2A, while the ratio of the rates if given in Figure 2B. Both transferases are assumed to follow Michealis-Menten kinetics.

glucuronosyltransferase enzymes on one hand, and the activation of the carboxylic group to a Co-A derivative as first step towards amino acid conjugation, on the other hand. Although little data is available on the enzymology of these two enzyme systems for the substrates, the in vivo data clearly show that activation to a Co-A derivative is very sensitive to steric hindrance by groups at the α-C atom; glucuronidation is much less or not at all inhibited by these groups. These results were confirmed by some in vitro experiments in mitochondrial (Co-A activation) and microsomal (UDP-glucuronosyltransferase) fractions from rat liver (Table 2). The results show that the presence of substituents at the α-C position, changes the balance from amino acid conjugation to glucuronidation.

Table 2. Substrate specificity of glucuronidation and Co-A activation of phenylacetic acid derivatives.

R	Glucuronidation (nmol/30 min)	Co-A activation (nmol/30 min)
- H	0	89
- methyl	14	0
- phenyl	28	0

Data taken from Dixon et al., 1977.

The K_m for glucuronidation and sulphation of a series of p-substituted phenols (Table 3) showed that the affinity for sulphation was, in most cases five- to a hundred-fold higher than that for glucuronidation (Mulder and Meerman, 1978).

PHARMACOKINETICS OF THE SUBSTRATE

In vivo, in perfused organs and in intact cells the pharmacokinetics of drug distribution, membrane transfer into the cell, and elimination by excretion or biotransformation determine the substrate concentration available to the transferases at the site of conjugation. The ease with which the substrate passes membranes (either by diffusion, or by carrier-mediated transport) determined its initial distribution volume while eventual

Table 3. K_m values for some phenols for glucuronidation and sulphation.

Para substituent	K_m glucuronidation (mM)	K_m sulphation (mM)
- H	3.25	0.14
- F	2.34	0.05
- Br	0.11	0.02
- CN	1.69	0.04
- CH_3	0.27	0.28
- $C(CH_3)_3$	0.11	1.56
- OCH_3	2.60	0.03

Data taken from Mulder and Meerman, 1978.

sequestration processes in a certain tissue or an organ (accumulation in fat tissue of lipid soluble drugs etc) determine the final distribution volume at steady state. The rates of these distribution processes determine the substrate concentration and substrate availability at the site of conjugation by a particular enzyme. This implies that a single dose of a substrate will result in continuously changing concentrations of the substrate inside a cell, and that the (changes in) concentration in different cells may be very different. As the concentration of the substrate increases, some pathways will become saturated, and others that are still unsaturated "take over" from that point. For instance, saturation of sulphation of harmol in the rat liver perfusion does not result in a decreased extraction of this substrate, because glucuronidation has enough "spare capacity" to ensure that the extraction of harmol remains approximately 85-95% (Pang et al., 1981).

A continuously changing pattern of products with time will result when a single dose is given that saturates one of the competing pathways (Figure 2). Steady state infusion experiments at various rates will demonstrate unambigously that such a situation exists (as long as no depletion of co-factors occurs). For a substrate, the dependence of the intracellular concentration in various organs on the blood concentration may be very different, so that saturation of a conjugation in one organ or cell type does not necessarily mean that also in another cell type saturation has already occurred. Moreover, the intracellular substrate concentration may not be linear with the extracellular (blood) concentration (Koster and Mulder, 1982), which lead to apparent anomalies in enzyme kinetics.

The route of administration is an important determinant of the time course for the substrate concentration in blood. When the substrate is given orally, it has to be absorbed, and blood concentrations will never reach those which result from intravenous administration of the same dose of the substrate. If competition is determined by K_m values of competing transferases, this implies that after oral administration the chance of saturation is less than after i.v. dosage, and oral administration will tend to favour conjugation with the highest affinity. Obviously, another difference between these routes of administration is first pass conjugation in gut mucosa and the liver after oral dosage. When, for some reason, oral absorption is slowed down, this may result in a changed outcome of a competition, between two pathways, because of the lower blood level of the substrate. This happens also when the same dose of a substrate is administered over a longer period of time, since then also the resulting blood levels will be lower.

The above implies that dose-dependent shifts in conjugation are expected if the competing transferases have different K_m's. This has been observed, for example, for phenol in the rat (Weitering et al., 1979) and for salicylamide in the dog (Waschek et al., 1984).

COMPETITION FOR CONJUGATION IN THE SAME CELL.

The conjugating enzymes are localised in various cell compartments : some in the cytosol (sulphotransferases, glutathione transferases, acetyltransferases), some in the endoplasmic reticulum (UDP-glucuronosyl-transferase, glutathione transferases) some in the mitochondria (CoA activation for amino acid conjugation). This may imply that in some cases the transferases involved, if they are in different cellular compartments, may draw their substrate from different intra-cellular pools, and, in fact, may operate at different substrate concentrations. For instance, there are indications that the substrate for glucuronidation is more readily available if it is in the lipid phase of the endoplasmic reticulum rather than freely dissolved in the cytosol (Zakim and Vessey, 1977; Whitmer et al., 1984). Certainly a high lipid solubility favours

glucuronidation (Mulder and van Doorn, 1975; Schaefer <u>et
al.</u>, 1981). Interestingly, Fry and Paterson (1985) show<u>ed</u>
that sulphation is not influenced by lipid-solubility
(Figure 3).

**Figure 3. Rates of glucuronidation (G) and sulphation (S)
of a series of substituted phenols in isolated rat
hepatocyte as a function of their lipid-solubility.**

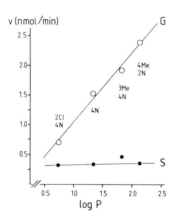

Date are taken from Fry and Paterson (1985). P represents
the octanol/0.1M phosphate buffer, pH7.4 partition
coefficient. The rate of conjugation is given as
nmol/min/2 x 10^6cells; In the figure the position of the
substituents is given; Me is methyl, N is nitro and Cl is
chloro.

High lipid-solubility does not necessarily mean that a
compound will be glucuronidated rather than sulphated. For
instance, p-nitrophenol generated from p-nitroanisol by
cytochrome P-450, is sulphated rather than glucuronidated,
in spite of its high lipid-solubility and the fact that it
is generated at the endoplasmic reticulum (Minck <u>et al.</u>,
1973). The reason probably is that the distances at the
sub-cellular level are so small, that diffusion out of the
membrane phase is very rapid, in spite of a certain
preference of the substrate for the lipid phase.
     When the substrate supply is relatively slow, it is
possible that a substrate never reaches certain sites for
conjugation deeper in the cell interior because it has
already been totally converted directly after entry into
the cell before it could reach those sites (Tipping and

Ketterer, 1981). The cytosol, after all, is rather a compartmentalised "soup" than a solution (Wheatley, 1985), and diffusion may be limited due to the extremely high concentration of solutes (high and low molecular weight) and membranes in the cytosol.

Yet, when two competing transferases are within the same cell, they must draw ultimately from the same total pool of substrate available within the cell. Therefore, unavoidably, one conjugation will compete with the other for the common substrate, and K_m and V_{max} values will decide the final outcome, although anomalies may be observed (Koster and Mulder, 1982).

CO-SUBSTRATE AVAILABILITY; DIET

Efficient conjugation requires an ample supply of the co-substrate; depletion of a co-substrate may, therefore, change the balance between two competing pathways. Under normal conditions the co-substrates are readily available, as long as a sufficient diet is provided, and no large doses of a substrate are given (Mulder and Krijgsheld, 1984). For the biosynthesis of some of the co-substrates the nutritional supply of a component may become rate-limiting. For instance, L-cysteine may be depleted if there is a high demand for glutathione; the same applies to sulphation, where sulphate-availability is limited. On the other hand, for glucuronidation, no special nutritional supplies are required. If a substrate for both glucuronidation and sulphation, for instance paracetamol, is given at high dose, its sulphation will deplete inorganic sulphate, and even UDPGA may be depleted (Howell et al., 1986). At the same time, glutathione is depleted at those high doses by the reactive intermediate generated from paracetamol by cytochrome P450 activity, so that cell toxicity occurs (Mitchell et al., 1976). This demonstrates that co-substrates may be depleted by a high dose of a substrate. It occurs in particular, with sulphur-containing substances like "active sulphate" (PAPS), taurine and glutathione which are dependent on cysteine and methionine supplies. Acetylation, methylation and amino acid conjugation will be much less affected, as long as coenzyme A is not depleted, since this is regenerated after conjugation it is not lost. The protein content of the diet is very important for the sulphur-containing cosubstrates, in particular PAPS and glutathione. Recently, Jung (1985) has shown that rats on a protein-deficient diet (5% instead of 23% protein) excreted only 41% of a dose of paracetamol as sulphate conjugate, this was 70% at 23% protein; for glucuronidation the opposite occurred: 35% (at 5% protein in diet), versus 12% (at 23% protein in diet).

The concentration of the various co-substrates for conjugations in the various organs or cell types is not the same. Very big differences have been noted in different organs (Mulder and Krijgsheld, 1984). Besides the concentration, also (or even more) important is the maximum bio-synthetic capacity of the organ for that co-substrate. Thus it is possible that a particular conjugation in an organ becomes deficient due to co-substrate exhaustion, while in another organ this same conjugation reaction can still be unimpaired due to a high bio-synthetic capacity for the co-substrate. It seems (but much hard data is lacking) that the liver has a very high capacity for bio-synthesis of all co-substrates. For instance, the PAPS concentration in the liver is only approx. 30 nmol/g, while sulphation rates of 100 nmol/g/min for harmol could be reached in the perfused liver (Pang et al., 1981).

The availability of the co-substrates will affect the ratio between competing conjugation: when at high dose, a co-substrate is depleted, obviously only the other reaction can take place after that point.

EXCRETION OF CONJUGATES : CAUSE OF MISINTERPRETATIONS

When the competition for conjugation of a substrate is studied by the excretion pattern of the conjugates only in urine, this may result in misinterpretations, especially when the experiments are done in rats. The reason is that some conjugates are preferentially excreted in bile. For instance, in the rat, glucuronide conjugates are excreted to a high extent in bile, while sulphate conjugates will be found much more in urine (See for instance, Mulder, 1986, Figure 2). If a glucuronide is excreted in bile, it may be hydrolyzed in the gut, and subsequently it may become available again for conjugation. At that time it will be present in the body at a lower concentration than initially. Since sulphation has a lower K_m than glucuronidation, the chances are high that the second time that the molecule is conjugated, it becomes sulphated. If that occurs, and if only what (ultimately) comes out in urine is being measured, the conclusion would be that such a compound is little glucuronidated, while, in fact, an appreciable part of the dose may have been glucuronidated initially. This can be compared to glutathione conjugation, followed by excretion of the glutathione conjugate in bile, and of the mercapturate in the urine.

Very little of the glutathione conjugate will be found in the urine (since it is excreted primarily in bile) although the presence of mercapturate indicates that it has been formed. However, the presence of sulphate conjugates does not tell whether glucuronides have been formed initially that have subsequently been hydrolyzed. Therefore, in studies on the formation of primary metabolites one has to collect bile in order to ascertain that any primary metabolites excreted in bile are also obtained. This is especially important in the rat since this animal has a high biliary excretory activity.

Another possibility is the further metabolism of a conjugate, once it has been synthesised. The further metabolism of glutathione conjugates has already been mentioned. Other examples are the labile sulphate conjugates. They may be metabolically labile because they are readily hydrolysed by sulphatases in the body (Powell and Olavesen, 1981) or they may be chemically labile like the sulphate conjugates of many hydroxamic acids, that, upon synthesis, break down almost instantanously to form reactive nitrenium ions (Mulder, 1981). Such labile sulphate conjugates obviously will be missed, and only secondary metabolites may be measured. For instance, sulphation of N-hydroxyl-2-acetylaminofluorene can only be detected indirectly by its selective inhibition, and the resulting increase in glucuronidation (Meerman et al., 1980).

ORGAN SPECIFICITY

Within the same animal the various organs may show a different conjugation pattern for the same substrate, which is due to factors as already discussed for species differences. For instance, Rush et al (1983) showed that in the rat p-nitrophenol, at a certain dose level, is mainly sulphated in the whole animal, while the contribution of the kidney is mainly glucuronidation (Table 4). Furthermore, in the rat for most substances the gut mucosa contributes virtually only glucuronidation (both during absorption from the gut and during conjugation of drugs that have been given intravenously, but may be conjugated in the intestinal area, outside the liver), while the liver may actively convert them to sulphates (Koster, 1985). Such differences can be studied by isolated cells or perfused organs (liver, lung, kidney, gut) or in vivo by administering drugs at various sites. However, one must keep in mind that in different systems, the rate of substrate presentation to the transferases

Table 4. Conjugation of p-nitrophenol by the rat during
infusion of p-nitrophenol: total conjugation and contribution by the kidney in males and females.

	IN KIDNEYS	OUTSIDE KIDNEYS	TOTAL
	nmol/min/kg (ratio G/S)		
Male Rats			
Glucuronide	76	640	716
	(= 2.92)	(= 0.70)	(= 0.76)
Sulphate	26	911	937
Female Rats			
Glucuronide	199	712	911
	(= 4.85)	(= 0.66)	(= 0.81)
Sulphate	41	1078	1119

Data taken from Rush et al, (1983); p-nitophenol infusion:
2.0 μmol/min/kg; steady state, p-nitrophenol plasma
concentration: females $27 \pm 7 \mu M$, males $33 \pm 5 \mu M$.

inside the cell may be very different even at the same
substrate concentration. If the cells in the organ are
exposed to the same concentration in the surrounding medium
it will depend on the rate of the uptake processes
(diffusion, carrier transport) how high the concentration
inside the cell becomes. Thus, the same perfusion medium
concentration may lead to different intracellular substrate
concentrations in different organs. Furthermore, not all
cells are equal within an organ. It has been shown for the
substrate harmol (sulphation and glucuronidation compete
for this phenolic substrate) that within the liver there is
a gradient for glucuronidation relative to sulphation due
to the fact that hepatocytes in zone 1 in the liver have a
higher sulphation activity than those in zone 3 (relative
to glucuronidation which is rather constant). This may be
related to oxygen availability (required for PAPS and UDPGA
synthesis) in zone 1 and 3, since sulphation requires
somewhat higher oxygen levels than glucuronidation (Aw and
Jones, 1982). Alternatively, it may be due to different

transferase levels in zone 1 and 3. Substrate availability most likely is not the reason (Pang et al., 1981; 1983; Dawson et al., 1985).

REFERENCES

Aw, T.Y. and Jones, D.P. (1982). J. Biol. Chem, 257, 8997.

Caldwell, J. (1978) in: "Conjugation Reactions in Drug Bio-transformation" (ed. Aitio, A). Elsevier Biomedical Press, Amsterdam, 111.

Caldwell, J. (1982) in "Metabolic Basis of Detoxication: Metabolism of Functional Groups" (ed. Jacoby, W.B., Bend, J.R. and Caldwell, J), Academic Press, New York, N.Y. 292.

Dawson, J.R., Weitering, J.G., Mulder, G.J., Stillwell, R.N. and Pang, K.S (1985). J. Pharm. Exp. Ther. 234, 691.

Dixon, P.A.F., Caldwell, J. and Smith, R.L. (1977). Xenobiotica 7, 727.

Fry, J.R. and Paterson, P. (1985). Brit. J. Pharmacol, 84, 133P.

Howell, S.R., Hazelton, G.A. and Klaassen, C.D. (1986). J. Pharm. Exp. Ther, 236, 610.

Jacoby, W.B. (ed) (1980). "Enzymatic Basis of Detoxication", vol 2, Academic Press, New York, N.Y.

Jung, D. (1985). J. Pharm. Exp. Ther, 232, 178.

Koster, A.S. (1985). Glucuronidation in the rat intestinal wall in vitro and in vivo. PhD Thesis, University of Utrecht, The Netherlands.

Koster, H. and Mulder, G.J. (1982) Drug Metab. Dispos. 10, 330.

Meerman, J.H.N., Van Doorn, A.B.D. and Mulder, G.J. (1980). Cancer Res, 40, 3772.

Minck, K., Schupp, R.R., Illing, H.P.A., Kahl, G.F. and Netter, K.J. (1973) Naun. Schm. Arch. Pharmacol, 279, 347.

Mitchell, J.R., Hinson, J.A. and Nelson, S.D. (1976) in "Gluathione Metabolism and Function" (eds. Arias, I.M. and Jacoby, W.B.) Raven Press, New York, N.Y. 357.

Mulder, G.J. (1981). "Sulfation of Drugs and Related Compounds", CRC Press, Boca Raton, FL.

Mulder, G.J. (1982) in "Metabolic Basis of Detoxication : Metabolism of Functional Groups"(eds. Jacoby, W.B., Bend, J.R. and Caldwell, J.). Academic Press, New York, N.Y. 247.

Mulder, G.J. (1985) in "Progress in Drug Metabolism" (eds. Bridges, J.W. and Chasseaud, L.F), vol 8, Taylor and Francis Ltd, London, UK., 35.

Mulder, G.J. (1986). Fed. Proceed, 45, July issue.

Mulder, G.J. and Krijgsheld, K.R. (1984). "Drugs and Nutrients" (eds. Roe, D.A. and Campbell, T.C). Marcel Dekker, New York, N.Y. 119.

Mulder, G.J. and Meerman, J.H.N. (1978). in "Conjugation Reactions in Drug Biotransformation" (ed. Aitio, A). Elsevier Biomedical Publ., Amsterdam, 389.

Mulder, G.J. and van Doorn, A.B.D. (1975). Biochem. J. 151, 131.

Pang, K.S., Koster, H., Halsema, I.C.M., Scholtens, E. and Mulder, G.J. (1981). J. Pharm. Exp. Ther, 219, 134.

Pang, K.S., Koster, H., Halsema, I.C.M., Scholtens, E., Mulder, G.J. and Stillwell, R.N. (1983). J. Pharm. Exp. Ther, 224, 647.

Powell, G.M. and Olavesen, A.H. (1981) in "Sulfation of Drugs and Related Compounds" (ed. Mulder, G.J), CRC Press, Boca Raton, FL, 187.

Rush, G.F., Newton, J.F. and Hook, J.B. (1983). J. Pharm. Exp. Ther, 227, 658.

Schaefer, M., Okulicz-Kozaryn, I., Batt, A.M., Siest, G. and Loppinet, V. (1981). Eur. J. Med. Chem, 16, 461.

Tipping, E. and Ketterer, B. (1981). Biochem. J. 195, 441.

Waschek, J.A., Rubin, G.M., Tozer, T.N., Fielding, R.M., Couet, W.R., Effeney, D.J. and Pond, S.M. (1984). J. Pharm. Exp. Ther, 230, 89.

Weitering, J.G., Krijgsheld, K.R. and Mulder, G.J. (1979). Biochem. Pharmac, 28, 757.

Wheatley, D.N. (1985). Life Sci, 36, 299.

Whitmer, D.I., Ziurys, J.C. and Gollan, J.L. (1984). J. Biol. Chem, 259, 11969.

Zakim, D. and Vessey, D.A. (1977). J. Biol. Chem, 252, 7534.

SUBCELLULAR LOCALISATION OF DRUG METABOLIZING ENZYMES IN RELATION TO THEIR FUNCTION

Benedicte Antoine, Gerard Siest, Sylvie Fournel, AthanaseVisvikis and Maria-Monika Wellman-Bednawska.

Centre Du Medicament, Unite Associee C.N.R.S. No 597, 30 rue Lionnois - 54000 NANCY, France.

INTRODUCTION

It stands to reason from a pharmacological and toxicological point of view that a fundamental and functional role is played by plasma and nuclear membranes in the cell. The plasma membrane constitutes not only a sort of mechanical filter towards drug and xenobiotic entrance but also a receiver-transmitter of external messages inside the cell. Identically, nuclear membranes receive and transmit the information addressed to the genetic material then return its coded responses. Other organelles such as mitochondria, dictyosomes and lysosomes demarcate territories for specific functions.

The majority of metabolism of drugs and endogenous compounds occurs in the endoplasmic reticulum (ER). Nevertheless this compartment can no longer be considered as the sole site for drug metabolising enzyme-mediated biotransformations. A few years ago oxidative metabolic processes were investigated in nuclear membranes and found to be genuine to the nuclei (Romano et al., 1983). A specific isozyme of cytochrome P-450, the cytochrome P-448 was shown to be present in the nuclei as early as 1979 (Bresnick et al., 1979). Recently, metabolism of benzo(a)pyrene was compared between nuclear and microsomal fractions in rat liver (Oesch et al., 1985) and in the rhesus monkey liver (Pacifici et al., 1986). These data argue for the real participation of other membranes than ER in drug metabolism. In the monkey, nuclei differ from microsomes in the lack of formation of quinones, In the rat, the metabolite pattern of benzo(a)pyrene obtained by incubation with nuclear fractions differed slightly from that produced by the fractions of ER, but plasma membranes (PM) and mitochondria produced markedly different patterns. This was regarded by Oesch as an indirect trace of a potentially different pattern of cytochrome P-450 isozymes present in the individual membranes. Moreover, it was shown that liver mitochondria possess a cytochrome P-450 system, which plays an important role in a major function of this tissue, i.e. the synthesis of bile acids and steroids (Bresnick, 1984).

In the same way, different epoxide hydrolases exist in the cytosol (Hammock et al., 1980) and in several membrane fractions (Stasiecki et al., 1980). Besides the microsomal epoxide hydrolase, with a broad specificity for many xenobiotic epoxides, there is a cytosolic epoxide hydrolase more specialised for trans-substituted oxiranes and a cholesterol-5,6-oxide hydrolase which is differentially regulated in the nuclear envelope than in ER (Carubelli et al., 1986) and may be responsible for the metabolism of endogenously formed steroidal epoxides (Batt et al., 1984).

In the case of UDP-glucuronosyltransferases, few studies have been done until now on particular locations of specific isoforms, mainly because of the extreme difficulty in purifying this lipid dependent family of enzymes. Nevertheless, in a recent commentary (Siest et al., 1986), we underlined the potential existence of at least one UDPGT form more specialised in protection against toxic compounds, and whose sublocation seems to be restricted to the ER and the nuclear envelope.

Indeed, just as the tissue-specific pattern of activity tends to be associated with the metabolic advantages of such separate positioning, so the subcellular distributions of activity tend to reflect intracellular organisation and compartmentation of cellular functions. Simply on the basis of the structural divergences of multiple enzyme forms it would not be surprising to find that differential subcellular distributions of isozymes are a relatively common occurrence. Until now, few studies have been done in this respect, the reasons for this limited development may arise from :
i) the difficulty to purify isozymes and then to obtain antibodies recognising epitopes of molecular forms which were coded by a same subfamily of genes, i.e. UDP glucuronosyltransferases.
ii) the technical difficulties related to the preparation of subcellular organelles and the lability of their enzymatic system.
iii) the necessity for very sensitive and specific analytical methods for monitoring their activity.
iv) suspicion that ER contamination could account for the activities observed in other membranes.
The detection of specialised reactions catalysed by

specific isozymes in a particular location would argue for
their genuine presence in other membranes than ER, as
already shown in nuclear envelope and in mitochondria. On
the contrary, the observation of a similar isozyme pattern
between two membranes could be interpreted, as either the
result of ER-contamination or being the result of breakdown
residues.

Our purpose consists of a synthetic review of major
drug metabolising enzyme subcellular localizations in the
liver, namely to underline the lack of knowledge concerning
specific localisations of isozymes in relation to their
function. We choose to consider the plasma membranes which
play a crucial part in the regulation of cellular
metabolism and which are nevertheless not widely
investigated. We propose a comparison between specific
mono-oxygenase capacities and UDP-glucuronic acid
conjugation in different subcellular membranes of the
liver.

SUBCELLULAR DISTRIBUTION OF PHASE I ENZYMES

We present in Table 1 a brief report of published data
about the distribution of cytochrome P-450 and its
reductase and of cytochrome b_5 between the various liver
endomembranes. These data clearly confirm the predominance
of phase I enzymes in the smooth ER but also suggest their
genuine presence in the other endomembranes. Most authors
agree that the respective amounts in nuclear envelope,
Golgi and plasma membranes were too high to only be the
result of smooth ER contamination. Nevertheless, only
screening of the different membranes for the various
isozymes would result in confirmation of the real meaning
of such a specific isozyme in relation to its function.
The arguements in favour of endogenous cytochrome P-450 and
P-420, cytochrome b_5, NADH and NADPH dehydrogenases in
plasma membranes (Jarasch et al., 1979; Goldenberg, 1982)
concern the relatively high amounts or differential
stability of the proteins in this liver subfraction.
Before attempting a systematic immunodetection of different
isozymes, we wanted to initially proceed by measuring some
mono-oxygenase activities, each being specific for one
cytochrome P-450 isozyme before and after administration of
its preferential inducer (Table 2).

Gamma glutamyltransferase was measured as a marker for
bile canalicular PM. Its enrichment in PM, compared with
the homogenate is around 15 and this is of the same order
as previously reported (Magdalou et al., 1982; Antoine et
al., 1986). In the same way, the plasma membrane RNA

Table 1. Comparison of the monooxygenase capacities of rat liver membranes.

NE	RER	SER	GA	PM	REFERENCE
		Cytochrome P-450			
	115	100	50	30	Sandberg et al., 1980
24	105	100	32	21	Jarasch et al., 1979
16	75	100	22	18	Stasiecki et al., 1980
	87	100	12	17	Von Bahr et al., 1972
20	91	100			Gonzalez et al., 1982
	59	100	2.5		Tsuji et al., 1977
	59	100	33	37	Antoine et al., 1986
NADPH cytochrome c reductase					
	111	100	28	16	Sandberg et al., 1980
16	72	100	13	9	Jarasch et al., 1979
6	77	100	11	14	Stasiecki et al., 1980
	80	100	27	17	Von Bahr et al., 1972
32	92	100			Gonzalez et al., 1982
	64	100	8-13	11	Fleisher et al., 1967
	70	100	4		Tsuji et al., 1977
	69	100	41	10	Antoine et al., 1986
		Cytochrome b_5			
	78	100	56		Sandberg et al., 1980
35	70	100	38	27	Stasiecki et al., 1980
	84	100	28	28	Von Bahr et al., 1972
28	76	100			Gonzalez et al., 1982
	58	100	5		Tsuji et al., 1977
	71	100	35	39	Antoine et al., 1986

NE : nuclear envelope, RER and SER : rough and smooth endoplasmic reticulum, PM : plasma membrane, GA : Golgi apparatus.

Values represent percentage of SER amount or activity.

Table 2. Comparison of phase I activities in rat liver microsomes and plasma membranes, before and after induction.

Enzyme Activity or Content	CONTROL RATS		PM/ER	PHENOBARBITAL TREATED RATS	
	ER	PM		ER	PM
Cytochrome P-450[a]	0.85±0.23	0.23±0.07	0.27	2.17±0.11	0.32±0.06
7-ethoxyresorufin 0-deethylase[b]	5.20±0.90	3.10±1.10	0.60	ND	ND
Benzphetamine-N demethylase[c]	5.37±1.16	0.91±0.34	0.17	9.25±0.58	0.93±0.16
Lauric acid 12-hydroxylase[c]	0.17±0.07	0.04±0.01	0.24	ND	ND
Benzopyrene 4,5 oxide/epoxide hydrolase[c]	7.18±1.56	0.65±0.13	0.09	22.4 +4.3	1.68±0.17
Gamma glutamyl-transferase[c]	1.58±0.48	11.41±2.35	7.22	1.92±0.31	ND
RNA[d]	0.108±0.007	0.021±0.004	0.19	0.102±0.008	0.019±0.003

Methods used are, in the same decreasing order as in the table, Matsubara et al (1976), Burke and Mayer (1975), Yang and Strickhart (1974), Fournel et al (1985), Dansette et al (1979), Szasz (1969) and Fleck and Begg (1965).

cont'd

Table 2 (Cont'd)

Enzyme Activity or Content	3MC TREATED RATS		CLOFIBRATE TREATED RATS	
	ER	PM	ER	PM
Cytochrome P-450[a]	1.82+0.63	0.30+0.12	0.79+0.04	0.13+0.00
7-ethoxyresorufin 0-deethylase[b]	1,010+280	89.0 +55.0	ND	ND
Benzphetamine-N demethylase[c]	ND	ND	ND	ND
Lauric acid 12-hydroxylase[c]	ND	ND	1.59+0.29	0.11+0.06
Benzopyrene 4,5 oxide/ epoxide hydrolase[c]	7.67+0.75	0.80+0.35	8.97+2.35	0.70+0.18
Gamma glutamyl- transferase[c]	1.62+0.65	12.06+6.56	1.33+0.34	4.20+0.72
RNA[d]	0.116+0.010	0.025+0.003	0.089+0.007	0.011+0.002

a nmol/mg protein; b pmol/min/mg protein; c nmol/min/mg protein; d mg/mg protein. ND not determined. Values are means of three different subfractionations. ER and Pm were isolated according to Amar-Costesec et al (1974) and Neville (1968) from male Wistar rat livers. Maximal induction levels were obtained with: one IP injection of PB (100 mg/kg bodyweight then 1 g/l drinking water (decapitation on the fifth day); one IP injection of 3MC (100mg/kg bodyweight), decapitation on the fifth day and one daily gastric intubation, for 9 days, at a dose of 200mg/kg bodyweight for clofibrate acid treatment.

content is in good agreement with other authors (Stasiecki et al., 1980). Previous analysis of our PM fraction has shown that it was contaminated by no more than 10% of rough and smooth endoplasmic reticulum (RER and SER). (These data were based on RNA amount and NADPH cytochrome c reductase activity measured in PM (Antoine et al., 1986).

Results obtained on sublocalization of benzopyrene 4,5-oxide/epoxide hydrolase (EH) confirms previous findings (Galteau et al., 1985) which suggested an exclusive location of this EH isoform in the SER. Our PM fraction only contained 9% of the microsomal EH activity (whatever the inducer used), thus our PM appeared to be only 9% contaminated by SER. Stasiecki et al., have even mentioned a benzopyrene 4,5-oxide/EH in PM which represented 25% of the SER activity. Based on the previous remarks, we can reasonably consider that each PM activity exceeding 10% of the respective microsomal activity, could reflect its genuine presence in PM. This would be the case for cytochrome P-450, benzphetamine N-demethylase and lauric acid 12-hydroxylase representing in PM 17 to 27% of the microsomal values. Calculating the microsomal contamination of PM, it was suggested that 50 to 80% of measured b-type cytochromes were endogenous to this subfraction (Goldenberg, 1982).

Firstly, taking into account that microsomes contained only 77% of their total protein amount as endoplasmic reticulum (de Duve, 1976) and, secondly that PM are 10% contaminated by ER, we have estimated the PM endogenous content to be : (in nmol/mg protein or nmol/min/ mg protein) 0.14 for total cytochrome P-450, 0.0024 for 7-ethoxyresorufin O-deethylase, 0.21 for benzphetamine N-demethylase and 0.018 for lauric acid 12-hydroxylase ; these PM endogenous values representing respectively 61%, 78%, 23% and 45% of the measured data.

The different mono-oxygenase activities were chosen to be respectively more representative of specific cytochrome P-450 isoforms. The 7-ethoxyresorufin O-deethylase, benzphetamine N-demethylase and lauric acid 12-hydroxylase activities would be more related to the 3-MC induced (P450c), phenobarbital-induced (P450b) and clofibrate-induced cytochrome P-450 isoforms (Ryan et al., 1979, Tamburini et al., 1984) respectively. In this context, our results would show that the endogenous total cytochrome P-450 of PM is more enriched in 3-MC induced-cytochrome P-450 isozymes than in phenobarbital- or clofibrate-induced ones.

Another interesting point to mention is the weak inducibility of these phase 1 activities in PM compared with the situation observed in microsomes, as we already

observed after a single phenobarbital injection (Antoine et
al., 1986). Such differences in inducibility between two
subcellular fractions were reported as an arguement in
favour of the endogenous presence of the same enzyme in
each membrane (Gontovnick and Bellward, 1981).

SUBCELLULAR LOCALIZATION OF UDP-GLUCURONOSYLTRANSFERASES

The UDP-glucuronosyltransferases (UDPGT EC.2.4.1.17)
are a family of membrane-bound enzymes involved in the
conjugation of various exogenous substrates (such as drugs)
or endogenous ones (such as bilirubin or steroid hormones)
with UDP-glucuronic acid (UDPGA). The existence of at
least seven or eight molecular forms of the enzyme is
suggested on the basis of physiological criteria (such as
perinatal development, or induction) or physico-chemical
properties (such as the structure of their substrates and
the pI of more or less specific purified preparations). A
summary of the characteristics of the different UDPGT
molecular forms is presented in Table 3. Because of its
extreme phospholipid dependence and perhaps because of an
unique gene family (i.e. coding for very homologous
proteins), the identification of UDPGT isozymes has not
enjoyed the same development and success as the cytochrome
P-450 dependent mono-oxygenase complex. However, the first
characterizations of different cDNA coding sequences for
UDPGTs were described very recently by two teams, Mackenzie
et al (1984a) and Jackson and Burchell (1986). The
molecular biology will permit the real basis of the UDPGT
functional heterogeneity to be investigated.

The existence of two distinct populations of UDPGT, one
for endogenous compounds and the other for xenobiotics is
reasonable to envisage (Siest et al., 1986). For example,
endogenous compounds and "natural" xenobiotics (such as
monoterpenoid alcohols)/UDPGT activities generally show low
capacities (low Vmax) but higher affinity (low Km) in
conjugating their substrates, their high specificity
providing for regular elimination of physiological
molecules. Conversely, xenobiotic/UDPGTs seem to
compensate for their low affinity (low specificity) towards
a diversity of substrate structures by a high velocity to
efficiently detoxify these various drugs, as well as
greater inducibility (Antoine et al., 1984; Thomassin et
al., 1985 and Boutin et al., 1985).

Very few studies have been done until now in regard to
the subcellular localization of different UDPGT activities,
in relation to their function. Table 4 summarises the
published data. Despite the diversity of the methods and

Table 3. Characteristics of the Different UDPGT Molecular Forms.

Substrate Specificity	Specific Induction	Ontogenic Development	UDPGT Form	Subcellular Localization[d]
Aromatic flat <0.4nm, group 1 substrates	TCDD, 3MC B-naphtho-flavone	late fetal	GT_1/ pnp GT	ER, NE (mitochon-dria)
Bulky molecules >0.4nm, group 2	PB[a] TSO	neonatal	GT_2	ER, GA, PM
Monoterpenoid alcohols[c]	PB[b]	-	GT_2A	ER, PM
Bilirubin	Clofibrate and related hypolipid-aemic agents	neonatal	Bili-rubin GT/GT_3	ER, GA
Digitoxigenin, monodigitoxo-side[c]	Spirono-lactone	neonatal	-	ER
3α hydroxy-steroid Estrone Androsterone	Aroclor 1254	neonatal	-	ER
17 hydroxy-steroid Testosterone	PB	neonatal	-	ER, GA, PM

(From Siest G, 1986).

[a]considered as specific inducer of group 2 substrate conjugation, but also induces other forms of UDPGT. [b]specific inducer in the guinea pig. [c]considered to be a separate form on the basis of selective induction. [d]other subcellular locations are mentioned when specific activity in percentage of microsomal activity is higher than 50%.

Table 4. Presence of UDP-Glucuronosyltransferase in Sub-cellular Membranes of Rat Liver.

3 MC INDUCIBLE SUBSTRATES	Specific activity (% of microsomes)			
	NE	GA	PM	References
4-methyl-	100			Zaleski, 1982
umbelliferone		21	18	Antoine, 1983
p-nitrophenol	100			Zaleski, 1982
	100			Gorski, 1977
	89			Bansal, 1981
	75			Elmamlouk, 1981
	49			Gonzalez, 1982
		11	39	Von Bahr, 1972
		30	25	Antoine, 1983
1-naphthol	222			Wishart, 1980
	116			Zaleski, 1982
	149	73	61	Stasiecki, 1982
PB INDUCIBLE SUBSTRATES				
Eugenol	19	26	21	Antoine, 1983
Borneol	24	38	45	Antoine, 1983
Morphine	25	67	100	Antoine, 1983
Chloramphenicol	50	88	105	Antoine, 1983
Testosterone	15	77	105	Antoine, 1983
Bilirubin	22	65	-	Hauser, 1984
		41	15	Antoine un-published data

of substrate concentrations used, two conclusions can be drawn: (i) the existence of a carcinogen-induced UDPGT (GT_1), mainly located in the ER and the nuclear envelope, perhaps in relation to its function, i.e. to protect genetic material against carcinogenic compounds, which often bind to DNA, (ii) UDPGTs that act on "natural" xenobiotics or endogenous substrates seem to be distributed more widely inside the hepatocyte. We chose to study the response of different UDPGT activities to several inducers both in microsomes and PM (Table 5). The distribution of UDPGT activities between ER and PM in control rats is in accordance with the summarised data of Table 4. Endogenous UDPGT activities in the PM, calculated as mentioned for phase 1 enzymes, give specific activities (nmol/min/ mg protein) of 7.6 for 4-methylumbelliferone, 8.7 for 4-nitrophenol and 0.03 for bilirubin. Bilirubin/UDPGT (GT_3) was found to be absent from the PM by Hauser et al., 1984). Our results lead to the same conclusion in regard to the weak estimated endogenous activity found in PM. Another argument could consist of the non-inducibility of PM bilirubin/UDPGT by phenobarbital and clofibrate, in contrast with the situation observed in microsomes.

The weak amount of $GT_1(S)$ (4-methylumbelliferone and 4-nitrophenol/UDPGTs) found in the PM (respectively 11 and 21% of microsomal values) is confirmed by its specific inducibility by 3-methylcholanthrene in contrast to the situation observed with phenobarbital.

GT_{2a} (monoterpenoid alcohol, i.e. borneol/UDPGT) is found to be ubiquitous in ER, Golgi and plasma membranes, as assessed by Vmax determination (Antoine et al., 1984). Surprisingly, borneol/UDPGT does not seem to be inducible by phenobarbital in PM, in our experimental conditions. GT_{2b} (morphine/UDPGT) was found to be at least equally distributed between ER and plasma membranes.

Similarly, Pacifici et al (1986) reported a broad distribution of morphine/UDPGT between microsomes, nuclei and mitochondria in human liver; and in human intestinal mucosa, morphine/UDPGT is mainly associated with the nuclear fraction. Keeping in mind that PM exhibited a nucleo-microsomal distribution during a classical microsome fractionation procedure (Amar-Costesec et al, 1974), it could be suggested that morphine/UDPGT is preferentially located in the canalicular PM to conjugate the molecule close to its excretion pathway, the bile (Brock and Vore, 1982). Finally, steroid/UDPGTs, either testosterone or androsterone/UDPGT were shown to also conjugate some bile acids (Matern et al., 1982; Kirkpatrick et al., 1984). This suggests that their presence in bile canalicular PM

The questions that come to mind in a discussion of sublocalization are what are the mechanism and control of such intracellular traffic of some proteins?

We attempted to trace the possible migration of different newly synthesised UDPGT forms after a single phenobarbital injection (Antoine et al., 1986). These preliminary results suggested that, in contrast to GT_1 (4-nitrophenol) which seems to be sequestered in its site of synthesis (ER), morphine/UDPGT may migrate to Golgi

**Table 5. UDPGT activities in microsomes and plasma
membranes in control and induced rat livers.**

Substrate	Control Rats			Phenobarbital-treated Rats	
	ER	PM	PM/ER	ER	PM
4-methyl umbelli-ferone	69.4+12.5	16.6+1.3	0.24	148.6+18.3	18.2+2.3
4-nitro-phenol	42.1+ 7.3	14.2+1.0	0.34	90.8+12.8	17.4+2.0
Borneol	8.2+ 1.9	10.5+1.6	1.28	14.7+3.9	6.9+2.8
Morphine	4.0+ 0.8	10.3+1.8	2.58	6.9+1.6	10.1+0.3
Bili-rubin	0.91+ 0.08	0.15+0.6	0.16	1.72+0.28	0.18+0.04

Substrate	3-Methylcholanthrene treated Rats		Clofibrate treated rats	
	ER	PM	ER	PM
4-methyl umbelliferone	335.6+41.9	58.5+19.3	51.3+12.0	9.7+0.9
4-nitro-phenol	193.4+31.0	37.2+ 9.5	29.4+ 3.9	10.6+0.5
Borneol	8.1+ 2.9	3.0+ 2.2	7.7+ 2.6	7.0+1.5
Morphine	3.5+ 0.7	6.1+ 2.3	5.0+ 1.6	6.2+0.4
Bilirubin	0.77+0.17	0.14+0.03	1.72+0.27	0.17+0.04

Activities (expressed in nmol/min/mg protein) were
measured by the method of Mulder and Van Doorn modified by
Colin-Neiger (1984) [UDPGA] = 4.5mM, [Substrates] =
0.5mM, after maximal Triton X-100 activation.

Values are means+SD of three different subfractionations.

ER and PM isolation and inducer treatments, were performed
as in the legend of Table 2.

membranes, where an increase of activity was observed following its increase in ER. These findings should be compared with those of Mackenzie (1984b, 1986) who showed firstly, the glycosylation of some UDPGTs with specificity towards testosterone and morphine (this raised the question of their eventual passage in the Golgi) and secondly, the proteolytic cleavage of at least one phenobarbital-induced UDPGT form (that exhibits a similarity with the secretory protein pathway). Thus, UDPGT should be the first drug-metabolizing membrane-bound enzyme which has been found to be cleaved proteolytically in the ER (Kreibich et al., 1983). Though this information is not evidence that some UDPGT forms migrate, it is surprising enough to deserve mention.

ARE PLASMA-MEMBRANES INVOLVED IN DRUG OR ENDOGENOUS COMPOUND METABOLISM?

We underlined the potential presence of some specific cytochrome P-450 isozymes and some UDPGT molecular forms in the liver PM. Despite being partial and preliminary results, they seem to be worthy of further interest particularly when molecular biology will permit the real distinction between the different isozymes of an enzyme family. Such an investigation will permit evaluation of the pharmacological role of PM and other liver organelles.

Another plasma membrane-bound enzyme whose real function is not fully known is the gamma-glutamyl-transferase (GGT EC.2.3.2.2). Several physiological functions have been suggested for GGT including mediation of amino acid transport, uptake of gamma glutamyl compounds, oligopeptide group translocation, participation in secretory processes and involvement in mercapturic acid synthesis.

It is also involved in the metabolism of xenobiotics and endogenous compounds such as prostaglandins and leuko-trienes (Anderson et al., 1982). However, its relation with drug-metabolizing enzymes is not fully understood, except its participation in the first step of the degradation of free and conjugated glutathione.

Interestingly, the major location of GGT is not the ER but the PM. This could suggest a potential function of PM in at least some endogenous compounds metabolism. For example, both a cytochrome P-450 and GGT are involved in the metabolism of leukotrienes. This raises the question if these two proteins could be space-related.

Similarly, as phenobarbital induces specific molecular

forms of drug metaolizing enzymes, we observed the appearance of a new GGT polypeptide in PM after phenobarbital (Antoine et al, 1986). Though the meaning of induction processes still remains obscure from a pharmacological point of view, this example illustrates a parallel behaviour of GGT with drug metabolizing enzymes by new isoforms synthesis in response to an inducer. Are these isoforms specific and or space-related for a complementary pharmacological response?

To further define its structural and functional features and also to study its behaviour during induction and its relationship with drug metabolising enzymes, we have attempted to clone specific cDNAs for hepatic GGT coding sequences.

We screened a rat liver cDNA library constructed in the E.coli expression vector λ gtll, using specific antibodies as probes. We have isolated and partially characterised eight putative positive clones. Further characterisation and sequencing of these clones as well as the search for other positive clones are in progress.

Molecular biology and immunological characterisation of the enzymes in the different membranes in relation to specific pharmacological activity are the necessary steps before general acceptance of the presence of drug metabolising enzymes in these locations.

ACKNOWLEDGEMENTS

The authors thank M.W.H. Coughtrie for English correction of the manuscript.

REFERENCES

Amar-Costesec, A., Beaufay, H., Wibo, M., Thines-Sempoux, D., Feytmans, E., Robbi, M. and Berthet J. (1974). J. Cell. Biol., 61, 201.

Anderson, M.E., Allison, R.D. and Meister, A. (1982). Proc. Natl. Acad. Sci. USA, 79, 1088.

Antoine, B., Magdalou, J. and Siest, G. (1983). Biochem. Pharmacol., 32, 2629.

Antoine B., Magdalou, J. and Siest, G. (1984). Xenobiotica, 14, 575.

Antoine B., Rahimi-Pour, A., Siest, G., Magdalou, J. and Galteau, M.M. (1986). Cell. Biochem. Function (in press).

Bansal, S.K., Zaleski, J. and Gessner, T. (1981). Biochem. Biophys. Res. Commun, 91, 131.

Batt, A.M., Siest, G. and Oesch, F. (1984).

Carcinogenesis, 5, 1205.

Boutin, J.A., Thomassin, J., Siest, G. and Cartier, A. (1985). Biochem. Pharmacol, 34, 2235.

Bresnick, E., Boraker, D. and Hassuk, B. (1979). Molecular Pharmacology, 16, 324.

Bresnick, E. (1984). In "Drug metabolism" (ed. by Siest, G). Pergamon Press, Paris, p.77

Brock, W.J. and Vore, M. (1982). Drug Metab Disp, 10, 336.

Burke, M.D. and Mayer, R.T. (1975). Drug Metab. Disp, 3, 245.

Carubelli, R., Palakodety, R.B. and Griffin, M.J. (1986). Chem. Biol. Interact, 58, 125.

Colin-Neiger, A., Kaufmann, I., Boutin, J.A., Fournel, S., Siest, G., Batt, A.M. and Magdalou, J. (1984). J. Biochem. Biophys. Methods, 9, 69.

Dansette, P.M., Dubois, G.C. and Jerina, D.M. (1979). Anal. Biochem, 97, 340.

De Duve, C. (1976). Pontificae academiae scientarium scripts varia, 40, 47.

Elmanlouk, T.H., Mukhtar, H. and Bend, J.R. (1981). J. Pharmacol. Exp. Therap, 219, 27.

Fleisher, S. and Fleisher, B. (1967). in "Methods in Enzymology" (ed. Estabrook, R.W. and Pollman, M.E). Academic Press, Publ, New York, p.406.

Fleck, A. and Begg, D. (1965). Biochim. Biophys. Acta, 108, 333.

Fournel, S., Magdalou, J., Thomassin, J., Villoutreix, J., Siest, G., Caldwell, J. and Andre, J.C. (1985). Biochim. Biophys. Acta, 842, 202.

Galteau, M.M., Antoine, B. and Reggio, H. (1985). The EMBO J., 4, 2793.

Goldenberg, H. (1982). Enzyme, 27, 227.

Gontovnick, L.S. and Bellward, G.D. (1981). Drug Metab. Dispos, 9, 265.

Gonzales, F.J. and Kasper, C.B. (1982). Mol. Pharmacol, 21, 511.

Gorski, J.P. and Kasper, C.B. (1977). J. Biol. Chem, 252, 1336.

Hammock, B.D., Gill, S.S., Mumby, S.M. and Ota, K. (1980). in Molecular basis of environmental toxicity (ed. Bhatnagar R.S), Ann Arbor Science Publishers, Ann Arbor, p. 229.

Hauser, S.C., Ziurys, R.C. and Gollan, J.L. (1984). J. Biol. Chem, 259, 4527.

Jackson, M.R. and Burchell, B. (1986). Nucleic Acid Res, 14, 779.

Jarasch, E.D., Kartenbeck, J., Bruder, G., Fink, A., Morre, D.J. and Franke, W.W. (1979). J. Cell. Biol, 80, 37.

Kirkpatrick, R.B., Falany, C.N. and Tephly, T.R. (1984). J. Biol. Chem, 259, 6176.

Kreibich, G., Sabatini, D.D. and Adesnik, M. (1983). in "Methods in Enzymology" (ed. Fleisher, S.B). Academic Press Inc, New York, 96, p530.

Mackenzie, P.I., Gonzales, F.J. and Owens, I.S. (1984a). J. Biol. Chem, 259, 12153.

Mackenzie, P.I., Gonzales, F.J. and Owens, I.S. (1984b). Arch. Biochem. Biophys, 230, 676.

Mackenzie, P.I. (1986). J. Biol. Chem, 261, 6119.

Magdalou, J., Antoine, B., Ratanasavanh, D. and Siest, G. (1982). Enzyme, 28, 41.

Matern, H., Matern, S. and Gerok, W. (1982). J. Biol. Chem, 257, 7422.

Matsubara, T., Koike, M., Touchi, A., Tochino, Y. and Sugeno, K. (1976). Anal. Biochem, 75, 596.

Neville, D. M. Jr (1968). Biochim. Biophys. Acta, 154, 540.

Oesch, F., Bentley, P., Golan, M. and Stasiecki, P., (1985). Cancer Res, 45, 4838.

Pacifici, G.M., Bencini, C. and Rane, A. (1986). Xenobiotica 16, 123.

Pacifici, G.M., Blanck, A., and Rane, A. (1986). Acta Pharmacol et Toxicol, 58, 1.

Romano, M., Facchinetti, T. and Salmona, M. (1983). Drug Metabolism Reviews, 14, 803.

Ryan, D.E., Thomas, P.E., Korzeniowski, D. and Levin, W. (1979). J. Biol. Chem, 254, 1365.

Sandberg, P.O., Marzella, L. and Glauman, H. (1980). Exp. Cell. Res, 130, 393.

Siest, G., Magdalou, J., Antoine, B., Fournel, S. and Thomassin, J. (1986). Biochem. Pharmcol (in press).

Stasiecki, P., Oesch, F., Bruder, G., Jarasch, E.D. and Franke, W.W. (1980). Eur. J. Cell. Biol, 21, 79.

Szasz, G. (1969). Clin. Chem, 15, 124.

Tamburini, P.P., Masson, M.A., Bains, S., Makowski, R.J., Morris, B. and Gibson, G.G. (1984). Eur. J. Biochem, 139, 235.

Thomassin, J., Boutin, J.A. and Siest, G. (1985). Pharmacol. Res. Commun, 17, 1005.

Tsuji, H., Hattori, N., Yamamoto, T. and Kato, K. (1977). J. Biochem, 82, 619.

Von Bahr, C., Hietanen, E. and Glauman, H. (1972). Acta Pharmacol. Toxicol, 31, 107.

Wishart, G.J. and Fry, D.J. (1980). Biochem. J. 186, 687.

Yang, C.S. and Strickhart, F.S. (1974). Biomed. Pharmacol, 23, 3129.

Zaleski, J., Bansal, S.K. and Gessner, T. (1982). Can. J. Biochem, 60, 972.

THE ROLE OF CONJUGATING ENZYMES IN TOXIC METABOLITE FORMATION

Peter J. Van Bladeren, Irene M. Bruggeman, Wim M.F. Jongen, Annehieke G. Scheffer and Johan H.M. Temmink.

Department of Toxicology, Agricultural University, De Dreijen 12, 6703 BC, Wageningen, The Netherlands.

INTRODUCTION

In the last few years, examples have accumulated of compounds transformed into more reactive and/or more toxic derivatives by conjugating enzymes. In principle two modes of action can be distinguished : i) the conjugate exerts its toxic effect via interaction with a receptor, and ii) conjugation transforms (or is a step in the transformation of) a relatively unreactive compound into an electrophilic species which may react with cellular macromolecules.

The best example of the first group is formed by the leukotrienes. An epoxide (formed via a hydroperoxide) from arachidonic acid is conjugated with glutathione, to give leukotriene C_4 or SRSA (slow reacting substance of anaphylaxis), a compound with a potent pharmacological activity (Samuelsson, 1982). A number of related derivatives with similar activities have also been recognised (Samuelsson, 1983). Organic nitrates require activation for their vasodilatory activity. Thionitrites, such as S-nitrosoglutathione of the cysteine derivative, have been suggested as the proximal activators of guanylate cyclase, resulting in the relaxation of vascular smooth muscle (Yeates et al., 1985; Ignarro et al., 1981). Furthermore, a number of steroid glucuronides are known to have cholestatic activity. Although the exact mechanism is still unknown, it is not the result of reactive intermediates being formed (Mulder et al., 1986).

The second group, where reactions of electrophilic derivatives with cellular macromolecules form the basis of the toxic action, is the subject of the present chapter. In most cases the initial conjugates are the reactive intermediates and the electrophilic character obtained after conjugation is the decisive factor. In the case of sulphation, a hydroxyl group is turned into a relatively

good leaving group (Mulder et al., 1986). Replacement of a
bromide atom by sulphur during the conjugation of 1,2-
dibromoethane with glutathione results in a more reactive
species, due to the neighbouring group effect of the
sulphur (van Bladeren, 1983). In some cases however,
conjugation is just a step on the way to the ultimate
reacting species. Such is the case for hexachlorobutadiene, where the initial glutathione conjugate is
transformed in several steps into a thiol derivative which
is responsible for the (nephro) toxic action (Green and
Odum, 1985). Still another type of toxic (but not
reactive) conjugate was recently recognised. In the case
of benzyl and allyl isothiocyanate, formation of a
glutathione conjugate is a reversible reaction. The
reactive isothiocyanates may thus be released at some other
site in the cell or body.

FORMATION OF TOXIC CONJUGATES BY SULPHATION AND GLUCURONIDATION

Formation of sulphates and glucuronides are the main
conjugation reactions for compounds possessing a hydroxyl
group and amines may also be substrates for this reaction.
In general these conjugates are end products of metabolism
and are excreted into urine. In some cases, however, the
conjugates are more reactive than their parent compounds.
They break down to form carbenium or nitrenium ions that
can bind to cellular macromolecules and thus cause cell
death or tumour formation. The basis for the reactivity of
these conjugates is the fact that sulphates and to a lesser
degree glucuronides are better leaving groups than the
hydroxyl moiety.

In reactions of electrophiles with cellular
macromolecules, a number of factors are important including
i) leaving group ability, ii) stability of the remaining
cation, iii) steric hindrance and iv) what might be termed
nucleophile selectivity,i.e. which sulphur, nitrogen or
oxygen groups in which macromolecules are the preferred
target. It will be clear that the first two of these
factors influence each other strongly, and these factors
are especially important when considering reactive
sulphates and glucuronides.

The classical example of a reactive sulphate is the one
derived from N-hydroxy-2-acetylaminofluorene (N-hydroxy-2-
AAF). In Figure 1 a number of derivatives are depicted
that could all give rise to a nitrenium ion and thus react
with nuc leophiles. However, the sulphate is the only
derivative that can be considered a reactive

conjugate. At pH 7 in buffer it breaks down rapidly (Meerman et al., 1986), whereas the glucuronide is stable under these conditions (Mulder et al., 1986). In spite of this, the actual involvement of this sulphate ester in 2-AAF induced liver carcinogenesis has still not conclusively been shown (Mulder et al., 1986).

Figure 1. Formation of the nitrenium ion from N-hydroxy-2-acetylaminofluorene.

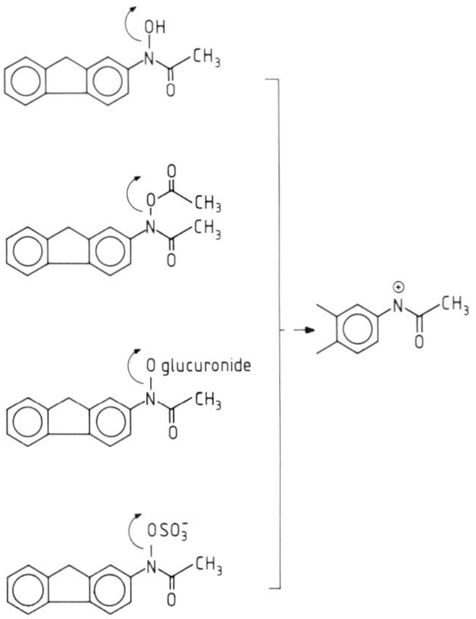

In principle, all four derivatives depicted might give rise to this cation. In reality only the sulphate is a good enough leaving group for this reaction to occur.

For other examples of reactive sulphate esters of hydroxamic acids or hydroxylamines, the interested reader is referred to the recent review by Mulder et al (1986).
The influence of the remaining cation can be amply demonstrated for sulphates formed from alcohols. The reactive esters known are all derived from benzylic or allylic alcohols. In these compounds, the positive charge of the carbenium ion is stabilised by delocalisation. In Figure 2, several examples of this phenomenon are given. From a number of simple benzylic alcohols, mercapturic acids are formed (Rietveld et al., 1983) and the corresponding benzyl sulphate is mutagenic in Salmonella typhimurium TA98 and TA100 (Watabe et al., 1982).

Figure 2.   Formation of carbenium ions from sulphate esters.

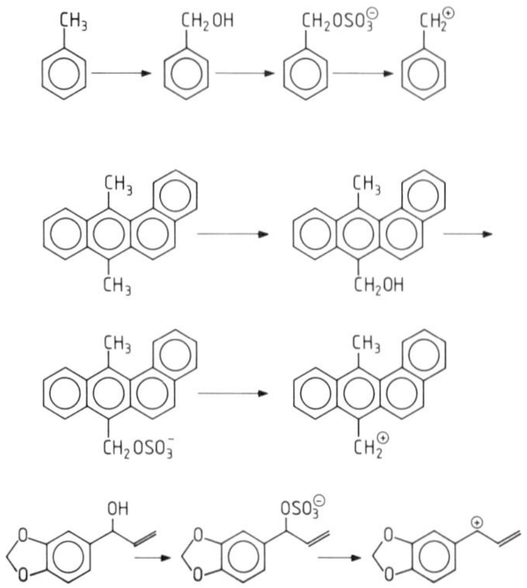

This reaction appears to be limited to benzylic and allylic alcohols.   For toluene see Rietveld et al (1983), for dimethylbenz(a)anthracene, Watabe et al (1983) and Cavalieri (1979), for hydroxysafrole, Boberg et al (1983).

The sulphate ester derived from 7-hydroxymethyl-12-methylbenz(a)anthracene is also mutagenic towards Salmonella TA98, much more even than the corresponding bromomethyl derivative (Cavalieri et al., 1979), and also reacts rapidly with glutathione at pH 7.4 (Watabe et al., 1982).   Similarly the sulphate of 1'-hydroxysafrole (activated both by a benzyl and allyl configuration) is held responsible for the covalent binding to protein, RNA and DNA and the carcinogenic activity of 1'-hydroxysafrole (Boberg et al., 1983).   Simple aliphatic alcohols are clearly not reactive enough for such reactions to occur.
   With these considerations in mind, one could try to predict when, for example, glucuronides would be toxic conjugates: to make up for the lower activity of the glucuronyl moiety as a leaving group, the remaining cation ought to be much more stable, i.e. better able to accommodate a positive charge.   The presence of electron donating groups on the benzene nucleus in benzylic alcohols might turn benzylic glucuronides into toxic conjugates - always provided of course that such conjugates are formed at all.

FORMATION OF TOXIC CONJUGATES BY GLUTATHIONE CONJUGATION

Conjugation with glutathione, usually catalyzed by the glutathione S-transferases is an important detoxification reaction for electrophilic substances. All substrates for the enzymatic conjugation will to some extent also react spontaneously. Depending on a number of factors, some conjugates may still be toxic, or even more toxic than the parent compound. Three groups of toxic glutathione conjugates have now been recognised (Figure 3).

Figure 3. The three classes of reactive glutathione conjugates.

Formation of reactive intermediates by glutathione conjugation

I   conjugate is reactive

e.g. $Br{-}CH_2CH_2{-}Br \longrightarrow Br{-}CH_2CH_2{-}SG$

II conjugate is transformed into reactive intermediate

e.g. $\underset{R}{\overset{Cl}{>}}C{=}\underset{Cl}{\overset{Cl}{<}} \rightarrow \underset{R}{\overset{Cl}{>}}C{=}\underset{Cl}{\overset{SG}{<}} \rightarrow \underset{R}{\overset{Cl}{>}}C{=}\underset{Cl}{\overset{SH}{<}}$

III Conjugate releases reactive intermediates

e.g. $R{-}N{=}C{=}S + GSH \rightleftarrows R{-}NH{-}\overset{\overset{\textstyle S}{\|}}{C}{-}SG$

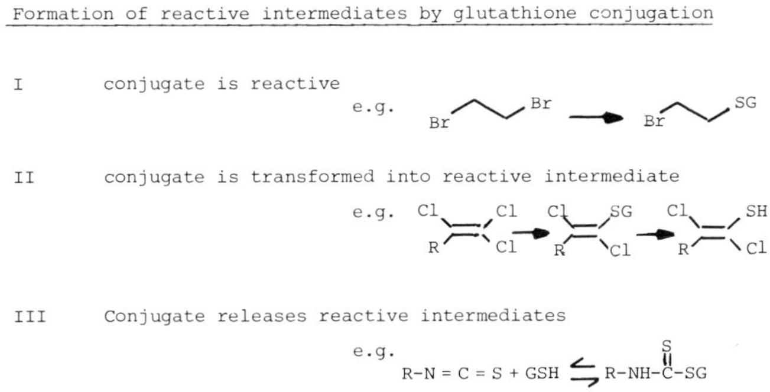

The best example of the first group, where the conjugate is reactive by itself is 2-bromoethylglutathione, formed from 1,2-dibromoethane (Van Bladeren, 1983). Compounds like hexachlorobutadiene give rise to glutathione conjugates, which can be further transformed into alkylating species (Wolf et al., 1984). The second group thus comprises glutathione conjugates that need further metabolic activation. Recently a third category was recognised : compounds for which the reaction with glutathione is reversible (Bruggeman et al., 1986; Temmink et al., 1986).

REACTIVE GLUTATHIONE CONJUGATES

After the initial discovery by Rannug (Rannug et al., 1979) that rat liver cytosol (containing the glutathione S-transferases) enhanced the mutagenic activity of 1,2-dichloroethane, numerous reports have appeared on the role of glutathione in the toxic action of vicinal dihalogenoalkanes. Most attention has been given to the known carcinogen 1,2-dibromoethane. The primary product of the conjugation of this compound with glutathione, S-2-bromoethylglutathione (see Figure 4), possesses a reactivity similar to sulphur mustard.

Figure 4. Formation of cyclic sulphonium ions from 1,2-dibromoethane (e.g. van Bladeren, 1981) and 1,4-dibromobutane (Buys et al., 1986).

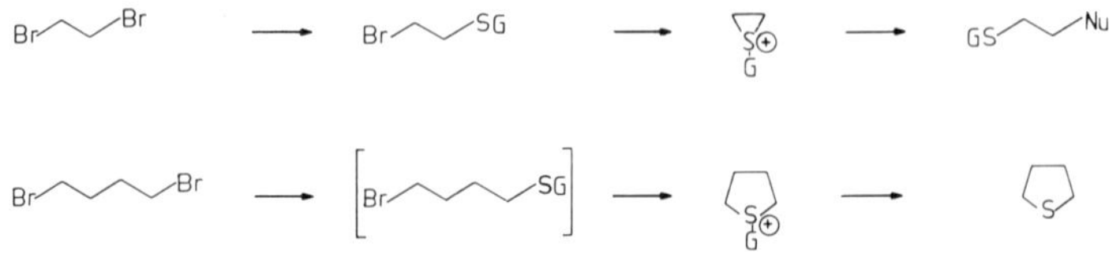

Br~~Br ⟶ Br~~SG ⟶ [S⊕ G] ⟶ GS~~Nu

Br~~~Br ⟶ [Br~~~SG] ⟶ [S⊕ G] ⟶ [S]

In the latter case, the sulphonium ion forms so rapidly that the intermediate bromobutylsulphide cannot be isolated. However, only the three membered ion reacts with nucleophiles. The five-membered ion only gives rise to tetrahydrothiophene.

Reactions of such β-halothioethers take place via an intermediate thiiranium or episulphonium ion (Bland and Stammer, 1983) : the lone electron pairs of the sulphur substituent attack the carbon bearing the halogen substituent. The mutagenicity of 1,2-dibromoethane can be enhanced considerably by the addition of rat liver cytosol to the incubation mixture (Table 1), and in agreement with this result, S-2-bromoethyl-N-acetyl-L-cysteine methyl ester was shown to be a potent mutagen (Van Bladeren et al., 1980).

Since that time the glutathione pathway has been shown to be involved in the induction of DNA repair in rat spermatocytes and hepatocytes (Working et al., 1986) and induction of DNA single strand breaks in rat hepatocytes (White et al., 1984). The same type of genotoxicity was found in vivo (Storer and Conolly, 1983).

1,2-Dibromoethane can also be metabolised via an oxidative pathway. Cytochrome P-450 dependent oxidation, followed by loss of hydrogen bromide results in the formation of bromoacetaldehyde, a reactive compound in its own right. This derivate should in principle be able to react with DNA (see e.g. Banerjee and van Duuren, 1979), even though the kinetics of binding were found to be relatively slow (Guengerich et al., 1981). However Sundheimer et al (1982) reported that binding of ^{14}C-labelled 1,2-dibromoethane to DNA in isolated hepatocytes

Table 1. Mutagenic activity of α,ω-dibromoalkanes towards
S. typhimurium TA 100[a]

Compound	Concentration (mM)	his[+]rev/plate		
		No added activating system	microsomes	S 100
Dibromoethane	1	99	144	343
	2	203	245	520
	3.5	279	340	861
	5	230	346	1026
Dibromopropane	1	-[b]	-	-
	2	-	38	-
	3.5	-	-	64
	5	-	52	132
Dibromobutane	1	85	-	-
	2	221	-	-
	3.5	290	-	-
	5	372	35	-

[a]Data taken from Buys et al, 1986. Test compounds were
incubated with bacteria, activating system and co-factors
where appropriate, for 6 hours. Bacteria were washed,
resuspended and plated.
[b] No enhancement above background his[+]colonies (mean:35)
observed.

was decreased by the glutathione depleting agent
diethylmaleate, and not influenced by the cytochrome P-450
inhibitor SKF 525A. Subsequently Ozawa and Guengerich
(1983) very elegantly demonstrated that a near-
stoichiometric binding of labels to DNA occurred when both
^{14}C-1,2-dibromoethane and ^{35}S- or ^{3}H-labelled glutathione
were used. The same type of binding was observed with
cytosol plus exogenous DNA and in rat hepatocytes. From
both studies it appeared as if the bromoethylglutathione
had a much higher affinity for DNA than for protein.
Recently the structure of the major DNA adduct both in vivo
and in isolated hepatocytes was conclusively elucidated
(Koga et al., 1986; Inskeep et al., 1986). It turns out

that the full glutathione moiety is still present in the
adduct (Figure 5) meaning that no breakdown of the
conjugate to the cysteine derivative or even further is
necessary for binding to occur.

**Figure 5. DNA adduct formed from 1,2-dibromoethane, S-2-
(N[7]-guanyl)ethyl glutathione. The structure was recently
elucidated by Koga et al (1986).**

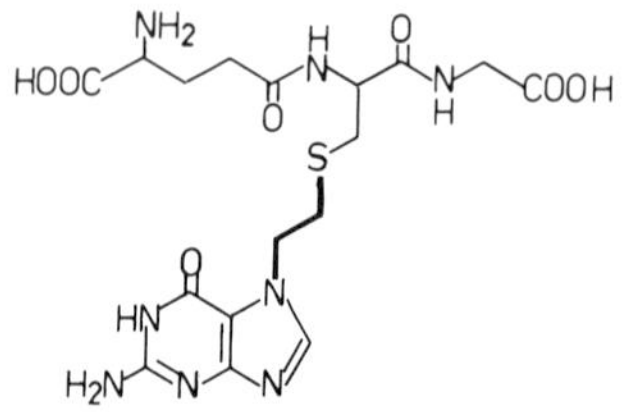

Interestingly, it was also found that the reactive
glutathione conjugate can leave the cell and react with
added extracellular DNA (Inskeep et al., 1986). These
results are highly significant with regard to the
postulated role of the glutathione conjugate in 1,2-
dibromoethane-induced carcinogenesis. With the aid of
deuterated 1,2-dibromoethane, it was demonstrated that the
ratio of conjugative and oxidative pathways in vivo (in
rats) is 1:4. In agreement with these numbers, inhibition
of oxidative metabolism in vivo, with 1-phenylimidazole or
disulphiram results in an 80% lower excretion of
mercapturic acids from 1,2-dibromoethane (van Bladeren et
al., 1981a and b), but co-treatment of rats with
disulphiram results in an increase in the occurrence of
1,2-dibromoethane induced tumour formation (Plotnick et
al., 1979; Wong et al., 1982).

1,2-Dibromoethane seems to have exactly the right
chemical properties for the formation of a reactive
glutathione conjugate. 1,2-Dichloroethane for instance is
mutagenic only at much higher doses (van Bladeren et al.,
1981c) even though the S-2 chloroethyl model conjugate is
highly mutagenic (Figure 6).

A glutathione-containing DNA adduct is also much harder
to demonstrate, and there is a question of whether it is
formed at all (Lin et al., 1985). Chlorine is not as good
a leaving group as bromine, and the specific activity of
rat liver glutathione S-transferases towards this compound
is much lower than toward 1,2-dibromoethane (van Bladeren
et al., 1981c). Similarly, introducing a small amount of
steric hindrance, such as a methyl group into the molecule

Figure 6. Mutagenicity towards Salmonella typhimurium TA100 of several 2-chloroethyl model conjugates (R=N-acetyl-L-cysteine methyl ester).

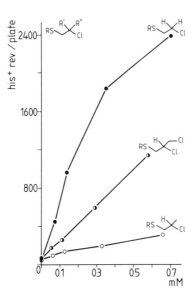

Data taken from Van Bladeren (1981b).

almost abolishes the mutagenic activity of a model conjugate (Figure 6). On the other hand, introduction of a second chlorine molecule as in S-2,3-dichloropropyl-N-acetyl-L-cysteine increases the mutagenic activity again, perhaps because a possibility for the formation of cross-links now exists, by formation of two consecutive episulphonium ions. However, the relevance of such a pathway in vivo is still in doubt.

1,2-Dibromo-3-chloropropane, for instance, where such a conjugate might be expected to occur, gave only a very small amount of glutathione-related covalent binding to DNA (Inskeep and Guengerich, 1984).

Recently, a study on the effect of chain-length between the two halogen atoms was completed (Buys, 1985). Based on the known properties of the sulphur atoms in anchimeric assistance it might be expected that 1,4-dibromobutane could also be activated via a cyclic sulphonium ion (Figure 4). 1,4-Dibromobutane is indeed a substrate for the transferases, and gives rise to the formation of sulphur containing metabolites in vivo (Onkenhout, 1985). In studies on synthetic conjugates it was found however, that the sulphonium ion forms so quickly that the intermediate bromobutyl derivative could not be demonstrated. The sulphonium ion is in fact stable enough not to be mutagenic (Table 1, Buys et al., 1986) and also unreactive towards nucleophiles.

In vivo tetrahydrothiophene and oxidised derivatives are indeed formed as the major metabolite. Interestingly, Roberts and Warwick (1961) have already demonstrated the occurrence of the same metabolites after treatment of rats with Busulfan, an analogous four-carbon compound possessing two leaving groups. In agreement with these results, no increase in glutathione-related binding to DNA could be demonstrated (Inskeep and Guengerich, 1984). Apart from the vicinal dihalogenoalkanes, activation via conjugation with glutathione seems to be important only for geminal dihalogeno alkanes such as methylene chloride (Jongen et al., 1982) and methylene bromide (van Bladeren et al., 1980b).

GLUTATHIONE CONJUGATES THAT REQUIRE METABOLIC ACTIVATION

The nephrotoxicity of S-1,2-dichlorovinyl)-L-cysteine has been known for a long time (e.g. Derr and Schulze, 1963; McKinney et al., 1959). This particular compound was formed during trichloroethylene extraction of soybean meal. Interest in such derivatives was renewed, when it was found that they might also be formed metabolically from a number of poly-halogeno vinyl compounds. Chlorotrifluoroethylene (Dohn et al., 1985) and hexachlorobutadiene are the best studied examples to date. Interestingly for both compounds, microsomal gluathione S-transferase is important in catalysing the conjugation reaction: hexachlorobutadiene is exclusively conjugated via the microsomal enzyme (Wolf et al., 1984), while chlorotrifluoroethylene is a substrate for both cytosolic and microsomal enzymes (Dohn and Anders, 1982). In the first case an addition/elimination reaction occurs resulting in a vinyl-glutathione adduct (Wolf et al., 1984), while for the fluorinated compounds an addition takes place (Dohn and Anders, 1982; Odum and Green, 1984). For vinyl compounds having only two fluorine atoms both types of products have been found synthetically (Sachdev et al., 1980). The pathway for activation of these conjugates is depicted in Figure 7. For the trichloroethylene-derived adduct (Stevens, 1986), two enzymes are very important: γ-glutamyl transpeptidase, responsible for removing the γ-glutamic acid moiety and cysteine conjugate; β-lyase (Stevens and Jacoby, 1983; Stevens, 1985) an enzyme that catalyses the β-elimination of an electrophilic sulphur-containing fragment from the cysteine derivative. These two enzymes combine in targeting these conjugates to the kidney, thus explaining the selective nephrotoxicity observed (Hassal et al., 1983; Elfarra et al., 1986; Gandolfi et al., 1981; Nash et al., 1982).

Figure 7. The general pathway for formation of reactive compounds from S-halogeno-vinyl-glutathione conjugates.

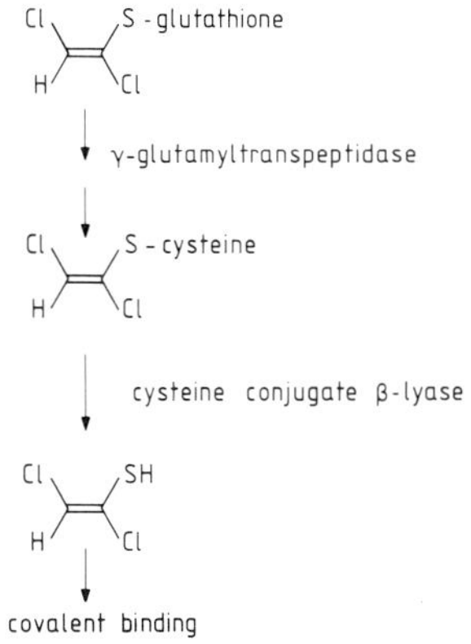

$$Cl\diagdown\quad\diagup S\text{-glutathione}$$
$$H\diagup\quad\diagdown Cl$$

↓ γ-glutamyltranspeptidase

$$Cl\diagdown\quad\diagup S\text{-cysteine}$$
$$H\diagup\quad\diagdown Cl$$

↓ cysteine conjugate β-lyase

$$Cl\diagdown\quad\diagup SH$$
$$H\diagup\quad\diagdown Cl$$

↓ covalent binding

The structure shown is derived from trichloroethylene (Stevens et al, 1986), but the same pathway is followed for hexachlorobutadiene (Green and Odum, 1985).

The vinyl-thiol is electrophilic and can react covalently with cellular macromolecules (Stevens et al., 1986). The exact mechanism is still a matter of speculation, since compounds like this have never been synthesised, but there is a clear resemblance to the enolic form of an α-chloro ketone, which could certainly explain the reactivity (Green and Odum, 1984).

The mutagenicity of hexachlorobutadiene was also studied. Initially a report appeared showing an increased mutagenic effect in Salmonella typhimurium TA100 only under conditions that favoured oxidative metabolism, perhaps epoxide formation (Reichert et al., 1984).

Even though these results were also found by others (van Bladeren et al., 1986) the in vivo relevance is questionable, since by far the main metabolic pathway for this compound is conjugation with glutathione (Wolf et al., 1984) and the glutathione derivatives are also mutagenic (Green and Odum, 1985). As an example, the mutagenic activity of the N-acetyl-L-cysteine derivative or hexachlorobutathione is shown in Figure 8.

Figure 8. Mutagenic activity of the N-acetyl-L-cysteine derivative of hexachlorobutadiene towards Salmonella typhimurium TA100 and NG57.

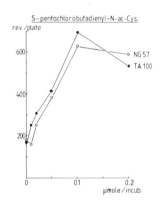

NG57 is a glutathione-deficient (<10%) derivative of TA100 (Kerklaan et al., 1985). Tests were performed in the presence of rat liver 9000g fraction, using a two-hour preincubation (Data taken from van Bladeren et al., 1986).

This compound does need the presence of a metabolizing system for the expression of mutagenicity (van Bladeren et al., 1986; Wild et al., 1986), but its only function appears to be deacetylation of the mercapturic acid to the cysteine derivative, to prepare it as a substrate for the β-lyase. The corresponding cysteine derivative is mutagenic by itself (Green and Odum, 1984), presumably because the bacteria possess similar β-lyase activities (Tomisawa et al., 1984). As can be seen in Figure 7 bacterial glutathione does not play a role in the mutagenic activity of the mercapturic acid. The glutathione deficient strain NG57 is derived from TA100 (Kerklaan et al., 1984) and possesses less than 10% of the glutathione content of TA100. This seems to indicate that the electrophilic vinyl-thiol is not detoxified efficiently by glutathione.

The major factors determining the toxic potential of this group of glutathione conjugates are thus i) their suitability as substrate for the cysteine conjugate β-lyases, and ii) the reactivity of the thiol products.

GLUTATHIONE CONJUGATES THAT ARE IN EQUILIBRIUM WITH THE PARENT COMPOUNDS

Allyl and benzyl isothiocyanate are both naturally occurring compounds (Fenwick et al., 1982). The latter is best known for its anticarcinogenic activity (e.g. Wattenberg, 1981), while the former has recently been shown to be a bladder carcinogen in male rats (Dunnick et al., 1982). The in vivo metabolism has been studied fairly extensively and conjugation with glutathione is the most important pathway (Brusewitz et al., 1977; Mennicke et al., 1983). Brusewitz et al (1977) observed that the mercapturic acid derived from benzyl isothiocyanate was unstable and in urine containing this compound, the free isothiocyanate was released. Isothiocyanates are known to react reversibly with thiols (Drobnica, 1977), i.e. the product dithiocarbamate is in equilibrium with the parent compounds. This is not the case for reactions with other nucleophiles. The products from the reaction with alcohols or amines are stable. In Figure 9 the time course of the reaction between equimolar amounts of glutathione and allyl and benzyl isothiocyanate is depicted.

Figure 9. Reaction between benzyl or allyl isothiocyanate (ITC) and glutathione (GSH).

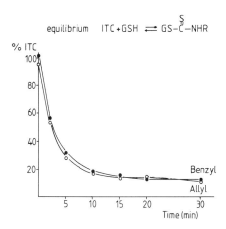

An equimolar amount of GSH was added to a solution of ITC in phosphate buffer pH 7.4. At different time points the reaction mixture was extracted with cyclohexane and the remaining amount of ITC determined spectrophotometrically (Bruggeman et al., 1986).

In 10-15 minutes, an equilibrium situation is reached where 15-20% of the isothiocyanates is still present in the unconjugated form. The position of this equilibrium can of course be influenced by conditions of pH and the concentration of the reactants (Bruggeman et al., 1986). In agreement with these results it was shown that the conjugates of these isothiocyanates display toxicities very similar to the parent compounds (Bruggeman et al., 1986; Temmink et al., 1986). In Figure 10 an experiment is shown where the cytotoxicity of all derivatives in the mercapturic acid pathway is compared. In general the benzyl derivatives are slightly more toxic than the allyl derivatives and, while the cysteine conjugates are more toxic than the glutathione adducts, the mercapturic acids are the least toxic. The implications of this finding for the in vivo situation are not easy to estimate, but it seems very possible that the isothiocyanates are detoxified at first, but could be released at some other site, where glutathione concentrations are lower or conditions of pH are different.

Figure 10. Cytotoxicity of benzyl and allyl isothiocyanate (AITC and BITC) conjugates with glutathione (GSH), cysteine (cys) and N-acetyl-L-cysteine (N-ac-cys).

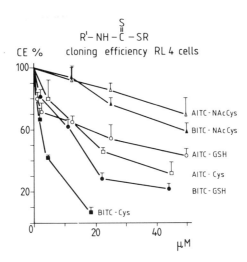

Cells in monolayer were exposed for two hours to the conjugates added in F10 medium. Cloning efficiency was determined after 10 days. (Bruggeman et al., 1986). Means+SD of 3-5 experiments are given.

Table 2. The inhibition of rat liver glutathione S-transferase by benzyl isothiocyanate and its glutathione
conjugate [a]

Treatment	Activities towards chlorodinitrobenzene[b]	
	before gel filtration	after gel filtration
none (n=6)	100+4.0%	100+4.0%
0.5mM BITC (n=4)	38.1+7.4%[c]	81.0+9.2%[c]
0.5mM BITC-GSH (n=4)	38.8+7.7%[c]	85.2+4.6%[c]
1.5mM BITC (n=2)	-	72.1+1.9%[c]
3.0mM BITC (n=2)	-	72.7+4.5%[c]

[a]Purified rat liver glutathione S-transferases (obtained
from Sigma) were incubated for 30 min with benzyl
isothiocyanate (BITC) or its glutathione conjugate (BITC-
GSH). Activity towards chlorodinitrobenzene was determined
directly or after the transferases were separated from
lower molecular weight compounds using a Biogel P-6 DG
column.
[b]Activity was determined according to Habig and Jacoby
(1981).
[c]P < 0.005 using student's t test

In this respect it is interesting that allyl isothiocyanate
exerts its carcinogenic effect in the bladder of the rat
(Dunnick et al, 1982), where the pH is usually basic, thus
favouring release of the isothiocyanate.

In order to further characterise the interaction of the
isothiocyanates with glutathione, the role of the
glutathione S-transferases has been studied. The reaction
can be followed spectrophotometrically, and in spite of the
fact that the isothiocyanates are highly reactive
compounds, catalysis by the transferases could be clearly
demonstrated (van Bladeren and Scheffer, manuscript in
preparation). In Table 2 the characteristics of the
reaction are given. Benzyl isothiocyanate has a higher
affinity for the enzymes than the allyl derivative. The
presence of glutathione S-transferases has no influence on
the equilibrium concentrations, but it was noticed that a
considerable amount of isothiocyanates became covalently
bound to the transferases. No difference was observed
between benzyl and allyl isothiocyanate in this respect.

Since we were interested in the effect of this binding, the inhibition of the conjugation of chlorodinitrobenzene (CDNB) was studied (Table 3). Glutathione conjugates are usually effective inhibitors of the glutathione S-transferases (Jacobson et al., 1979). In agreement with this fact, the glutathione conjugate of benzyl isothiocyanate is also an inhibitor of CDNB conjugation. Benzyl isothiocyanate by itself inhibits the reaction to the same extent, but this might be due to its rapid reaction with glutathione. The conjugate would then again act as the inhibitor. From Lineweaver-Burke plots it is evident that this inhibition is comparative (results not shown). However, when the transferases were separated from benzyl isothiocyanate and its glutathione conjugate by gel filtration, part of the inhibition remained. Increasing the concentrations of benzyl isothiocyanate did not result in increased inhibition. Allyl isothiocyanate, which binds to the transferase to the same extent did not cause a similar inhibition, in keeping with the observed lower affinity for the active site of the transferases. Further research into the origin of this effect is in progress.

Table 3. Michaelis-Menton parameters for the conjugation of isothiocyanates with glutathione catalysed by rat liver glutathione S-transferases [a]

Substrate	K_M apparent (mM)[b]	V_{max} apparent[b] mol/min/mg protein
AITC[c]	0.943 ± 0.0206	74.2 ± 10.6
BITC[c]	0.157 ± 0.019	50.7 ± 6.1

[a]Initial reaction rates were determined spectrophometrically at 275nm, a wavelength where the isothiocyanates do not absorb, but the conjugates do. Spontaneous reaction rates are 20-50% of total rates.
[b]AITC allylisothiocyanate; BITC benzylisothiocyanate.
[c]Means$\pm$SD of at least 5 experiments are given.

Thus far, the isothiocyanates are the only known examples of this type of toxic glutathione conjugate. Based on chemical considerations, one might envisage other classes of chemicals showing this types of behaviour, e.g. $\alpha \beta$- unsaturated ketones, where a reversible Michael addition might occur. It is certainly possible that more examples will come to light in the near future.

CONCLUSIONS

In general, conjugations are important detoxifying reactions. Depending on a number of special structural characteristics of the substrate, an activation by conjugation can sometimes occur. As the chemical rules governing such toxic conjugates are becoming better understood, the number of examples will continue to grow. On the other hand, in the interaction of reactive intermediates with cellular macromolecules and the effects thereof, more subtle factors than simple chemical reactivities also seem to play a role. The emphasis of future research will probably shift to the study of these factors, because only then meaningful structure-activity relationships might be developed.

REFERENCES

Banerjee, S. and Van Duuren, B.L. (1979). J. Nat. Cancer Inst, 63, 707.

van Bladeren, P.J., Breimer, D.D., Rotteveel-Smijs, G.M.T., de Jong, R.A.W., Buijs, W. and van der Gen, A. (1980a). Biochem. Pharmacol, 29, 2975.

van Bladeren, P.J., Breimer, D.D., Rotteveel-Smijs, G.M.T. and Mohn, G.R. (1980b). Mut. Res, 74, 341.

van Bladeren, P.J., Breimer, D.D., van Huijgevoort, J.A.C.T.M., Vermeulen, N.P.E. and van der Gen, A. (1981a). Biochem. Pharmacol, 30, 2499.

van Bladeren, P.J., Hoogeterp, J.J., Breimer, D.D. and van der Gen, A. (1981c). Biochem. Pharmacol, 30, 2983.

van Bladeren, P.J., Breimer, D.D., Rotteveel-Smijs, G.M.T. de Knijff, P., Mohn, G.R., van Meeteren-Walchli, B., Buijs, W. and van der Gen, A. (1981b). Carcinogenesis, 2, 499.

van Bladeren, P.J. (1983). J. Am. College Toxicol, 2, 73.

van Bladeren, P.J., van der Haar, R., van Welie, R. and Jongen, W.M.F. (1986). submitted.

Bland, J.M. and Stammer, C.H. (1983) J. org. Chem, 48, 4393.

Boberg, E.W., Miller, E.C., Miller, J.A., Poland, A. and Liem, A. (1983). Cancer Res 43, 5163.

Bruggeman, I.M., Temmink, J.H.M. and van Bladeren, P.J. (1986a). Tox. Appl. Pharmacol, 83, 349.

Bruggeman, I.M., Temmink, J.H.M. and van Bladeren, P.J. (1986b). Human Toxicol in press.

Brusewitz, G., Cameron, B.D., Chasseaud, L.F., Gorler, K., Hawkins, D.R., Koch, H. and Mennicke, W.H. (1977). Biochem, J. 162, 99.

Buijs, W. (1985). PhD Thesis, Leiden University, The Netherlands.

Buijs, W., van Meeteren-Walchli, B., de Smidt, P.C., Vermeulen, N.P.E., Booister-Schrijnemakers, J.G.M., van der Gen, A. and Mohn, G.R. (1986). Mut. Res in press.

Cavalieri, E., Roth, R. and Regan, R. (1979). in "Polynuclear Aromatic Hydrocarbons" (Jones, P.W. and Leber, P. eds) p.517, Ann Arbor Science, Ann Arbor.

Derr, R.F. and Schulze, M.O. (1963). Biochem. Pharmacol, 12, 465.

Dohn, D.R. and Anders, M.W. (1982). Biochem. Biophys. Res. Comm, 109, 1339.

Dohn, D.R., Leininger, J.R., Lash, L.H., Quebbeman, A.J. and Anders, M.W. (1985). J. Pharmacol. Exp. Ther, 235, 851.

Drobnica, L. and Gemeiner, P. (1975). Collect. Czech. Chem. Comm, 40, 3346.

Dunnick, J.K., Prejean, J.D., Haseman, J., Thompson, R.B., Giles, H.D. and McConnell, E.E (1982). Fundam. Appl. Toxicol, 2, 114.

Elfarra, A.A., Jacobsen, I. and Anders, M.W. (1986). Biochem. Pharmacol. 35, 283.

Fenwick, G.R., Heaney, R.K. and Mullin, W.J. (1982). CRC Crit. Rev. Food Sci. Nutr, 18, 123.

Gandolfi, A.J., Nagle, R.B., Soltis, J.J. and Plescia, F.H. (1981). Res. Comm. Chem. Pathol. Pharmacol, 33, 249.

Green, T. and Odum, J. (1985) Chem. Biol. Interact, 54, 25.

Guengerich, F.P., Mason, P.S., Stott, W., Fox, T.R. and Watanabe, P.G. (1981). Cancer Res, 41, 4391.

Habig, W.H. and Jacoby, W.B. (1981) Methods Enzymol 77, 231.

Hassell, C.D., Gandolfi, A.J. and Brendel, K. (1983). Toxicology, 26, 285.

Inskeep, P.B., Koga, H., Cmarik, J.L. and Guengerich, F.P. (1986). Cancer Res 46, 2839.

Inskeep, P.B. and Guengerich, F.P. (1984). Carcinogenesis 5, 805.

Ignarro, L.J., Lippton, H., Edwards, J.C., Baricos, W.H., Hyman, A.L., Kadowitz, P.I. and Gruetter, C.A. (1981). J. Pharmacol. Exp. Ther, 218, 739.

Jongen, W.M.F., Harmsen, E.G.M., Alink, G.M. and Koeman, J.H. (1982). Mut. Res, 95, 183.

Jacobson, I., Warholm, M. and Mannervik, B. (1979). Biochem, J. 177, 861.

Kerklaan, P.R.M., Zoetemelk, C.E.M. and Mohn, G.R. (1985). Biochem. Pharmacol, 34, 2151.
Koga, M., Inskeep, P.B., Harris, T.M. and Guengerich, F.P. (1986). Biochemistry, 25, 2192.
Lin, E.L.C., Mattox, J.K. and Pereira, M.A. (1985). Tox. Appl. Pharmacol, 78, 428.
Nash, J.A., King, L.J., Lock, E.A. and Green, T. (1984). Tox. Appl. Pharmacol, 73, 12.
McKinney, L.L., Picker, J.C., Weakley, F.B., Eldridge, A.C., Campbell, R.E., Cowaz, J.C. and Biester, H.E. (1959).J. Am. Chem. Soc, 81, 909.
Mennicke, W.H., Gorler, K. and Krumbiegel, G. (1983). Xenobiotica 13, 203.
Mulder, G.J., Meerman, J.H.H. and van den Goorbergh, A.M. (1986).in "Xenobiotic Conjugation Chemistry"(Paulson, G.D., Caldwell, J., Hutson, D.H. and Menn, J.J. eds). p. 282, Am. Chem. Soc. Washington DC.
Odum, J. and Green, T. (1984). Toxicol. Appl. Pharmacol, 76, 306.
Onkenhout, W. (1985). PhD Thesis, University of Leiden, The Netherlands.
Ozawa, H. and Guengerich, F.P. (1983). Proc. Natl. Acad. Sci. USA, 80, 5266.
Plotnick, H.B. (1978).J. Am. Med. Assn, 239, 1609.
Rannug, U., Sundvall, A. and Ramel, C. (1978). Chem. Biol. Interact, 20, 1.
Reichert, D., Neudecker, T. and Schutz, S. (1984). Mut. Res, 137, 89.
Rietveld, E.C., Plate, R. and Seutter-Berlage, F. (1983). Arch. Toxicol, 52, 199.
Roberts, J.J. and Warwick, G.P. (1961). Biochem. Pharmacol, 6, 217.
Sachdev, K., Cohen, E.M. and Simmon, V.F. (1980). Anesthenol, 53, 31.
Samuelson, B. (1982). Angew. Chem. Int. Ed. Engl, 21. 902.
Samuelson, B. (1983). Science, 220, 568.
Stevens, J.L. and Jacoby, W.R. (1983). Mol. Pharmacol, 23, 761.
Stevens, J.L. (1985). J. Biol. Chem, 260, 7945.
Stevens, J.L., Hayden, P. and Taylor, G. (1986). J. Biol. Chem, 261, 3325.
Storer, D.W., Conolly, R.B. (1983) Carcinogenesis, 4, 1491.
Sundheimer, D.W., White, R.D., Brendel, K. and Sipes, I.G. (1982). Carcinogenesis, 3, 1129.
Temmink, J.H.M., Bruggeman, I.M. and van Bladeren, P.J. (1986). Arch. Toxicol, in press.
Tomisawa, H., Suzuki, S., Ichihara, S., Fukuzawa, H. and

Tateishi, M. (1984). J. Biol. Chem, 259, 2588.

Watabe, T., Ishizuka, T., Isobe, MN., Ozawa, N. (1982). Science 215, 403.

Watabe, T., Ishizuka, T., Hakamata, Y., Aizawa, T. and Isobe, M. (1983). Biochem. Pharmacol, 32, 2120.

Wattenberg, L.W. (1981). Cancer Res, 41, 2991.

White, R.D., Petry, T.W. and Sipes, I.G. (1984). Chem. Biol. Interact, 49, 225.

Wild, D., Schutz, S. and Reichert, D. (1986). Carcinogenesis, 7, 431.

Wolf, C.R., Berry, P.M., Mash, J.A., Green, T. and Lock, E.A. (1984). J. Pharmacol. Exp. Ther, 228, 202.

Wong, L.C.K., Winston, J.M., Hong, C.B. and Plotnick, H. (1982). Toxicol. Appl. Pharmacol, 63, 155.

Working, P.K., Smith-Oliver, T., White, R. and Butterworth, B.E. (1986). Carcinogenesis, 7, 467.

Yeates, R.A., Lanten, H. and Leitold, M. (1985). Molec. Pharmacol, 28, 555.

CHARACTERISATION OF THE INHERITED DEFICIENCY OF
UDP-GLUCURONYL TRANSFERASE ACTIVITIES IN THE GUNN RAT

Michael W.H. Coughtrie[1], Brian Burchell[1] and John R. Bend[2]

[1]Department of Biochemistry, The University, Dundee, DD1 4HN, Scotland. [2] Laboratory of Pharmacology, NIH/NIEHS, Research Triangle Park, N.C. 27709, USA.

INTRODUCTION

UDP-glucuronyltransferases (UDPGT) are a family of closely related isoenzymes, of broad but overlapping substrate specificity, responsible for the glucuronidation of a wide range of xenobiotics, as well as endogenous compounds such as steroid hormones and bilirubin (Dutton, 1980; Burchell, 1981).

Gunn (1938) described a mutant strain of Wistar rat exhibiting inherited unconjugated hyperbilirubinaemia, and this has recently been shown to be due to the absence of the hepatic microsomal UDPGT isoenzyme catalysing bilirubin glucuronidation (Scragg et al., 1985). Similar clinical manifestations which exist in man are known collectively as Crigler-Najjar syndrome (Crigler and Najjar, 1952), and although the nature of this lesion remains unknown, the Gunn rat has been used as a model for the investigation of Crigler-Najjar syndrome (Cornelius and Arias, 1972).

Here we have used immunoblot analysis, with two polyclonal antibodies of different specificity, to determine that the Gunn rat lacks at least three UDPGT isoenzymes catalysing the conjugation of bilirubin and planar phenols.

EXPERIMENTAL

Wistar and Gunn rats (male, 10-11 weeks old) were maintained in the animal unit, University of Dundee. UDPGT enzyme assays (see Scragg et al., 1985 for references) were performed on liver microsomes in the presence of optimally-activating concentrations of Lubrol PX, determined for each substrate. SDS-polyacrylamide gel electrophoresis was performed as described by Laemmli (1970) on 7% gels and immunoblot analysis carried out as outlined by Domin et al. (1984).

RESULTS AND DISCUSSION

Comparison of UDPGT activities towards a range of substrates showed that activity towards bilirubin was not detectable, and that conjugation of 1-naphthol, 2-amino-phenol and β-estradiol was severely impaired (Table 1).

Table 1. Comparison of UDP-Glucuronyltransferases acti-vities in Wistar and Gunn rat liver microsomes

Substrate	UDPGT Activity (nmol/min/mg)[1]		
	Wistar	Gunn	Gunn/Wistar(%)
1-Naphthol	52.4+12.9	8.81+2.32	17
2-Aminophenol	1.74+0.52	0.09+0.01	5
2-Aminophenol +10mM 3-pentanone	3.22+0.34	1.45+0.15	45
Bilirubin	0.66+0.11	0[2]	0
Testosterone	2.95+0.35	1.99+0.27	68
β-Estradiol	0.66+0.06	0.18+0.03	11

1. Values represent mean+SD of at least 3 separate experiments assayed in the presence of optimally-activating concentrations of Lubrol PX.
2. Not detectable within the limits of the assay (> 0.02 nmol/min/mg).

Glucuronidation of digitoxigenin monodigitoxoside has also been demonstrated to be absent from the Gunn rat (Watkins and Klaassen, 1982). Activity towards testosterone was present in the Gunn rat at near-normal levels (Table 1), as was morphine UDPGT (not shown).

Differential inducibility has been used to investigate the heterogeneity of UDPGTs (e.g. Lilienblum et al., 1982). UDPGT activities which are β-naphthoflavone (BNF) inducible in Wistar rats (e.g. 1-naphthol, 2-aminophenol) are not sensitive to this treatment in Gunn rats (Figure 1). However, the phenobarbital (PB) inducible activities (testosterone and β-estradiol) appear to be further enhanced in the Gunn rat by PB treatment (Figure 1).

Figure 1. Induction of UDPGT activities in Wistar and Gunn rats by treatment with BNF and PB.

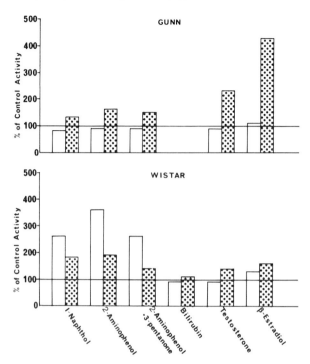

Animals received : filled bars - PB (100mg/kg i.p. in 0.9% NaCl 48 hrs prior to sacrifice, and 2g/l in drinking water for seven days prior to sacrifice); open bars - BNF (200mg/kg i.p. in corn oil 4 days and 2 days before sacrifice). Control animals received the vehicle only. Values represent the mean of at least three separate experiments.

Figure 2 shows the immunoblot analysis of Wistar and Gunn rat liver microsomes prepared from animals pretreated with either PB or BNF (a 3-MC type inducer). Blots were stained using anti-rat liver testosterone/ 4-nitrophenol UDPGT (Burchell et al., 1984) or with the more specific anti-rat kidney bilirubin/1-naphthol UDPGT, which recognises only bilirubin UDPGT (54kDa), phenol UDPGT (54kDa) and to a lesser extent an unidentified 56kDa immuno-reactive polypeptide (Figure 2 and M. Coughtrie et al, unpublished work). The immun-reactive polypeptide in Wistar rats, molecular weight 53kDa, has been identified as

Figure 2. Immunoblot analysis of xenobiotic-treated Wistar
and Gunn rat liver microsomes.

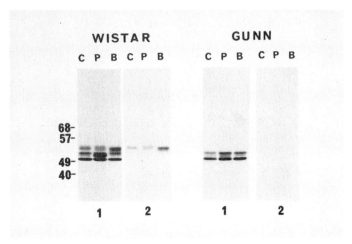

Microsomes were subjected to electrophoresis on 7% SDS-
polyacrylamide gels, and transferred to nitrocellulose.
Blots labelled "1" were immunostained with anti-rat liver
UDPGT, and those labelled "2" were stained with anti-rat
kidney UDPGT. Immuno-reactive polypeptides were visualised
using the immunoperoxidase method, with 4-chloro-1-naphthol
as substrate. C, microsomes from untreated animals; P,
microsomes from PB-treated rats and B, microsomes from rats
treated with BNF. The mobility of molecular weight
standards (40, 49, 57 and 68 kDa respectively) is shown.

phenol UDPGT (Scragg et al., 1985). This polypeptide
(Figure 2, Wistar 1B) appears to be increased in rats
receiving BNF, corresponding to a 3-fold increase in UDPGT
activity towards 1-naphthol and 2-aminophenol (Figure 1).
The greater specificity of the anti-rat kidney UDPGT
antibody clearly demonstrates this induction (Figure 2,
Wistar 2B). This polypeptide, and the 54kDa protein
identified as bilirubin UDPGT (Scragg et al., 1985) are
both absent from Gunn rat liver microsomes, as is a minor
immuno-reactive polypeptide at 56 kDa (Figure 2, Wistar
1C).
    Analysis of microsomes from developing Wistar and Gunn
rat livers demonstrated a) the absence of the 53kDa phenol
UDPGT in foetal Gunn liver and b) the absence of the 53, 54
and 56kDa polypeptides during every stage of Gunn rat
development (not shown). These findings suggest that
planar phenols are conjugated by another UDPGT isoenzyme(s)

in the Gunn rat, and also indicate a small contribution of this UDPGT(s) towards the in vitro glucuronidation of phenolic substrates in Wistar rats. Evidence that this may be testosterone UDPGT comes from the activation of 2-aminophenol UDPGT activity by 3-pentanone (Lalani and Burchell, 1979, and Table 1). Purified Gunn rat testosterone UDPGT activity towards 2-aminophenol was activated by 3-pentanone (not shown) and 2-aminophenol glucuronidation in foetal Wistar liver and adult Wistar kidney microsomes (neither of which exhibit testosterone UDPGT activity) were insensitive to 3-pentanone (M. Coughtrie et al., unpublished observations).

Here, we report the use of sensitive and specific immunoblot analysis to determine the extent of the inherited UDPGT deficiencies in the Gunn rat. The results show that at least 3 UDPGT isoenzymes are absent from the Gunn rat, a situation which could be due to deletion of the area(s) of the genome encoding these polypeptides. This proposal is currently under investigation in our laboratory.

ACKNOWLEDGEMENTS

M.W.H.C is in receipt of a S.E.R.C. studentship. B.B. is a Wellcome Trust Senior Lecturer.

REFERENCES

Burchell, B. (1981). Rev. Biochem. Toxicol, 3, 1.
Burchell, B., Kennedy, S.M.E., Jackson, M.R. and McCarthy, L.R. (1984). Biochem. Soc. Trans. 12, 50.
Cornelius, C.E. and Arias, I.M. (1972). Am. J. Pathol. 69, 369.
Crigler, J.F. and Najjar, V.A. (1952). Pediatrics 10, 169.
Domin, B.A., Serabjit-Singh, C.J. and Philpot, R.M. (1984). Anal. Biochem. 136, 390.
Dutton, G.J. (1980). in "Glucuronidation of drugs and other compounds" CRC Press, Boca Raton, FL.
Gunn, C.J.H. (1938). Heredity. 29, 137.
Laemmli, U.K. (1970). Nature (London). 227, 680.
Lalani, E-N.M.A. and Burchell, B. (1979). Biochem. J. 177, 993.
Lilienblum, W., Walli, A.K. and Bock, K.W. (1982). Biochem. Pharmacol. 31, 907.
Scragg, I., Celier, C. and Burchell, B. (1985). FEBS Lett. 183, 37.
Watkins, J.B. and Klaassen, C.D. (1982). Drug. Metab. Dispos. 10, 590.

STEREOSELECTIVE GLUCURONIDATION OF ORCIPRENALIN AND FENOTEROL IN RAT INTESTINAL AND HEPATIC CELLS AND MICROSOMES.

Andries Sj. Koster[1], Ank C. Frankhuijzen-Sierevogel[1], Peter A.L. Goossens[1] and Anton Mentrup[2].

[1]Department of Pharmacology, Faculty of Pharmacy, University of Utrecht, Catharijnesingel 60, 3511 GH Utrecht, The Netherlands. [2]Department of Pharmacochemistry, Boehringer-Ingelheim K.G., 6507 Ingelheim/Rhein, Federal Republic of Germany.

INTRODUCTION

A large proportion of drugs consists of a mixture of one (or more) pair(s) of enantiomers. Ample evidence indicates that the enantiomers should be treated as separate drugs with respect to almost every aspect of drug action (Ariens, 1986), metabolism (Testa, 1986) and pharmacokinetics (Walle and Walle, 1986). Stereoselective glucuronidation of propranolol (Thompson et al., 1981; Wilson and Thompson, 1984), oxazepam (Sisenwine et al., 1982) and morphine (Gawronska-Szklarz et al., 1985) has been described (note that morphine is normally administered as the pure (-)enantiomer). We decided to investigate the possible stereoselective glucuronidation of the β_2-sympathomimetics, orciprenalin and fenoterol. The data concerning fenoterol are reported in detail elsewhere (Koster et al., 1986a).

RESULTS AND DISCUSSION

Orciprenalin and fenoterol (Figure 1) are glucuronidated in the rat liver and intestine (Koster et al., 1985a; 1985b). More recently we established that fenoterol is glucuronidated by an enzyme form which is not induced by phenobarbital, 3-methylcholanthrene or Aroclor-1254, and which is not present in the rat kidney (Koster et al, 1986b). Fenoterol does, therefore, not belong to either the GT-1 or GT-2 group of UDP-glucuronosyltransferase substrates (Bock et al, 1980). An extra complication is added because fenoterol is conjugated to two different glucuronides (Pook et al., 1976; Koster et

Figure 1. Schematic representation of the microsomal glucuronidation of orciprenalin and fenoterol.

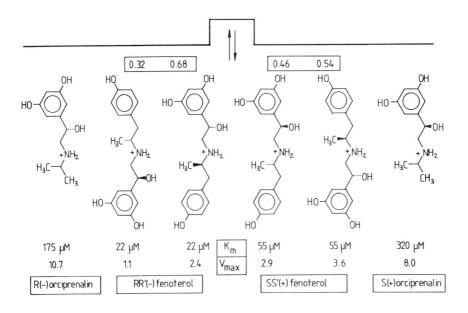

	175 μM	22 μM	22 μM	K_m	55 μM	55 μM	320 μM
	10.7	1.1	2.4	V_{max}	2.9	3.6	8.0

R(-)orciprenalin	RR'(-) fenoterol	SS'(+) fenoterol	S(+)orciprenalin

We suggest that for fenoterol, the fraction of para-glucuronide formed (indicated in boxes at the top) is dependent on the chance that the molecule is entering the active site of the enzyme (top of figure) "head first" (middle two drawings) or "tail first". This chance as well as the affinity and maximum reaction velocity (indicated at the bottom; V_{max} in nmole/min/mg) is influenced by the configuration at the optical active C-atoms. Note that the asymmetric centres are well away from the hydroxyl-group being conjugated.

al., 1986a), a para-glucuronide (FPG) and a meta-glucuronide (FMG). Orciprenalin forms only a meta-glucuronide (Figure 1).

The formation of glucuronides from the orciprenalin- and fenoterol-enantiomers in liver and intestinal microsomes is represented in Table 1.

It can be seen that statistically significant differences are present for V_{max} and K_m^{app}. In general the (-)enantiomers are conjugated with higher affinity than the (+)enantiomers. (+)-Fenoterol is metabolised with higher

Table 1. Glucuronidation of orciprenalin and fenoterol enantiomers in liver and intestinal microsomes.

Aglycone	para-glucuronide		meta-glucuronide	
	V_{max} (nmol/min/mg)	K_m^{app} (µM)	V_{max} (nmole/min/mg)	K_m^{app} (µM)
LIVER MICROSOMES				
S(+)-orciprenalin	-	-	11.4+1.2	266+62
R(-)-orciprenalin	-	-	13.6+0.6	135+21
SS'(+)-fenoterol	4.1+0.4*	75+15*	3.0+0.3	57+13*
RR'(-)-fenoterol	1.2+0.1*	26+7*	2.5+0.2	25+6*
INTESTINAL MICROSOMES				
S(+)-orciprenalin	-	-	4.6+0.6*	387+84
R(-)-orciprenalin	-	-	7.7+0.5*	214+26
SS'(+)-fenoterol	3.1+0.2*	47+7*	2.7+0.2	52+9*
RR'(-)-fenoterol	1.0+0.1*	19+3*	2.3+0.1	19+2*

Glucuronidation was measured in microsomes fully activated with Brij-58 under conditions linear with time and protein concentration in the presence of 10mM $MgCl_2$ and 3mM UDP-glucuronic acid.
*Significantly different ($p<0.05$) from the same parameter for the (+)enantiomer.

V_{max} than (-)fenoterol; for orciprenalin the reverse is true. A remarkable observation is that the fraction of para-glucuronide formed is independent of the concentration of fenoterol used. Fenoterol-para-glucuronide and fenoterol-meta-glucuronide are formed with different V_{max} but identical K_m^{app}. However, the fraction of para-glucuronide differs for the (+)enantiomer (0.54+0.01) and the (-) enantiomer (0.32+0.01) (Figure 1). The fraction of para-glucuronide as well as the overall V_{max} could not be changed by pretreatment of the animals with phenobarbital, 3-methylcholanthrene or Aroclor 1254 (data not shown).

We also investigated the glucuronidation of the orciprenalin- and fenoterol-enantiomers in isolated hepatocytes and intestinal epithelial cells. In isolated cells no differences in K_m^{app} were seen. Statistically significant differences were seen in the V_{max} for fenoterol in hepatocytes (0.17 ± 0.01 nmol/min/mg and 0.15 ± 0.01 nmol/min/mg; (+) and (-)enantiomer respectively) and enterocytes (0.44 ± 0.06 nmol/min/mg and 0.37 ± 0.05 nmol/min/mg; (+) and (-)enantiomer respectively) and for orciprenalin in hepatocytes (0.64 ± 0.04 nmol/min/mg and 1.06 ± 0.15 nmol/min/mg; (+) and (-)enantiomer respectively).

The results indicate that in vivo, the (+)enantiomer of fenoterol and the (-)enantiomer of orciprenalin may be more effectively metabolised by the liver and the intestine. Stereoselective first-pass metabolism in the intestinal wall and the liver may be a consequence. In that case the plasma racemate levels after oral and i.v. administration will not represent the plasma levels of the pharmacologically active (-)enantiomers (Walle and Walle, 1986). Our earlier studies concerning the first-pass metabolism of fenoterol (Koster et al., 1985b) will then be reduced to "sophisticated nonsense" (Ariens, 1986).

REFERENCES

Ariens, J.E. (1986). Tr. Pharmacol. Sci. 7, 200.

Bock, K.W., Clausbruch, U.C.von., Kaufmann, R., Lilienblum, W., Oesch, F., Pfeil, H. and Platt, K.L. (1980). Biochem. Pharmacol. 29, 495.

Gawronska-Szklarz, B., Svensson, J.O., Widen, J. and Rane, A. (1985). in "Advances in Glucuronide Conjugation" (Ed. by Matern, S., Bock, K.W. and Gerrok, W.). MTP-Press, Lancaster (UK), p.355.

Koster, A.Sj., Frankhuijzen-Sierevogel, A.C. and Noordhoek, J. (1985a). Drug Metab. Dispos. 13, 232.

Koster, A.Sj., Frankhuijzen-Sierevogel, A.C. and Mentrup, A. (1986a). Biochem. Pharmacol. 35, 1981.

Koster, A.Sj., Hofman, G.A., Frankhuijzen-Sierevogel, A.C. and Noordhoek, J. (1985b). Drug Metab. Dispos, 13, 464.

Koster, A.Sj., Schirmer, G. and Bock, K.W. (1986b). Biochem. Pharmacol (in press).

Pook, K.H., Rominger, K.L. and Arndts, D. (1976). J. Pharm. Sci. 65, 1513.

Sisenwine, S.F., Tio, C.O., Hadley, F.V., Liu, A.L., Kimmel, H.B. and Ruelius, H.W. (1982). Drug Metab. Dispos. 10, 60.

Thompson, J.A., Hull, J.E. and Norris, K.J. (1981). Drug Metab. Dispos. 9, 466.

Walle, T.H. and Walle, U.K. (1986). Tr. Pharmacol. Sci. 7, 155.

Wilson, B.K. and Thompson, J.A. (1984). Drug Metab. Dispos. 12, 161.

PHARMACOKINETICS OF GLUTATHIONE CONJUGATION IN THE RAT IN VIVO

J.M. te Koppele, E.J. van der Mark and G.J. Mulder.

Division of Toxicology, Center for Bio-Pharmaceutical Sciences, University of Leiden, The Netherlands.

INTRODUCTION

Although glutathione conjugation has been extensively studied in vitro, little insight has been gained into its kinetics in vivo, due to the absence of suitable model substrates. An ideal model substrate for such kinetic studies has to meet several requirements :
- it should be metabolised mainly by conjugation with glutathione, without appreciable competition by other metabolic routes.
- glutathione conjugation should be the rate-limiting factor in the elimination of the compound from blood. Experiments should be done in the linear dose range, where saturation of the transferase does not yet occur. To ensure that the clearance does not become limited by blood flow to organs, a low to intermediate extraction compound is preferred. High protein binding and slow transport processes of parent drug and/or metabolites should, be avoided.
- toxicity or pharmacological activities that influence the physiology or biochemistry of the conjugation system or animal should be absent.
- to circumvent administration problems of poorly water soluble substrates (as many in vitro substrates are), the model substrate should have a satisfactory water solubility.
- the metabolites should preferably be excreted in urine to enable convenient quantitation of the amount of substrate metabolised by glutathione conjugation.
     We chose the hypnotic drug α -bromoisovalerylurea (BIU; Figure 1) to study the pharmacokinetics of glutathione conjugation in vivo, since it seems to meet most of the requirements of an ideal model substrate. It is conjugated to a high extent with glutathione in man, resulting

Figure 1. Structure of α-bromoisovalerylurea (BIU).

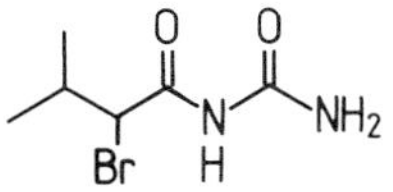

α-bromoisovalerylurea.

in excretion of 45 to 65% of the dose as mercapturates in urine within 24 hours (Niederwieser et al., 1978). BIU is reasonably water soluble and, as a registered drug, has little toxicity. In the rat BIU is also conjugated with glutathione: two glutathione conjugates were excreted in bile, whereas in urine two mercapturates were identified (te Koppele et al., 1987a). In both cases these were diastereomeric conjugates which were formed from the two enantiomers of the racemic BIU administered. However, no quantitative data on BIU metabolite formation in the rat were available. Therefore, we studied the excretion of BIU metabolites and the pharmacokinetics of BIU with respect to its requirements as model substrate.

After intravenous administration of [^{14}C-] BIU to unrestrained rats, 89% of the dose was recovered in urine within 24 hours, mainly as the (diastereomeric) mercapturates. This demonstrated that BIU was mainly metabolised by glutathione conjugation. In pentobarbital-anesthetised rats with a bile duct catheter, equal amounts of metabolites were excreted in bile and urine after intravenous administration of BIU. The metabolites found in bile were almost exclusively the two diastereomeric glutathione conjugates of BIU, which were formed to equal extents. In urine most of the metabolites were accounted for by the two diastereomeric mercapturates; they were formed in equal amounts (Figure 2).

Whereas no difference in the cumulative excretion of the diastereomeric metabolites was observed, a distinct stereoselectivity was found in the rates of excretion of the two diastereomeric glutathione conjugates: their half-lives of excretion in bile differed two- to three-fold. This was observed in anesthetised rats with a bile duct catheter, as well as in the perfused rat liver preparation. Similar differences in excretion rates were found for the excretion of the diastereomeric mercapturates in urine; in bile duct catheterised rats as well as rats with a ligated bile duct, a two-fold to three-fold difference was observed (Figure 3).

Figure 2. Cumulative excretion of radioactivity after i.v.
administration of [^{14}C-] BIU to anesthetised rats with a
bile duct and urine bladder catheter.

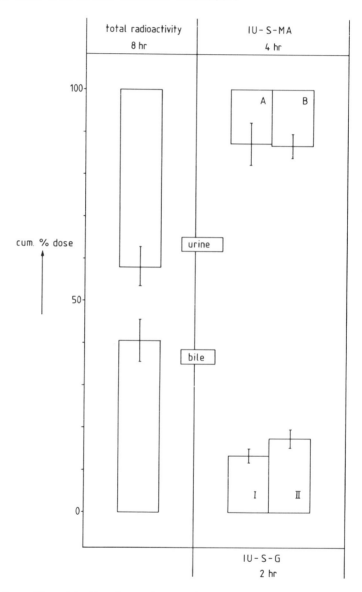

Total radioactivity in urine and bile is presented over a 8
hr period, whereas the amounts of glutathione conjugates
(bile) and mercapturates (urine) apply to periods of 2 and
4 hrs, respectively.

Figure 3. Excretion half-lives of the diastereomeric BIU glutathione conjugates (in bile) and BIU mercapturates (in urine).

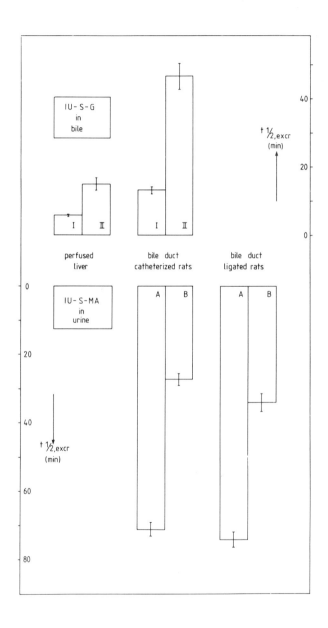

In the perfused liver preparation a low (initial) extraction ratio was found: E_H = 0.23. This suggests that hepatic clearance is not limited by liver blood flow. Furthermore, protein binding (40% was bound in plasma), and enzyme saturation (linear pharmacokinetics in the dose range studied: 22 to 270µmol/kg), are not likely to be limiting factors in the clearance of BIU from blood at these doses (te Koppele et al., 1987b).

Thus, α-bromoisovalerylurea is a promising substrate for studies of the pharmacokinetics of glutathione conjugation in vivo, in animals as well as man. The observed stereoselectivity in metabolite excretion rates indicates that BIU can be used to investigate the stereoselectivity of the processes involved.

REFERENCES

Niederwieser, A., Steinman, B. and Matasovic, A. (1978). J. Chromatogr. 147, 163.

te Koppele, J.M., van der Mark, E.J., Olde Boerrigter, J.C., Brussee, J., van der Gen, A., van der Greef, J., Mulder, G.J. (1987a). J. Pharmacol. Exp. Ther, accepted for publ.

te Koppele, J.M., Dogterom, P., Vermeulen, N.P.E., Meijer, D.K.F., van der Gen, A. and Mulder, G.J. (1987b). J. Pharmacol. Exp. Ther. accepted for publ.

THE SPONTANEOUS AND ENZYMIC REACTION OF N-ACETYL-BENZOQUINONE-IMINE WITH GLUTATHIONE : A STOPPED-FLOW KINETIC STUDY

B. Coles[1], I. Wilson[2], J. Hinson[3], S. Nelson[4], P. Wardman[2] and B. Ketterer[1].

[1]Middlesex Hospital Medical School, London, W.1, U.K. [2]Cancer Research Campaign, Gray Laboratory, Northwood, Middlesex, UK., [3] National Center for Toxicological Research, Jefferson, Arkansas, USA., [4]Department of Medicinal Chemistry, University of Washington, Seattle, Washington, USA.

INTRODUCTION

Paracetamol (acetaminophen) is a widely used pharmaceutical with valuable analgesic and antipyretic properties. In overdose however, it can cause severe hepatic necrosis, suggesting that either paracetamol itself or a metabolite is toxic. In experimental animals where similar toxicity is observed at high doses, this is associated with glutathione (GSH) depletion and covalent binding to hepatic proteins, a phenomenon associated, at least in part, with the production of an electrophile (Hinson, 1980).

A candidate electrophilic metabolite which is produced by hepatic oxidation of paracetamol is N-acetyl-benzoquinone imine (Q), the biological importance of which is evident from the presence of its GSH conjugate 3-glutathion-S-yl paracetamol ($QSGH_2$) in quantity in the bile of experimental animals given paracetamol (Dahlin et al, 1984; Hinson et al, 1982).

In the present paper we show that the rapid non-catalytic reaction of Q with GSH is apparently kinetically simple even though three products $QSGH_2$, paracetamol (QH_2) and oxidised glutathione (GSSG) are produced. We also show that GSH transferase isoenzymes catalyse the formation of $QSGH_2$ and, taking into account the intracellular compartmentation and protein binding of Q intrahepatically, consider what circumstances of paracetamol dosage and GSH concentration favour the enzymic reaction.

METHODS

The spontaneous reaction was conducted with a stopped-

flow mixer-drive unit under conditions which gave pseudo
first-order kinetics, using 5-20μM Q (Dahlin and Nelson,
1982), 0.1-10mM GSH and 50mM sodium phosphate in the pH
range 5-8 at 25°C. The pseudo first-order rate constants
were computed from the increase in transmittance at 260nm.
Conditions for the catalytic reaction were similar to those
above with the addition of 0.1 or 0.2mg GSH transferase 3-3
per ml. Initial rates were calculated from the linear
(several μs.) portion of the curves of T_{260} against time
and the spontaneous rate deducted to obtain a catalytic
rate.

For the competition between glutathione and cysteine as
nucleophiles, 5-20μM Q was reacted with a mixture of 0.1mM
GSH and 0.1mM cysteine in 50mM sodium phosphate pH 7.0, GSH
transferases (Ketterer et al, 1986) were added at 0.1 - 0.8
mg/ml. Reaction products were quantitated by HPLC, using a
Waters μ-Bondapak C-18 cartridge, the solvent 1% acetic
acid, 9% methanol, 90% water at a flow rate of 3ml/min.
Retention times were 3-S-cysteinyl paracetamol 5.4 min,
paracetamol 8.3 min and $QSGH_2$ 11.5 min. The molar ratio of
products was identical in the range 2-200μM quinone, 0.1-
10mM GSH and at pH 5.0, 7.0 and 9.0.

RESULTS

The Non-Enzymic Reaction
The rate constant for the loss of Q was first order in
GSH and Q in the range studied and the logarithm of the
second order rate constant for the reaction was dependent
on pH indicating that GS⁻ was the species involved in the
reaction. At pH 6.5, k=3.4 x $10^4 M^{-1} s^{-1}$. Although the
kinetics of reaction are simple, the products are $QSGH_2$,
QH_2 and GSSG, formed in a constant ratio of 3:2:2 (see also
Albano et al, 1985; Potter and Hinson, 1986) which is
independent of GSH and Q concentrations and pH.

The Enzymic Reaction
The relative catalytic effectiveness of GSH
transferase isoenzymes was determined by an indirect method
in which Q was reacted with a mixture of cysteine (CySH)
and GSH in the presence and absence of enzyme and the ratio
of GSH to CySH conjugates determined in each case. It is
seen from Table 1 that enzymic activity is associated with
the subunits composing the homodimers such that 3 > 4 > 1 [2]
2 > 6. In this paper where the effect of GSH transferases
on the hepatotoxicity of paracetamol is under consideration
GSH transferase 3-3 was chosen as an appropriate example
for our studies.

Table 1. The effect of GSH transferase on the reaction of Q with GSH and CySH.

ENZYME	GSH CONJUGATE	CySH CONJUGATE	RATIO
(0.1mg/ml)	molar %		
None	33.0	34.5	0.96
3-3	54.0	23.0	2.35
4-4	39.0	16.0	2.18
1-2	37.0	26.0	1.43
4-6	36.0	30.5	1.18

Data for the enzymic reaction at pH 6.5 plotted according to Lineweaver and Burke gave an apparent K_m of 2.8 μM and an apparent V_{max} of 27nmols^{-1}mg^{-1} i.e. an apparent k_{cat} of 1.4s^{-1}. These kinetic constants are described as apparent because neither substrate was present in saturating amounts.

DISCUSSION

The non-enzymic rate is extremely rapid and increases with pH indicating that GS$^-$ is the nucleophile responsible for reaction. The mechanism which yields three products, $QSGH_2$, QH_2 and GSSG in the ratio 3:2:2, regardless of the concentration of the reactants and the pH is not clear. It is not due to the reduction of $QSGH_2$ by GSH since $QSGH_2$ is stable in GSH. The ratio of $QSGH_2$ to Q however increases with increasing enzyme concentration suggesting that the product of the enzymic reaction is $QSGH_2$ alone. The rapid spontaneous rate has restricted information we have been able to obtain about the enzymic reaction with GSH transferase 3-3 since in order to differentiate the two in our experiments we have used pH 6.5 which is non-physiological and 10^{-3}M GSH which, since it is approximately the K_m for GSH transferase 3-3, does not saturate the enzyme (Ketterer et al, 1986).

A very important consideration in the distribution of xenobiotics such as paracetamol and its metabolites in the cell is the effect of compartmentation. The aqueous phases, lipid phases and protein-binding sites in the whole cell should all be considered, but for present purposes, the factors taken into account have been restricted to aqueous and lipid phases of the cytoplasm and substrate binding sites on the GSH transferases, since then we can draw analogies with other molecules of similar polarity, in which the ratio of Q_{free}, $Q_{protein\ bound}$, $Q_{lipid\ bound}$ is in the region of 0.01:1:1 (Tipping and Ketterer, 1981). The effect of this type of compartmentation is to reduce the non-enzymic rate of reaction by two orders of magnitude while reducing the enzymic rate to one half. Using the kinetic constants determined here and the compartmentation of reactants shown above it can be deduced that it is only at low doses of Q (μM) that the enzymic reaction predomibnates. At higher doses (e.g. 100μM) the non-enzymic reaction predominates resulting in the formation of QH_2 and GSSG in addition to $QSGH_2$. As long as the GSH reductase system remains adequate, effective detoxification may still take place. However, if the dose of Q is sufficient to cause GSH depletion covalent binding to protein may occur and the GSSG ratio in the cell may increase to detrimental levels.

REFERENCES

Albano, E., Rundgren, M., Harvison, P.J., Nelson, S.D. and Moldeus, P. (1985). Mol. Pharmacol, 28, 306.

Dahlin, D.C., Miwa, G.T., Lu, A.Y.H. and Nelson, S.D. (1984). Proc. Natl. Acad. Sci. USA, 81, 1327.

Dahlin, D.C. and Nelson, S.D. (1982). J. Med. Chem, 25, 885.

Hinson, J.A. (1980). in "Rev. Biochem. Toxicol" (E. Hodgson, J.R. Bend and R.M. Philpot, ed). Elsevier/ North Holland, New York, vol 2, 103.

Hinson, J.A., Monks, T.J., Hong, M., Highet, R.J. and Pohl, L.R. (1982). Drug. Metab. Dispos, 10, 47.

Ketterer, B., Meyer, D.J., Coles, B., Taylor, J.B. and Pemble, S. (1986). in "Anticarcinogenesis and anti-mutagenesis mechanisms" (D.M. Shankel., P.E. Hartman., T. Kada and A. Hollaender, eds). Plenum Press, N.Y. 103.

Potter, D.W. and Hinson, J.A. (1986). Mol. Pharmacol, 30, 33.

Tipping, E. and Ketterer, B. (1981). Biochem, J, 195, 441.

4. Techniques in drug analysis.

THE DETECTION OF DRUG METABOLITES IN BIOLOGICAL SAMPLES BY HIGH RESOLUTION PROTON NMR SPECTROSCOPY.

J.K. Nicholson[1] and I.D. Wilson[2]

[1]Department of Chemistry, Birkbeck College, University of London, Malet Street, London, WC1E 7HX, UK and [2]Department of Safety of Medicines, ICI Pharmaceutical Division, Meerside, Alderley Park, Macclesfield, Cheshire, ST5 4TG, UK.

INTRODUCTION

With the advent of the lastest generation of high field pulsed Fourier transform NMR spectrometers, increasingly complex biochemical problems can now be studied by high resolution NMR spectroscopy. In recent years we have been concerned with applications of proton NMR spectroscopy in the analysis of urine and plasma samples for both endogenous and drug metabolites (Iles et al, 1983; Nicholson et al, 1983; Bales et al, 1984a & b; Everett et al, 1984; Nicholson et al, 1984a & b; Bales et al, 1985; Nicholson et al, 1985b; Coleman and Norton, 1986; Tulip et al, 1986; Wilson and Ismail, in press; Wilson et al, in press). Although NMR is a relatively insensitive technique when compared with most other spectroscopic or chromatographic methods, there are several intrinsic advantages that make NMR-based analytical approaches attractive. For instance, rapid multi-component analysis can often be effected with a minimal sample pre-treatment. Furthermore, it is not necessary to make assumptions as to the identity of compounds present in the sample prior to analysis, as the chemical information content of NMR spectra is very high. This is in marked contrast to most other analytical methods, particularly chromatography, where in general the analyst sets out to devise highly specific methods where sample preparation, chromatography and detection are deliberately optimised to detect a limited number of closely related compounds. However, in order for NMR to be able to detect them, analytes must be present in relatively large amounts, i.e. at concentrations of $> 50\mu M$, and must have suitable proton signals, usually from CH, CH_2 or CH_3 groups. Ideally, resonances from the drug metabolites should lie in regions of proton NMR spectrum which we have previously described as being low in chemical noise, i.e. they are relatively free of signals from interferring endogenous components (Wilson <u>et al</u>, in press).

One of the factors limiting the more widespread use of proton NMR for the study of drug metabolism is that, hitherto, it has been assumed that such studies required the use of spectrometers operating at very high magnetic field strengths e.g. 9.4 or 11.75 Tesla (corresponding to proton resonance frequencies of 400 and 500 MHz respectively) to give maximal sensitivity and signal dispersion. Although such instrumentation is becoming more common in research laboratories, it is still not widely available due to the very high capital costs involved. However, we have now demonstrated with the aid of some very simple and rapid sample preparation procedures that drug metabolism and excretion studies can be performed effectively using "routine" instruments operating at much lower frequencies such as 200-250 MHz, so making the technique more widely available.

In particular we have found that disposable solid phase extraction can effect rapid sample clean-up prior to NMR analysis for drug metabolites. With this technique, the compounds of interest are selectively retained on an adsorbent (contained in a small disposable column) from which they can be recovered by elution with a suitable solvent. The results described here show the application of solid phase extraction chromatography with nuclear magnetic resonance (SPEC-NMR) for the analysis of urine samples containing a range of commonly used drugs such as trental (oxpentifylline), ibuprofen, and naproxen.

MATERIALS AND METHODS

<u>NMR spectroscopy</u> ^{1}H HMR spectra were measured at ambient probe temperature (25°) on Varian EM360 (60 MHz Continuous Wave) and Jeol FX90, Bruker WM200, WM250, WH400 and AM500 pulse Fourier transform spectrometers operating at 90, 200, 250, 400 and 500 MHz respectively. Measurements at 400 and 500 MHz involved the collection of 32-64 Free induction decays (FIDs) after 30-40° pulses into 16384 computer points. A total recycle time of at least 5s was used to allow full T_1 relaxation, 90, 200 and 250 MHz spectra were acquired with 90° pulses and typically 350 FIDs were collected, spectra were again fully T_1 relaxed. The signal from the residual water protons was suppressed where necessary by the application of a pre-saturating secondary

irradiation field at the water resonance frequency with the decoupler coils, the irradiation being gated off during acquisition of the FID.

Sample preparation : 400 and 500 MHz ^{1}H NMR spectra were obtained from untreated urine samples containing added ^{2}H$_2$O to 20% as an internal field frequency lock, containing a known amount of sodium-d$_4$-(trimethylsilyl) propionate, as both a chemical shift and concentration standard. 90, 200 and 250 MHz ^{1}H NMR spectra were obtained from on selected samples by freeze drying 2ml of urine and reconstituting in 1ml of ^{2}H$_2$O and from solid phase extracted samples redissolved in deuterated solvents (see below).

Solid Phase Extraction Chromatography with NMR (SPEC-NMR) For the experiments involving solid-phase sample preparation the following procedure was adopted : Samples of acidified urine (2ml) were loaded into 3ml capacity C18 Bond-Elut columns which had been activated by washing with 5ml of methanol and then 5ml of water. In most experiments the urine samples were acidified with 10μl/ml of 99% formic acid. At this point the column was washed with 5ml of $C^2H_3O^2H$ or mixtures of $C^2H_3O^2H$ and ^2H_2O. Column eluates were collected into 20 ml scintillation vials. Solvents were then removed using a stream of nitrogen, and freeze drying if necessary.

In order to further clean up or fractionate metabolites present in some samples, stepwise elution procedures were employed. Urine samples were applied to the C18 columns as previously described and after washing with acidified water were eluted with methanol-water mixtures starting with 20:80 and progressing through 40:60, 60:40, and 80:20 steps to 100% methanol. The methanol fractions after removal of solvent, were redissolved in ^{2}H$_2$O and placed in 5mm outside diameter NMR tubes prior to ^{1}H NMR analysis (see below). The aqueous fractions were freeze dried, and then redissolved in ^{2}H$_2$O.

RESULTS AND DISCUSSION

General Characteristics of NMR Spectra of Human and Rat Urine
Figure 1 shows typical 400 MHz ^{1}H NMR spectra of untreated urine from a normal human subject and a laboratory rat. Reasonable signal to noise ratios were usually obtained with 48 accumulations, but very dilute urine samples required more. Therefore, even allowing for a long T_1 relaxation delay between pulses, spectra could usually be obtained within five minutes, without any sample pre-treatment. Resonances from a wide range of endogenous

Figure 1.   Typical 400 MHz NMR spectra of human and rat urine.

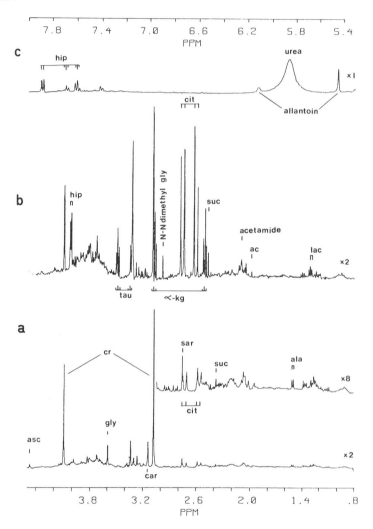

a : aliphatic region of a 400 MHz NMR spectrum obtained from control human urine
b : aliphatic region of a 400 MHz NMR spectrum obtained from a normal laboratory rat (Fischer 344)
c : aromatic region of the same 400 MHz NMR spectrum as b
Ac, acetate; ala, alanine; asc, ascorbate; car, carnitine; cit, citrate; Cr, creatinine; gly, glycine; hip, hippurate; α-kg, α-ketoglutarate; lac, lactate; sar, sarcosine; suc, succinate; tau, taurine.

compounds were observed and identified by making standard
additions of candidate compounds and by considering their
chemical shifts and coupling patterns (Bales et al 1984;
Nicholson et al, 1984a). Many of these compounds are of
considerable physiological importance and, furthermore,
their urinary concentrations often reflect the
physiological metabolic, or pathological status of the
animal or subject.

Observation of signals from compounds at low
concentrations (millimolar range) in the presence of the
very large water signal (>100 molar in protons) can pose
severe dynamic range problems in Fourier transform
spectrometers. All such instruments utilise analogue to
digital converters, which can introduce digitisation errors
into spectra if large signals are present. Without
adequate suppression of the water signal, the information
to be obtained on metabolites in biological materials is
greatly limited due to inadequate digitisation of their
signals (Bales et al, 1984a). The simple expedient of
freeze drying urine and reconstituting it in a smaller
volume of ^2H_2O largely overcomes this problem, but may
result in the loss of volatile components and the selective
deuteration of exchangeable protons. In this way we were
able to detect and quantify the acidic metabolite of the
drug oxpentifylline without difficulty (Wilson et al, in
press). However, the interpretation of spectra of freeze
dried urine samples obtained at 260 MHz was still
complicated to some extent by interference from endogenous
urinary components, and there is a limit to the amount by
which urine samples may be concentrated before the
increased ionic strength of the solution adversely affects
the quality of the spectra obtained. We have therefore
explored other simple methods of preparing samples for NMR
analysis for xenobiotic metabolites, in particular, the use
of solid phase extraction columns to effect rapid clean up
of urine samples.

DRUG METABOLITE ANALYSIS IN URINE SAMPLES WITH HIGH FIELD NMR SPECTROMETERS

If very high field NMR spectrometers are available,
drug metabolite analysis in urine samples can often be
achieved with little or no sample preparation (Bales et al
1984a and b; Nicholson et al, 1984b). A typical 500 MHz 1H
NMR spectrum of urine collected 6 hours after paracetamol
ingestion is shown in Figure 2 and serves for discussion of
the peak assignments (see also Bales et al, 1984b; Bales et
al, 1985). These were aided by first recording and

Figure 2.   A 500 MHz spectrum obtained from the urine of a
normal human volunteer following ingestion of 1g of
paracetamol.

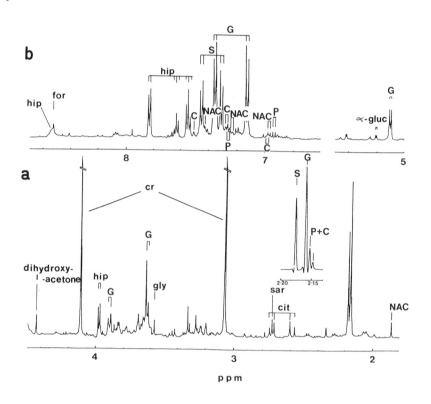

a -   Aliphatic region; b-aromatic region; C, cysteinyl
conjugate of paracetamol; G, glucuronide conjugate of
paracetamol; α -gluc, α-anomeric proton of glucose; for,
formate; NAC, N-acetyl cysteinyl conjugate of paracetamol;
S, sulphate conjugate of paracetamol; otherwise as for
Figure 1.

assigning peaks for paracetamol and its major metabolites
(A major advantage of NMR is that "fingerprints" of
molecules often consist of more than one resonance, each
with characteristic chemical shifts, relative intensities
and sometimes spin-spin coupling patterns.   In favourable
cases this allows unambiguous identification of the
substance.   This is in contrast to traces from liquid-
chromatographic effluents, obtained with electronic
absorption of fluorescence detectors which gave only a

single peak for each metabolite. The acetanilide N-acetyl groups of the metabolites all gave sharp signals in the narrow range from 2.13 to 2.19 ppm. These were well resolved at 400 or 500 MHz if the resolution was enhanced by application of a Gaussian function to the FID before Fourier transformation. Paracetamol metabolites have other characteristic ^{1}H NMR resonances (Bales et al, 1984a & b). In addition to the N-acetyl resonances, the aromatic ring protons give rise to resonances with clearly identifiable coupling patterns spread over about 0.6ppm (Figure 2). In the case of the glucuronide, the β-anomeric proton of the sugar ring has a further characteristic doublet resonance at 5.11ppm (J = 6 Hz) and also resonance between 3.6 and 3.9ppm corresponding to other sugar ring protons. An additional assignment aid for the N-acetyl-L-cysteinyl conjugate, was the sharp singlet for the side-chain N-acetyl group at 1.84ppm. In a detailed NMR study of the metabolism and excretion of paracetamol by man, we found that there was good agreement between NMR and conventional liquid chromatographic measurements on paracetamol metabolite concentrations (Bales et al, 1984b).

Clearly there is considerable potential for very high field ^{1}H NMR in studies of drug metabolism and excretion. Other workers have recently shown that these techniques can be applied to study completely different classes of drugs such as penicillins (Everett et al, 1984 and metronidazole (Coleman and Norton, 1986). In the first case Everett and co-workers were able to identify a previously unknown metabolite of the β-lactam ampicillin, i.e. diketopiperazine, using predominantly spin-echo Fourier transform methods to analyse untreated urine samples. Spin-echo pulse sequences are also required for matrices containing significant quantities of protein as this significantly attenuates their broad resonances and so minimises interferences (Nicholson et el, 1983; 1984b). Furthermore, NMR is a non-equilibrium perturbing and non-invasive technique and so is uniquely suited to the study of drug metabolism in isolated but fully intact biochemical systems such as cell suspensions (Nicholson et al, 1985a).

STUDIES WITH LOW TO MEDIUM FIELD STRENGTH NMR SPECTROMETERS

If very high field NMR instrumentation is not available then at least some sample preparation steps are necessary before drug metabolite analysis can be affected. However, these procedures can be simple and rapid enough not to render the NMR approach unattractive for studies of xenobiotic metabolism. The simplest of these methods is to

freeze dry the sample. This allows both concentration of
metabolites and removal of the water by redissolution in a
reduced volume of deuterated solvent, hence also
eliminating problems emanating from the very high dynamic
range of biological samples. The 250 MHz ^{1}H NMR spectrum
of a freeze dried control urine sample with the signals
from many endogenous metabolites assigned is shown in
Figure 3. The spectrum contains several frequency
"windows" in which there are few resonances from endogenous
compounds and in which signals from drug metabolites may be
observed with relatively little interference. NMR spectra
measured at higher field strengths are less prone to
interferences from endogenous compounds or chemical noise
(Wilson et al, in press) as signals have a greater
frequency dispersion and overlap less with each other.

A more selective and flexible method of sample
preparation, involves the use of disposable solid phase
columns with bonded C18 moieties. After loading an aliquot
of the urine sample shown in Figure 3 onto a C18 Bond-Elut
column it was possible to show that only urinary pigments
were retained in the matrix without acidification of the
sample. On lowering the pH with formic acid to
approximately pH 2, the bulk of the urinary aromatic acids
(e.g. hippurate, indoxyl sulphate, tyrosine and
phenylalanine) were selectively retained on the column,
whilst most of the non-aromatic organic and amino acids
passed through the column into eluate. The aromatic
compounds were then recovered on washing the column with
methanol. Indeed, 20% methanol was sufficiently elutropic
to give complete recovery of these components. The use of
solid phase extraction chromatography on acidified urine
samples following dosing with a variety of drugs was then
instigated as described below.

FURTHER STUDIES WITH SOLID PHASE EXTRACTION COLUMNS AND NMR (SPEC-NMR)

Trental (Oxpentifylline). We have recently
investigated the quantitative analysis of 1-(3'-
carboxypropyl)-3,7-dimethylxanthine, CPDX which is the
major metabolite of oxpentifylline excreted in urine
following oral dosing with 600mg of the drug. In the
freeze dried urine of a subject treated with this drug,
signals for the two N-methyl groups at the N3 and N7
positions and the C8H proton are clearly visible even in
the 250 MHz ^{1}H NMR spectrum (Figure 4a). However, signals
for the side chain methylene groups are subject to
considerable overlap with resonances from endogenous

Figure 3. A typical 250 MHz NMR spectrum obtained for the urine of a normal human subject. The urine was freeze dried and redissolved in ^2H_2O for NMR analysis.

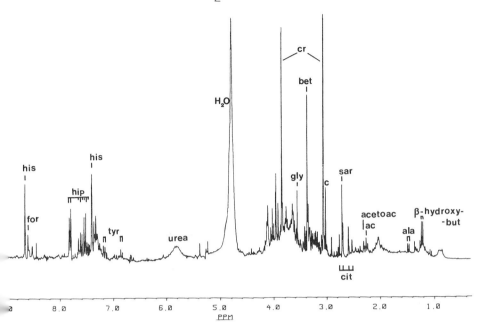

acetoac, acetoacetate; c, creatinine;β-hydroxybut,β-hyd-roxybutyrate; bet, betaine; his, histidine; tyr, tyrosine; otherwise as for Figure 1.

metabolites. A very significant improvement in this respect was obtained by concentrating the metabolite onto a C18 cartridge and then eluting with methanol. Whilst the purification achieved by this simple procedure might suffice for unequivocal assignment in most cases, superior separation could be obtained by washing the cartridge with methanol-water 20:80 (v/v) prior to eluting the CPDX with 100% methanol. This approach gave a virtually clean preparation of CPDX (Figure 4b).

Naproxen. The spectrum shown in Figure 5a was obtained from a urine sample covering the period 0-5.5h after a single oral dose of the non-steroidal anti-inflammatory drug naproxen (d-2[6-methoxy-2-napthyl]-propionic acid). A prominant doublet is observed at 5.5ppm corresponding to the β-anomeric proton of the naproxen glucuronides. Signals from the α-methyl protons from the propionyl side chain together with a number of aromatic signals between 7

Figure 4.   250 MHz NMR spectra (in ^2H_2O) obtained for the
urine of a normal human volunteer for the period 8 to 10h
following an oral dose (600mg) of oxpentifylline (trental).

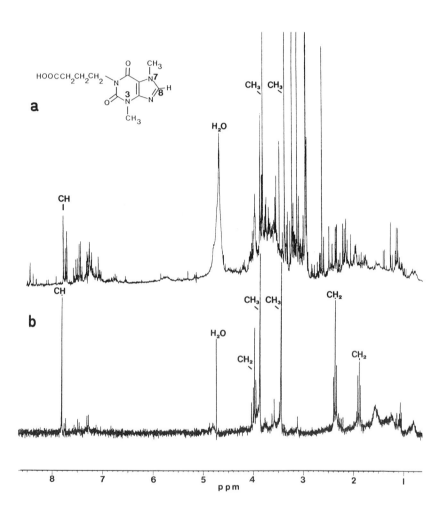

a : The sample was freeze dried and redissolved in ^2H_2O
prior to analysis.
b : ^{C}18 Bond Elut Cartridge. After loading the acidified
urine the catridge was washed with 20% methanol-water (pH2)
to elute endogenous contaminants. The metabolite (see
inset) was recovered by elution with methanol.

Figure 5. A 250 MHz NMR spectra (in ^2H_2O) of urine for the period 0 to 5.5h after an oral dose (500mg) of naproxen.

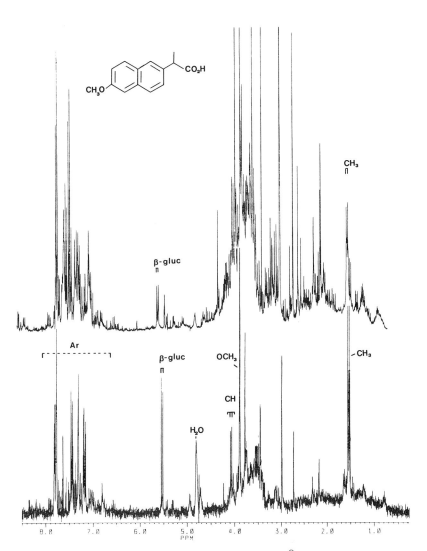

A - Freeze dried urine reconstituted in ^2H_2O.
B - The same sample following SPE on a C18 Bond Elut cartridge, and elution with methanol. The sample was acidified to pH2 with formic acid prior to SPE. Note the enhancement of the signals due to drug related material compared to A.

and 8ppm are also observed. However, the signals from the naproxen metabolites were weak in comparison to those of the endogenous urinary components. Concentration of the metabolites onto a C18 cartridge, followed by elution with methanol, gave the spectrum shown in Figure 5b (after removal of the solvent and redissolution in ^2H_2O). In this spectrum signals due to the drug related material were greatly enhanced. When this procedure was repeated with sequential washing of the cartridge with a stepwise gradient of increasing methanol content, it allowed the complete removal of most endogenous components, and the separation of the drug metabolites into fractions that gave readily interpretable ^1H NMR spectra, i.e. for the 40% methanol wash, 0-desmethyl naproxen plus parent compound, both as glucuronides (Figure 6a), whilst the 60% methanol wash gave only naproxen glucuronide (Figure 6b).

Ibuprofen. The NMR spectrum shown in Figure 7a was obtained from a urine sample collected 2-4h after a single oral dose of 400mg of ibuprofen (2-[4-isobutylphenyl]-propionic acid. After drug treatment many new resonances were observed. These included a broad envelope of overlapping aromatic resonances centred at about 7.25ppm, and a prominent doublet at 5.4ppm from the β-anomeric proton of ibuprofen and its metabolites (present as glucuronide conjugates). The spectral region from 0.8 to 1.5ppm also contained several signals of drug origin including a large singlet at 1.18ppm (methyl group from a metabolite with a hydroxylated isobutyl side chain, i.e. 2-[4-(2-hydroxy-2-methylpropyl)-phenyl] propionic acid, HMPPP). Application of 2ml of acidified urine to a C18 column, followed by elution of the retained material with methanol produced the result shown in Figure 7b. As seen with the CPDX metabolite of oxpentifylline and the naproxen metabolites, the signals from the ibuprofen metabolites were much more prominent in this spectrum. Using the stepwise gradient elution techique, it was possible to further fractionate the ibuprofen metabolites into two groups each of two metabolites both essentially free of endogenous compounds. The first group, eluting with 40% methanol, appeared by NMR to contain HMPPP, and the side chain oxidised metabolite 2-[4-(2-carboxy-2-methylpropyl)-phenyl] propionic acid both present as glucuronide conjugates. Elution with 60% methanol led to the recovery of ibuprofen (as its glucuronide) and the 2-[4-(1-hydroxy-2-methylpropyl)-phenyl] propionic acid metabolite (also as a glucuronide). A small amount of contamination of the 60% fraction with metabolites predominently eluting in the 40% wash was also observed. Thus in this way the metabolites

Figure 6. Fractionation of naproxen metabolites (from Figure 5A) on a C18 Bond Elut cartridge using stepwise gradient elution with acidified methanol-water in 20% increments.

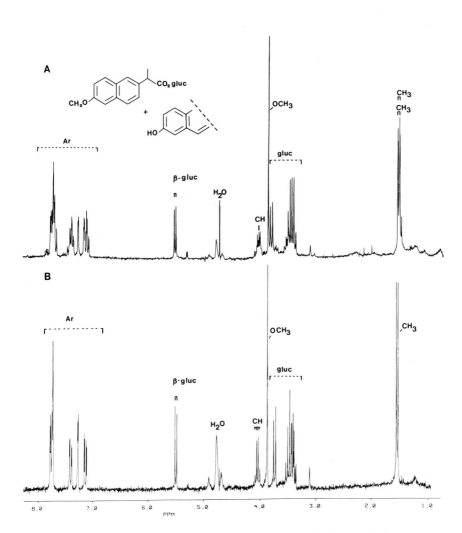

A : a mixture of naproxen glucuronide and O-desmethyl naproxen glucuronide eluting with 40% methanol-water.

B : Naproxen glucuronide eluted with 60% methanol-water.

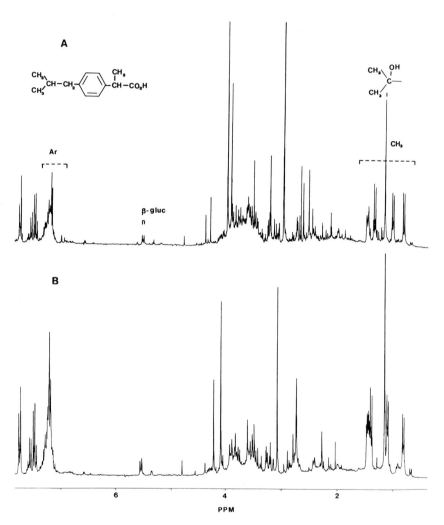

Figure 7.   A 250 MHz NMR spectra (in ^2H_2O) of a urine
sample from a healthy human volunteer following oral
administration of ibuprofen (400mg).

A - Freeze-dried urine for the period 2 to 4h post dose.
B - Following SPE of acidified urine from 7A on a C18 Bond
Elut column and elution with methanol.   Note the
enhancement of the drug related signals compared to those
of the endogenous metabolites.

may first be concentrated and only partially purified of endogenous components as an aid to quantification and identification, whilst gradient elution enables some statement as to the structure of the metabolites to be made.

In order to test the effectiveness of lower field NMR instrumentation for the detection of ibuprofen metabolites after using a C18 column to concentrate the compounds from a urine sample, we redissolved the dry residue from a methanolic eluate in d_6 DMSO and obtained spectra from 400, 200, 90 MHz and 60 MHz spectrometers. We found that 200 MHz spectra allowed the identification of all metabolites, and that signals from the major metabolites were adequately resolved even at 90 MHz after collection of 300 scans on a Fourier transform (FT) machine. 60 MHz Continuous Wave spectroscopy proved inadequate for the task both in terms of sensitivity and signal dispersion, indicating that a 90 MHz FT spectrometer at least must be used in order for this approach to be successful in drug metabolite detection.

We also investigated the capacity of the C18 cartridge for ibuprofen metabolites by gradually increasing the amounts of urine loaded onto the column until no further retention of drug related substances occurred. There was very little breakthrough of the metabolites until about 15 ml of urine was loaded to a 3ml C18 Bond Elut column. At 20ml some drug related material was not retained and passed straight through the column. However, elution of the retained material with methanol gave very concentrated samples containing primarily drug metabolites and consequently allowed superior quality NMR spectra, with very good signal to noise ratios, to be obtained after the collection of only 16-32 FIDs. Figure 8 shows the spectrum obtained following the elution with methanol of a cartridge to which 12ml of urine had been applied (i.e. insufficient to cause metabolite breakthrough). The columns appear to have a greater capacity or affinity for drug metabolites of this type than the endogenous components. Thus few signals from endogenous components are observed even though no attempt has been made to remove them by stepwise procedures. In this case the high loading of the column is beneficial both in terms of purification and ease of NMR detection.

At present NMR spectroscopy is an insensitive technique when compared with chromatographic analysis methods. So urinary drug excretion studies by NMR are limited to compounds which are used in fairly large amounts and excreted rapidly. However a major advantage in using ^{1}H NMR as a tool for directly analysing the low molecular

Figure 8. Concentration of ibuprofen metabolites from 12ml
of the urine shown in Figure 7A onto a C18 Bond Elut
cartridge and elution with methanol. Note the virtual
absence of signals due to endogenous urinary components.

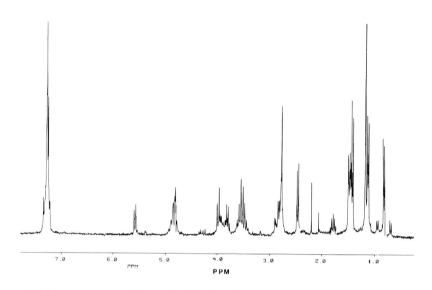

weight components of biological materials, is that
toxicological information of mechanistic significance can
be obtained, by interpreting the changing patterns and
concentrations of endogenous metabolites in reponse to a
xenobiotic challenge. This case is well illustrated by
reference to our ^{1}H NMR work on the effects of mercuric
chloride on the urinary composition of rats (Nicholson et
al, 1985b). In this study it was possible to use NMR as a
multi-parametric indicator of acute nephrotoxicity that in
addition to being at least as sensitive as conventional
biochemical measurements also gave information on basic
mechanisms of mercury toxicity, particularly those relating
to inhibitory effects on citric acid-cycle enzymes.
Finally, it should be stressed that NMR spectroscopy is a
technique that is still developing rapidly, and major
advances in the methodology, in particular data processing,
are occurring in quick succession, so that the range of NMR
applications in drug metabolism and toxicity studies will
be expected to widen in the next few years.

In previous studies we have shown that high field [1]H
NMR spectroscopy of biological fluids such as plasma and
urine can provide qualitatative and quantitative data on
contained drug and endogenous metabolites. This work

involved the use of very high frequency measurements on biological samples, thus minimising peak overlap and allowing the interpretation of very complex patterns of partially overlapping resonances from structurally similar metabolites. Lower field measurements on such complex matrices normally require some type of preliminary clean up of the sample in order to aid interpretation of the resulting NMR spectrum. The present study has extended the methodology to include a simple and rapid procedure for sample preparation leading to NMR analysis of drug metabolites in urine samples after therapeutic doses of several commonly used (and sometimes abused) drugs given at normal therapeutic doses, i.e. solid phase extraction chromatography and NMR (SPEC-NMR). Each compound studied has its own NMR fingerprint of signals making a positive identification of the parent or metabolite in an unknown sample a possibility. SPEC-NMR seems to offer several useful features. At one level this method can greatly simplify NMR spectra of urine samples by the selective removal of many of the endogenous components that are not retained on the column. The method is also valuable in that considerable concentration of metabolites can be achieved very easily. This is of particular importance as NMR spectroscopy is an inherently insensitive technique in comparison to most other analytical methods, although the information content of NMR spectra is very high. A more sophisticated use of the C18 columns involves employing stepwise elution procedures to fractionate complex mixtures of metabolites, which further simplifies interpretation of the NMR spectra, and is of particular value if only modest NMR instrumentation is available. Indeed, this approach has proved to be very powerful in that under certain circumstances we have been able to obtain essentially pure metabolites (e.g. naproxen glucuronide) very rapidly, as such SPEC-NMR may be competitive to preparative HPLC for certain applications. The source of analytical power in this method is the use of the NMR spectrometer to provide a multi-frequency (or multi-component) detector for the chromatographic process. Obtaining information in this way relies only on the compound under study having observable protons and being present in sufficient concentrations in the final measured sample (typically > 0.1 mM). SPEC-NMR has many of the advantages of directly linked experimental LC-NMR systems with none of the disadvantages. LC-NMR is intrinsically very difficult as the two techniques have very different sample treatment and handling characteristics, e.g. LC: often uses mixed solvents, a flowing system, and operates with relatively low

concentrations of substances; NMR: single, preferably
deuterated solvent, a static sample (in the flow sense) but
sample should be spinning to obtain highest possible
resolution, and high concentrations of compounds
(millimolar concentration range). LC-NMR systems also
render the (very expensive) spectrometer part of the system
unavailable for other uses during operation. Direct
matching of these requirements is currently very difficult
with most desired separation procedures.

Using a SPEC-NMR approach complete separation of
metabolites appears to be unnecessary in most cases, as the
NMR "detector" effectively "separates" the metabolites on
the basis of the magnetic and hence chemical properties of
their protons. This new philosophy requires only
sufficient physical separation of metabolites in order for
the NMR spectrum to be unambiguously interpretable, and so
does not necessitate the rigorous chromatographic
procedures that are normally required in drug metabolism
work, i.e. the chromatography may be quick and simple.
There may also be applications of SPEC-NMR in preparative
scale chromatographic separations, as unlike conventional
preparative LC, SPEC-NMR method development is very fast
and relatively inexpensive. To date our studies with SPEC-
NMR have been limited to C18 bonded phase and to urine
samples. However, it should be possible to use this
approach to other biological fluids such as plasma and also
to tissue extracts, and to use other types of silica-bonded
moieties to extend the range of drugs that can be studied.

ACKNOWLEDGEMENTS

We are grateful to the National Kidney Research Fund,
for supporting this and related work.

REFERENCES

Bales, J.R., Higham, D.P., Howe, I., Nicholson, J.K. and
    Sadler, P.J. (1984a). Clin. Chem. 30, 426.
Bales, J.R., Nicholson, J.K. and Sadler, P.J. (1985).
    Clin. Chem, 31, 757.
Bales, J.R., Sadler, P.J., Nicholson, J.K. and Timbrell,
    J.A. (1984b). Clin. Chem, 30 (10, 1631.
Coleman, M.D. and Norton, R.S. (1986). Xenobiotica, 16, 69.
Everett, J.R., Jennings, K., Woodnut, G. and Buckingham,
    M.J. (1984). J. Chem. Soc. Chem. Commun, 14, 894.
Iles, R., Buckingham M.J. and Hawkes, G.E. (1983).
    Biochem. Soc. Trans, 11, 374.
Nicholson, J.K., Bales, J.R., Sadler, P.J., Juul, S.M.,

Macleod, A. and Sonksen, P.H. (1984a). The Lancet, ii, 751.

Nicholson, J.K., Buckingham, M.J. and Sadler, P.J. (1983). Biochem J. 211 (3), 605.

Nicholson, J.K., O'Flynn, M., Sadler, P.J., Macleod, A., Juul, S.M. and Sonkson, P.H. (1984b). Biochem. J. 217, 365.

Nicholson, J.K., Timbrell, J.A., Bales, J.R. and Sadler, P.J. (1985a). Mol. Pharmacol, 27, 634.

Nicholson, J.K., Timbrell, J. and Sadler, P.J. (1985). Mol. Pharmacol, 27, 644.

Tulip, K., Wilson, I.D., Troke, J., Nicholson, J.K. and Timbrell, J.A. (1986). Drug Met. Disp (in press).

Wilson, I.D. and Ismail, I.M. J. Pharm. Biomed. Analysis, (in press).

Wilson, I.D., Ismail, I.M., Fromson, J. and Nicholson, J.K. J. Pharmaceut. Biomed. Analysis (in press).

RAPID METABOLIC PROFILING USING THERMOSPRAY LC-MS/MS

Patrick Rudewicz and Kenneth Straub

Smith Kline and French Laboratories, 709 Swedeland Road,
Swedeland, Pennsylvania, 19479, USA.

INTRODUCTION

The combination of a "thermospray" HPLC-MS interface and a tandem mass spectrometer provides a unique tool for the rapid elucidation of drug metabolite structures. Many classes of compounds including polar and thermally labile conjugates can be efficiently ionised to yield molecular species which can subsequently be collisionally dissociated to yield structurally informative fragment ions. In the past, work in this laboratory has been aimed at designing specific tandem mass spectrometry (MS/MS) scan sequences that can be used to characterise common classes of drug conjugates. Neutral loss scans have been shown to give high specificity for the detection of O-glucuronides (176 amu) and aryl sulphate esters (80 amu). By combining neutral loss scans that are specific for conjugating groups together with precursor ion scans that are specific for substructural features of a given drug, both primary and secondary metabolites can be rapidly identified within a complex sample matrix.

The use of this methodology for the characterisation of drug metabolites is illustrated by the HPLC-MS/MS analysis of a catecholamine drug, ibopamine (SK&F 100168; epinine diisobutyric ester), a positive inotropic agent currently under investigation for treatment of patients with congestive heart failure (Dei Cas et al., 1983). Previous studies have shown that when ibopamine is administered, the isobutyryl groups are rapidly hydrolyzed and epinine (N-methyldopamine) is released into the circulation (Boyce et al, 1984). The major urinary metabolites of ibopamine in both the rat and the dog have been identified (Hwang et al, 1984) using conventional methodologies and are shown in Figure 1. Studies with monkeys indicated the possible presence of novel metabolic pathways, prompting us to explore the use of HPLC-MS/MS for the identification of the metabolites of ibopamine in this species.

Figure 1. Major metabolites of ibopamine identified in the rat and the dog (^{14}C label is denoted by).

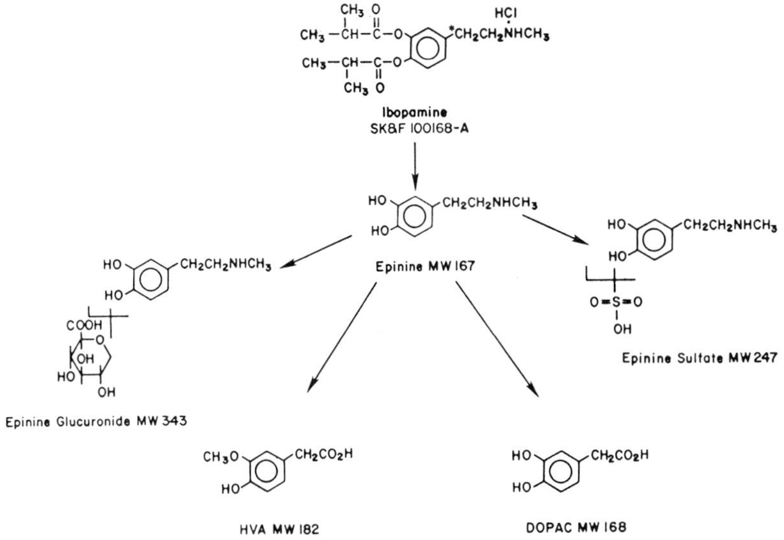

EXPERIMENTAL

Mass Spectrometry. HPLC-MS/MS experiments were carried out on a tandem quadrupole mass spectrometer ("TSQ-15", Finnigan-MAT, San Jose, CA), equipped with a Finnigan thermospray ion source. Typical operating temperatures were : vaporizer 140°C; jet 190-200°C aerosol 220-240°C. An electron filament was not employed. A Beckman "Ultrasphere" octadecyl-silanecolumn (4.6mm x 25cm, 5μ particle size) was used for all separations. A linear gradient of 50 mM ammonium acetate (pH 4.0) and methanol was used (2% organic for 5 min then 2% --> 30% in 20 min) at a flow rate of 1.2 ml/min. HPLC-MS/MS analyses were carried out on 20μl samples of filtered urine obtained from male Cynomolgus monkeys which had received 350 or 35 mg/kg of SK&F 100168-A-[14]C (ibopamine; "A" refers to the hydrochloride salt) in distilled water by gavage. The urine samples were injected directly onto the HPLC column without prior extraction and were determined by liquid scintillation counting to contain between 10ng and several μg of each component.

RESULTS AND DISCUSSION

By designing an appropriate set of precursor and neutral loss scans, a relatively complete characterisation of the metabolic fate of a given drug can be achieved during a single chromatographic analysis. In effect, the MS/MS instrument can work as a specific detector for glucuronides or other conjugates. For example, figure 2 shows the total ion current (TIC) and four reconstructed ion chromatograms (RIC) obtained when an experiment that is diagnostic for 0-glucuronides (a neutral loss scan of 176 amu) is carried out using a 20µl injection of monkey urine. The TIC indicates the presence of a major component with a retention time similar to that of epinine glucuronide, as well as a number of additional minor components. The mass spectrum of the major component consists primarily of two ions, m/z 168 amd m/z 18. The precursor ion to m/z 168 is (168 + 176) = m/z 344, which corresponds to protonated epinine glucuronide. The ion at m/z 18 (NH_4^+) is derived from (18 + 176) = m/z 194, which corresponds to an ammoniated glucuronic acid ion. A reconstructed ion chromatogram for m/z 18 is also shown in Figure 2, and it is evident that the intensity of this ion parallels that of the TIC observed with this experiment; hence, co-maximisation of m/z 18 with another ion under the conditions of a neutral loss of 176 provides strong evidence for the presence of an 0-glucuronide. This is demonstrated by a consideration of two other components that are evident in Figure 2, with retention times of ca. 6.5 min and 13 min. The component at 13 min. has a neutral loss spectrum which consists principally of two ions, of m/z 18 and m/z 200. This is consistent with a glucuronide of homovanillic acid (HVA) or its isomer (3-hydroxy-4-methoxy-phenylacetic acid) and the full scan (Q1) mass spectrum of this component confirms the presence of an ion corresponding to $(M+NH_4)^+$ for this conjugate at m/z 376. The second minor component (A_1) evident in Figure 2, eluting immediately after epinine glucuronide, gives a neutral loss spectrum consisting of the ions m/z 18 and m/z 182; this is consistent with an 0-methyl-epinine glucuronide. The full scan mass spectrum of this component gives the expected protonated molecular ion at m/z 358. There are additional components which are evident in the neutral loss 176 amu TIC of Figure 2 that appear to be glucuronides, but a detailed analysis of their mass spectra, and the absence of ^{14}C radiolabel peaks, suggest that they are not drug-related.

Oxidative deamination is a common metabolic pathway for

Figure 2. Reconstructed ion chromatograms for a TSP-MS/MS experiment (neutral loss 176 amu) obtained with a 20μl sample of monkey urine : m/z 18, 168, 200, total ion current (TIC).

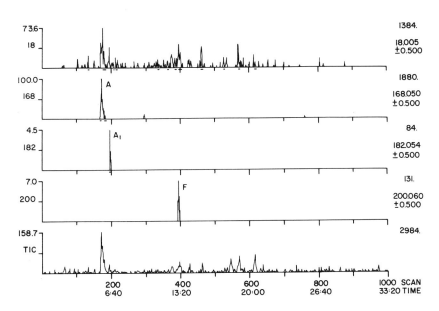

amines and the presence of metabolites which contain a carboxylic acid can be detected by a neutal loss scan of 44 amu in the negative ion mode. This scan results in two major peaks with neutral loss spectra consisting of m/z 123 and m/z 137. These ions are derived from precursor ions at m/z 167 and m/z 181 which correspond to the (M-H)$^-$ ions of dihydroxyphenylacetic acid (DOPAC) and HVA, respectively. A comparison of their retention times and CAD spectra with synthetic standards confirms their identification. HPLC-MS/MS was also used to identify two sulphate conjugates of epinine. Reconstructed ion chromatograms (RIC) of daughter ion spectra of m/z 248 (MH$^+$ for epinine sulphate) show two major components that give identical CAD spectra, both of which are identical to those obtained for synthetic epinine sulphate. Comparison of LC retention times with synthetic standards confirms that both the 3 and the 4 isomers are present.

These results demonstrate the utility of HPLC-MS/MS for the rapid identification of metabolites in an unextracted biological sample. Using this technique, all of the major urinary metabolites (> 98% of the ^{14}C radiolabel) of ibopamine in the monkey were identified and shown to be qualitatively similar to those isolated from both the rat and the dog.

REFERENCES

Boyce, M., Dalton, N., Goodwin, B., Walker, P., Weg, M., Sandler, M. (1985), Br. J. Clin. Pharmacol, 19, 143P.

Dei Cas, L., Bolognesi, R., Cucchini, F., Fappani, A., Riva, S. (1983). J. Cardiovascular Pharmacol, 5, 249.

Hwang, B.Y-H., Kuo, G.Y., Lynn, R.L. (1984). IUPHAR 9th Internatl. Congress of Pharmacology, London, Abstract No. 523P.

HPLC PROCEDURES FOR DRUG METABOLISM STUDIES : THE POTENTIAL OF COLUMN SWITCHING.

J. Schmid and W. Roth

Department of Biochemistry, Dr. Karl Thomae GmbH,
D-7950 Biberach, FRG.

INTRODUCTION

The growing importance of the understanding of drug action and toxicity in different species has resulted in an increased pressure and need for analytical methods which provide a basis for the quantification of drug and metabolites in biological fluids. It is the aim of this paper to outline some principles of HPLC with column switching for metabolic studies (Roth et al, 1981).

MATERIALS AND METHODS

HPLC Equipment

A diagram of the equipment is given in Figure 1. An isocractic pump 1 model 300B (Gyncotek Munich FRG) transfers the contents (urine, plasma) of the loop (2 ml) with a flow rate of 1.5 ml/min (0.1M ammonium acetate) to the precolumn (40 mm x 4.6 mm i.d) filled with Bondapak C-18 Porasil (37-75μm). The switching values are type 7001 (Rheodyne).
Most of the metabolites are retained on the reverse-phase, whereas polar compounds such as salts and proteins are flushed from the column. This is monitored by a combination of diode-array- and radio-detector.
After two minutes, valve 2 (lower part of Figure 1) connects the precolumn to the main column 260 mm x 4.6 mm i.d filled with Hypersil ODS 5μm and the gradient pump 2 model 5060 (Varian) is beginning to transfer the sample (vice backflush) onto the main column. Simultaneously, valve 3 is switched to bring the effluent to the detector. After 7 minutes with 0.1M ammonium acetate a gradient is started to 100% methanol within 27 min. At the end of the run, the gradient pump 2 equilibrates the main column and the pump 1, the precolumn.

Figure 1. HPLC column switching unit.

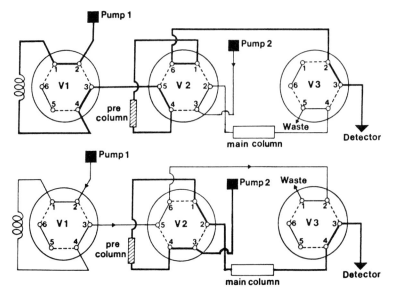

HPLC conditions for preparative runs : Precolumn conical
shape (Ruijten et al, 1984) length 40mm diameter 35mm (top)
16mm (bottom) filled with Porasil B 37-75µm, maincolumn 300
x 8 mm 5 µm Hypersil ODS. The precolumn is loaded with 200
ml urine with a flow of 10ml/min. The maincolumn is run
with a flow of 5ml/min and a gradient with solvents as
above over 120 min.
Sample preparation for faeces : 1g faeces is diluted with
3ml of methanol, mixed for 1 hour, the residue is spun
down, 0.2ml thereof is diluted with 0.8ml of buffer (as
above) [to reduce elution strength] and the whole sample is
injected onto the precolumn (further process as above).
Sample preparation for microsomes : 4ml buffer-solution (pH
7.4) containing up to 10mg microsomal protein are directly
injected onto the precolumn with a flow of 2ml/min (further
process as above).

Drug ^{14}C-labelled Pimobendan with a specific activity of
4.6 mCi/nMol was used (Formulae Figure 2).
Animals : 5 male baboons received an oral dose of 5mg/kg
Pimobendan.

RESULTS

    In Figure 2 the main metabolites of Pimobendan are
depicted: The demethylation product (M1), a sulphate

Figure 2. Pimobendan and its metabolites

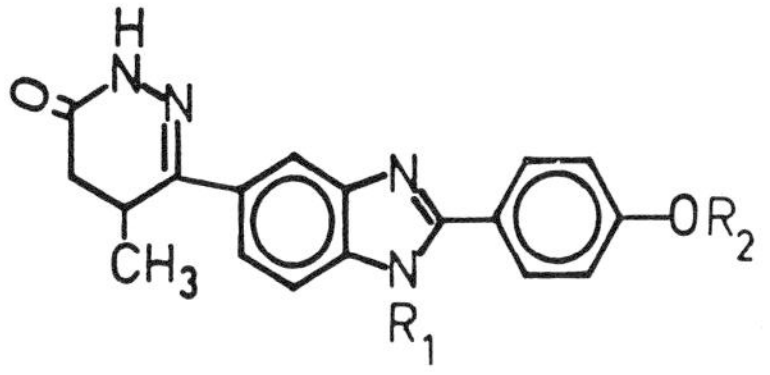

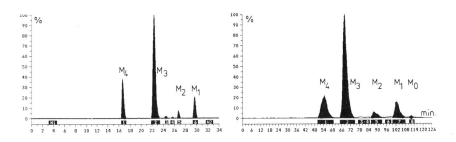

	R₁	R₂
Parent compound	H	CH₃
M₁	H	H
M₂	H	SO₃⁻
M₃	Gluc. acid	CH₃
M₄	Gluc. acid	H

conjugate thereof (M2) and interestingly two N-glucuronides of the parent compound (M3) and of the M1 (M4).

In Figure 3 the metabolic pattern of Pimobendan in urine is depicted. The analytical and preparative runs are very similar. All metabolites are retained on the precolumn and properly separated by the main column. The extraction ratio for urine is > 99%. For faeces we found with the technique described above 85% and for microsomes 98.5%.

Figure 3. Metabolic pattern in urine of baboons after p.o. administration of 5 mg/kg ^{14}C-Pimobendan.

A : Analytical method   B : Preparative method.

DISCUSSION

HPLC with column switching is superior to all other methods for <u>metabolic pattern analysis</u> due to :

- Minimal sample pretreatment (no artifacts);
- Automatic injection of sample (day and night operation)
- Gradient formation and combination of different detectors,

- Automatic quantification of extraction yield and data handling.

The following biochemical requirements must be kept in mind before isolation of metabolites :

- Study the dose-dependency of metabolic patternsbefore isolating metabolites.
- Compare single-dose pattern versus steady-state pattern to detect metabolites with long elimination half-life.

On the other hand the parameters of separation established by an analytical method can be easily adapted to semi-preparative runs :

- The first preparative run should be performed with separation material similar to the one used in the analytical run, but with bigger columns and flatter gradients,
- Start with volumes of less than 500ml and repeat the first step 10 to 20 times, remaining close to the analytical procedure,
- Recheck isolated pure products in the analytical system used at the beginning, to detect artifacts.

ACKNOWLEDGEMENTS

The excellent collaboration of S. Kaschke and K. Beschke is greatly appreciated.

REFERENCES

Roth, W. et al, (1981). J. Chromatogr, 222, 13.
Ruijten, H.M. et al, (1984). J. Chromatogr, 314, 183.

N-METHYLACETAMIDE, UNLIKE N-METHYLFORMAMIDE, IS NOT A HEPATOTOXIN IN THE MOUSE : THE ROLE OF METABOLISM

Philip Kestell, Michael D. Threadgill and Andreas Gescher.

CRC Experimental Chemotherapy Group, Pharmaceutical Sciences Institute, Aston University, Birmingham. B4 7ET.

N-Alkylformamides are industrial solvents and recent investigations have shown some of them to be hepatotoxic. N-Methylformamide (NMF, $HCONHCH_3$) has attracted interest since apart from being a hepatotoxin it possesses anti-neoplastic properties (Gate et al, 1986). However, N-methylacetamide (NMA, $CH_3CONHCH_3$) a close structural analogue, has neither antineoplastic properties nor is it hepatotoxic at doses up to 3 g/kg in the CBA/CA mouse (Kestell et al, unpublished). It has been suggested that NMF is metabolised to a reactive intermediate which may be responsible for the liver damage (Whitby et al, 1984; Pearson et al, 1986 unpublished). As yet the precise mechanism of NMF toxicity has not been elucidated, partly due to the lack of appreciable biotransformation in vitro. However, NMF undergoes extensive metabolism in vivo and the major urinary metabolites have been identified as methylamine and S-(N-methylcarbamoyl)N-acetylcysteine (Kestell et al, 1985; 1986a). Little is known about the metabolism of NMA and so in an attempt to explain the difference in biological properties between NMA and NMF the metabolism of NMA was investigated in vivo.

Male CBA/CA mice (20-25g) received NMA (400 mg/kg) in saline by the i.p. route and urine was collected during a 24hr period both before and after administration. For the analysis of urinary methylamine, urine samples were treated with 2,4-dinitrofluorobenzene and extracted with ether. The extracts were examined by HPLC (Baba et al, 1984). The amount of methylamine excreted after NMA administration did not exceed the amount of methylamine found in control urine. Urine samples were also analysed by TLC according to the method described by Kestell et al, (1985, 1986a,b). There was no evidence of the formation of a drug-derived mercapturate. However when TLC plates were developed in a solvent consisting of benzene : acetone : acetic acid (3 :

2 : 2, v/v) and sprayed with phenylhydrazine/ferric chloride reagent (Nair and Francis, 1980), a material (Rf = 0.48) was detected by colour reaction. This metabolite was absent from control urine samples. It was isolated by preparative TLC and analysed by 400mHz ^{1}H-NMR using D_2O as solvent. In the resulting spectrum three major signals were observed: 2.03 (s,3H), 4.69 (s,2H) and 4.92 (s,DOH). Authentic N-(hydroxymethyl)acetamide gave an identical spectrum. Quantitation of this metabolite by GLC (Gescher et al, 1982) revealed that 54±10% (mean± s.d, n=5) of the dose was excreted as the carbinolamide within 24 hrs after administration.

   The results of this study suggest that NMA is extensively metabolised in vivo with C-hydroxylation at the N-methyl group to give N-(hydroxymethyl)-acetamide ($CH_3CONHCH_2OH$). It is noteworthy that dimethylformamide also undergoes N-methyl C-hydroxylation as a major metabolic pathway (Kestell et al, 1986b). This is in contrast to NMF which undergoes oxidative metabolism predominantly in the formyl group. Whereas formyl oxidation may well be the prelude to hepatotoxicity, N-methyl C-hydroxylation appears to be a detoxification reaction.

REFERENCES

Baba, S., Watanabe, F., Gejyo, F. and Arakawa, M. (1984). Clin. Chim. Acta, 136, 49.

Gate, E.N., Threadgill, M.D., Stevens, M.F.G., Chubb, D., Vickers, L.M., Langdon, S.P., Hickman, J.A. and Gescher, A. (1986). J. Med. Chem (in press).

Gescher, A., Gibson, N.W., Hickman, J.A., Langdon, S.P., Ross, D. and Atassi, G. (1982). Br. J. Cancer, 45, 843.

Kestell, P., Gescher, A. and Slack, J.A. (1985). Drug Metab. Dispos, 13, 587.

Kestell, P., Gledhill, A.P., Threadgill, M.D. and Gescher, A. (1986a). Biochem. Pharmacol, in press.

Kestell, P., Gill, M.H., Threadgill, M.D., Gescher, A., Howarth, O.W. and Curzon, E.H. (1986b). Life Sci, 38, 719.

Nair, B.R. and Francis, J.D. (1980). J. Chromatog, 195, 158.

Whitby, H., Gescher, A. and Levy, L. (1984). Biochem. Pharmacol, 33, 295.

5. Probes for
drug metabolizing enzymes.

SUBSTRATES AND INHIBITORS AS PROBES OF INDIVIDUAL FORMS OF DRUG METABOLISING SYSTEMS

M. Danny Burke[1] and C. Roland Wolf[2]

[1]Department of Pharmacology, University of Aberdeen, Aberdeen, AB9 1AS, UK., [2]Imperial Cancer Research Fund, Laboratory of Molecular Pharmacology, Department of Biochemistry, Edinburgh, UK

INTRODUCTION

The majority of the enzymes involved in drug metabolism exist as multiple forms or isozymes. In many studies, for example the effects of a disease or a chemical on drug metabolism, it is, therefore, essential to distinguish, identify and measure the individual enzyme forms. Substrates and inhibitors have been used for this purpose ever since the discovery of the multiplicity of drug metabolising enzymes, but the success of this approach depends on the degree of specificity shown by each of the different forms of an enzyme. This paper reviews the substrates and inhibitors that have been commonly employed to measure individual forms of drug metabolising enzymes and assesses the extent to which their use has been successful. It concentrates on studies with rat liver in order to provide some continuity between enzymes and is highly selective in its coverage, dealing mainly with the cytochromes P-450 but also discussing briefly the epoxide hydrolases, glutathione transferases and UDP-glucuronyl-transferases.

The history of the use of substrates as probes for individual forms of drug metabolising enzymes encompasses the history of the discovery and developing understanding of these enzymes. Observations that inducing agents, such as phenobarbitone (PB) and 3-methylcholanthrene (3MC), selectively increased some drug metabolism reactions rather than others were among the first clues that there are multiple forms of the enzymes (Lu and West, 1979). The finding that a particular reaction is selectively induced by one agent rather than by others is still amongst the most persuasive that the reaction is a selective probe for

the form of the drug metabolising enzyme induced by that
agent. More recently the study of drug metabolism has
acquired, in antibodies, a new method of probing the
individual enzyme forms. The combined use of isozyme-
selective substrates and isozyme-specific inhibitory
antibodies gives the most powerful means yet of measuring
functionally active individual forms of drug metabolising
enzymes.

     This Workshop celebrates the career of Dennis Parke and
this year is the twentieth anniversary of the publication
by Dennis V. Parke and his then student, Paddy Creaven, of
a paper that was probably the first report of a substrate
showing regio-selectivity for two different forms of a drug
metabolising enzyme, cytochrome P-450 (Creaven and Parke,
1966). The paper reported the differential induction by PB
and 3MC of the 2- and 4-hydroxylations of biphenyl.
Remarkably, it was published two years before a paper
asking whether cytochrome P-450 was one haemoprotein or
many (Hildebrandt et al, 1968) and another nine years
elapsed before the different biphenyl hydroxylase
specficities of pure PB-induced and 3MC-induced forms of
cytochrome P-450 were demonstrated conclusively (Burke and
Mayer, 1975). As well as providing possibly the first
indication that there was more than one form of cytochrome
P-450, Dennis Parke also published the first report that
isosafrole (ISF) induces yet a different form of the
haemoprotein (Parke and Rahman, 1971).

EPOXIDE HYDROLASES

     Four different forms of epoxide hydrolase have been
identified and three of them have very different
specificities for substrates and inhibitors (Table 1). The
nomenclature of the four forms in Table 1 is not an agreed
system, merely a convenient one of our own, and EH 1 is the
form most commonly measured as "the" epoxide hydrolase.
Substrates and inhibitors can act as very specific probes
for these multiple forms of epoxide hydrolase.

UDP-GLUCURONYLTRANSFERASES

     Although it is agreed that there are multiple forms of
UDP-glucuronyltransferases, there is no consensus as to how
many exist. The categorisation of UDP-glucuronyltransferases relies heavily on differences in substrate
specificity. Five forms are listed in Table 2, based on
differences in substrate specificity and isoelectric point
of the purified enzymes and on differences in the

Table 1. Specificities of rat liver epoxide hydrolase.

EPOXIDE HYDROLASE	SUBSTRATES	INHIBITORS
EH I microsomal pH opt 8.5-9	cis-mono- and di-substituted oxiranes, styrene 7,8-oxide, benzo(a)pyrene 4,5-oxide, phenanthrene 9,10-oxide	TCPO (trichloro- propeneoxide)
EH II microsomal pH opt. 6.8-7.2	trans-1,2-disubstituted oxiranes, trans-stilbene oxide	4PCO (4-phenyl- chalcone oxide)
EH III microsomal	Δ5-steroid epoxides cholesterol 5,6-oxide	α-imino- cholesterol
EH IV cytosolic	trans-1,2-disubstituted oxiranes, trans-stilbene oxide	4PCO

Table compiled from Guengerich (1983), Guenthner (1986), Guenthner and Oesch (1983), Hammock and Hasagawa (1983), Levin et al (1983), Mullin and Hammock (1982) and Oesch et al (1984).

inducibility of microsomal reactions by PB and 3MC. The isoelectric point data are from mice, whilst the specificity and induction data are from rats, and it may not be valid to combine this information from two species. Transferase forms A (ii) and C are apparently constitutive, non-inducible forms in mice and rats respectively. Except for bilirubin glucuronyltransferase, it is doubtful whether substrate specificity differences are sufficiently great to allow the use of substrates alone to distinguish between forms of UDP-glucuronyltransferase.

GLUTATHIONE TRANSFERASES

At least ten isozymes of rat glutathione transferase have been identified (Mannervik, 1985) and the substrate selectivities of the major hepatic, cytosolic forms are summarised in Table 3. The differences in substrate selectivity are probably large enough to distinguish

Table 2. Specificities of liver microsomal UDP-glucuronyl-transferases.

UDP-GLUCURONYL TRANSFERASE	SUBSTRATE	INDUCTION[1]	IEP[2]
A	1-Naphthol	0.4	8.5
	3-OH-Benzo(a)pyrene	0.3	8.5
A (ii)	1-Naphthol	control	6.7
B	Bilirubin	2.2	ND
C	Oestrone	(nil)	8.5
	Phenolphthalein	(nil)	8.5
D	4-Hydroxybiphenyl	3.4	6.7
	Chloramphenicol	3.3	ND

[1]Ratio of inducibility by PB (PB-induced specific activity/control specific activity) to inducibility by 3MC (3MC-induced specific activity/control specific activity) for rat liver microsomes. Control = results apply to control microsomes only. Nil = reaction not inducible by PB or 3MC.
[2]Isoelectric point measured in mouse liver microsomes. ND = not determined.
Table compiled from Burchell (1981), Mackenzie et al (1985) and Ullrich and Bock (1984).

experimentally between certain of these, and other (Hayes and Chalmers, 1983) isozymes. Mannervik et al (1985) have proposed that glutathione transferases can be grouped into three classes, distinguishable by a combination of their substrate and inhibitor specificities. Class alpha (rat isozymes 1-1, 1-2 and 2-2) is distinguished by high activity with cumene hydroperoxide and a lower IC_{50} value for inhibition by haematin than for inhibition by Cibacron blue. Class pi (rat isozyme 7-7 present in kidney) shows substrate selectivity for ethacrynic acid and a higher IC_{50} with haematin than with Cibacron blue. Class mu (rat isozymes 3-3 and 4-4) shows substrate selectivity for phenylbutenone and a low IC_{50} with triphenyltin chloride.
Glutathione transferase reactions are induced by PB, 3MC, trans-stilbene oxide (TSO) and propylthiourea (PTU), but the degrees of induction are small and there is no clearly selective induction of particular reactions that could be

Table 3. Specificities of the major rat liver glutathione transferases.

SUBSTRATE	GLUTATHIONE TRANSFERASE ISOZYME					
	1-1	1-2	2-2	3-3	3-4	4-4
	activity of pure isozyme (μ moles/min/mg protein)					
Chlorodi-nitrobenzene	33	28	19	38	28	18
Dichloro-nitrobenzene	0.05	0.03	0.05	4	3	0.2
Phenylbutenone	0	0	0	0.05	0.05	1.4
Ethacrynic acid	0.2	0.6	1.3	0.2	0.4	0.8
Androstenedione	4	2	0.4	0.02	0.01	0.002
Bromosulpho-phthalein	0	0	0	0.8	0.3	0.03
Cumene hydro-peroxide	3	4	7	0.5	0.6	1.0

For each substrate the rate with the most active isozyme is underlined.
Table compiled from Jakoby and Habig (1980), Jakoby et al (1984), Mannervik (1985), Mannervik and Jensson (1982) and Mannervik et al (1985).

used to indicate the substrate specificities of individual induced isozymes (Table 4).

CYTOCHROMES P-450

The number of identified forms of cytochrome P-450 is growing all the time. Some forms of cytochrome P-450 are involved in physiological reactions, e.g. steroid and prostaglandin synthesis. These "physiological cytochromes P-450" are generally highly substrate-specific, allowing substrates to be used as probes for them. The majority of cytochromes P-450, however, are able to participate in the metabolism of many different foreign compounds and substrates are far less adequate probes for these "xenobiotic cytochromes P-450". Table 5 lists several forms of cytochrome P-450 for which highly distinctive substrates have been suggested.
    Inducibility is one of the most characteristic features

Table 4. Induction of glutathione transferase activities[1]

Substrate	PB	3MC	TSO	PTU
	(fold induction over control)			
Chlorodinitrobenzene	2.3	1.8	4.0	1.7
Dichloronitrobenzene	2.1	1.4	3.3	1.2
Ethacrynic acid	1.5	1.5	ND	1.8
Butylene oxide	1.1	1.5	ND	ND

[1] Results show the induction by PB, 3MC, trans-stilbene oxide (TSO) or propylthiouracil (PTU), based on specific activities for rat liver cytosol.
Table compiled from Baars et al (1978), Clifton and Kaplowitz (1978), Guthenberg et al (1980) and Lee et al (1986).

of many forms of "xenobiotic cytochrome P-450" and the differential induction of microsomal monooxygenase reactions (i.e. induction of a reaction primarily by one category of agent and induction of a different reaction primarily by another category of agent) has been key evidence for the classification of multiple forms of the enzyme. A microsomal reaction that is induced by an agent is probably catalysed by the form(s) of cytochrome P-450 induced by the same agent. The greater the degree of induction and the fewer the number of different types of agent that induce the reaction, the more specific the reaction probably is for one form (or family of co-induced forms) of cytochrome P-450. In view of the large degree of overlap in specificity between different purified forms of cytochrome P-450, however, selectivity is probably a more correct term than specificity. Metabolic selectivity takes the form of either compound-selectivity or regio-selectivity. A substrate showing compound-selectivity is metabolised by only one reaction (or at least only one reaction is measured) and this is catalysed by one form of cytochrome P-450 in preference to others; the most selective (and therefore most useful) examples of such substrates are each probes for only one form of cytochrome P-450. A compound showing regio-selectivity is metabolised at more than one position on the molecule and the reaction at each different position is catalysed preferentially by a

Table 5. Reaction selectivities of individual cytochrome P-450 forms.

P-450 FORM[1]	DISTINCTIVE REACTION
2c (h, UT-A)	Testosterone 2α-hydroxylation
	Androstenedione 16α-hydroxylation
2d (i, UT-I)	Steroid disulphate 15β-hydroxylation
3 (a, UT-F)	Testosterone 7α- hydroxylation
	Androstenedione 7α- hydroxylation
UT-H	Debrisoquine 4-hydroxylation
PB-1 (PB-C)	S-Warfarin 7-hydroxylation
PB-2a (PCN-E)	Androstenedione 6β-hydroxylation
	Triacetyloleandomycin complexation
PB-4 (b, PB-B)	Androstenedione 16β- hydroxylation
	Pentoxyresorufin O-dealkylation
BNF-B (c)	Ethoxyresorufin O-deethylation
ISF-G (d)	Methoxyresorufin O-demethylation
	Oestradiol 2-hydroxylation
P-452	Lauric acid 12-hydroxylation
Vitamin D_3 25-hydroxylase	
Cholesterol 7α- hydroxylase	
Steroid synthetases	
Prostaglandin synthetases	

[1]Equivalent forms are shown in parentheses.
Table compiled from Burke, Mayer and Wolf (unpublished),
Ryan et al (1982), Tamburini et al (1984), Waxman et al
(1985) and Waxman (1986).

different form of cytochrome P-450; such substrates are
probes for several forms of cytochrome P-450. Tables 6-9
list commonly used substrates showing compound- or regio-
selectivity for cytochrome P-450, as evidenced either from
differential induction of their microsomal reactions or
from direct study of the major purified constitutive and
induced froms of cytochrome P-450.
    Harmine hydroxylation and harmol oxidation are
reactions that we have recently found to be good indicators

for 3MC-induced cytochrome P-450 (Tweedie and Burke, 1986;
Figure 1). Noteworthy substrates additional to those
listed in Tables 6-9 are p-nitrophenol and 1-[3-
(diethylamino)propyl]amino-9-methoxyellipticine, which are
compound-selective for ethanol- and 3MC-induced cytochrome
P-450 respectively, and lauric acid, which is regio-
selective at the 12-position for clofibrate- induced
cytochrome P-450. The relative microsomal specific
activities of p-nitrophenol hydroxylation are 16%
(control), 100% (ethanol-induced), 28% (PB-induced) and 25%
(β-naphthoflavone [BNF]-induced) (Reinke and Moyer, 1985).
1-[3-(diethylamino)propyl]amino-9-methoxyellipticine is O-
demethylated by 3MC-induced but not by control or PB-
induced microsomes, whereas neither 9-methoxyellipticine
nor ellipticine differentiate clearly between these types
of induction (Lesca et al., 1977; Roy et al., 1985). The
relative microsomal specific activities of laurate 12-
hydroxylation are 3% (control), 100% clofibrate-induced
and 10% (PB-induced) (Orton and Parker, 1982). In
contrast, the differences in the rate of laurate 11-
hydroxylation between control, clofibrate- and PB-induced
microsomes are less than 2-fold (Orton and Parker, 1982),
whilst BNF induces neither the 11- nor the 12-hydroxylation
(Okita and Masters, 1980).

In studies of, for example, the ability of a disease or
a chemical to increase or decrease drug metabolism, it is
probably adequate and valid to interpret a differential
effect on the microsomal metabolism of compound-selective
and regio-selective model substrates as evidence that the
effect on cytochrome P-450 is "selective among the
different forms". With the exception of the "physiological
cytochromes P-450" it is probably not valid, however, to
define, on the basis of substrate probes alone, precisely
which forms of cytochrome P-450 are affected. The
following few lines indicate some of the problems commonly
encountered in the interpretation of results. An agent may
induce several different forms of cytochrome P-450 to
differing extents and in such instances it may not be clear
which induced forms are primarily responsible for an
increase in a reaction rate measured in microsomes (e.g.
PB-induced ethylmorphine N-demethylation : Elshourbagy and
Guzelian, 1980; Guengerich et al., 1982). Alternatively a
microsomal reaction may be inducible by several agents each
known to induce a different form of cytochrome P-450 (e.g.
ethoxycoumarin O-deethylase: Tables 6 and 8): in such a
case it would be difficult to decide into which category of
inducing agent to place a newly investigated compound.
Conversely, sometimes, as with the ISF-, troleandomycin

Figure 1. Differentially induced metabolism of harmine and harmol.

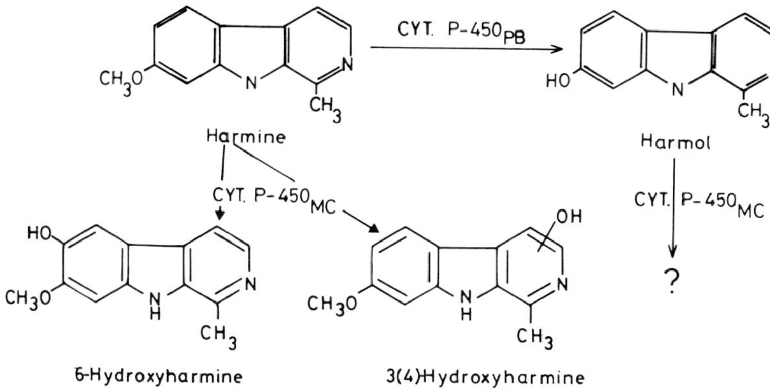

Harmine

Harmol

6-Hydroxyharmine

3(4)Hydroxyharmine

The arrow labels show whether the rate of production of the metabolite by rat liver microsomal cyt. P-450 is induced primarily by PB or by MC. The identity of the product of 3MC-induced harmol metabolism is not known.

(TAO)- and SKF 525A-induced forms of cytochrome P-450, the induced form is inhibited by a stable complex formed with a metabolite of the inducing agent, and in these cases an increase in microsomal reaction rate is often not seen (Delaforge et al., 1983; Dickins et al., 1979; Pershing and Franklin, 1982: Synder and Remmer, 1982). In the early days of the study of cytochrome P-450 an induction of 2- or 3-fold in a microsomal reaction rate was considered a highly significant effect, but more recently it has become clear that inductions of 50- to 200- fold can occur in the immuno-quantifiable levels of individual forms of cytochrome P-450 protein (although both metabolically active haemoprotein and inactive apoprotein may be included in the measurement). In many instances a probable explanation for an induction of less than 10-fold in a microsomal reaction is that the reaction is catalysed significantly by both constitutive and induced form(s), e.g. benzphetamine N-demethylation (Tables 6 and 8). Sometimes, when studied with purified cytochrome P-450 a reaction is highly selective for one induced form of the enzyme, yet the same reaction measured in microsomes shows evidence of only weak inducibility and no clear selectivity as to which agents it is induced by (e.g. aminopyrine N-

Table 6. Compound-selectivity with induced liver
microsomal cytochrome P-450.

SUBSTRATE	UT	PB	INDUCER[1] PCN (relative activity)	BNF/3MC	ISF	
Acetanilide	22	41	46	100	59	a
Aldrin	24	68	100(F)	12	ND	b
Aminopyrine	54	100	85	42	63	a
Aniline	29	44	34	29	100	a
Benzo(a)pyrene	19	31	19	100	43	a
Benzphetamine	28	100	39	17	42	a
4-Butoxybiphenyl	14	25	ND	100	ND	c
4-Methoxybiphenyl	38	100	ND	54	ND	c
Cyclohexane	16	100	ND	12	ND	d
Dichloro-p-nitroanisole	4	100	ND	5	ND	e
Erythromycin	25	ND	100	ND	ND	f
Ethoxycoumarin (high [s])	7	32	12	100	34	a
Methoxycoumarin	48	100	ND	39	35	g,h
Ethoxyresorufin	1	10	8	100	21	i
Benzyloxyresorufin	1	100	4	13	39	i
Methoxyresorufin	2	59	5	100	14	i
Pentoxyresorufin	1	100	6	1	11	i
Ethylmorphine (M)	44	100	91	24	91	a
Ethylmorphine (F)	10	44	100	22	ND	j
p-Nitroanisole	10	100	8	56	46	a
Theophylline	16	27	20	100	ND	k
Zoxazolamine	25	32	40	100	ND	l

[1]Relative activities in liver microsomes from untreated
(UT) rats and rats induced with PB, pregnenolone 16 -
carbonitrile (PCN), BNF or MC (BNF/MC) or isosafrole (ISF).
Results along rows are relative percentages of the activity
in the most active type of microsomes. Comparisons are
valid along rows but not down columns. Results for any
particular substrate are for the same reaction measured
with all the different types of microsomes.
ND= not determined.
F = specifically female rats. M = specifically male rats.
a - Guengerich et al (1982)   b - Wolff and Strecker (1985)
c - Davies and Creaven (1967) d - Ullrich (1969)
e - Hultmark et al (1979)   f - Wrighton et al (1985)
g - Kamataki et al (1980)   h - Matsubara et al (1983)
i - Burke et al (1985)   j - Lu et al (1972)
k- Lohmann and Miech (1976)   l- Tomaszewski et al (1976)

Table 7. Regio-selectivity with induced liver microsomal cytochrome P-450.

SUBSTRATE	METABOLITE	UT	PB	PCN	3MC	ISF	
				(relative activity)			
Androstenedione	6β-OH	28	80	100	20	93	a
	7α-OH	43	83	52	57	100	
	16α-OH	100	80	65	42	30	
	16β-OH	4	100	7	2	24	
Antipyrine	3-OHMe	100	85	ND	76	ND	b
	4-OH	44	100	ND	54	ND	
	2-Nor	37	100	ND	30	ND	
Biphenyl	2-OH	4	12	21	100	87	c
	3-OH	4	100	4	25	ND	
	4-OH	21	100	13	36	100	
Harmine	harmol	24	100	ND	39	ND	d
	6-OH	4	5	ND	100	ND	
	3(4)-OH	3	9	ND	100	ND	
n-Hexane	1-OH	21	70	26	100	ND	e
	2-OH	15	100	16	8	ND	
	3-OH	11	100	32	58	ND	
Testosterone	6β-OH	27	60	100	26	ND	f
	7α-OH	41	100	92	96	ND	
	16α-OH	2	100	3	3	ND	
R-Warfarin	7-OH	12	100	14	7	9	g
	8-OH	5	50	5	100	36	
	10-OH	9	59	100	4	32	

The INDUCER[1] column spans UT, PB, PCN, 3MC, ISF.

[1]Footnotes and abbreviations as for Table 6.

a - Waxman et al (1985)
b - Kahn et al (1982)
c - Billings and McMahon (1978); Lake et al (1973)
d - Tweedie and Burke (1986)
e - Frommer and Ullrich (1974); Toftgard and Nilsen (1982)
f - Lu et al (1976)
g - Guengerich et al (1982)

Table 8. Compound-selectivity with purified forms of rat cytochrome P-450.

SUBSTRATE	UT-A	PB-B	FORM[1] PCN-E (relative	BNF-B activity)	ISF-G	
Acetanilide	13	9	11	100	9	a
Aminopyrine	20	100	11	26	34	a
Aniline	32	95	5	32	100	a
Benzo(a)pyrene	40	34	13	100	22	a
Benzphetamine	40	100	3	18	15	a
p-Nitroanisole	2	61	2	100	5	a
Ethoxycoumarin (high [s])	9	34	3	100	13	a
Ethylmorphine	100	54	4	20	11	a[2]
Methoxyresorufin	11	3	ND	33	100	b
Ethoxyresorufin	2	<1	<1	100	10	a,b
Pentoxyresorufin	<1	100	ND	7	7	b
Benzyloxyresorufin	3	100	ND	77	19	b

[1]Relative activities with a purified constitutive form of rat liver cytochrome P-450 (UT) and the major forms induced by phenobarbitone (PB-), pregnenolone 16α-carbonitrile (PCN-), β-naphthoflavone (BNF-) or isosafrole (ISF-). Results along rows are relative percentages of the activity in the most active type of microsomes. Comparisons are valid along rows but not down columns. Results for any particular substrate are for the same reaction measured with all the different types of microsomes. ND = not determined.

[2]123% relative ethylmorphine N-demethylase activity is given by form PB-C.

a - Guengerich et al (1982)
b - Burke, Mayer and Wolf (unpublished).

demethylation; Figure 2). Such a discrepancy might be due to the involvement of unidentified forms of cytochrome P-450 in the reaction or a loss of activity upon purification of certain forms, e.g. the major PCN induced form loses ethylmorphine N-demethylation and TAO complexation activity

Table 9. Regio-selectivity with purified forms of rat cytochrome P-450.

SUBSTRATE	METABOLITE	UT-A	PB-B	PBN-E	BNF-B	ISF-G	
				(relative activity)			
Warfarin	(S)7-OH	4	9	9	100	2	a[2]
	(R)8-OH	5	5	0	100	5	a
	(R)10-OH	100	12	56	6	3	a
Testosterone	7α-OH	100[3]	<1	ND	2	<1	b
	16α-OH	<.1	100	ND	5	3	b
	6β-OH	19	19	ND	86	100	b

The header FORM[1] spans UT-A PB-B PBN-E BNF-B ISF-G.

[1]Footnotes and abbreviations as for Table 8.
[2]509% relative (S)-warfarin 7-hydroxylase activity is given by form PB-C.
[3]Testosterone results are for a constitutive form equivalent to UT-F, which has a different selectivity from UT-A.
a - Guengerich et al (1982)   b - Ryan et al (1980)

(Elshourbagy and Guzelian, 1980; Wrighton et al., 1985). In other instances observed induced microsomal reaction rates are much less than the theoretical rates calculated from turnover numbers of purified cytochrome P-450 forms and their immunologically determined microsomal content (e.g. p-nitroanisole 0-demethylation; Figure 3). A likely explanation for this is that there is more catalytically inactive (but nevertheless antigenic) cytochrome P-450 apoprotein than there is active holoprotein.

It appears that, even for the most selective substrates, the correlations between results with purified cytochrome P-450 and results with microsomes are not yet good enought to allow the confident use of substrates alone as probes for many individual forms of "xenobiotic cytochrome P-450".

INHIBITORS OF CYTOCHROME P-450.

The major inhibitors used to differentiate between functionally active forms of cytochrome P-450 are listed in

Figure 2. Aminopyrine N-demethylase activities of different forms of purified cytochrome P-450 and differently induced microsomes from rat liver.

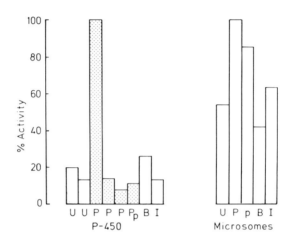

The 100% values for P-450 and for microsomes are <u>not</u> comparable with each other. U = two constitutive forms of cytochrome P-450 or microsomes from untreated rats. P = three different PB-induced forms of cytochrome P-450 or PB-induced microsomes. Pp = a cytochrome P-450 form induced by either PB or PCN. p = PCN-induced microsomes. B = the major BNF-induced form of cytochrome P-450 or BNF-induced microsomes. I = the major ISF-induced form of cytochrome P-450 or ISF-induced microsomes. Results from Guengerich <u>et</u> <u>al</u> (1982).

Table 10. The inhibitors are unlikely to identify individual cytochrome P-450 forms, but more probably characterise families of cytochrome P-450 forms having the same relevant reaction characteristics in common. It should not be assumed that the effects of an inhibitor reported for one reaction in a particular tissue or species will be the same when tested with a different reaction, tissue or species. α-Naphthoflavone (ANF) can very clearly distinguish polycyclic aromatic hydrocarbon (PAH, e.g. 3MC and BNF)-induced forms of cytochrome P-450 from constitutive or otherwise induced forms, but with the other inhibitors distinctions between forms of cytochrome P-450 are based on much smaller differences in IC_{50} values. In our opinion ellipticine and 9-hydroxyellipticine do not, as inhibitors, differentiate as clearly as ANF between PAH-

Figure 3. P-nitroanisole O-demethylase activities of differently induced microsomes from rat liver.

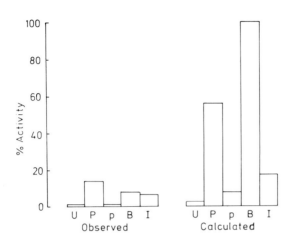

The 100% values for P-450 and for Observed and Calculated are comparable with each other. U = microsomes from untreated rats. P = PB-induced microsomes. p = PCN-induced microsomes. B = BNF-induced microsomes. I = ISF-induced microsomes. Observed = activities measured with microsomes. Calculated = activities for microsomes calculated from activities of pure constitutive or induced forms of cytochrome P-450 and the level of each form in microsomes. Results from Guengerich et al (1982).

induced and PB-induced forms of cytochrome P-450 (Delaforge et al., 1980; Lesca et al., 1978; 1979). However, a very clear distinction between PAH-induced and PB-induced cytochrome P-450 is given by a comparison of the apparent dissociation constants (Ks) of ellipticine and metyrapone for dithionite-reduced cytochrome P-450 (Lesca et al., 1980). Inhibitors are most able to identify particular types of cytochrome P-450 when used with substrates showing high selectivity for individual forms of the enzyme.

ALKOXYRESORUFINS

Ethoxyresorufin was introduced as a highly selective substrate for 3MC-induced cytochrome P-450 (Burke and Mayer, 1974, 1975). More recently certain members of a

homologous series of ethers based on ethoxyresorufin have
been synthesised and shown to be highly selective for other
induced forms of cytochrome P-450 (Tables 6 and 8; Burke
and Mayer, 1983; Burke et al., 1985). The coordinated use
of the parent compound, phenoxazone, and the methoxy,
ethoxy, pentoxy and benzyloxy ethers is especially powerful
in distinguishing cytochrome P-450 forms (Figure 4; Wolf et
al, 1986; Burke, Mayer and Wolf, unpublished).

When measuring induced microsomal alkoxyresorufin 0-
dealkylation rates it is essential not to use too high a
concentration of microsomal protein, otherwise although a
linear reaction rate may be seen, the true initial rate
will have been missed in the first few seconds and the
induced rate will be severely underestimated. When an
alkoxyresorufin is metabolised by microsomes containing
only a low concentration of the form of cytochrome P-450
for which the substrate is selective, i.e. from a rat
induced by the "wrong" type of agent, an initial lag-phase
or dip may be seen in the reaction time-curve. This is
probably due to reduction of the substrate, at the carbonyl
oxygen, to a non-fluorescent metabolite, catalysed by
NADPH-cytochrome P-450 reductase and occuring initially at
a faster rate than the cytochrome P-450 mediated 0-
dealkylation to fluorescent resorufin. We do not know
whether the "true" substrate for cytochrome P-450 is the
keto or the enol form of the alkoxyresorufin. The
reduction and accompanying decrease in fluorescence can be
seen by reacting an alkoxyresorufin with purified NADPH-
cytochrome P-450 reductase in the presence of NADPH: when
the NADPH is exhausted the reduced alkoxyresorufin
spontaneously reoxidises and the fluorescence returns to
the original level (Figure 5). With monooxygenase systems
reconstituted from purified cytochrome P-450 and NADPH-
cytochrome P-450 reductase three alternative patterns of
alkoxyresorufin reaction time-curve can be seen. If the
substrate is not metabolised by the form of cytochrome P-
450 used, an initial decrease of fluorescence and return to
the original level will occur, as in the solid line in
Figure 5. If the substrate is metabolised by the
cytochrome P-450, but only slowly, an initial decrease in
fluorescence will be followed by a steady increase beyond
the initial level, as in the dashed line in Figure 5. If
the substrate is metabolised more rapidly by the cytochrome
P-450 used, there will be an immediate rise in fluorescence
without any preceeding fall. The molar ratio between
cytochrome P-450 and its reductase will influence these
time-curves. Another problem when measuring
alkoxyresorufin 0-dealkylation with purified cytochrome P-

Table 10. Inhibitors of rat liver microsomal cytochrome P-450.

INHIBITOR	SELECTIVITY[1]	SUBSTRATE	
α-Naphtho flavone	3MC/BP>control>=PB	Benzo(a)pyrene[2]	a,b
		Ethoxyresorufin	c
		Ethoxycoumarin	
Metyrapone	PB>=control>3MC/BP	Ethoxycoumarin	d
		Ethoxyresorufin	c
		Benzo(a)pyrene	a
	PB>3MC>control	Dichloronitroanisole	e
SKF-525A	PB=control>3MC	Methylaminoazobenzene	f
		Benzo(a)pyrene[3]	g
	PB=control=3MC	Ethylmorphine	f
		Ethoxyresorufin	c
Tetrahydro- furan	Control=EtOH>PB=MC	Ethoxycoumarin	d
DMSO	Control >> 3MC	Benzo(a)pyrene	b
Ethanol	Control = 3MC>PB	Dichloronitroanisole	e
	Control > 3MC	Benzo(a)pyrene	b
	3MC > PB	Aldrin	h

[1]The relative sensitivities of different induced states or rat liver microsomal reactions are shown (i.e. PB > 3MC signifies that the reaction in PB-induced microsomes is inhibited to a greater extent that the reaction in 3MC-induced microsomes). Inducers: PB, phenobarbitone; 3MC, 3-methylcholanthrene; BP, benzo(a)pyrene; EtOH, ethanol.
[2]0.1mM α-naphthoflavone inhibits 3MC-induced microsomes but stimulates control microsomes (Ref. b).
[3]Results are for mouse liver microsomes.
a - Lesca et al (1978);   b - Wiebel et al (1971)
c - Burke et al (1977);   d - Ullrich et al (1975)
e - Hultmark et al (1979);   f - Sladek and Mannering (1969)
g - Goujon et al (1972);   h - Wolff (1980)

450 is that the type and concentration of buffer greatly influences the reaction rate (Figure 6; Burke, Mayer and Wolf, unpublished). To complicate matters further, the buffer effect is not the same for all the alkoxyresorufins or for all forms of cytochrome P-450.

Figure 4. Alkoxyresorufin O-dealkylase activities of purified forms of rat liver cytochrome P-450.

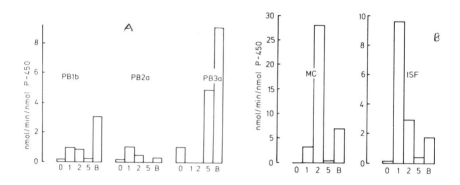

A : PB-induced forms 1b, 2a and 3a (the major PB-induced form).   B : the major MC-and ISF-induced forms.   The numbers below the bars indicate the substrate used: 0=phenoxazone (the unsubstituted parent compound of the homologous series of ethers); 1=methoxyresorufin; 2=ethoxyresorufin; 5=pentoxyresorufin; B=benzyloxyresorufin. Results from Burke, Mayer and Wolf (unpublished) and Wolf et al (1986).

Figure 5. Time course of ethoxyresorufin reduction and O-deethylase.

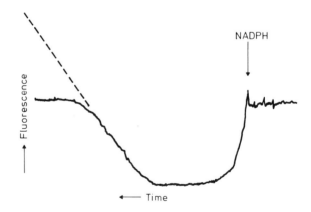

The figure shows a tracing from a chart recorder connected to a fluorimeter set to measure the fluorescence of

resorufin (the product of the O-deethylation reaction).
Solid line tracing: the reaction mixture contained
ethoxyresorufin and pure NADPH-cytochrome c reductase and
the reaction was started with NADPH at the time indicated
by an arrow. Dashed line tracing: the reaction mixture
contained ethoxyresorufin, pure NADPH-cytochrome c
reductase and a pure form of cytochrome P-450 having low
ethoxyresorufin O-deethylase activity. The tracing for the
reaction in the presence of cytochrome P-450 is the same as
the solid line until the dashed line diverges. The solid
line shows changes in ethoxyresorufin fluorescence, which
is weak but measurable at the wavelength settings for
resorufin. The dashed line shows the increase in resorufin
fluorescence. Results from Burke, Mayer and Wolf
(unpublished).

**Figure 6. Buffer effect on ethoxyresorufin O-deethylase by
purified cytochrome P-450.**

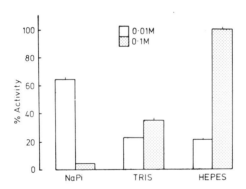

The monooxygenase was reconstituted using the pure major
MC-induced form of cytochrome P-450 and NADPH-cytochrome c
reductase. Reaction mixtures contained sodium-potassium
phosphate, Tris or HEPES buffer at either 0.01M or 0.1M
concentration. Results from Burke, Mayer and Wolf
(unpublished).

INHIBITORY ANTIBODIES AGAINST CYTOCHROME P-450

Evidence has been presented above that there are
serious reservations to the use of substrates alone or
substrates plus inhibitory chemicals for identifying
individual forms of cytochrome P-450, either in microsomes
or in purified preparations. This problem may have been
solved by the growing availability of inhibitory polyclonal
and monoclonal antibodies specific for individual

cytochrome P-450 forms. The use of antibodies to quantify
total antigenic cytochrome P-450, i.e. both active
holoprotein and metabolically inactive apoprotein, is
described elsewhere in these Proceedings. However,
antibodies can also identify the presence of specifically
functional forms of cytochrome P-450 - arguably a much more
important achievement (Ryan et al., 1982). The extent to
which an antibody specific for one form of cytochrome P-450
inhibits a reaction in, for example a microsomal suspension
or a whole cell or tissue homogenate, indicates the extent
to which that form is present and is contributing to that
reaction. The demonstration of potent antibody-inhibition
of reactions in microsomes may, in fact, be more reliable
than the use of purified cytochrome P-450 in reconstituted
systems as a way of finding out the reaction specificity of
an individual form of cytochrome P-450. This is because
microsomes probably contain the mono-oxygenase system in a
largely physiologically "correct" state, whereas there is
now ample published evidence that the metabolic activity of
purified cytochrome P-450 can be greatly influenced by the
ratios of NADPH-cytochrome P-450 reductase, cytochrome b_5
and lipid in a reconstituted system, and even by the method
of reconstitution itself (Gorsky and Coon, 1986; Gutt et
al., 1986; Jansson et al., 1985).

Newman and Guzelian (1983) demonstrated the power of
the antibody approach in the course of discovering that the
major PCN-induced form of rat liver cytochrome P-450
catalyses aldrin epoxidation: the microsomal reaction was
inhibited by a specific antibody, whereas the purified
enzyme was devoid of aldrin epoxidation activity. We have
used the same approach to answer the question of which
form(s) of cytochrome P-450 are responsible for
ethoxyresorufin O-deethylation (EROD) in liver microsomes
of untreated rats. Amongst purified forms of cytochrome P-
450 ethoxyresorufin is a highly selective substrate for the
major 3MC-induced form (Table 8 and Figure 4). Inhibitory
antibodies showed that, as expected, EROD in 3MC-induced
rat liver microsomes was catalysed primarily by the major
3MC-induced form of cytochrome P-450 (Burke, Mayer and
Wolf, unpublished). Control microsomes have very low EROD
activity, which could be due to the small amount of highly
active 3MC inducible cytochrome P-450 present. However,
control microsomal EROD was powerfully inhibited by
antibodies to a form of cytochrome P-450, cytochrome P-450-
PB1A, that is marginally inducible by PB but not inducible
by 3MC, whereas the antibody to the major 3MC-inducible
form, cytochrome P-450-MC1B, was much less inhibitory
(Figure 7; Burke, Mayer and Wolf, unpublished). This

suggests that form PB1A was mainly responsible for EROD in control microsomes, even though purified form PB1A had only 1.5% of the EROD activity of purified form MC1B.

CONCLUSIONS

i. The use of selective substrates alone to distinguish between different forms within families of drug metabolising enzymes is most successful with epoxide hydrolases and with forms of UDP-glucuronyltransferase and cytochrome P-450 having a narrow specificity for "physiological" substrates. It also successfully differentiates between classes of glutathione transferases. It is least successful with those forms of UDP-glucuronyltransferase and cytochrome P-450 having broad

Figure 7. Effect of antibodies against cytochrome P-450 on ethoxyresorufin O-deethylation by liver microsomes of untreated rats.

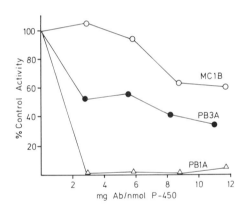

Microsomes were preincubated with ammonium sulphate-precipitated polyclonal antibodies against cytochrome P-450-MC1B (the major MC-induced form of cytochrome P-450), cytochrome P-450-PB3A (the major PB-induced form of cytochrome P-450) or cytochrome P-450-PB1A (a form of cytochrome P-450 that is marginally induced by PB). Results from Burke, Mayer and Wolf (unpublished).

specificities for xenobiotic substrates.
ii. The use of inhibitory chemicals can improve the ability of selective substrates to probe for particular types of drug metabolising enzymes.
iii. Substrates and inhibitory chemicals probably identify

families of drug metabolising enzyme forms with certain reaction characteristics in common, rather than identifying individual forms of the enzymes. This can be advantageous, compared with the immunoquantitation of individual forms, however, since the measurement will include previously unidentified forms and forms for which antibodies are not available.

iv. The combination of inhibitory antibodies and selective substrates is the most powerful way of identifying functionally active individual forms of drug metabolising enzymes.

v. The selective induction of a reaction at least 10-fold by only one category of inducing agent is a useful guide that the reaction can be used as a probe for those forms of the drug-metabolising enzyme that are induced by that same category of agent. If a reaction is selectively induced to a large extent, say 20-fold, by its "definitive" inducer then it should not be assumed, however, that a small increase in the reaction, say 2-fold, by another agent represents a specific induction of the same type.

vi. A reaction that is proven to be highly selective for one induced family of forms of a drug-metabolising enzyme can probably be used confidently to identify other instances of the same type of induction in tissue preparations, for example microsomes. It is not valid, however, to assume that the reaction is a selective probe for the same inducible forms of the enzyme in preparations from untreated animals or animals treated with other categories of inducing agent.

REFERENCES

Baars, A.J., Jansen, M. and Breimer, D.D. (1978). Biochem. Pharmacol, 27, 2487.

Billings, R.E. and McMahon, R.E. (1978). Mol. Pharmacol, 14, 145.

Burchell, B. (1981). in "Reviews in Biochemical Toxicology", vol 3 (Ed. by Hodgson, E., Bend, J.R. and Philpot, R.M). Elsevier, New York, p.1.

Burke, M.D. and Mayer, R.T. (1974). Drug Metab. Disp, 2, 583.

Burke, M.D. and Mayer, R.T. (1975). Drug Metab. Disp, 3, 245.

Burke, M.D. and Mayer, R.T. (1983). Chem-Biol Interactions, 45, 243.

Burke, M.D., Prough, R.A. and Mayer, R.T. (1977). Drug Metab. Disp, 5, 1.

Burke, M.D., Thompson, S., Elcombe, C.R., Halpert, J.,

Haaparanta, T. and Mayer, R.T. (1985). Biochem. Pharmacol, 34, 3337.

Clifton, G. and Kaplowitz, N. (1978). Biochem. Pharmacol, 27, 1284.

Creaven, P.J. and Parke, D.V. (1966). Biochem. Pharmacol, 15, 7.

Davies, W.H. and Creaven, P.J. (1967). Biochem. Pharmacol, 16, 1839.

Delaforge, M., Ioannides, C. and Parke, D.V. (1980). Chem. Biol. Interactions, 32, 101.

Delaforge, M., Jaouen, A. and Mansuy, D. (1983). Biochem. Pharmacol, 32, 2309.

Dickins, M., Elcombe, C.R., Moloney, S.J., Netter, K.J. and Bridges, J.W. (1979). Biochem. Pharmacol, 28, 231.

Elshourbagy, N.A. and Guzelian, P.S. (1980). J. Biol. Chem, 225. 1279.

Frommer, U. and Ullrich, V. (1974). FEBS Lett, 41, 14.

Gorsky, L.D. and Coon, M.J. (1986). Drug Metab. Disp, 14, 89.

Goujon, F.M., Nebert, D.W. and Gielen, J.E. (1972). Mol. Pharmacol, 8, 667.

Guengerich, F.P. (1983). in "Reviews in Biochemical Toxicology", vol 4 (Ed. by Hodgson, E., Bend, J.R. and Philpot, R.M.). Elsevier, New York, p.5.

Guengerich, F.P., Dannan, G.A., Wright, S.T., Martin, M.V. and Kaminsky, L.S. (1982). Biochemisty, 21, 6019.

Guenthner, T.M. (1986). Biochem. Pharmacol, 35, 839.

Guenthner, T.M. and Oesch, F. (1983). J. Biol. Chem, 258, 15054.

Guthenberg, C., Morganstern, R., De Pierre, J.W. and Mannervik, B. (1980). Biochim. Biophys. Acta, 631, 1.

Gutt, J., Catin, T., Dayer, P., Kronbach, T., Zanger, U. and Meyer, U.A. (1986). J. Biol. Chem, in press.

Hammock, B.D. and Hasagawa, L.S. (1983). Biochem. Pharmacol, 32, 1155.

Hayes, J.D. and Chalmers, J. (1983). Biochem. J. 215, 581.

Hilderbrandt, A., Remmer, H. and Estabrook, R.W. (1968). Biochem. Biophys. Res. Commun, 30, 607.

Hultmark, D., Sundh, K., Johansson, L. and Arrhenius, E. (1979). Biochem. Pharmacol, 28, 1587.

Jakoby, W.B. and Habig, W.H. (1980). in "Enzymatic Basis of Detoxification". Vol 1 (Ed. by Jakoby, W.B.). Academic Press, New York, p.63.

Jakoby, W.B., Ketterer, B. and Mannervik, B. (1984). Biochem. Pharmacol, 33, 2539.

Jansson, I., Tamburini, P.P., Favreau, L.V. and Schenkman, J.B. (1985). Drug Metab. Disp, 13, 453.

Kahn, G.C., Boobis, A.R., Murrary, S. and Davies, D.S.

(1982). Xenobiotica, 12, 509.

Kamataki, T., Ando, M., Yamazoe, Y., Ishii, K. and Kato, R. (1980). Biochem. Pharmacol. 29, 1015.

Lake, B.G., Hopkins, R., Chakraborty, J., Bridges, J.W. and Parke, D.V. (1973). Drug Metab. Disp, 1, 342.

Lee, E., Okuno, S. and Kariya, K. (1986). Biochem. Pharmacol, 35, 1835.

Lesca, P., Lecointe, P., Paoletti, C. and Mansuy, D. (1977). Biochem. Pharmacol, 26, 2169.

Lesca, P., Lecointe, P., Paoletti, C. and Mansuy, D. (1978). Biochem. Pharmacol, 27, 1203.

Lesca, P., Rafidinarivo, E., Lecointe, P. and Mansuy, D. (1979). Chem.Biol. Interactions, 24, 189.

Levin, W., Michaud, D.P., Thomas, P.E. and Herina, D.M. (1983). Arch. Biochem. Biophys, 220, 485.

Lohmann, S.M. and Miech, R.P. (1976). J. Pharmacol. Expt. Therap, 196 213.

Lu, A.Y.H. and West, S.B. (1979). Pharmacol. Rev. 31, 277.

Lu, A.Y.H., Levin, W., Ryan, D., West, S.B., Thomas, P., Kawalek, J., Kuntzman, R. and Conney, A.H. (1976). in "Anticonvulsant Drugs and Enzyme Induction" (Ed. by Richens, A. and Woodford, F.P). Associated Scientific Publishers, Amsterdam, p. 169.

Lu, A.Y.H., Somogyi, A., West, S., Kuntzman, R. and Conney, A.H. (1972). Arch. Biochem. Biophys, 152, 457.

Mackenzie, P.I., Joffe, M.M., Munson, P.J. and Owens, I.S. (1985). Biochem. Pharmacol, 34, 737.

Mannervik, B. (1985). in "Advances in Enzymology", vol 57 (Ed. by Meister, A). Interscience, John Wiley and Sons, New York, p. 357.

Mannervik, B. and Jensson, H. (1982). J. Biol. Chem, 257, 9909.

Mannervik, B., Alin, P., Guthenberg, C., Jensson, H., Tahir, M.K., Warholm, M. and Jornvall, H. (1985). Proc. Natl. Acad. Sci, 82, 7202.

Matsubara, T., Otsubo, S. and Yoshihara, E. (1983). Jap. J. Pharmacol, 33, 1065.

Mullin, C.A. and Hammock, B.D. (1982). Arch. Biochem. Biophys, 216, 423.

Newman, S.L. and Guzelian, P.S. (1983). Biochem. Pharmacol, 32, 1529.

Oesch, F., Timms, C.W., Walker, C.H., Guenthner, T.M., Sparrow, A., Watabe, T. and Wolf, C.R. (1984). Carcinogenesis, 5, 7.

Okita, R.T. and Masters, B.S.S. (1980). Drug Metab. Disp, 8, 147.

Orton, T.C. and Parker, G.L. (1982). Drug Metab. Disp, 10, 110.

Parke, D.V. and Rahman, H. (1971). Biochem. J. 123, 9p.
Pershing, L.K. and Franklin, M.R. (1982). Xenobiotica, 12, 687.
Reinke, L.A. and Moyer, M.J. (1985). Drug Metab. Disp, 13, 548.
Roy, M., Monsarrat, B., Cros, S., Lecointe, P., Rovalle, C. and Bisagni, E. (1985). Drug Metab. Disp, 13, 497.
Ryan, D.E., Thomas, P.E. and Levin, W. (1980). J. Biol. Chem, 255, 7941.
Ryan, D.E, Thomas, P.E., Reik, L.M. and Levin, W. (1982). Xenobiotica, 12, 727.
Sladek, N.E. and Mannering, G.J. (1969). Mol. Pharmacol, 5, 186.
Snyder,R.and Remmer, H. (1982). in "Hepatic Cytochrome P-450 Monoxygenase system" (Ed. by Schenkman J.B. and Kupfer, D), Pergamon Press, Oxford, p.227.
Tamburini, P.P., Masson, H.A., Bains, S.K., Makowski, R.J., Morris, B. and Gibson, G.G. (1984). Eur. J. Biochem, 139, 235.
Toftgard, R. and Nilsen, O.G. (1982). Toxicology, 23, 197.
Tomaszewski, J.E., Jerina, D.M., Levin, W. and Conney, A.H. (1976). Arch. Biochem. Biophys, 176, 788.
Tweedie, D.J. and Burke, M.D. Drug Metab. Disp, in press.
Ullrich, V. (1969). Hoppe-Seyler's Z. Physiol. Chem, 350, 357.
Ullrich, D. and Bock, K.W. (1984). Biochem. Pharmacol, 33, 97.
Ullrich, V., Weber, P. and Wollenberg, P. (1975). Biochem. Biophys. Res. Commun, 64, 808.
Waxman, D.J. (1986). in "Cytochrome P-450", (Ed. by Ortiz de Montellano, P.R). Plenum Press, New York, p. 525.
Waxman, D.J., Dannan, G.A. and Guengerich, F.P. (1985). Biochemistry, 24, 4409.
Wiebel, F.J., Leutz, J.C., Diamond, L. and Gelboin, H.V. (1971). Arch. Biochem. Biophyds, 144, 78.
Wolf, C.R., Seilman, S., Oesch, F., Mayer, R.T. and Burke, M.D. Biochem. J. in press.
Wolff, T. (1980). in "Biochemistry, Biophysics and Regulation of Cytochrome P-450" (Ed. by Gustafsson, J.A., Carlstedt-Duke, J., Mode, A. and Rafter, J). Elsevier, Oxford, p.137.
Wolff, T. and Strecker, M. (1985). Biochem. Pharmacol, 34, 2593.
Wrighton, S.A., Schuetz, E.G., Watkins, P.B., Maurel, P., Barwick, J., Bailey, B.S., Hartle, H.T., Young, B. and Guzelian, P. (1985). Mol. Pharmacol, 28, 312.

BIOLOGICAL ACTIVITIES OF MODIFIERS OF CYTOCHROME P-450 ACTIVITIES *

Hugo Vanden Bossche and Paul A.J. Janssen

Janssen Pharmaceutica Research Laboratories, B-2340 Beerse, Belgium.

INTRODUCTION

The importance of cytochrome P-450 isozyme containing systems in catalysing, the hydroxylation and dealkylation of xenobiotics is widely recognised. The discovery by Estabrook et al (1963) that a cytochrome P-450 participated in the 21-hydroxylation of progesterone opened an exponentially expanding field for research of the role cytochrome P-450 isozymes play in the metabolism of key endobiotics. This discovery was also at the onset for the search of cytochrome P-450 specific inhibitors.

The aim of this overview is to provide data on specific inhibitors of cytochrome P-450 isozymes and their therapeutic applications.

ERGOSTEROL BIOSYNTHESIS INHIBITORS AS POTENT ANTIFUNGAL AGENTS

Cytochrome P-450 isozymes :

The presence of cytochrome P-450 in cell extracts from Saccharomyces cerevisiae was first observed by Lindenmayer and Smith (1964). In their study on cytochromes and other pigments of baker's yeast they reported the presence of a 450-CO-pigment resembling that seen in liver microsomes. Alexander et al (1974) first assumed the involvement of this cytochrome P-450 in the conversion of lanosterol to zymosterol during ergosterol biosynthesis, thus similar to the system involved in the oxidative metabolism of lanosterol in mammalian liver (Gibbons and Mitropoulos, 1973). The requirement for a heme in oxygenation reactions between lanosterol and ergosterol was proven by studies of Trocha et al (1977). These authors found in a nystatin resistant mutant of S. cerevisiae lanosterol as well as 4,14-dimethyl cholesta-8,24-dien-3β-ol, 4,14-dimethyl-ergosta-2,24(28)-dien-3β-ol, and 14-methylergosta-8,24(28)-

dien-3β-ol. This indicates a block in removal of the methyl group at C-14 of lanosterol. An ergosterol requiring derivative of the mutant, which also carried a mutation in heme biosynthesis, did not require ergosterol for growth when a heme was added to the medium. Ohba et al (1978) showed that the conversion of lanosterol to 4,4'-dimethylzymosterol by a microsomal fraction of S.cerevisiae is oxygen and NADPH dependent and inhibited by antibodies to yeast cytochrome P-450. These observations led the authors to conclude that in yeast microsomes, cytochrome P-450 (cytochrome P-450$_{14-DM}$) is involved in the oxidative removal of the 14α-methylgroup (C-32 methylgroup attached to C-14 of the sterol framework) from lanosterol. This conclusion was confirmed by incubating lanosterol with a reconstituted system consisting of cytochrome P-450$_{14-DM}$ and NADPH-cytochrome P-450 reductase, both purified from yeast microsomes, in the presence of molecular oxgyen (Aoyama and Yoshida, 1978; Aoyama et al, 1984). This resulted in the formation of 4,4'-dimethyl-5α-cholesta-8,14,24-trien-3β-ol, proving the 14α-demethylation of lanosterol. Furthermore this study proved that in yeast the hydroxylation of the 14-methyl group, the oxidation of the 14-hydroxymethyl to an aldehyde and the oxidative elimination of the aldehyde as formic acid with the concomitant introduction of a 14,15 double bond are mediated by cytochrome P-450.

So far, the oxygenated intermediates of lanosterol, lanost-8-en-3β, 32-diol and 3β-hydroxylanost-8-en-32- al, have not been identified in yeast. However, Trzaskos et al (1984) using a reconstituted system of a homogeneous lanosterol demethylase cytochrome P-450 from rat liver and NADPH-cytochrome c reductase found three metabolites: lanost-8-en-3β-32-diol, 3β-hydroxylanost-8-en-32-al and 4,4-dimethyl-5α-cholesta-8,14-dien-3β-ol. The chemical structure of these metabolites has been recently proven (Shafiee et al, 1986). This suggests that in liver a single cytochrome P-450 isozyme is responsible for the entire demethylation reaction. These results also suggest that an NAD-dependent enzyme is not required for the oxidation of the 14-hydroxymethyl to an aldehyde as suggested previously (Pascal et al, 1980).

In both yeast and liver microsomes a cytochrome P-450 independent reduction of the 14-desaturated derivative is needed. An AY-9944 (trans, 1-4-bis-(2-chlorobenzylamino-ethyl)-cyclohexane dihydrochloride)-sensitive 14-reductase has been isolated from rat liver microsomes (Paik et al, 1984) and identified in yeast microsomes (Aoyama and Yoshida, 1986).

The outline of the 14-demethylation reaction sequence is presented in Figure 1. It is interesting to note that a second cytochrome P-450 isozyme seems to be involved in the biosynthesis of ergosterol from lanosterol. Studying the Δ 22-desaturation of ergosta-5,7-dien-3β-ol in a microsomal fraction of S. cerevisiae, Hata et al (1981) found that this stage in the biosynthesis was carbon monoxide and metyrapone sensitive and insensitive to cyanide or azide. This suggests the involvement of a cytochrome P-450-containing monooxygenase system in the reaction. Since the Δ 22-desaturation was not inhibited by the 14$^\alpha$-demethylase inhibitor, buthiobate, nor by rabbit antibodies against cytochrome P-450$_{14-DM}$ it was concluded that the Δ 22-desaturation cytochrome P-450 isozyme is different from that involved in the 14α-demethylation (Hata et al, 1983). According to Ortiz de Montellano and Reich (1986) cytochrome P-450 inhibitors can be divided into three categories :

1. Agents that bind reversibly, competing in this way with substrates for occupancy of the active site.
2. Agents that form quasi-irreversible complexes with the heme iron atom and simultaneously bind to lipophilic regions of the protein.
3. Agents that bind irreversibly to the protein or the prosthetic heme group or that accelerate the degradation of the prosthetic heme group.

Pyridine, pyrimidine, imidazole and triazole derivatives are effective inhibitors that interact strongly with both the protein and the prosthetic heme iron. A number of these lipophilic nitrogen heterocycles are isozyme-specific inhibitors of the lanosterol 14-demethylation, others are more specific inhibitors, e.g. of the 11-hydroxylase, 17,20-lyase, aromatase or thromboxane synthase. For the latter especially, the pyridine-based inhibitors are highly selective whereas triazole derivatives seem to have high affinity for the cytochrome P-450 dependent lanosterol 14α-demethylation in yeast microsomes.

A great number of the triazole and imidazole derivatives are important antifungal agents. Some of them are breakthroughs in antifungal therapy in human and veterinary medicine, others show excellent activity against phytopathogenic fungi. Examples of these compounds are given in Figure 2.

Addition of the azole derivatives to microsomal suspensions prepared from S. cerevisiae or Candida albicans yielded type II spectra with a Soret maximum at about 420 nm and a minimum at about 398 nm (Vanden Bossche et al,

Figure 1. 14α-Demethylation of lanosterol. P-450$_{14DM}$ represents the cytochrome P-450-dependent hydroxylase system.

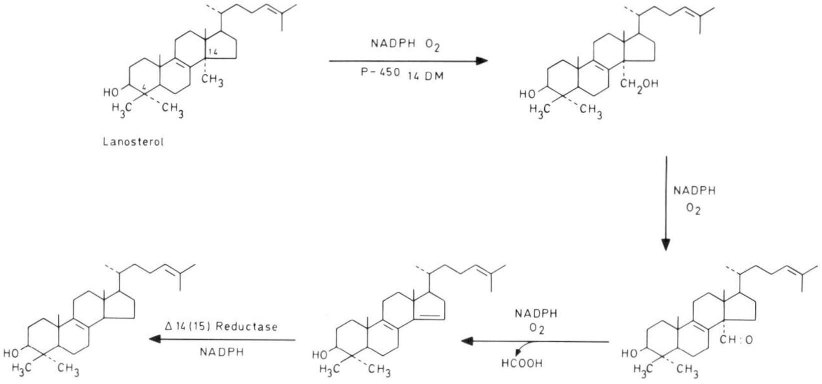

1984a, 1986). Using cytochrome P-450 purified from S. cerevisiae, Yoshida and Aoyama (1986) found that the triazole antifungal triadimefon caused similar type II spectral changes. A type II spectral change suggests binding of the unhindered nitrogen (N$_3$ in the imidazole ring, N$_4$ in the triazole ring) to the heme iron atom at the site occupied by the exchangable sixth ligand, i.e. the site of dioxygen binding. Dioxygen binding is a step prior to the formation of the oxygen radical needed to hydroxylate the 14α-methyl group of lanosterol. As expected, these azole derivatives also compete with carbon monoxide for binding to the 6th coordination place of the reduced iron atom (Vanden Bossche and Willemsens, 1982; Vanden Bossche et al, 1984a,b, 1986; Vanden Bossche, 1985). After reduction with dithionite and saturation with CO of microsomal suspensions of S.cerevisiae or Candida albicans, the reduced cytochrome P-450-CO complex was stable over the 60min. measurement period (Vanden Bossche et al, 1986). When the cytochrome P-450 isozymes present in the microsomal fraction were titrated with N-phenylimidazole (up to 5 x 10^{-3}M), ketoconazole (up to 10^{-5}M) or itraconazole (up to 5 x 10^{-6}M, i.e. at the limit of solubility), then reduced and bubbled with CO, the absorption peak at 448nm was decreased by 64%, 90% and 91% respectively. After 60 min, CO seemed to be able to replace N-phenylimidazole almost completely and

Figure 2. Imidazole and triazole antifungals of clinical and agriculture use.

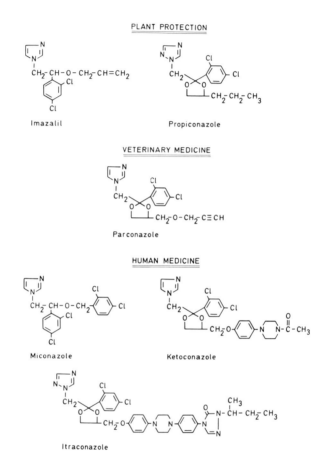

ketoconazole partly, whereas the cytochrome P-450-itraconazole complex was stable (Vanden Bossche et al, 1986). Studies of Yoshida and Aoyama (1986) with purified cytochrome P-450 from S. cerevisiar indicated that the cytochrome P-450-triademefon-complex was readily converted into the CO-complex whereas the itraconazole-complex was stable. Since the affinity of the unhindered N_4 for the heme iron is similar for both N_1-substituted triazoles, the differences observed might result from differences in affinity of their nonligating portion for the apoprotein. It is of interest to note that the ability of a compound to form a type I spectrum (absorption peak at about 385 nm and

a trough at about 420 nm) with microsomal cytochrome P-450
from livers is determined primarily by its lipophilicity.
Indeed a good correlation between binding and the apparent
partition coefficient between octanol and water (log P) has
been found (Al-Gailany et al, 1978). Type I spectral
changes are generally accepted to arise as a consequence of
substrate binding to the apoprotein. Based on the results
obtained by Al-Gailany et al (1978) it can be assumed that
the interaction domain is a hydroprobic portion of this
apoprotein. It is likely that the lipophilicity of the
nonligating portion of type II inducers also contributes to
their interaction with cytochrome P-450. Indeed the log
P's of N-phenylimidazole, ketoconazole and itraconazole are
1.93, 3.7 and 5.7 respectively, this corresponds with the
differences in affinity of the 3 azole derivatives for
cytochrome P-450 isozymes in C. albicans microsomes (Vanden
Bossche et al, 1986).

Sterol biosynthesis :
Triarimol, a pyrimidine derivative, shown above to
interfere with the cytochrome $P-450_{14-DM}$ was the first
fungitoxic agent found to interfere with ergosterol
synthesis. Indeed, triarimol at a concentration of 2µg/ml
was found to decrease the ergosterol content of sporidia of
Ustilago maydis by almost 95%. A concomitant accumulation
of the 14α-methylsterols 24-methylenedihydrolanosterol,
obtusifoliol and 14α-methylfecosterol was found (Ragsdale,
1975). The inhibition of ergosterol biosynthesis in
U.avenae by triadimefon and another triazole derivative
fluotrimazole (Buchenauer, 1976; Buchenauer and Grossmann,
1977) led Motolcsy et al (1977) to propose ergosterol
biosynthesis as a potential target for selective antifungal
action. A number of studies have shown that the imidazole
antifungals miconazole, imazalil, parconazole and
ketoconazole and the triazole propiconazole and
itraconazole interfere selectively at low concentrations
with the 14α-demethylation of lanosterol in yeast and
fungi. Table 1 presents examples of yeast and fungi in
which the inhibitory effects of these azole derivatives
have been proven.
    The inhibitory effects on ergosterol biosynthesis and
the concomitant accumulation of 14α-methyl sterols observed
at much lower concentrations than those needed to affect
growth. For example, a 50% inhibition of ergosterol
synthesis in exponentially growing C. albicans (strain ATCC
44859) was achieved at 5.5×10^{-10}M of itraconazole after
1h of contact whereas more than 10^{-8}M was needed to achieve
a similar effect on growth (Vanden Bossche et al, 1984a).

Table 1.   Imidazole and triazole antifungals inhibiting ergosterol synthesis in fungi.

SPECIES	AZOLE DERIVATIVES	REFERENCE
Aspergillus fumigatus	Ketoconazole Itraconazole	Marichal et al, 1985
Aspergillus nidulans	Imazalil	Siegel & Ragsdale (1978), Siegel & Solel (1981)
Botrytis cinerea	Imazalil	Leroux & Gredt (1978)
	Propiconazole	Leroux & Gredt (1981)
Candida albicans	Ketoconazole	Vanden Bossche et al (1979, 1980)
	Imazalil	Marriott (1980)
	Itraconazole	Vanden Bossche et al (1984a,b, 1986)
	Miconazole	Vanden Bossche et al (1978)
	Parconazole	Pye & Marriott (1982)
Candida tropicalis	Propiconazole	Sanglard (1985)
Penicillium spp	Imazalil	Leroux & Gredt (1978)
	Propiconazole	Vanden Bossche et al (1984b)
Pityrosporum ovale	Ketoconazole Itraconazole	Vanden Bossche (unpublished results)
Saccharomyces cerevisiae	Ketoconazole	Vanden Bossche (unpublished results
	Imazalil	Vanden Bossche et al (1984a)
	Miconazole	Vanden Bossche (unpublished results)
	Propiconazole	Leroux & Gredt (1981)
Saccharomyces uvarum	Propiconazole	Sanglard (1985)
Trichopyton mentogrophytes	Miconazole	Morita et al (1985)
Ustilago spp	Imazalil	Buchenauer (1977), Leroux & Gredt (1978)
	Propiconazole	Leroux & Gredt (1981)

When the same strain of C. albicans was grown for 4h in the presence of parconazole, 50% inhibition of ergosterol

biosynthesis was achieved at 5 x 10^{-9}M. Under the same
conditions a slight effect on growth was observed at 10^{-5}M
only. After 24h of incubation a 50% decrease in growth was
found at 3 x 10^{-8}M. Therefore the interaction of the azole
derivatives with the cytochrome P-450 dependent 14α-
demethylase may contribute to their effects on growth. It
should be noted that the azole derivatives completely
inhibit ergosterol synthesis at low concentrations.
Indeed, taking itraconazole as an example, it was found
that, by using TLC to separate the different sterols,
contact photography to localise them and gas chromatography
combined with mass spectrometry to identify the sterols, no
ergosterol was found in C. albicans incubated for 24h in
the presence of 5 x 10^{-9}M itraconazole (Vanden Bossche et
al, 1984a). The presence of 14α-methylfecosterol and 14α-
methyl-ergosta-8,24(28)-dien-3β,6α-diol in C. albicans
incubated in the presence of imidazole and triazole
antifungals indicate that the cytochrome P-450 isozyme
involved in the Δ22-desaturation is not affected by these
azole derivatives. The presence of a 3,6-diol derivative
suggests the availability of a 6-hydroxylase that is
insensitive to azole antifungals.

Effects of ergosterol depletion and accumulation of
14α-methylsterols:
According to Bloch (1979) the minimal requirements for a
sterol to function as a membrane compound are a free
equatorial hydroxyl group at C-3, flatness and preferred
dimensions of the molecule. Since the 14α-methyl group of
lanosterol for example is axially orientated and increases
the thickness of the molecule by approximately 0.2nm,
differences in membrane effects between ergosterol and
lanosterol could be expected. Using differential scanning
calorimetry (D.S.C) it was shown that ergosterol, when
incorporated in 1,2-dipalmitoyl-L-phosphatidylcholine
multilamellar vesicles, decreased the enthalpy of melting.
At an ergosterol concentration of 15 mol % the enthalpy
reached zero (Vanden Bossche et al, 1984b). When
ergosterol was replaced by lanosterol a much smaller effect
on the enthalpy was observed indicating that lanosterol was
fluidising the membrane to a lower degree than ergosterol.
By using glucose permeability as a parameter it was found
that the incorporation of ergosterol into unilamellar
vesicles composed of phosphatidylcholine, phosphatidyl-
ethanolamine and diphosphatidylglycerol, reduced the
release of trapped glucose by 57%. When lanosterol was
used instead of ergosterol the release of trapped glucose
was almost similar to that observed with the vesicles

composed of the phospholipids only (Vanden Bossche et al, 1982).

Using a yeast sterol auxotroph it was found that growth on cholesterol is precluded until small amounts of ergosterol are available (Rodriguez et al, 1985). This phenomenon was called the sparking of growth in which cholesterol satisfies an overall membrane function and ergosterol fulfils a sparking function (Rodriguez et al, 1985). Dahl and Dahl (1986) further proved that minute amounts of ergosterol are needed in S. cerevisiae to stimulate cell proliferation.

It is tempting to speculate that inhibition of growth may result as a consequence of the azole antifungal-induced depletion of ergosterol and the concomitant accumulation of 14α-methylsterols functional changes in the yeast and fungal membranes, e.g. permeability changes, membrane leakiness, changes in the activities of membrane bound enzymes (Vanden Bossche, 1985). Thus, the described interaction with the 14α-demethylase cytochrome P-450 isozyme might be at the origin of, for example, itraconazole's activity in candidosis, pityriasis, sporotrichosis, chromomycosis, aspergillosis, paracocci-dioidomycosis, meningeal cryptococcosis and dermatophytoses (Cauwenbergh et al, 1986).

Selectivity of azole derivatives :
Recent studies (Vanden Bossche et al, 1986) have shown that, unlike ketoconazole, itraconazole does not significantly affect in vitro androgen, gluco- and mineralocorticoid steroidogenesis. Itraconazole also does not affect the cytochrome P-450 dependent aromatase nor the 1-hydroxylase of 25-hydroxy-vitamin D_3 in a microsomal fraction of human placenta and kidney mitochondria respectively (unpublished results). To obtain 50% inhibition of the 14α-demethylation of lanosterol in phytohemagglutinin stimulated human peripheral lymphocytes, 4×10^{-7}M itraconazole is needed (Vanden Bossche et al, 1986). A similar inhibition of cholesterol synthesis in subcellular fractions of rat liver was reached at 7×10^{-6}M (Vanden Bossche et al, 1984a).

Ketoconazole affects certain cytochrome P-450 isozymes in microsomal and mitochondrial fractions of mammalian cells at higher concentrations than those needed to interfere with the cytochrome P-450 isozyme in yeast microsomes. When the effects of ketoconazole on the absorbance increment (ΔA) between 450nm and 490nm of the reduced cytochrome P-450-CO-complex of phenobarbital induced liver was measured, a 50% decrease (I_{50}-value) in the ΔA (450-490) was found at 4×10^{-6}M (Vanden Bossche et al, in press). This high concentration of ketoconazole corresponds with the Ki value of 8.5×10^{-6}M found by Meredith et al (1985) for the aminopyrine N-demethylation in rat liver microsomes and with the 1.2×10^{-6}M needed to obtain 50% inhibition of the ethylmorphine N-demethylase activity in liver microsomes from rats pretreated with phenobarbital (Sheets and Mason, 1984).

In man, the metabolism of theophylline and chlordiazepoxide was slightly affected only after repetitive dosing with 400mg ketoconazole for 5 days (Brown et al, 1985). Daneshmend et al (1983) were unable to find a significant effect of ketoconazole (200mg twice daily for 5 days) on the antipyrine clearance. After a 7 day, 400mg per day course of oral ketoconazole, a decrease of 25% in the total body clearance of antipyrine was found (D'Mello et al, 1985).

In vitro experiments indicate that ketoconazole at concentrations between 2×10^{-7}M and 10^{-5}M inhibits cytochrome P-450 dependent steroidogenic enzymes in mitochondria and/or microsomes of placenta, testicular and adrenal cortex cells (Santen et al, 1983; Vanden Bossche et al, 1985a,b in press). For example when bovine adrenal cortex mitochondria were incubated for 30 min, a 50% inhibition of the 11-hydroxylase mediated synthesis of cortisol and corticosterone was achieved at 3.8×10^{-7}M and 7.5×10^{-7}M ketoconazole respectively (Vanden Bossche et al, in press). 50% inhibition of pregnenolone synthesis was obtained when the side chain cleavage cytochrome P-450, adrenodoxin and adrenodoxin reductase (all three isolated from bovine adrenal cortex mitochondria), were incubated for 30 min at 37°C in the presence of 1.7×10^{-6}M ketoconazole (Willemsens and Vanden Bossche, 1985). It should be noted that in vivo, the partial block of cortisol biosynthesis (Pont et al, 1982) induces a feed-back increment of plasma adrenocorticotropic hormone (ACTH) levels. This increase keeps the basal cortisol levels within the normal range (Pont et al, 1984; Heyns et al, 1985).

Ketoconazole only inhibits slightly the cytochrome P-450-dependent aromatase in pig testes and human placenta microsomes. An I_{50} value of 7.5×10^{-6}M and $> 10^{-5}$M was found (unpublished results). Of great interest is ketoconazole's effect on testis microsomal cytochrome P-450 isozmyes. A 50% decrease in the ΔA (450-490) is achieved at 1.3×10^{-6}M (Vanden Bossche et al, 1984a) and 3.9×10^{-7}M (Vanden Bossche et al, 1985b) respectively for dog and piglet testis microsomes.

ANDROGEN BIOSYNTHESIS AND AROMATASE INHIBITORS

For most fungal infections a daily dose of 200mg ketoconazole is effective. However for some systemic infections e.g. coccidiodomycoses a daily dose of 200mg ketoconazole is usually too low and higher doses of 400 to 1200 mg daily have been administered for prolonged periods (Graybill and Craven, 1983). A small number of patients treated with these high doses developed gynecomastia and/or loss of libido (Graybill and Craven, 1983; Pont et al, 1982; 1984; 1985). The gynecomastia appears to be the result of an elevated estradioltestosterone ratio.

Decreased plasma testosterone levels have been shown in rats and dogs receiving ketoconazole. This effect was found to be transient and reversible (Trachtenberg, 1984, De Coster et al, 1984).

Ketoconazole also suppressed testosterone production in dispersed rat testicular cells (Pont et al, 1982; Vanden Bossche et al, in press). A 50% decrease was observed at 2 x 10^{-6}M (Vanden Bossche et al, in press). Endocrinological studies on male patients and healthy young male volunteers receiving ketoconazole doses from 200 to 600mg (Pont et al, 1982; Santen et al, 1983; De Coster et al, 1985) demonstrated a transient lowering of plasma testosterone levels. Plasma testosterone decreased maximally to 14% of basal values 8h after an oral dose of 600mg. A complete recovery was observed 24h after treatment (Pont et al, 1982).

In normal men receiving a single dose of 200mg ketoconazole, the total and free plasma testosterone fell to levels to 60% below basal within 4-8h and returned to control values by 24h after drug administration (Santen et al, 1983). The decrements of plasma testosterone levels may result from ketoconazole's effects on the testes microsomal cytochrome P-450 isozymes described above. In view of these results we studied the effects of ketoconazole on pregnenolone and progesterone metabolism in subcellular fractions of rat testis (Vanden Bossche et al, 1985a,b; Lauwers et al, 1985). As shown in Figure 3 the formation of the androgens dehydroepiandrosterone, androstenediol, androstenedione and testosterone is catalysed by two microsomal cytochrome P-450-dependent enzymes, i.e. the steroid 17α- monooxygenase (17α-hydroxylase) and the 17,20-lyase (C21-steroid side chain cleavage enzyme or P-450$_{sccII}$). The results obtained indicate that ketoconazole is an inhibitor of the 17,20-lyase. A subcellular fraction containing the microsomes and cytosol (S10-fraction) of the rat testes incubated in

Figure 3.   Testosterone synthesis in testes (Δ5-Pathway).

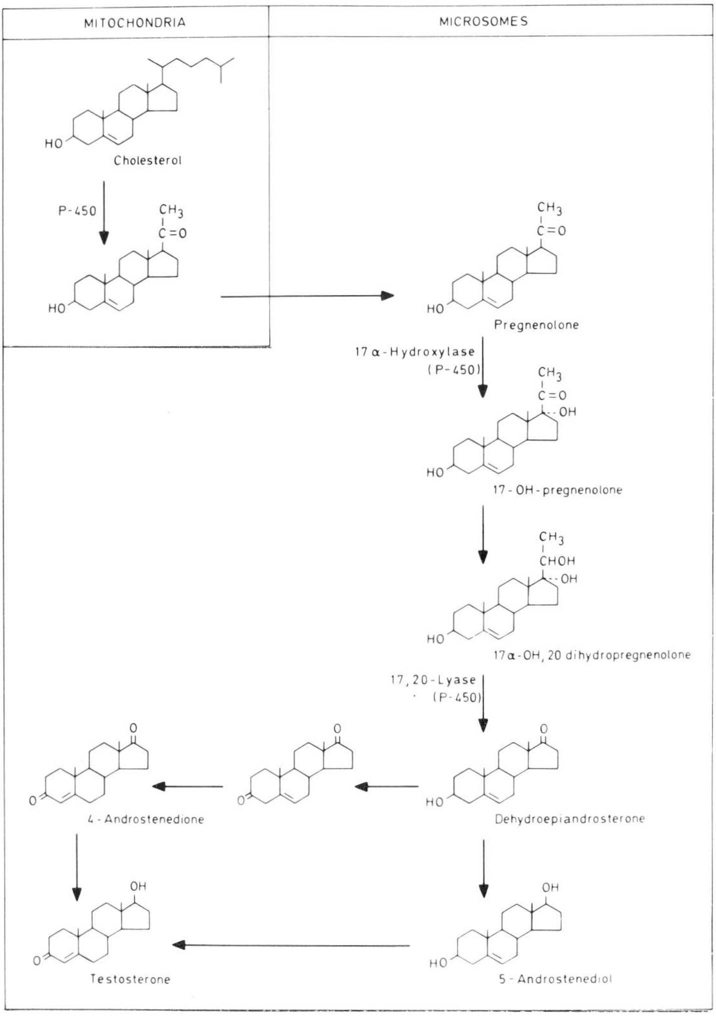

the presence of NADPH converted [^{14}C]-pregnenolone into
androgens.   In the presence of ketoconazole the decreased
androgen synthesis resulted in the accumulation of 17α-OH,
20-dihydropregnenolone (previously called 17α,20α-diOH-
pregnenolone). Maximum accumulation was reached at 5 x
10-^{7}M ketoconazole.   At concentrations > 10^{-6}M an
accumulation of pregnenolone was observed with a
concomitant decrease in the 17α-OH, 20-dihydropregnenolone

content. Similar results were obtained with progesterone as substrate. Indeed at concentrations $\geqslant 5 \times 10^{-7}$M an accumulation of 17$\alpha$-OH, 20-dihydroprogesterone was observed. Of interest is that at concentrations $\geqslant 5 \times 10^{-6}$M, an increase in 17$\alpha$-OH progesterone was measured. This indicates a feed-back inhibition of the 20-reductase. At concentrations $\geqslant 10^{-5}$M an increase in the progesterone content was found indicating a feed back inhibition of the 17α-hydroxylase.

The interaction of ketoconazole with the cytochrome P-450-dependent 17,20-lyase was further proven by incubating an S10-fraction of rat testes with tritium labelled 17α-OH, 20-dihydroprogesterone and NADPH. A 50% inhibition of the androgen synthesis was seen at about 2×10^{-7}M; 100% inhibition was reached at a ketoconazole concentration of 5×10^{-5}M.

The mitochondrial cytochrome P-450 dependent cholesterol side-chain cleavage in a reconstituted system containing cytochrome P-450 isolated from pig testis mitochondria and adrenodoxin plus adrenodoxin reductase isolated from bovine adrenal cortex mitochondria is much less sensitive to ketoconazole than the 17,20-lyase. Indeed 3×10^{-6} M is needed to obtain 50% inhibition. Thus the preferential target seems to be the 17,20-lyase.

Using the microsomes of bovine adrenal cortex, a 50% decrease in the synthesis of dehydroepiandrosterone and androstenedione was found at a ketoconazole concentration of 4×10^{-7}M. Evidence is available that this decreased androgen synthesis also results from an inhibition of the 17α-hydroxylase or 17,20-lyase (Vanden Bossche et al, in press).

An inhibition of the androgen biosynthesis in both the testicular and adrenal cortical cells make ketoconazole a suitable candidate for the treatment of androgen dependent diseases, mainly prostate carcinoma (Amery et al, 1986). By administering 400mg ketoconazole orally t.i.d (every 8h), serum-testosterone levels within the castrate range were obtained within one day in prostrate cancer patients. As could be predicted from the in vitro studies, the adrenal androgens androstenedione and dihydroepiandrosterone levels were reduced too. Clinical improvement and a lowering of acid phosphatase were achieved within the first days in previously untreated patients who no longer responded to previous therapies. Thus, the observation of a rare side effect during antifungal treatment with ketoconazole, i.e. gynecomastia, has offered new perspectives for the treatment of prostrate carcinoma.

The limited number of studies reviewed already indicate

the possibility to develop cytochrome P-450 isozyme specific inhibitors that are potent antifungal agents and androgen biosynthesis inhibitors of use in the treatment of prostate carcinoma. Other cytochrome P-450 isozymes are also interesting targets for specific inhibitors. An example is the aromatase catalysing the conversion of androgens to estrogens. The sequence of reactions in this biosynthesis involved three enzymatic hydroxylations (Figure 4). The aromatisation requires NADPH and O_2. A number of experiments suggest the involvement of a cytochrome P-450 isozyme (Waterman et al, 1986).

Figure 4. The Aromatase System.

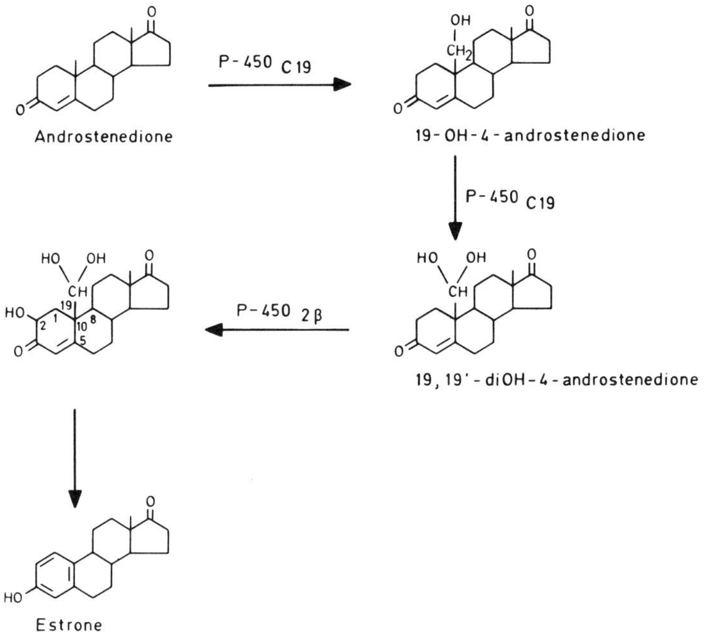

Androstenedione

P-450 C19

19-OH-4-androstenedione

P-450 C19

19,19'-diOH-4-androstenedione

P-450 2β

19,19'-diOH-4-androstenedione

Estrone

Because some breast tumours are estrogen-dependent, a specific inhibitor of the aromatase is of great interest. Aminoglutethimide (3-(4-aminophenyl)-3-ethyl-piperidine-2,6-dione) is becoming increasingly used for the treatment of hormone-dependent metastatic breast cancer (Santen et al, 1982a; Harris et al 1982; Troner, 1982). It binds to cytochrome P-450 complexes, showing a type II spectrum, and blocks several steps in steroid hydroxylation (Uzgiris et al, 1977). The binding affinity is 2.6 times greater for the d- than for the l-isomer. The former is 2.5 times more potent as an inhibitor of the cytochrome P-450-dependent cholesterol side-chain cleavage than the l-isomer (Uzgiris et al, 1977). A similar stereoselectivity of the active center of the 11-hydroxylase was found with etomidate (Vanden Bossche et al, 1984c). Aminoglutethimide inhibits the aromatase in e.g. human breast tumour homogenates, human placental microsomes and rat brain (Santen et al, 1982b). However, its poor selectivity causes a wide range of metabolic effects in patients (Santen et al, 1982b) that compromise its utility. Investigations by Foster et al, (1985) showed that replacement of the aniline group in aminoglutethimide by a more basic pyridine (pKa : 5.23 as compared with 4.58 for the aniline) yielded a compound (3-ethyl-3-(4-pyridil)-piperidine-2,6-dione) that competitively inhibits the aromatase in human placental microsomes but is non-inhibitory towards the cholesterol side-chain cleavage enzyme. These results indicate the possibility to improve the selectivity of cytochrome P-450 inhibitors by simple chemical modification.

EPILOGUE

The examples given in this paper indicate that cytochrome P-450 dependent enzyme systems can be exploited in the construction of important antifungals and agents that may play a central role in the therapy of steroid mediated cancers. The list of isozymes discussed here can be extended to those involved in the synthesis of e.g. thromboxane, of bile acids, of ent-7α-hydroxykaurenoic acid, a key-step in the synthesis of giberellins, the plant growth promotors, and of trans-p-coumaric acid, an intermediate in the biosynthesis of the plant cell wall component, lignin.

Further studies of this superfamily of hemoproteins first recognised in the later fifties will provide unequalled opportunities to develop important cytochrome P-450 isozyme selective inhibitors of use in medicine and agriculture.

ACKNOWLEDGEMENTS

The authors are grateful to D. Bellens, W. Cools, J. Gorrens, W. Lauwers, P. Marichal, H. Verhoeven and G. Willemsens for their collaboration. Grateful appreciation is expressed to K. Donne for typing the test and to L. Leijssen for preparing the figures. This work was supported by a grant from the "Instituut voor Aanmoeding van het Wetenschappelikj Onderzoek in Nijverheld en Landbouw".

REFERENCES

Alexander, K.T.W., Mitropoulos, K.A. and Gibbons, G.F. (1974). Biochem. Biophys. Res. Commun, 60, 460.

Al-Gailany, K.A.S., Houston, J.B. and Bridges, J.W. (1978). Biochem. Pharmacol, 27, 783.

Amery, W.K., De Coster, R. and Caers, L.I. (1986). Drug. Develop. Res, 6, in press.

Aoyama, Y. and Yoshida, Y. (1978). Biochem. Biophys. Res. Commun, 85, 28.

Aoyama, Y., Yoshida, Y. and Sato, R. (1984). J. Biol. Chem, 259, 1661.

Aoyama, Y. and Yoshida, Y. (1986). Biochem. Biophys. Res. Commun, 134, 659.

Bloch, K. (1979). Crit. Rev. Biochem, 7, 1.

Brown, M.V., Maldonada, A.L., Meredith, C.G. and Speeg, K.V. (1985). Clin. Pharmacol. Therap, 37, 290.

Buchenauer, H. (1976). Z. Pflanzenkr Pflanzenschutz, 83, 363.

Buchenauer, H. (1977). Z. Pflanzenkr Pflanzenschutz, 84, 440.

Buchenauer, H. and Grossmann, F. (1977). Neth. J. Plant Pathol, 83 (suppl) 93.

Cauwenbergh, G., De Doncker, P., Stoops, K., De Dier, A., Goyvaerts, H. and Schuermans, V. (1986). Rev. Infect. Dis, in press.

Dahl, J.S., Dahl, C.E. (1986). Biochem. Biophys. Res. Commun, 133, 844.

Daneshmed, T.K., Warnock, D.W., Ene, M.D., Johnson, E.M., Parker, G., Richardson, M.D. and Roberts, C.J.C. (1983). J. Antimicrob. Chemother, 12, 185.

De Coster, R., Beerens, D., Dom, J. and Willemsens, G. (1984). Acta Endocrinol, 107, 275.

De Coster, R., Caers, I., Haelterman, C. and Debroye, M. (1985). Eur. J. Clin Pharmacol, 29, 489.

D'Mello, A.P., D'Souza, M.J. and Bates, T.R. (1985). The Lancet, July 27, 209.

Estabrook, R.W., Cooper, D.Y. and Rosenthal, O. (1963). Biochem. Zeit, 338, 741.

Foster, A.B., Jarman, M., Leung, C.S., Rowlands, M.G., Taylor, G.N., Plevey, R.G. and Sampson, P. (1985). J. Med. Chem, 28, 200.

Gibbons, G.F. and Mitropoulos, K.A. (1973). Eur. J. Biochem, 40, 267.

Graybill, J.R. and Craven, P.C. (1983). Drugs, 25, 41.

Harris, A.L., Powles, T.J. and Smith, I.E. (1982). Cancer
Res (Suppl) 42, 34055.
Hata, S., Nishino, T., Komori, M. and Katsuki, H. (1981).
Biochem. Biophys. Res. Commun, 103, 272.
Hata, S., Nishino, T., Katsuki, H., Aoyama, Y. and Yoshida,
Y. (1983). Biochem. Biophys. Res. Commun, 116, 162.
Heyns, W., Drochmans, A., Van der Schueren, E. and
Verhoeven, G. (1985). Acta Endocrinol, 110, 276.
Lauwers, W.F.J., Le Jeune, L., Vanden Bossche, H. and
Willemsens, G. (1985). Biomed. Mass Spectro, 12, 296.
Leroux, P. and Gredt, M. (1978). Ann. Photopathol, 10, 45.
Leroux, P. and Gredt, M. (1981). Neth. J. Plant Pathol, 87,
240.
Lindenmayer, A., Smith, L. (1964). Biochim. Biophys. Acta,
93, 445.
Marichal, P., Gorrens, J. and Vanden Bossche, H. (1985). J.
Med. Vet. Mycol, 23, 13.
Marriott, M.S. (1980). J. Gen Microbiol, 117, 253.
Matolcsy, G., Kavacs, M., Tuske, M. and Toth, B. (1977).
Neth. J. Plant Pathol, 83 (Suppl) 39.
Meredith, G.G., Maldonado, A.L. and Speeg, K.V. (1985).
Drug Met. Dispos, 13, 156.
Morita, T. and Nozawa, Y. (1985). J. Invest. Dermatol, 85,
434.
Ohba, M., Sato, R., Yoshida, Y., Nishino, T. and Katsuki,
H. (1978). Biochem. Biophys. Res. Commun, 85, 21.
Ortiz de Montellano, P. and Reich, N.O. (1986). in
"Cytochrome P-450 : structure, mechanism and bio-
chemistry" (Ed by Ortiz de Montellano, P.R). Plenum
Press, New York, 273.
Paik, Y.-K., Trzaskos, J.M., Shafies, A. and Gaylor, J.
(1984). J. Biol. Chem. 259, 13413.
Pascal, R.A., Chang, P. and Schroepfer, G.J. (1980). J. Am.
Chem. Soc, 102, 6599.
Pont, A., Graybill, J.R., Craven, P.C. and Galgiani, J.N.
(1984). Arch. Intern. Med, 144, 2150.
Pont, A., Goldman, E.S. and Sugar, A.M. (1985). Arch.
Intern. Med. 145, 1429.
Pont, A., Williams, P.L., Loose, D.S., Feldman, D., Reitz,
R.E., Bochra, C. and Stevens, D.A. (1982). Ann. Intern.
Med, 97, 370.
Pye, G.W. and Marriott, M.S. (1982). Sabouraudia, 20, 325.
Ragsdale, N.N. (1975). Biochim. Biophys. Acta, 380, 81.
Rodriguez, R.J., Low, C., Bottema, C.D.K. and Parks, L.W.
(1985). Biochim. Biophys. Acta, 837, 336.
Santen, R.J., Worgul, T.J., Samojlik, E., Boucher, A.E.,
Lipton, A. Harvey, H. (1982a). Cancer Res (Suppl) 42,
3397s.

Santen, R.J., Santner, S.J., Tilsen-Mallett, N., Rosen, H.R., Samajlik, E. and Veldhuis, J.D. (1982b). Cancer Res (Suppl) 42, 3353s.

Santen, R.J., Vanden Bossche, H., Symoens, J., Brugmans, J. and De Coster, R. (1983). J. Clin. Endocrinol. Metab, 57, 732.

Sanglard, D. (1985). Dis. ETH No. 7814, ADAG Administration and Druck AG, Zurich, 57.

Shafiee, A., Trzaskos, J.M., Paik, Y.-K. and Gaylor, J.L. (1986). J. Lipid Res, 27, 1.

Sheets, J.J. and Mason, J.I. (1984). Drug. Met. Dispos, 12, 603.

Siegel, M.R., Ragsdale, N.N. (1978). Pestic. Biochem. Physiol, 9, 48.

Siegel, M.R., Solel, Z. (1981). Pestic. Biochem. Physiol, 15, 222.

Trachtenberg, J. (1984). J. Urology, 132, 599.

Trocha, P.J., Jasne, S.J. and Sprinson, D.B. (1977). Biochemistry, 16, 4721.

Troner, M.B. (1982). Cancer Res (Suppl) 42, 3402s.

Trzaskos, J.M., Kawata, S., Daulerio, A. and Gaylor, J.L. (1984). Fed. Proceed, 43, 2034 (Abstract 3586).

Uzgiris, V.I., Whipple, C.A. and Salhanick, H.A. (1977). Endocrinology, 101, 89.

Vanden Bossche, H. (1985). in "Current topics in medical mycology" (Ed. by McGinnis, M.R) vol. 1, Springer-Verlag, New York, 313.

Vanden Bossche, H., Willemsens, G., Cools, W., Lauwers, W.F.J. and Le Jeune, L. (1978). Chem. Biol. Interact, 21, 59.

Vanden Bossche, H., Willemsens, G., Cools, W., Cornelissen, F., Lauwers, W.F. and Van Cutsem, J.M. (1980). Antimicrob. Ag. Chemother, 17, 922.

Vanden Bossche, H. and Willemsens, G. (1982). Archiv. Int. Physiol. Biochem, 90, B218.

Vanden Bossche, H., Ruysschaert, J.-M., Defrise-Quertain, F., Willemsens, G., Cornelissen, F., Marichal, P. and Cools, W. (1982). Biochem. Pharmacol, 31, 2609.

Vanden Bossche, H., Willemsens, G., Marichal, P., Cools, W. and Lauwers, W. (1984a). in "Mode of action of antifungal agents" (Ed. by Trinci, A.P.J. and Ryley, J.F). Cambridge University Press, Cambridge, 321.

Vanden Bossche, H., Lauwers, W., Willemsens, G., Marichal, P., Cornelissen, F. and Cools, W. (1984b). Pestic. Sci, 15, 188.

Vanden Bossche, H., Willemsens, G., Cools, W. and Bellens, D. (1984c). Biochem. Pharmacol, 33, 3861.

Vanden Bossche, H., Lauwers, W., Willemsens, G. and Cools,

W. (1985a). in "Microsomes and drug oxidations" (Ed. by Boobis, A.R., Caldwell, J., de Matteis, F. and Elcombe C.R). Taylor and Francis, London, 63.

Vanden Bossche, H., Lauwers, W., Willemsens, G. and Cools, W. (1985b). EORTC Genitourinary group, monograph 2, Part A : Therapeutic principles in metastatic prostate cancer (Ed. by Schroeder, F.H. and Richards, B). Alan, R. Liss, New York, 187.

Vanden Bossche, H., Bellens, D., Cools, W., Gorrens, J., Marichal, P., Verhoeven, H., Willemsens, G., De Coster, R., Beerens, D., Haelterman, C., Coene, M.-C., Lauwers, W. and Le Jeune, L. (1986). Drug Develop. Res, 6, in press.

Vanden Bossche, H., De Coster, R., Amery, W.K. (in press). in "Pharmacology and clinical use of inhibitors of hormone secretion and action" (Ed. by Furr, B. and Wakeling, A.E). Praeger, Eastbourne.

Waterman, M.R., John, M.E. and Simpson, E.R. (1986). in "Cytochrome P-450, structure, mechanism and biochemistry" (Ed. by Ortiz de Montellano, P.R). Plenum Press, New York, 345.

Willemsens, G. and Vanden Bossche, H. (1985). in "Cytochrome P-450 biochemistry biophysics and induction" (Ed. by Vereczkey, L. and Magyar, K). Akademiae Kiado, Budapest, 203.

Yoshida, Y., Aoyama, Y. (1986). in "In vitro and in vivo evaluation of antifungal agents" (Ed. by Iwata, K. and Vanden Bossche, H). Elsevier Science Publishers, Amsterdam, 123.

ANTIBODIES AS PROBES FOR DRUG METABOLISING ENZYMES

Philip Bentley, Willy Staubli, Francoise Bieri and Felix
Waechter.

Central Toxicology Unit, CIBA-GEIGY Limited, CH-4002, Basel,
Switzerland.

INTRODUCTION

Antibodies potentially provide very specific probes for
individual drug metabolising enzymes and isoenzymes. This
specificity is a consequence of the recognition by the
antibody molecules of defined regions, epitopes, within the
enzymes. Principally two types of antibody preparation may
be distinguished - polyclonal and monoclonal.

Polyclonal antibodies are prepared in whole animals,
usually rabbits or goats, and consequently contain a
mixture of immunoglobin molecules directed against
different epitopes within an antigen.

Monoclonal antibodies, on the other hand, are prepared
in vitro from hybridoma cells resulting from the fusion of
myeloma cells and B-lymphocytes isolated from the spleens
of immunized animals, generally mice or rats (Kohler and
Milstein, 1975). Since each such antibody results from a
single cell clone the immunoglobin molecules are all
directed against a single epitope within the antigen.
Consequently many different monoclonal antibodies may be
prepared against a single antigen.

Both types of antibody have been used as probes for
drug metabolising enzymes, each has its advantages and
disadvantages, some of which are listed in Table 1. It is
apparent that the preparation of choice will depend upon
the intended use and upon the properties of the available
antigen preparation. The various ways in which antibodies
have been used for drug metabolising enzymes are listed in
Table 2.

REACTION PHENOTYPING

This term implies the use of antibodies to determine
the contribution of an enzyme, or isoenzyme, to a specific
reaction or metabolic process. This may be achieved either

Table 1. Types of antibody preparation

A. Monoclonal Antibodies

    Advantages
- Defined molecular species
- Several different antibodies may be prepared against the same protein
- Supply indefinite
- Antigen need not be pure for immunization
- Large amounts available
- Required properties may be selected

    Disadvantages
- Often will not precipitate antigen
- Preparation and screen time consuming
- Selected epitopes may not be specific for one protein

B. Polyclonal Antibodies

    Advantages
- Easily prepared
- Generally precipitate antigen

    Disadvantages
- Require pure antigen preparation for immunization
- Supply limited and animal specific
- Require more extensive purification

---

by immunoprecipitating the enzyme from complex mixtures or proteins (e.g. solubilised membrane fractions) or by using antibodies which specifically inhibit the enzyme under investigation and then determining the effect of such precipitation or inhibition upon the metabolic process in question. For example, using polyclonal antibodies raised against rat liver microsomal epoxide hydrolase to immunoprecipitate the enzyme from solubilised microsomal fractions, Oesch and Bentley (1976) were able to show that the hydration of styrene oxide and benzo(a)pyrene 4,5-oxide were catalysed by the same microsomal enzyme. An extension of these studies showed that the same enzyme catalysed the hydration of several other substrates (Bindel et al, 1979; Bogel-Bindel 1982). Immunoinhibition studies have been extensively used to determine the contribution of different cytochrome P-450 isoenzymes towards the oxidation of various substrates and to investigate the regio- and stereo- selectivity of the individual isoenzymes involved in the metabolism of e.g. warfarin (Kaminsky et al, 1980; 1984), testosterone (Ryan et al, 1982; Reik et al, 1985) progesterone (Reubi et al, 1984) and N-acetylaminofluorene (Fujino et al, 1984). Both monoclonal and polyclonal antibodies have been used for such experiments. Monoclonal antibodies have the advantage that inhibitory antibodies may be selected (Reik et al, 1985). Using monoclonal antibodies to a 3-methylcholanthrene inducible cytochrome P-450, Park et al (1982) could demonstrate that at least two isoenzymes were responsible for aryl hydrocarbon hydroxylase and ethoxycoumarin O-de-ethylase activities in control and phenobarbital-induced microsomes, whereas only a single form seemed to catalyse these two reactions in microsomal fractions from 3-methylcholanthrene-induced rats. However, care must be taken when working with monoclonal antibodies to cytochrome P-450 because they are not always mono-specific (Levin et al, 1985), despite their ability to distinguish closely related isoenzymes (Reik et al, 1985).

Reaction phenotyping helps to define the substrate specificity of the individual enzymes and isoenzymes and thus contributes not only to our understanding of the enzymes themselves, but may permit predictions to be made concerning the effects of enzyme inducers and inhibitors on foreign compound metabolism, thus assisting in our understanding of unexpected drug-drug interactions.

ANTIGEN DETECTION

The most common use of antibodies is as specific tools to detect the corresponding antigens. As shown in Table 2 this may vary from the detection within a cell or tissue section (immunohistochemistry) to the detection of the antigen as the product of in vitro protein synthesis or as a means of screening a c-DNA library as an aid to cloning the specific gene. In many cases the antibodies must be labelled before they can be visualised, some typical labelling methods are shown in Table 3. Appropriate labels may be coupled directly to the immunoglobin molecules, but in this case care must be taken to ascertain that the ability of the antibody to bind the antigen is not impaired by the chemical modification. For this reason indirect labelling methods are often used; in this case the label is attached to a protein with a high affinity for the immunoglobin, for example an anti-anti-body, or protein A.

Table 2. Uses of Antibodies

A. Reaction Phenotyping
                 Immunoinhibition
                 Immunoprecipitation

B. Antigen Detection
                 Comparison of Proteins
                         Immunodiffusion
                         Immunoelectrophoresis
                 Immunoassay
                         Quantitative Immunoprecipitation
                         Radial Diffusion
                         Quantitative Electrophoresis
                         RIA
                         ELISA
                 Immunohistochemistry
                         Tissue Distribution
                         Analysis of cell cultures
                 Immunocytochemistry
                 Immunoelectronmicroscopy
                 Blotting analysis
                 c-DNA Library Screening
                 In Vitro Protein Synthesis

C. Immunoaffinity Purification

Table 3. Labelling methods for antibodies.

METHOD	EXAMPLE	USES
Radio Labelling	I ^{131}	RIA, Immunoautoradiography
Fluorescence Labelling	Fluorescence	Immunohistochemistry
Enzyme Labelling	Peroxidase Alkaline Phosphatase	Immunohistochemistry Immunoblotting ELISA USERA
Electron Dense Labelling	Colloidal Gold Ferritin	Immunohistochemistry Immunocytochemistry Immunoelectronmicroscopy

Antibodies provide very powerful tools to distinguish between individual proteins and have been extensively used to compare isoenzymes of cytochrome P-450. Thus it has been shown that some isoenzymes are immunologically related to one another, whilst others are immunologically unique (Thomas et al, 1983; Ryan et al, 1982; Reik et al, 1985; Levin et al, 1985). Comparisons are possible between isoenzymes from different species or from different organs. Cytochromes P-450 isolated from rat and rabbit lungs are immunologically cross-reactive with their liver counterparts (Kaminsky et al, 1979; Serabjit-Singh et al, 1979) and microsomal epoxide hydrolases from rat liver, kidney, lung and testis are all immunologically related (Guengerich et al, 1979). On the other hand, the microsomal epoxide hydrolases of rat and human livers are immunologically distinct (Lu et al, 1979).

Immunological methods have been extensively used to quantitate individual drug metabolising enzymes or isoenzymes in subcellular fractions. Several different methods have been used (Table 4). In all cases the validity of the results will depend upon the specificity of the antibodies used. Cross-reactivity is particularly problematic with cytochrome P-450 where in some cases addition of the estimated concentrations of the individual isoenzymes has yielded values greater than that estimated spectrophotometrically.

Quantitative immunoprecipitation has also been used to study the maintenance and induction of cytochrome P-450 isoenzymes in hepatocyte cultures, for example Schuetz et al (1984) demonstrated that glucocorticoids induce de novo synthesis of a cytochrome P-450 isoenzyme in primary cultures of rat hepatocytes. Moreover, specific immunoprecipitation is essential for studies on the bio-synthesis of drug metabolising enzymes in cell free systems; as with human cytochromes P-450 (Guengerich et al, 1986) and rat liver cytochrome b5, cytochrome b5 reductase, cytochrome P-450 reductase, and epoxide hydrolase (Okada et al, 1982). In a similar manner antibodies may be used to screen c-DNA expression libraries, an essential part of the molecular cloning of the genes coding for the antigens (Guengerich et al, 1986; Tukey et al, 1985).

Extensive studies on the distribution of drug metabolism enzymes within various organs have been performed immunohistochemically. In most cases antibodies have been visualised using indirect peroxidase labelling (Sternberger et al, 1970). Such studies have shown that most of the enzymes are heterogeneously distributed within the liver and in some cases the distribution was altered by

Table 4.   Methods used for Immunoquantitation of Drug Metabolising Enzymes.

METHOD	ENZYME	REFERENCE
Radial Immuno Diffusion	Cytochromes P-450	Thomas et al, 1979;1981; 1983; Parkinson et al, 1983
	Glutathione transferases	Bhargava et al, 1982 Jennson et al, 1985 Somo et al, 1986
Rocket Electro- phoresis	Cytochromes P-450	Gasser et al, 1982 Dai et al, 1984
	Glutathione transferases	
Immuno- blotting	Cytochromes P-450	Dannan et al, 1983
Radioimmuno- assay	Cytochromes P-450	Park et al, 1984 Song et al, 1985 Phillips et al, 1983
	UDP-Glucuronyl transferases	Chowdhury et al, 1983
ELISA	Cytochromes P-450	Paye et al, 1984
	Epoxide Hydrolase	Wolf et al, 1983

enzyme induction. Microsomal epoxide hydrolase was concentrated mainly in centrilobular hepatocytes in livers from untreated rats, treatment with phenobarbital enhanced this heterogeneity, whilst induction with acetylamino-fluorene or nafenopin resulted in a more homogeneous immune staining pattern (Bentley et al, 1979; Staubli et al, 1984). These studies also showed that the enzyme was found only in hepatocytes, since very little staining was observed in the non-parenchymal cells. Similar studies have been performed with other drug metabolising enzymes (Table 5).

In general components of the mono-oxygenase system are more concentrated in centrilobular regions. The pheno-barbital inducible forms of cytochrome P-450 tend to show very little immunostaining in midzonal and periportal cells. The 3-methylcholanthrene inducible isoenzymes show

Table 5. Immuno histochemical determination of the localisation of some drug metabolising enzymes in the rat liver.

ENZYME	CONTROL DISTRIBUTION	INDUCERS	ALTERATION	REFERENCE
Cytochrome P-450 PB-B[1]	CL>MZ>PP	-	-	Baron et al, 1981
Cytochrome P-450 MC-B[1]	CL>MZ=PP	-	-	Baron et al, 1981
Cytochrome P-450 PB1[1]	CL>MZ*	PB,PCN,MC,BNF,Iso,Aro	Yes	Wolf et al, 1984
Cytochrome P-450 PB2	CL[2]	PB,PCN,MC,BNF,Iso,Aro	Yes	Wolf et al, 1984
Cytochrome P-450 MC1	CL[2]	PB,PCN,MC,BNF,Iso,Aro	Yes	Wolf et al, 1984
Cytochrome P-450 MC2	PO[2]	PB,PCN,MC,BNF,Iso,Aro	Yes	Wolf et al, 1984
Cytochrome P-450 reductase	CL=MZ>PP	PB,PCN,MC,BNF,Iso,Aro	Yes	Taira et al, 1980 a,b; Dees et al, 1980; Wolf et al, 1984
Expoxide Hydrolase	CL>MZ	PB,PCN,MC,BNF,Iso,Aro AAF,Naf,TSO	Yes	Bentley et al, 1979 Staubli et al, 1984
Glutathione S-transferase B	CL>MZ	PB,PCN,MC,BNF,Iso,Aro	Yes	Wolf et al, 1984
Glutathione S-transferase C	CL>MZ	PB,PCN,MC,BNF,Iso,Aro	No	Wolf et al, 1984
UDP-lucuronyl-transferase	CL>MZ>PP	PB,MC	Yes	Ullrich et al, 1984

CL=Centrilobular, MZ=Midzonal, PP=Periportal, PB=Phenobarbital, PCN=Pregnenolone carbonitrile, MC=Methylcholanthrene, BNF= -naphthoflavone, Iso=Isosafrole, Aro=Aroclor, AAF=Acetylaminoflourene, Naf=Nafenopin.
1 Terms may refer to the same isoenzyme   2 Only minor staining in this zone.

a more homogenous distribution (Baron et al 1981; Wolf et al, 1984). An exception was P-450MC2 (P-450c). This isoenzyme could only be demonstrated in periportal cells in liver sections from control and β-naphthoflavone-induced animals, but was homogenously distributed after phenobarbital treatment (Wolf et al, 1984). A similar marked change in the distribution upon enzyme induction has been reported for the 3-methylcholanthrene inducible form of UDP-glucuronyl transferase. This enzyme was found mainly in centrilobular cells of control and 3-methylcholanthrene induced rats, but was more concentrated in periportal regions following phenobarbital treatment (Ullrich et al, 1984).

Immunohistochemistry has also been performed to study the distribution of drug metabolising enzymes in extrahepatic tissues including lung (Dees et al, 1980; Serabijit-Singh et al, 1980) and exocrine pancreas (Kawabata et al, 1984). In these tissues the enzymes were shown to be concentrated in a particular cell type rather than distributed evenly throughout the organ, accounting for the sensitivity of these cells to chemically induced toxicity.

Further marked heterogeneities in the distribution of some drug metabolising enzymes have been observed in the liver following treatment of rats with hepatocarcinogens and tumour promotors. Enzymes which have been shown to be over expressed in enzyme altered foci include epoxide hydrolase, UDP-glucuronyltransferase, cytochrome P-450 and glutathione transferase (Staubli et al, 1984; Buchmann et al, 1985; Kraus et al, 1984; Fischer et al, 1983; Schulte-Hermann et al, 1986). The reason for the over expression of these enzymes in the foci, which are thought to be precursors of liver tumours, is unclear.

The demonstration by immunohistochemistry of small numbers of cells with inordinately high enzyme contents is a good illustration of the power of such techniques, such effects would not be observed with the more commonly used biochemical methods. Similarly immunohistochemistry clearly indicates that the effects of enzyme inducers are more complex than apparent from simple measurement of enzyme activity. In this respect histochemical techniques may become increasingly important for studying responses in cultured cells (Ratanasavanh et al, 1986).

The ability to visualise the antigen using immunological techniques has proved valuable for investigations with subcellular fractions. In this case using biochemical determinations it is difficult to ascertain whether low levels of enzyme activity are genuinely associated with the fraction in question, or the result of contamination by small amounts of highly active organelles. Moreover, exhaustive purification of some subcellular organelles can be very. time consuming. Conjugation of antibodies with electron dense markers such as ferritin or colloidal gold permits detection of antigens using electron microscopy. By such methods it was possible to demonstrate that in rat liver, cytochrome P-450 and epoxide hydrolase were associated with the cytoplasmic surface of the nuclear envelope (Matsuura et al, 1981; Waechter et al, 1982). The nuclear antigen content was increased in both cases by treatment with enzyme inducers, indicating that the nuclear enzymes are also inducible. Quantitative immunoelectron-microscopy showed that both enzymes were present in smooth microsomal fractions at higher concentrations than in rough microsomal fractions; in agreement with biochemical measurements. With anti-epoxide hydrolase no specific labelling of intact mitochondria, lysosomes or peroxisomes was observed (Waechter et al, 1982).

From the above discussion it is apparent that antibodies provide a unique tool to study drug metabolising enzymes. Their uniqueness rests largely in the ability to visualise the immunoglobin molecules, thereby providing an important reinforcement of biochemical determinations at the tissue, cellular, subcellular and molecular level.

ENZYME PURIFICATION

Theoretically it should be possible to utilise the specificity of the antibody-antigen reaction for biospecific immunopurification of drug metabolising enzymes; particularly since immunoblotting experiments show that antibodies will often identify the antigen in complex mixtures of proteins. However, the affinity of the antibodies for their antigens is very high. Consequently, although it is straightforward to immobilise antibodies on an inert matrix and to bind the antigen to this matrix, it is generally not possible to dissociate the enzyme from this complex under conditions which maintain the enzymic activity. Recently (Friedman et al, 1985) have, however, made some progress towards biospecific affinity purification using specific antibodies. These authors demonstrated that a cytochrome P-450 isoenzyme maintained its antigenicity after elution from an immunoaffinity-chromatography matrix prepared using a monoclonal antibody. Thus, although the enzyme activity was lost, the epitope responsible for antibody binding remained intact.

Consequently the catalytically inactive cytochrome could be used in a second chromatography step to displace catalytically active cytochrome from the immobilised antibodies. Using similar techniques it may prove possible to purify other drug metabolising enzymes.

REFERENCES

Baron, J., Jedick, J.A. and Guengerich, F.P. (1981). J. Biol. Chem, 256, 5931.

Bentley, P., Waechter, F., Oesch, F. and Staubli, W. (1979). Biochem. Biophys. Res. Commun, 91, 1101.

Bhargava, M.M., Ohmi, N., Arias, I.M. and Becker, F.F. (1982). Oncology, 39, 378.

Bindel, U., Sparrow, A., Schmassmann, H., Golan, M., Bentley, P. and Oesch, F. (1979) Eur.J.Biochem, 97, 275.

Buchmann, A., Kuhlmann, W., Schwarz, M., Kunz, W., Wolf, C.R., Moll, E., Freidberg, T. and Oesch, F. (1985). Carcinogenesis, 6, 513.

Chowdhury, J.R., Chowdhury, N.R., Moscioni, A.D., Tukey, R., Tephly, T. and Arias, I.M. (1983). Biochem. Biophys. Acta, 761, 58.

Dannan, G.A., Guengerich, F.P., Kaminsky, L.S. and Aust, S.D. (1983). J. Biol. Chem, 258, 1282.

Dao, D.D., Patridge, C.A., Kurosky, A. and Awasthi, Y.C. (1984). Biochem. J. 221, 33.

Dees, J.H., Coe, L.D., Yasukochi, Y. and Masters, B.S. (1980). Science, 208, 1475.

Fischer, G., Ullrich, D., Katz, N., Bock, K.W. and Schauer, A. (1983). Virchows Arch (Cell Path) 42, 193.

Friedman, F.K., Robinson, R.C., Song, B.J., Park, S.S. and Gelboin, H.V. (1985). Biochemistry, 24, 7044.

Fujino, T., Est, D., Park, S.S. and Gelboin, H.V. (1984). J. Biol. Chem, 259, 9044.

Gasser, R., Hauri, H.P. and Meyer, U.A. (1982). FEBS Letts, 147, 239.

Guengerich, F.P., Distlerath, L.M., Reilly, P.E.B., Wolff, T., Shimada, T., Umbenhauer, D.R. and Martin, M.V. (1986). Xenobiotica, 16, 367.

Guengerich, F.P., Wang, P., Mason, P.S. and Mitchell, M.B. (1979). J. Biol. Chem, 254, 12255.

Jensson, H., Erikson, L.C. and Mannervik, B. (1985). FEBS Letts, 187, 115.

Kaminsky, L.S., Dannan, G.A. and Guengerich, F.P. (1984). Eur. J. Biochem, 141, 141.

Kaminsky, L.S., Fasco, M.J. and Guengerich, F.P. (1979). J. Biol. Chem, 254, 9657.

Kaminsky, L.S., Fasco, M.J. and Guengerich, F.P. (1980). J. Biol. Chem, 255, 85.

Kawabata, T.T., Guengerich, F.P. and Baron, J. (1983). J. Biol. Chem, 258, 7767.

Kawabata, T.T., Wick, D.G., Guengerich, F.P. and Baron, J. (1984). Cancer Res, 44, 215.

Kohler, G. and Milstein, C. (1975). Nature, 256, 495.

Kraus, P., Schulte-Hermann, R., Timmermann-Trosiener, I. and Schuppler, J. (1984). Toxicol. Pathol, 12, 344.

Levin, W., Thomas, P.E., Reik, L.M., Ryan, D.E., Bandiera, S., Haniu, M. and Shively, J.E. (1985). in "Microsomes and Drug Oxidations" (Ed. by Boobis, A.R., Caldwell, J., de Matteis, F. and Elcombe, C). Taylor & Francis, London, p.13.

Lu, A.Y.H., Thomas, P.E., Ryan, D., Jerina, D.M. and Levin, W. (1979). J. Biol. Chem, 254, 5878.

Matsuura, S., Masuda, R., Omori, K., Negishi, M. and Tashiro, Y. (1981). J. Cell. Biol, 91, 212.

Oesch, F. and Bentley, P. (1976). Nature 259, 53.

Okada, Y., Frey, A.B., Guenthner, T., Oesch, F., Sabatini, D.D. and Kreibich, G. (1982). Eur. J. Biochem, 122, 393.

Park, S.S., Fujino, I., West, D., Guengerich, F.P. and Gelboin, H.V. (1982). Cancer Res, 42, 1798.

Park, S.S., Fujino, T., Miller, H., Guengerich, F.P. and Gelboin, H.V. (1984). Biochem. Pharmacol, 33, 2071.

Parkinson, A., Safe, S.H., Robertson, L.W., Thomas, P.E., Ryan, D.E., Reik, L.M. and Levin, W. (1983). J. Biol. Chem, 258, 5967.

Paye, M., Beaune, P., Kremers, P., Guengerich, F.P., Letawe-Goujon, F. and Gielen, J. (1984). Biochem. Biophys. Res. Commun, 122, 137.

Phillips, I.R., Shephard, E.A., Bayney, R.M., Pike, S.F., Rabin, B.R., Heath, R. and Carter, N. (1983). Biochem. J. 212, 55.

Ratanasavanh, D., Beaune, P., Baffet, G., Rissel, M., Kremers, P., Guengerich, F.P. and Guillouzo, A. (1986). J. Histochem. Cytochem, 34, 527.

Reik, L.M., Levin, W., Ryan, D.E., Maines, S.L. and Thomas, P.E. (1985). Arch. Biochem. Biophys, 242, 365.

Reubi, I., Griffin, K.J., Raucy, J. and Johnson, E.F. (1984). Biochemistry, 23, 4598.

Ryan, D., Thomas, P.E., Reik, L.M. and Levin, W. (1982). Xenobiotica, 12, 727.

Schuetz, E.G., Wrighton, S.A., Barwick, J.L. and Guzelian, P.S. (1984). J. Biol. Chem, 259, 1999.

Schulte-Hermann, R., Timmermann-Trosiener, I. and Schuppler, J. (1986). Carcinogenesis, 7, 1651.

Serabjit-Singh, C.J., Wolf, C.R. and Philpot, R.M. (1979). J. Biol. Chem, 254, 9901.

Serabjit-Singh, C.J., Wolf, C.R. and Philpot, R.M. (1980). Science, 207, 1469.

Soma, Y., Satoh, K. and Sato, K. (1986). Biochim. Biophys. Acta, 869, 247.

Song, B.J., Gelboin, H.V., Park, S.S., Friedmann, F.K. (1985). Biochem, J. 231, 671.

Staubli, W., Bentley, P., Bieri, F., Frohlich, E. and Waechter, F. (1984). Carcinogenesis, 5, 41.

Sternberger, L.A., Hardy, P.H., Cuculis, J.J. and Meyer, H.G. (1970). J. Histochem. Cytochem. 18, 315.

Taira, Y., Greenspan, P., Kapke, G.., Redick, J.A. and Baron, J. (1980a). Mol. Pharmacol, 18, 304.

Taira, Y., Redick, J.A. and Baron, J. (1980b). Mol. Pharmacol, 17, 374.

Thomas, P.E., Koreniowski, D., Ryan, D. and Levin, W. (1979). Arch. Biochem. Biophys, 192, 524.

Thomas, P.E., Reik, L.M., Ryan, D.E. and Levin, W. (1981). J. Biol. Chem, 256, 1044.

Thomas, P.E., Reik, L.M., Ryan, D.E. and Levin, W. (1983). J. Biol. Chem, 258, 4590.

Tukey, R.H., Okino, S., Barnes, H., Griffin, K.J. and Johnson, E.F. (1985). J. Biol. Chem, 260, 13347.

Ullrich, D., Fischer, G., Katz, N. and Bock, K.W. (1984). Chem. Biol. Interactions, 48, 181.

Vogel-Bindel, U., Bentley, P. and Oesch, F. (1982). Eur. J. Biochem, 126, 425.

Waechter, F., Bentley, P., Germann, M., Oesch, F. and Staubli, W. (1982). Biochem. J. 202, 677.

Wolf, C.R., Moll. E., Friedberg, T., Oesch, F., Buchmann, A., Kulmann, W.D. and Kunz, H.W. (1984). Carcinogenesis, 5, 993.

Wolf, C.R., Oesch, F., Timms, C., Guenthner, T., Hartman, R., Marun, M. and Burger, R. (1983). FEBS Letts, 157, 271.

QUANTITATIVE CYTOCHEMISTRY

Joseph Chayen and Lucille Bitensky

Division of Cellular Biology, Kennedy Institute of Rheumatology, Bute Gardens, Hammersmith, London, W6 7DW.

THE NATURE OF QUANTITATIVE CYTOCHEMISTRY

In studies done by normal light microscopy there are two quite disparate forms of investigation that are often confused. The first is histochemistry which has been well defined by Barka and Anderson (1963) in their text book of Histochemistry. They said that histochemistry "is a system of chemical morphology that adds another dimension to histology but which shares the basically static character of the morphological sciences. Its contribution cannot be assessed in the dynamic, physiological terms of biochemistry .... finite measurement is not the immediate goal of microscopic histochemistry. Deriving its theoretical foundations from chemistry, histochemistry remains essentially a morphological tool". In complete contrast, quantitative cytochemistry is essentially a micro-form of rigorous biochemistry, done at the level of the individual cell. Because it involves relatively non-disruptive procedures, it can further extend conventional biochemical analyses (as will be considered later). This applies particularly with respect to membrane-bound activities which can be markedly altered by homogenisation in normal biochemical studies. However, when the activities can be compared, the activities recorded by quantitative cytochemistry agree closely with those found by conventional biochemistry (Chayen, 1978a as regards pentose-shunt dehydrogenase; Olsen et al, 1981 for β-glucuronidase). Even with such activities, the particular advantage of quantitative cytochemistry is that it measures activity in individual cells instead of that measurable by normal biochemistry in samples that must contain 10^6 cells (Olsen et al, 1981). This is of especial value in endocrinology and in toxicology where the active agent may have its major effect on specific tissue components that may constitute perhaps only 5-10% of the total mass of an organ (see later).

THE RANGE OF QUANTITATIVE CYTOCHEMISTRY

The best known techniques of quantitative cytochemistry involve chromogenic reactions, whether to disclose particular substances or active groups or to measure enzymatic activities. However the methodology of quantitative cytochemistry is virtually as extensive as is that of general biochemistry. Microfluorometry can be used for quantifying fluorescent compounds or fluorescent reactions and for measuring changes in the state of cellular and sub-cellular membranes; dry mass of individual cells, or of cellular organelles within cells, can be measured by microscopic interferometry (Chayen, 1967; Darracott-Cankovic et al, 1984 for the water content of biopsies of oedematous human heart); the orientation of molecules (e.g. changes in myosin in human heart biopsies: Chayen et al, 1985; changes in proteoglycans: Kent et al, 1983); and uptake and distribution of radioactive labels by quantitative autoradiography (e.g. Pelc, 1958).

PRECISION OF QUANTITATIVE CYTOCHEMISTRY

Probably the clearest evidence of the precision of this form of micro-biochemistry comes from the cytochemical bioassays (e.g. Chayen, 1978b; Chayen, 1980). In these bioassays, the target tissue is maintained for 5h in non-proliferative maintenance culture and then exposed to graded concentrations of the hormone (usually 10^{-15} to 10^{-12} g/ml) or to dilutions of the plasma ($1:10^2$ to $1:10^4$) that is to be assayed. The tissue is then chilled, sectioned, and reacted for a biochemical activity that is influenced by the hormone. The index of precision (λ) of such assays is as low as around 0.1 (a λ as high as 0.2 is normally acceptable in bioassays). These cytochemical bioassays have found wide acceptance (e.g. WHO Report, 1975; Chayen and Bitensky, 1983) since they are often far more sensitive than the equivalent immunoassays and have the additional advantage of defining the circulating concentration of biologically active hormone.

METHODOLOGY

The methods of quantitative cytochemistry differ in many critical aspects from those of histochemistry. They have been fully reviewed by Chayen et al (1973a), and by Chayen (1978b; 1980). The processes involve (i) briefly chilling the tissue rapidly to -70°C in hexane; (ii) cutting the block of tissue in a cryostat maintained at around -25°C with the knife chilled to around -70°C; (iii) flash-drying the section off the knife; and (iv) using protective colloid stabilisers, when necessary, for retaining the integrity of the section during the cytochemical reaction. The coloured reaction-product is measured in individual cells by microdensitometry.

APPLICATIONS OF QUANTITATIVE CYTOCHEMISTRY IN TOXICOLOGY

There are now many examples of the particular value of quantitative cytochemistry in toxicological problems. These may be grouped under three headings :
i. activities which can be nullified by severe preparatory procedures such as homogenization;
ii. the specific localisation of activity within a complex tissue
iii. activities which depend on the interaction of different cellular compartments.
(i) Activities which can be nullified by preparatory procedures. The typical example is the effect of homogenisation and isolation of mitochondria on the activity of, for example, mitochondrial glutamate dehydrogenase. Bendall and de Duve (1960) had shown that the activity of this enzyme increased with increasing times of homogenisation. Chayen and Bitensky (1968) showed that the early changes in activity, related to the effect of liver damage, were even lower than the changes found as a consequence of mild homogenisation so that the effect of homogenisation could mask changes likely to be induced by mild liver toxins.
(ii) The localisation of altered activity within a complex tissue. This has particular relevance to the assay of the biological activity of hormones and to the effect of toxic material that influences only a specific cell-type which may constitute only a small fraction of the mass of an organ. It is a phenomenon of such general pertinence that it merits elaboration. Suppose you have a tissue in which all the cells have a particular activity, such as glucose-6-phosphate dehydrogenase (G6PD) activity. Then per unit mass, you may have 1000 units of this activity. Let us suppose that a hormone, or a toxic substance, doubles this activity in specific target cells that constitute ten percent of the mass of this organ. The activity 'per gramme', of the tissue will change from 1000 to 1100, which may well be within the limits of measurement. However for each affected cell, the activity will be doubled, and this will be readily measurable by quantitative cytochemistry. This is the basis of the cytochemical bioassay of many

polypeptide hormones (Chayen, 1980; Chayen and Bitensky, 1983). For example, parathyroid hormone influences the distal convoluted tubules of the kidney (among others). These constitute about 5-10% of the cortex of the kidney. Low concentrations (up to 0.1 pg/ml) of the hormone may almost double the G6PD activity in these tubules: this is the basis of the cytochemical bioassay of this hormone which is now widely used (Kent and Zanelli, 1983). This principle has been used by Smith and Wills (1981a) in their studies on the effects of unsaturated lipids on the liver. Another specific example concerning the effect of phenobarbitone on the liver will be considered in more detail (below).

(iii) Interaction between different cellular compartments. Perhaps the most heuristic value of quantitative cytochemistry is that it allows the detection, and measurement, of metabolic interactions that may occur between different sub-cellular compartments within individual cells. These are of two types : the first deals with the disposition of reducing groups produced by the activity of cytosolic G6PD activity; the second is concerned with interactions between cytosolic and mitochondrial enzymatic activity. Both can be influenced by drugs but these effects cannot be appreciated in disrupted and isolated systems.

(a) The disposition of cytosolic reducing equivalents. It has been shown (Chayen, 1978a) that the estimation of the total activity of two of the main cytosolic, NADPH-producing enzymes, measured by quantitative cytochemistry is quantitatively identical to that measured by conventional homogenate biochemistry (in μmoles of hydrogen/cm^3). But quantitative cytochemistry can extend the analysis of this activity in that it can differentiate between the amount of the NADPH that can be utilised at high negative electrode-potential and that at low electrode-potential. That is, it can differentiate between NADPH used, for example, for biosynthetic activity and that used for the cytochrome P-450 system (Chayen and Bitensky, 1982; Chayen et al, 1986). Analysis of this type was used to elucidate the effect of dietary lipid on the liver (Smith and Wills, 1981a). It was also used to show the differential effect of steroids (Chayen et al, 1973b, 1974). For example, although progesterone in the reaction-medium had no effect on the total production of reducing equivalents derived from G6PD in rat liver, it markedly altered the disposition of these reducing equivalents towards the biosynthetic pathway. Similarly, in experimentally induced liver tumours in rats, although the total G6PD activity was unaffected, the proportion of reducing equivalents made available to the biosynthetic pathway was markedly increased in the tumours, with a concomitant decrease in the proportion available to the low electrode-potential pathway (Chayen et al, 1974). (b) **Interactions between cytosolic and mitochondrial activities.** The basis of these studies is as follows: triplicate sections are reacted either with a substrate for a mitochondrial enzyme (I), or with one for a cytosolic enzyme (II), or with both together (III). The activity recorded in the last group (III) would be expected to be equal to the sum of the activities recorded in I plus II. Where synergism occurs, activity III is considerably greater than the sum of the other two activities. For example, in sections of rat liver, reacted so as to give low levels of activity of succinate dehydrogenase (2µg formazan/mm^3/h) and moderate levels of G6PD activity (39µg formazan/mm^3/h), there was considerable enhancement of total activity when both substrates were included together (74µg formazan/mm^3/h). In the presence of progesterone or pregnenolone, this enhancement was virtually lost whereas cortisone did not alter the enhanced activity (Chayen et al, 1974). In recent studies, Bachelet et al (1986) showed that this type of synergistic activity, between mitochondrial and cytosolic systems, could be demonstrated in sections of rat kidney and that it was most marked in the pars recta which is the major site of 1α-hydroxylation of 25-hydroxyvitamin D$_3$. The evidence of these workers strongly supported the earlier finding (Chayen et al, 1974) that this enhanced activity was due to increased flow of reducing equivalents from succinate dehydrogenase activity synergistically abetted by the production of cytosolic reducing equivalents generated by the cytosolic G6PD activity.

MICROSPECTROPHOTOMETRIC ASSAY OF CYTOCHROMES P-450 AND P-448.

A particular application of quantitative cytochemistry is the definition of the localisation of a specific activity within a complex tissue. This is characterised by the microspectrophotometric analysis of cytochrome P-450 and P-448. For this work (Gooding et al, 1978; Chayen et al, 1979) the Zeiss double beam ultraviolet and visible microspectrophotometer (Zeiss UMSP) has been used (Figure 1) which, basically, is a conventional double-beam recording spectrophotometer built around a microscope. Rat liver was chilled and sectioned, normally at 40µm to give

reasonably strong signals. The sections were exposed first
to dithionite and then to carbon monoxide; they were
mounted in 20% polyvinyl alcohol (which stabilises and
protects the sections even at relatively neutral pH
values).

Validity of method and induction by phenobarbital : To test
the validity of such microspectrophotometric measurements
pellets were made from the same sample of microsomes as was
used for the conventional biochemical assay of cytochrome
P-450 from both normal rats and those fed with
phenobarbitone. The results by both procedures (μmol/l)
were in close agreement. Estimates of the P-450 content of
hepatocytes in sections of these livers showed double the
content found biochemically: this was found to be due to
the loss of cytosolic material during the biochemical
extraction of the microsomes, as shown by the glucose-6-
phosphatase content of the microsomal and of the total
liver samples. The particular advantage of the
cytochemical assay was that it demonstrated firstly that
the distribution of the cytochrome P-450 was not uniform
across the lobule but was higher close to the centrilobular
vein and secondly that feeding with phenobarbitone markedly
increased the concentration of cytochrome P-450
particularly centrilobularly (Gooding et al, 1978; Chayen
et al, 1979). Similar effects of phenobarbitone were
reported by Smith and Wills (1981b) who also showed, in
contrast, that dietary lipids caused uniform changes in the
concentration of cytochrome P-450 throughout the lobule.

Effect of other agents. The short-term effect of carbon
tetrachloride in rats (0.125 ml/100g body weight) before
obvious signs of necrosis (2 h after treatment), has been
investigated. It was clear (Table 1), that, in
phenobarbitone-treated rats, the major effect on the
cytochrome P-450 concentration per cell was on the cells of
the centrilobular region. In rats treated with 3-methyl
cholanthrene (0.075 mmol/kg daily for 3 days) the main
induction was found more towards the centre of the lobule
(Figure 2). The absorption maximum of the induced
cytochrome P-448, in these cells, could be readily
distinguished by direct microspectrophotometry (Figure 3).
Essentially similar results were found by Connelly (1983)
in more extended studies.

CONCLUSIONS

It is hoped that this brief review may indicate that
quantitative cytochemistry is a precise form of
microbiochemistry applied to individual cells within a

Figure 1. A Zeiss ultraviolet and universal microspectrophotometer.

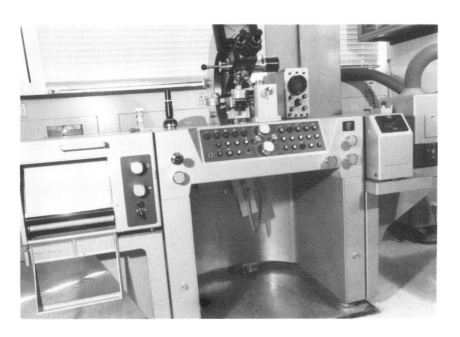

From the right there is the xenon arc in its housing, with
an exhaust pipe to remove gases; a conventional Zeiss
monochromator, the specimen microscope; the subsidiary
microscope tube for viewing the contol speciment that is
traversed by the second beam; and the chart recorder.

complex tissue. The most widely used aspect of this
methodology at present is in the assay of the biological
activity of hormones for which there was an immediate need
(WHO Report, 1975). In general, toxicological problems
seem to be capable of elucidation by conventional
biochemical procedures although we have attempted to show
that cytochemistry can clarify the particular cell-type or
location that is specifically influenced by an active
agent, such as phenobarbitone or 3-methylcholanthrene.
However, the real impact of quantitative cytchemistry may
well be found in the case of drugs, or toxic agents, that
involve the synergistic activities of different subcellular components within the target-cells.

Table **1.** Microspectrophotometric measurement of cytochrome P-450 content per cell (μmol/l) in intact liver sections.

TREATMENT	PERIPORTAL	CENTRILOBULAR
Phenobarbitone (n = 30; 3 rats)	33.4+3.2	113.9+4.6
Phenobarbitone + CCl_4 2hr (n = 39; 5 rats)	25.6+1.8	26.0+2.3
% decrease	23	77
	$0.05 > p > 0.02$	$p < 0.001$

Figure **2.** A trace of the maximum absorption at 448nm derived from full absorption traces of individual hepatocytes at defined positions across a single liver lobule of a rat fed with 3-methylcholanthrene.

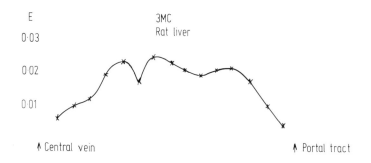

ACKNOWLEDGEMENT

We are grateful to Professor J.W. Bridges and Professor T.F. Slater, and to members of their Departments, for help with this work, and to the Arthritis and Rheumatism Council for Research for general support.

Figure 3. Absorption traces of individual hepatocytes in different sections from rats treated with either phenobarbitone or 3-methylcholanthrene. The resolution of the two peaks is apparent.

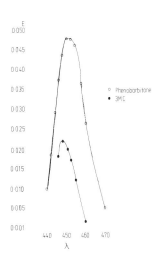

REFERENCES

Bachelet, M., Lair, M., Thomas, M., Monet, D., Ulmann, A. and Bader, C. (1986). Cell Biochem. Funct, 4, 227.

Barka, T. and Anderson, P.J. (1963). "Histochemistry", Harper and Row, New York.

Bendall, D.S. and de Duve, C. (1960). Biochem. J., 74, 444.

Chayen, J. (1967). in "In Vivo techniques in histology", (Ed. by Bourne, G.H). Williams and Wilkins, Baltimore, P. 40.

Chayen, J. (1978a). in "Biochemical Mechanisms of Liver Injury". (Ed. by Slater, T.F). Academic Press, London, p. 257.

Chayen, J. (1978b). Int. Rev. Cytol, 53, 333.

Chayen, J. (1980). "The Cytochemical Bioassay of Polypeptide Hormones", Springer, Berlin.

Chayen, J. and Bitensky, L. (1968). in "The Biological Basis of Medicine". (Ed. by Bittar, E.E. and Bittar, N). Academic Press, New York, Vol 1, p. 337.

Chayen J. and Bitensky, L. (1982). Rev. Pure Appl. Pharmacol. Sci, 3, 271.

Chayen, J. and Bitensky, L. ,Eds. (1983). "Cytochemical Bioassays: Techniques and Clinical Applications", Marcel Dekker, New York.

Chayen, J., Altman, F.P. and Butcher, R.G. (1973b). in "Fundamentals of Cell Pharmacology". (Ed., Dikstein, S). Chas. C. Thomas, Springfield, Illinois, p. 196.

Chayen, J., Bitensky, L., Braimbride, M.W. and Darracott-Cankovic, S. (1985). Cell Biochem. Funct, 3, 101.

Chayen, J., Bitensky, L. and Butcher, R.G. (1973a). "Practical Histochemistry", Wiley, London.

Chayen, J., Bitensky, L., Butcher, R.G. and Altman, F.P. (1974). Advs. Steroid Biochem. Pharmacol, 4, 1.

Chayen J., Bitensky, L., Johnstone, J.J., Gooding, P.E. and Slater, T.F. (1979). in "Quantitative Cytochemistry and its Applications". (Eds. Pattison, J.R., Bitensky, L. and Chayen, J). Academic Press, London, p. 129.

Chayen, J., Howat, D.W. and Bitensky, L. (1986). Cell Biochem. Funct, 4 (in the press).

Connelly, J.C. (1983). PhD Thesis, University of Surrey.

Darracott-Cankovic, S., Braimbridge, M.V., Kyosola, K., Bitensky, L. and Chayen J. (1984). Cell Biochem. Funct, 2, 57.

Gooding, P.E., Chayen, J., Sawyer, B. and Slater, T.F. (1978). Cell Biol. Interact, 20, 299.

Kent, G.N. and Zanelli, J.M. (1983). in "Cytochemical Bioassays : Techniques and Clinical Applications". (Eds. Chayen J. and Bitensky, L). Marcel Dekker, New York, p. 255.

Kent, G.N., Dodds, R.A., Bitensky, L., Chayen, J., Klenerman, L. and Watts, R.W.E. (1983). J. Bone Jt. Surg. 65B, 189.

Olsen, I., Dean, M.F., Harris, G. and Muir, I. (1981). Nature (Lond), 291, 244.

Pelc, S. (1958). in "General Cytochemical Methods". (Ed., Danielli, J.F). Academic Press, New York, p. 279.

Smith, M.T. and Wills, E.D. (1981a). Biochem. J. 200, 691.

Smith, M.T. and Wills, E.D. (1981b). FEBS Letts, 127, 33.

WHO Report (1975). WHO Expert Committee on Biological Standisation. 26th Report. WHO Tech. Rep. Ser, 565.

IN VIVO PROBES FOR DRUG METABOLISING ENZYMES

B. Kevin Park

Department of Pharmacology and Therapeutics, Liverpool
University, Liverpool, L69 3BX.

INTRODUCTION

Metabolism may be an important determinant of drug efficacy, duration of effect and toxicity in an individual (Park and Breckenridge, 1981). There is therefore a need to develop in vivo test systems with which to answer the following questions :-

1. Do individuals vary in their ability and capacity to metabolise a particular drug?
2. Can a particular drug modulate (by either inhibition or induction) the activity of the drug-metabolising enzymes?
3. Is the metabolism of a particular drug susceptible to inhibition or induction by another drug (or environmental factor)?
4. In what circumstances are changes or differences in metabolism of either clinical or toxicological relevance?

The versatility of the systems responsible for drug metabolism is partly based on the multiplicity of enzymes which can effect a particular biotransformation. This concept is particularly well established for the hepatic cytochrome P-450 mixed-function oxidase enzymes, which have been partly purified, and have been well characterised in in vivo studies (Boobis and Davies, 1984; Guengerich et al, 1986). We are therefore faced with the problem of monitoring the activities of a large, but as yet undefined number of enzymes which do not possess absolute substrate specificity.

The key consideration in the assessment of drug metabolising enzyme activity in man, is to classify the enzyme of interest using model compounds in vitro, or probe drugs in vivo, which may serve as representative substrates

for the individual forms of the enzyme of interest.
However, it must be noted at the outset, that only a small
number of compounds have the pharmacological, toxicological
and pharmacokinetic properties required of a probe drug,
that can be used safely in patient and volunteer studies.

PROBES FOR GENETIC VARIATION IN DRUG METABOLISM

It is important from both a therapeutic and a
toxicological viewpoint to recognise individuals who have a
genetically determined inability to perform a particular
biotransformation. The two classical examples of
polymorphic drug metabolism reactions are the acetylation
of various drugs and hydrolysis of succinylcholine. The
capacity of individuals to acetylate therapeutically
important drugs such as isoniazid, hydralazine and
procainamide can be assessed using the probe drug
sulphadimidine (Weber and Hein, 1985).

Until recently pharmacogenetic polymorphisms in drug
oxidation were considered rare, despite the fact that the
majority of lipophilic drugs are metabolised by the hepatic
cytochrome P-450 enzymes. A number of monogenically
controlled polymorphic drug oxidations have now been
discovered (Table 1).

Table 1. Polymorphic drug oxidation in man.

Debrisoquine	Mahgoub et al., 1977
Sparteine	Eichelbaum et al., 1979
Mephenytoin	Kupfer et al., 1981
Tolbutamide	Scott and Poffenbarger, 1979
Carboxymethylcysteine	Waring et al., 1982
Antipyrine	Penno and Vesell, 1983
Nifedipine	Kleinbloesem et al., 1984
Theophylline	Miller et al., 1984

The most extensively studied have been the debrisoquine
and sparteine polymorphisms, which are thought to be
identical pharmacogenetic entities (Smith, 1985; Eichelbaum
et al, 1986). These two compounds have been used
extensively as in vivo probes to 1) identify individuals as
either extensive metabolisers (EM) or poor metabolisers
(PM), 2) determine the metabolic relationship with other
drugs, using either population studies or smaller groups

(phenotyped panels), 3) to assess the pharmacological and physiological consequences of the polymorphic nature of human drug oxidation reactions.

The oxidation (O-demethylation) of dextromethorphan to dextrorphan is under the same genetic control as the 4-hydroxylation of debrisoquine (Schmidt et al, 1985). It has therefore been suggested that measurement of the urinary dextromethorphan/dextrophan ratio, is an attractive alternative pharmacogenetic probe, because of the innocuous pharmacological properties of the drug.

The genetic polymorphism in mephenytoin oxidation is independent of the debrisoquine/sparteine polymorphism; the frequency of Swiss subjects with an inherited deficiency in mephenytoin hydroxylation was found to be 4% (Jupfer and Preisig, 1984). A list of drugs associated with the mephenytoin polymorphism is short, and at present contains only nirvanol and mephobarbitone. Polymorphism in oxidation at a sulphur centre was discovered during studies of the metabolism of the mucolytic agent S-carboxymethyl-cysteine (Waring et al, 1982). One study has indicated that individuals with impaired sulphoxidation status are more susceptible to major adverse reactions to D-penicillamine (Emery et al, 1984).

PROBES FOR MODULATION OF DRUG-METABOLISING ENZYME ACTIVITY

Since its introduction by Vesell (reviewed, 1979) the antipyrine test has been widely used to determine the qualitative and quantitative effects of genetic factors, drugs and environmental factors, and of disease, on the activity of the mixed-function oxidase system. Antipyrine has most of the pharmacokinetic properties required of an ideal probe drug and, importantly, has little or no pharmacological or toxicological activity at the dose (600mg) routinely used in volunteer and patient studies. It must be noted, however, that antipyrine is an auto-inducer, and therefore must not be given too frequently within a particular study (Ohnhaus and Park, 1979).

Genetic variation may be eliminated in a particular study by using each subject as their own control, and measuring antipyrine clearance before, during and after imposition of the factor under consideration. Antipyrine clearance, has been used to investigate the enzyme inducing properties of all drugs which are known to stimulate drug oxidation in man. In addition, the effects of dietary factors (Anderson et al, 1982), age and cigarette smoking (Vestal and Wood, 1980) on drug oxidation have been explored using the antipyrine test.

Breimer and co-workers (1983) have shown that more qualitative data may be obtained by measuring the partial clearances of antipyrine to its three metabolites, norantipyrine, 4-hydroxyantipyrine and 3-hydroxymethylantipyrine. The metabolites are thought to represent products of individual enzymes. Thus rifampicin selectively induces the enzyme responsible for norantipyrine formation (Toverud et al, 1981) while, in contrast, phenytoin selectively increases the formation of 4-hydroxyantipyrine (Shaw et al, 1985).

Antipyrine has also been used extensively to investigate inhibition of human hepatic drug oxidation in vivo. For example, the antimalarial drug primaquine produced a marked, but time-dependent, inhibition of antipyrine metabolism after a single (45mg) dose (Back et al, 1983a). There was a reduction in clearance to all three phase I metabolites. However, the antipyrine test cannot be used to predict the effects of a putative inhibitor on other drugs. Thus, primaquine does not inhibit the oxidation of the steroids ethynylestradiol or cortisol (Back et al, 1984), which are thought to be metabolied by independent cytochrome P-450 enzymes.

The time-course of inhibition of antipyrine metabolism by cimetidine was investigated in an elegant experiment by Teunissen et al, (1985). The clearance to all three metabolites was measured under steady-state conditions, while antipyrine was administered continuously, by rectal infusion. The effect of cimetidine was similar for the three major pathways, and persisted for almost 48h after the last dose of the H_2-antagonist.

Tolbutamide has been used as a probe drug for investigation of polymorphism in drug oxidation, as well as for studies on enzyme induction and enzyme inhibition. Tolbutamide clearance provides a sensitive probe for changes in the activity of drug-oxidising enzymes because its plasma elimination is dependent upon a single oxidative biotransformation in the liver. The sulphonamide sulphaphenazole produces a five-fold decrease in tolbutamide plasma clearance, and a corresponding decrease in excretion of urinary metabolites (Pond et al, 1977). Although sulphaphenazole is a potent inhibitor of tolbutamide hydroxylation, it has no effect on the oxidation of antipyrine, cortisol and sparteine (Back et al, 1983b; Park et al, unpublished data). We presume from these in vivo studies that tolbutamide is oxidised by an enzyme distinct from those involved in the oxidation of antipyrine, cortisol and sparteine which are themselves representative substrates for individual forms of cytochrome P-450 (Figure 1). However, definitive classification of probe drugs, with respect to particular enzymes, awaits purification and full characterisation of human cytochrome P-450 enzymes.

Figure 1. Graphic representation of different forms of human cytochrome P-450 (adapted from Breimer).

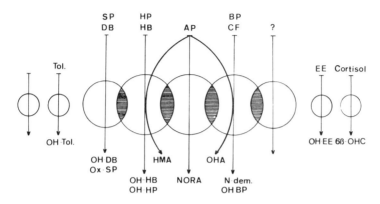

Key : Tol = tolbutamide; SP = sparteine; DB = debrisoquine; HP = heptobarbitone; HB = hexobarbitone; AP = antipyrine; HMA = 3-hydroxymethylantipyrine; NOR = norantipyrine; OHA = 4-hydroxyantipyrine; BP = benzpyrene; CF = caffeine; EE = ethynylestradiol. See text for details.

The activity of the hepatic mixed-function oxidase system can be monitored indirectly by analysis of isotopically (^{12}C or ^{14}C) labelled carbon dioxide in breath, after administration of a test drug labelled on an appropriate methyl group. Aminopyrine, which undergoes two successive N-demethylations in the liver, has been widely used for this purpose. The rate of breath output of labelled CO_2 is measured after enzyme induction with phenobarbitone, but is decreased by pretreatment with disulfiram, an inhibitor of the mixed-function oxidase system (Hepner and Vesell, 1975).

Theophylline and caffeine have been proposed as suitable probes for the human equivalent of the cytochrome P-448 (P_1-450) enzymes present in rat liver. The clearance of theophylline in smokers was greater that in non-smokers; total body clearance of theophylline showed a good correlation with serum thiocyanate concentrations, an index of exposure to cigarette smoke (Hunt et al, 1976).

Similarly, it was found that the rate of labelled CO_2 excretion after administration of ^{14}C-labelled caffeine to smokers was on average, twice that in non-smokers (Kotake et al, 1982).

NON-INVASIVE METHODS

Non-invasive methods for the assessment of drug-metabolising enzymes are defined as those which do not require administration of a probe drug such as antipyrine. Instead, the disposition of an endogenous substance is monitored. Numerous endogenous compounds, including steroids, fatty acids, and prostanoids, are metabolised by cytochrome P-450 enzymes, but only one compound, 6β-hydroxycortisol (6β-OHC), has been found useful in this respect.

6β-OHC is a minor metabolite of cortisol formed primarily by hepatic mixed-function oxidases and excreted, unchanged in urine (Park and Ohnhaus, 1983). The excretion of the steroid is reduced by cimetidine, an inhibitor of hepatic mixed-function oxidases, but the changes are small (<25%) and thus 6β-OHC excretion cannot be used as a measure of enzyme inhibition.

In contrast, urinary 6β-OHC provides a sensitive marker of enzyme induction. The excretion of the steroid is increased markedly by all therapeutic agents which produce a significant enzyme induction in man (Figure 2). However, cigarette smoking had no effect on 6β-OHC excretion in man, while, in animals, we have shown that induction of the aromatic hydrocarbon hydroxylase system occurs independently of cortisol 6β-hydroxylation.

The major advantage of a non-invasive method, as exemplified by urinary 6β-OHC, is of course that administration of a probe drug, which may in itself alter enzyme activity, is not necessary. Therefore, measurement of urinary 6β-OHC may be easily incorporated into any study of drug metabolism in man, alongside the probe drugs mentioned above, and can also be used to monitor the time-course of enzyme induction.

RELATIONSHIP BETWEEN THE METABOLISM OF PROBE DRUGS AND CLINICALLY IMPORTANT DRUGS

Much research in clinical pharmacology has been directed towards predicting the capacity of an individual to metabolise clinically important drugs, by measuring the pharmacokinetics of probe drugs. In some instances fairly good correlations have been obtained, but in most instances the results have been disappointing. This is not

Figure 2.   The effects of various drugs on urinary 6β-
hydroxycortisol excretion.

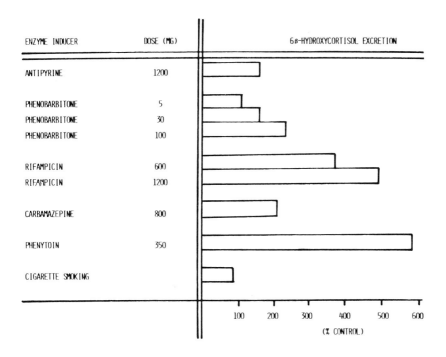

surprising given the multiplicity of human cytochrome P-450
enzymes, and the fact that many drugs are metabolised by
several enzymes simultaneously. However, probe drugs can
be used to indicate where factors which influence the
activity of the drug-metabolising enzymes may be of
clinical importance.
     One of the most striking examples of the clinical
importance of polymorphism in drug oxidation is illustrated
by the peripheral neuropathy and hepatotoxicity associated
with the anti-anginal drug perhexiline. The drug is
ampiphilic and thus forms stable, non-degradable complexes
with phospholipids which accumulate in certain cells and
thereby produce cytotoxicity. The metabolism of
perhexiline is associated with that of debrisoquine; poor
oxidisers of perhexiline are also poor metabolisers of
debrisoquine (Cooper et al, 1984). Shah et al, (1982) have
suggested that determination of debrisoquine oxidation
status might be of predictive value in controlling
(predicting) the neurotoxicity of this drug, the incidence
of which appears to be related to individual's half-life

(Singlas et al, 1978).   Given the wide variation in
exposure to the drug between PM and EM phenotypes, it would
seem appropriate to measure the pharmacokinetics of new
drugs in panels of volunteers phenotyped for known
polymorphisms in drug oxidation.

The clinical importance of polymorphism in drug
metabolism and therefore the importance of phenotyping
individuals taking a particular drug, is dependent upon the
fraction of the drug cleared via the pathway which exhibits
polymorphism.   The contribution of debrisoquine
polymorphism to the metabolism and actions of β -
adrenoceptor drugs has been actively investigated by
Lennard et al (1986).   The polymorphism is a major
determinant of the metabolism, pharmacokinetics and some of
the pharmacological actions of metoprolol, bufurolol and
timolol.   In contrast, the pharmacokinetics and
pharmacodynamics of propranolol are not related to
debrisoquine polymorphism, although PM phenotypes show a
deficiency in 4-hydroxypropranolol formation.

Phenotyping individuals may provide insight into the
aetiology of certain diseases.   A recent study suggests
that   patients   with   Parkinson's   disorder   are
disproportionate as a group with respect to the occurrence
of the allele which determines defective metabolism of
debrisoquine (Barbeau et al, 1985).

Adverse drug effects precipitated by changes, rather
than deficiences, in drug-metabolising enzyme activity are
generally restricted to drugs with a narrow therapeutic
range, where a relatively small change in elimination rate
may be associated with a change from a therapeutic to a
toxic response.   Numerous factors may alter the capacity of
an individual to metabolise drugs.   In practice, the most
important considerations are age, enzyme induction and
enzyme inhibition.   Probe drugs have been used to assess
the impact of these various factors on the ability of the
human liver to oxidise drugs (Park, 1982).   The question
that arises is, can we relate the changes observed in the
pharmacokinetics of a probe drug to changes in the
metabolism, and pharmacological effect, of a particular
therapeutic agent?

Drug interactions with oral anticoagulants provide
some useful examples in this respect.   Cimetidine is a
potent inhibitor of drug oxidation and reduces the
clearance of probe drugs such as antipyrine, theophylline
and tolbutamide (Somogyi and Gugler, 1982).   Co-
administration of the H_2-antagonist cimetidine increases
steady-state plasma concentration of warfarin and also
prolongs prothrombin time to a dangerous level (Serlin et

al, 1979). However, more recent work has shown that cimetidine only inhibits the metabolism of R-warfarin (Choonara et al, 1986). This stereoselective interaction may have a regioselective basis. In vitro studies (Kaminsky et al, 1984) have shown that R-warfarin is oxidised primarily in the 6-position, whereas S-warfarin undergoes extensive 7-hydroxylation. The two reactions are catalysed by distinct cytochrome P-450 enzymes.

Propranolol produced a small increase (14.7%) in steady state plasma warfarin concentrations in volunteers, but this change did not have a measurable dynamic effect as shown by the lack of significant change in prothrombin time (Scott et al, 1984). Propranolol is known to inhibit the elimination of several drugs which are metabolised by the hepatic mixed-function oxidase system including antipyrine (Greenblatt et al, 1978) and theophylline (Conrad and Nyman, 1980).

Thus, while probe drugs can be used to screen for potential sources of drug interactions, they cannot be used to predict, with certainty, either the biochemical nature or the pharmacological importance of such drug interactions.

For most drugs, metabolism represents a clearance mechanism and it is therefore quantitative, rather then qualitative, aspects of metabolism which are considered important. However, in certain circumstances, a normal biotransformation may lead to formation of a toxic metabolite. Chemically reactive metabolites are particularly important in this respect because their covalent binding with biopolymers in vivo might induce various forms of toxicity. There is therefore a need to develop test systems to monitor the formation of such metabolites in vivo.

One approach is to measure the degree of chemical conjugation to a macromolecule in vivo. Occupational exposure to ethylene oxide can be assessed by measurement of the levels of an amino acid adduct in haemoglobin (Calleman et al, 1978). Blood samples from humans exposed to ethylene oxide were analysed for the presence of N-3(2-hydroxyethyl)histidine by mass spectrometry and by iron exchange amino acid analysis. The long half-life of haemoglobin (60 days) make it a particularly attractive target macromolecule for monitoring chronic exposure (Neumann, 1984).

A second possible approach is to identify, and then quantify, novel urinary metabolites derived from chemical conjugates of target macromolecules formed in vivo. Autrup et al, 1985 have developed a method for monitoring exposure to the potent liver carcinogen aflatoxin B_1 by detection of 8,9-dihydro-(7'-guanyl)-9-hydroxyaflatoxin B_1 in human urine.

In this regard, we have used 2,4-dinitrofluorobenzene as a model chemically reactive metabolite (Maggs et al, 1986). After intravenous administration, the majority of the compound (90%) is detoxified by glutathione conjugation and excreted as the corresponding mercapturic acid. A small proportion 5-10% forms dinitrophenyl haptens on lysine residues in circulating proteins. These conjugates are taken up into Kupffer cells, hydrolysed and the dinitrophenyl group is excreted as a simple N-acetyl-lysine conjugate. Measurement of such novel amino acid conjugates, in urine, may provide a useful probe with which to monitor drug conjugation in vivo, in patients with drug allergy.

CONCLUSIONS

A limited number of in vivo probes are now available with which to assess the importance of various factors which may contribute to the wide inter-individual variation in capacity and ability to metabolise drugs. A better understanding of the use and the limitations of these probes will come from characterisation of the individual enzymes (isozymes) and their representative substrates, using a combination of in vitro and in vivo techniques. With these methods it is possible to anticipate, but not predict, which types of drugs will be subject to wide variation in metabolism and therefore pharmacological effects.

Measurement of the fractional clearance of a drug to its various metabolites provides a more rational basis for understanding factors which may influence the pharmacological and toxicological response to that drug. This is particularly relevant for drugs which produce their toxicity by formation of toxic metabolites.

REFERENCES

Anderson, K.E., Conney, A.H. and Kappas, A. (1982). Nutrition Reviews, 40, 161.
Autrup, H., Wakhisi, J., Vahakangas, K., Wasunna, A. and Harris, C.C. (1985). Environ. Health Perspect, 62, 105.
Back, D.J., Purba, H.S., Park, B.K., Ward, S.A. and Orme, M.L'E. (1983a). Brit. J. Clin. Pharmac, 16, 497.
Back, D.J., Park, B.K., Tjia, J.F. and Newby, S. (1983b). Brit. J. Clin. Pharmac, 16. 460.

Back, D.J., Maggs, J.L., Purba, H.S., Newby, S. and Park, B.K. (1984). Brit. J. Clin. Pharmac, 18, 603.

Barbeau, A., Roy, M., Paris, S., Cloutier, T., Plasse, L. and Poirer, J. (1985). Lancet 2, 1213.

Boobis, A.R. and Davies, D.S. (1984). Xenobiotica, 14, 151.

Breimer, D.D. (1983). Clin. Pharmacokinet, 8, 371.

Calleman, C.J., Ehrenberg, L., Jansson, B., Osterman-Gokkar, S., Segerback, D., Svensson, K. and Wachtmeister, C.A. (1978). J. Environ. Pathol. Toxicol, 2, 427.

Choonara, I.A., Cholerton, S., Haynes, B.P., Breckenridge, A.M. and Park, B.K. (1986). Brit. J. Clin. Pharmac, 21, 271.

Cooper, R.G., Price Evans, D.A. and Whibley, E.J. (1984). J. Med. Genetics, 21, 27.

Conrad, K.A. and Nyman, D.N. (1980). Clin. Pharmac. Ther, 28, 463.

Eichelbaum, M., Spannbrucker, N., Steincke, B. and Dengler, H.J. (1979). Eur. J. Clin. Pharmac, 16, 183.

Eichelbaum, M., Reetz, K.P., Schmidt, E.K. and Zekorn, C. (1986). Xenobiotica, 16, 465.

Emery, P., Hutson, G., Idle, J.R., Mitchell, S.C., Danayi, G.S., Smith, R.L. and Waring, R.H. (1984). Brit. J. Clin. Pharmac, 18, 286P.

Greenblatt, D.J., Franke, K. and Huffman, D.H. (1978). Circulation, 57, 1161.

Guengerich, F.P., Distlerath, L.M., Reilly, P.E.B., Wolff, T., Shimada, T., Umbenhauer, D.R. and Martin, M.V. (1986). Xenobiotica, 16, 367.

Hepner, G.W. and Vesell, E.S. (1975). Ann. Int. Med, 83, 632.

Hunt, S.N., Jusko, W.J., Yurchack, A.M. (1976). Clin. Pharmac. Ther, 19, 546.

Kaminsky, L.S., Dunbar, D.A., Wang, P.P., Beaune, P., Larrey, D., Guengerich, F.P., Schnellmann, R.G. and Sipes, I.G. (1984). Drug Metab. Disp, 12, 470.

Kleinbloesem, C.H., van Brummelen, P., Faber, H., Danhof, M., Vermeulen, N.P.E. and Breimer, D.D. (1984). Biochem. Pharmacol, 33, 3721.

Kotake, A.N., Schoeller, D.A., Lambert, G.H., Baker, A.L., Schaffer, D.D. and Josephs, H. (1982). Clin. Pharmac. Ther, 32, 261.

Kupfer, A., Dick, B. and Preisig, R. (1981). Hepatology, 1, 524.

Kupfer, A. and Preisig, R. (1984). Eur. J. Clin. Pharmacol, 26, 753.

Lennard, M.S., Tucker, G.T., Silas, J.H. and Woods, H.F. (1986). Xenobiotica, 16, 435.

Maggs, J.L., Kitteringham, N.R., Grabowski, P.S. and Park, B.K. (1986). Biochem. Pharmac, 35, 505.

Mahgoub, A., Idle, J.R., Dring, L.G., Lancaster, R. and Smith, R.K. (1977). Lancet 2, 584.

Neumann, H.G. (1984). Arch. Toxicol, 56, 1.

Ohnhaus, E.E. and Park, B.K. (1979). Eur. J. Clin. Pharmac, 15, 139.

Miller, C.A., Slusher, L.B. and Vesell, E.S. (1985). J. Clin. Invest, 75, 1415.

Park, B.K. (1982). Brit. J. Clin. Pharmac, 14, 631.

Park, B.K. and Breckenridge, A.M. (1981). Clin. Pharma- cokinet, 6, 1.

Park, B.K. and Ohnhaus, E.E. (1983). Arztl. Lab, 29, 53.

Penno, M.B. and Vesell, E.S. (1983). J. Clin. Invest, 71, 1698.

Pond, S.N., Birkett, D.J. and Wade, D.N. (1977). Clin. Pharmac. Ther, 22, 573.

Schmid, B., Bircher, J., Preisig, R. and Kupfer, A. (1985). Clin. Pharmac. Ther, 38, 619.

Scott, A.K., Park, B.K. and Breckenridge, A.M. (1984). Br. J. Clin. Pharmac, 17, 559.

Scott, J. and Poffenbarger, P.L. (1979). Diabetes, 28, 41.

Serlin, M.J., Sibeon, R.G., Mossman, S., Breckenridge, A.M., Williams, J.B.B., Atwood, J.L. and Willoughby, J.M.T. (1979). Lancet, 317.

Shah, R.R., Oates, N.S., Idle, J.R., Smith, R.L. and Lockhart, J.D.F. (1982). Br. Med. J, 284, 295.

Shaw, P.N., Houston, J.B., Rowland, M., Hopkins, K., Thiercelin, J.F. and Morselli, P.L. (1985). Br. J. Clin. Pharmac, 20, 611.

Singlas, E., Goujet, M.A. and Simon, P. (1978). Eur. J. Clin. Pharmac, 14, 195.

Smith, R.L. (1985). in "Microsomes and Drug Oxidations" (Eds. A.R. Boobis., J. Caldwell., F. de Matteis., C.R. Elcombe). Taylor and Francis, London, 349.

Somogyi, A. and Gugler, R. (1982). Clin. Pharmacokinet, 7, 23.

Teunissen, N.W.E., Kleinbloesem, C.H., de Leede, L.G.J. and Breimer, D.D. (1985). Eur. J. Clin. Pharmac, 28, 681.

Toverud, E-L., Boobis, A.R., Brodie, M.J., Murrary, S., Bennett, P.N., Whitmarsh, V.B. and Davies, D.S. (1981). Eur. J. Clin. Pharmac, 21, 155.

Vesell, E.S. (1979). Clin. Pharmac. Ther, 26, 275.

Vestal, R.E. and Wood, A.J.J. (1980). Clin. Pharmacokinet, 5, 309.

Waring, R.H., Mitchell, S.C., Shah, R.R., Idle, J.R. and Smith, R.L. (1982). Biochem. Pharmac, 31, 3151.

Weber, W.W. and Hein, D.W. (1985). Pharmacol. Rev, 37, 25.

cDNA AND COMPLETE AMINO ACID SEQUENCE OF RAT 3-METHYL-CHOLANTHRENE-INDUCIBLE NAD(P)H:MENADIONE OXIDOREDUCTASE

John A. Robertson and Daniel W. Nebert

Laboratory of Developmental Pharmacology, National Institute of Child Health and Human Development, National Institutes of Health, Bethesda, Maryland 20892, USA.

NAD(P)H:menadione oxidoreductase (NMOR, EC 1.6.99.2; also known as DT-diaphorase) plays a detoxifying role in drug metabolism, protecting against mutagenicity (Chesis et al, 1984; De Flora et al, 1985) and the covalent binding of reactive intermediates to proteins (Smart and Zannoni, 1984), as well as circumventing the oxidative stress and toxicity elicited by certain quinones (Lind et al, 1982; Thor et al, 1982; Di Monte et al, 1984a,b). NMOR activity is induced by treatment with a variety of xenobiotics, and induction is known to occur via transcriptional activation (Williams et al, 1984). Preliminary evidence has indicated control by the Ah locus for induced expression of at least one NMOR gene (Kumaki et al, 1977). Our group is interested in the identity, expression and regulation of the genes encoding Ah receptor-regulated drug-metabolising enzymes. We are now able to provide the complete cDNA and deduced amino acid sequences for the Ah receptor-regulated form of NMOR, designated $NMOR_1$ (Robertson et al, 1986).

$NMOR_1$ was isolated from 3-methylcholanthrene (MC)-treated rat hepatic cytosol by a rapid, two-step procedure using affinity gel purification (Hojeberg et al, 1981) and fast protein liquid chromatography (FPLC). Monospecific antiserum to $NMOR_1$ was raised in rabbits by intra-nodal injection. Cytosol from control and MC-treated Ah-responsive (B6) and Ah-nonresponsive (D2) mice and a Western (immuno)-blot procedure with this antiserum were used to confirm both the Ah receptor-regulated induction in mice and the affinity of this antiserum for the MC-induced form of NMOR. A cDNA expression library was constructed in λgt11 and screened with antiserum (Huynh et al, 1984). Antiserum-positive clones were plaque-purified and further characterised by showing enhanced hybridisation to MC-induced rat poly(A)$^+$RNA. The longest cDNA clone (approximately 1.6kb) was sequenced via the (35S) Sanger method. This shows an open-reading frame (bases 75 to 899) bounded by a 5' untranslated region of 74nt and 3' untranslated region of 602nt (Figure 1). The cDNA thus encodes a protein of 274 amino acids (Mr=30,946), which compares well with the size (32 kilodaltons) estimated by SDS-PAGE. Amin acid sequence analysis of FPLC-resolved peptides of $NMOR_1$, tryptic digests was used to confirm the identity of this cDNA by homology (at amino acids 81-90 and 263-271) with the amino acid sequence predicted from the cDNA sequence. FASTP computer program analysis (Lipman and Pearson, 1985) revealed no significant homology with any other protein sequenced to date, indicating that $NMOR_1$ is a member of a heretofore uncharacterised gene family. This study represents the first cloning and sequence of a cDNA encoding the complete amino acid sequence of an Ah receptor-regulated, Phase II drug-metabolising enzyme and should enable us to define the molecular biology of this gene and its product.

REFERENCES

Chesis, P.L., Levin, D.E., Smith, M.T., Ernster, L. and Ames, B.N. (1984). Proc. Natl. Acad. Sci, USA, 81, 1696.

De Flora, S., Morelli, A., Basso, C., Romano, M., Serra, D. and De Flora, A. (1985). Cancer Res, 45, 3188.

Di Monte, D., Bellomo, G., Thor, H., Nicotera, P. and Orrenius, S. (1984a). Arch. Biochem. Biophys, 235, 343.

Di Monte, D., Ross, D., Bellomo, G., Eklow, L. and Orrenius, S. (1984b). Arch. Biochem. Biophys, 235, 334.

Hojeberg, B., Blomberg, K., Stenberg, S. and Lind, C. (1981). Arch. Biochem. Biophys, 207, 205.

Huynh, T.U., Young, R.A. and Davis, R.W. (1984). in DNA Cloning Techniques : A Practical Approach (Ed. by Glover, D). IRL Press, Oxford, Vol 1. p. 49.

Kumaki, K., Jensen, N.M., Shire, J.G.M. and Nebert, D.W. (1977). J. Biol. Chem, 252, 157.

Lind, C., Hochstein, P. and Ernster, L. (1982). Arch. Biochem. Biophys, 216, 178.

Lipman, D.J. and Pearson, W.R. (1985). Science, 227, 1435.

Robertson, J.A., Chen, H.C. and Nebert, D.W. (1986). J. Biol. Chem (submitted).

Smart, R.C. and Zannoni, V.G. (1984). Mol. Pharmacol, 26, 105.

Thor, H., Smith, M.T., Hartzell, P., Bellomo, G., Jewell, S. and Orrenius, S. (1982). J. Biol. Chem. 257, 12419.

Williams, J.B., Wang, R., Lu, A.Y.H. and Pickett, C.B. (1984). Arch. Biochem. Biophys, 232, 408.

Figure 1. Nucleotide and predicted amino acid sequence of a cDNA for NMOR.

```
NMOR1 CDNA:
                                 30                                60                                90
CAGGGTCGTCCTGGCAACCAGCTGCTCAGCCAATCAGCGCTTGACACTACGATCCGCCCCCAACTTCTGGAGCCATGGCGGTGAGAAGAGCCCTGATTGTATTGGCCC
                                                                             M  A  V  R  R  A  L  I  V  L  A
      120                           150                           180                           210
ACGCAGAGAGGACATCATTCAACTATGCCATGAAGGAGGCTGCTGTGGAGGCTCTGAAGAAGAAAGGATGGGAGGTGGTCGAATCTGACCTCTATGCTATGAACTTTA
H  A  E  R  T  S  F  N  Y  A  M  K  E  A  A  V  E  A  L  K  K  K  G  W  E  V  V  E  S  D  L  Y  A  M  N  F
                     240                           270                           300
ACCCCCTCATTTCCAGAAACGACATCACAGGGGAGCCGAAGGACTCGGAGAACTTTCAGTACCCTGTTGAGTCATCTCTGGCGTATAAGGAAGGCCGCCTGAGCCCGG
N  P  L  I  S  R  N  D  I  T  G  E  P  K  D  S  E  N  F  Q  Y  P  V  E  S  S  L  A  Y  K  E  G  R  L  S  P
  330                           360                           390                           420
ATATTGTAGCTGAACAGAAAAAGCTGGAAGCTGCAGACCTGGTGATATTTCAGTTCCCATTGTATTGGTTTGGGGTGCCCGCCATTCTGAAAGGCTGGTTTGAGAGAG
D  I  V  A  E  Q  K  K  L  E  A  A  D  L  V  I  F  Q  F  P  L  Y  W  F  G  V  P  A  I  L  K  G  W  F  E  R
              450                           480                           510                           540
TGCTTGTAGCAGGATTCGCCTACACGTATGCCACCATGTATGACAAGGGTCCTTTCCAGAATAAGAAGACCTTGCTTTCCATCACCACCGGGGGCAGCGGCTCCATGT
V  L  V  A  G  F  A  Y  T  Y  A  T  M  Y  D  K  G  P  F  Q  N  K  K  T  L  L  S  I  T  T  G  G  S  G  S  M
                           570                           600                           630
ACTCTCTGCAGGGTGTCCACGGGGACATGAACGTCATTCTCTGGCCAATTCAGAGTGGCATTCTGCGCTTCTGTGGCTTCCAGGTCTTAGAACCTCAACTGGTGTACA
Y  S  L  Q  G  V  H  G  D  M  N  V  I  L  W  P  I  Q  S  G  I  L  R  F  C  G  F  Q  V  L  E  P  Q  L  V  Y
      660                           690                           720                           750
GCATTGGCCACACCCCACCCGATGCCCGCGTGCAGGTCCTGGAAGGGTGGAAGAAGCGTCTGGAGACTGTCTGGGAGGAGTCACCACTCTACTTTGCTCCAAGCAGCT
S  I  G  H  T  P  P  D  A  R  V  Q  V  L  E  G  W  K  K  R  L  E  T  V  W  E  E  S  P  L  Y  F  A  P  S  S
                    780                           810                           840
TGTTTGACCTAAACTTCCAGGCAGGATTCTTACTGAAAAAAGAGGTTCAAGAGGAGCAGAAAAAGAACAAGTTTGGCCTTTCTGTGGGCCATCATTTGGGCAAGTCCA
L  F  D  L  N  F  Q  A  G  F  L  L  K  K  E  V  Q  E  E  Q  K  K  N  K  F  G  L  S  V  G  H  H  L  G  K  S
  870                           900                           930                           960
TTCCAGCCGACAACCAGATCAAAGCTAGAAAATAAGGTTTTCCATACCATGTAGTTAGACCCAGGTTTCTTTTTCCCCAGCTTGCCTGGCTTGCTTTCAGTTTTCGCC
I  P  A  D  N  Q  I  K  A  R  K  *
             990                           1020                          1050                          1080
TTTGTTCCACAAGGATAGGAAAAGGAGGAGGCTCGCCTCATGCGTTTTTGGATAGTTCTGCCACGGCGTGTGACAGCAAAATGAACGAGGTCAGATTAGGGGCCTCAG
                          1110                          1140                          1170
GTGGCCTGGGATATGAATCAGGGAGAGGTGTAGCCGCGAGCGGGGAAAATACTCTTCTAGGTCTTTTGTACACTATAAGCTTTTTTCTTCGGGCTAGCCTGGCTAAAT
      1200                          1230                          1260                          1290
GGCATCCAATCCTCCACCCACTTGTTGCTATTAGTTACCTCTCTGTGGTTTAGGGCAGGAGGGAATTGCTCAAACAATGGCTGAGGGACTAACTTGTTTAGCAGTTAG
                   1320                          1350                          1380
CTAAAGCCTGTTTATGATCCATCCTGGTTTCAATTACTGTGCAGTGACTGACAAGCCTCGGGGGATTGCTCTCCAGCTCTTCTCTGCCTTGTACATAGCACACCCAGG
  1410                          1440                          1470                          1500
TCCTGGGAAATGAATACAAAAACAGGTCTCCGCCTCATTCTTGCTATTCTTTCTTTGTGTGTGTGTGTGTGGAAATAAATGGATATTTCACACGTCA*
```

KINETICS OF DRUG INHIBITION: USE OF METABOLITE CONCENTRATION-TIME PROFILES TO ASSESS RELATIVE IMPORTANCE OF INHIBITOR POTENCY AND INHIBITOR PHARMACOKINETICS

P. Nicholas Shaw[1] and J. Brian Houston[2]

[1]Department of Pharmacy, University of Nottingham, University Park, Nottingham NG7 2RD and [2]Department of Pharmacy, University of Manchester, Oxford Road, Manchester M13 9PL.

Inhibition of drug metabolism is usually investigated in vitro but the information derived from such experiments does not permit the prediction of the extent of inhibition when the inhibitor is administered in vivo. In order for such extrapolations to be made, information is required not only on the affinity of the inhibitor for the enzyme but also the effective inhibitor concentration prevailing in vivo, i.e. a knowledge of the pharmacokinetics of the inhibiting agent (Shaw et al, 1986).

We have investigated, using a simple pharmacokinetic model, the role of various factors on the in vivo inhibition of a model compound metabolised by two parallel pathways. These pathways are of equal importance and both metabolites show formation rate limited pharmacokinetics (Houston, 1982). The description of inhibition is based on Michaelis-Menten kinetics and was first applied in vivo by Rowland and Matin (1978). Under conditions where the metabolism occurs by a first-order process, the equation is:

$$\text{Rate of metabolism} = \frac{k.A}{(I + I/K_I)} \qquad \text{Eq. 1}$$

where A = amount of drug, I = amount of inhibitor, k = first order rate constant for drug elimination, K_I = amount of inhibitor which diminishes the effective k (or total body clearance) by one-half.

Drug and metabolite concentration-time profiles were computer generated using the ISIS Interactive Simulation Language implemented on the Cyber 170-730 at UMRCC, UK. Simulations were performed over a time period equivalent to 1000 minutes and the following initial conditions were

used: unit doses of both drug and inhibitor, drug t1/2 of
111 mins and equal volumes of distribution for drug and
metabolites.
The following factors were investigated :-
(a) Changing the value of K_I at a steady state inhibitor
    concentration.
(b) Varying the elimination half-life of the inhibitor
(c) Varying the dose of inhibitor
(d) Inhibition of one or both metabolic pathways
(e) Observation of drug and metabolite under the above
    conditions.

   Initial simulations (Figure 1) were performed under
conditions where the inhibitor concentration was at steady-
state and the influence of K_I during non-selective
inhibition can be seen. Since the inhibitor is present at
a steady-state concentration there exists a constant
inhibitory effect which is solely dependent on K_I, as K_I
decreases there is a concurrent increase in drug half-life,
the corresponding percentages of inhibition are shown on
this figure. The profiles for the metabolites arising from
the drug demonstrate marked changes from the non-inhibited
state. Non-selective inhibition produces a large decrease
in Cmax whilst due to the formation rate-limited behaviour
of the metabolites, the half-life follows that of the
parent drug, i.e. increases with decreasing K_I. Selective
inhibition of one pathway also results in noticeable
changes in that particular metabolite profile, with
relatively small changes in half-life but large changes in
AUC and a pronounced decrease in Cmax.

   Figure 2 shows a series of computer simulations which
examined the effect of elimination half-life of the
inhibitor. Equation 1 was modified to include the
inhibitor pharmacokinetics, which were assumed to follow a
monoexponential decline.

   The pharmacokinetics of the inhibitor were included by
assuming its elimination to be mono-exponential in nature,
i.e. $I = I_0 e^{-kI.t}$
where k_I = rate constant for elimination of the inhibitor
      I_0 = amount of inhibitor in the body at time zero

These simulations were performed at two values of K_I (0.1,
0.01) corresponding to 90 and 99% inhibition respectively,
with K_I altered to provide changes in the inhibitor half-
life. Drug concentration-time profiles show a curvilinear
nature since the total amount of inhibitor, and hence
inhibitory effect, is decreasing with time. A tenfold
decrease in K_I from 0.1 to 0.01 appears only to have minor
effects on the drug profile. When the metabolites are

Figure 1. Effect of K_I on drug (left-panel) and metabolite (right-panel) concentration-time profiles, inhibitor concentrations are maintained at steady state and the inhibition is non-selective.

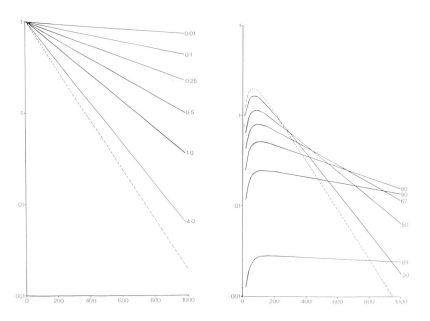

The following K_Is (percentage of inhibition) were investigated :- 4 (20%), 1 (50%), 0.5 (67%), 0.25 (80%), 0.1 (90%), 0.01 (99%).

examined however, a more pronounced sensitivity to changes both in K_I and inhibitor elimination rate with changes in both AUC and Cmax value is apparent. The action of the inhibitor with regard to pathway selectivity was also investigated under the same conditions, namely those of varying elimination rate of inhibitor. Selectivity of inhibition manifested the expected results, with much more significant changes noted in the metabolite profile during inhibition of that metabolite, when compared to the concentration-time curve for the non-inhibited metabolite. The effect of increasing dose size was also examined and tended to shift the metabolite curves to later time points whilst still retaining the general shape of curve. Parent drug profiles again displayed the time-dependent effect due to inhibitor elimination. For both the above cases the

Figure 2. Effect of inhibitor elimination half-life on the inhibition effect evident in drug (upper panel) and metabolite (lower panel) concentration-time profiles

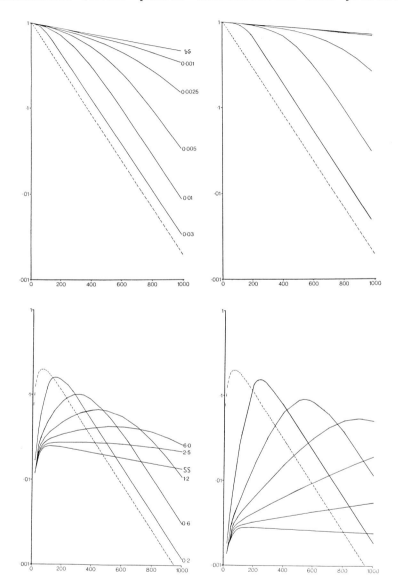

Inhibition is non-selective, K_I is 0.1 (left) or 0.01 (right). The following K_I's were investigated (inhibitor : drug half-life ratio) : 0.03 (0.2), 0.01 (0.6), 0.005 (1.2), 0.0025 (2.5), 0.001 (6).

metabolite profiles were much more sensitive in the detection of both extent and type (i.e. selectivity) of inhibition.

Two major conclusions are evident from these investigations :-

(a) metabolite concentration-time profiles are a more sensitive probe of inhibition than drug-concentration-time profiles

(b) the pharmacokinetics of the inhibitor are often more critical to the inhibitory response apparent in vivo than the inhibitor potency.

REFERENCES

Houston, J.B. (1982). Pharmacol. Therap, 15, 521.
Rowland, M., Matin, S.B. (1973). J. Pharmacokin. Biopharm, 1, 553.
Shaw, P.N., Tseti, J., Warburton, S., Adedoyin, A., Houston, J.B. (1986). Drug Metab. Dispos, 14, 271.

NITROIMIDAZOLE INHIBITION OF MOUSE AND HUMAN CYTOCHROME P-450 MEDIATED HYDROXYLATION OF THE CHLOROETHYLNITROSOUREA CCNU

P. Workman, F.Y.F. Lee, M.I. Walton, J.T. Roberts and N.M. Bleehen

MRC Unit and University Department of Clinical Oncology and Radiotherapeutics, MRC Centre, Hills Road, Cambridge, CB2 2QH.

INTRODUCTION

The chloroethylnitrosourea (CCNU [1-(2-chloroethyl)-3-cyclohexyl-1-nitrosourea] is widely used in the treatment of cancer in man. The principal elimination pathway in vivo involves metabolism of the cyclohexyl ring by cytochrome P-450 producing up to 5 or 6 monohydroxylated metabolites which differ in physicochemical and biological properties (May et al, 1974; Wheeler et al, 1977). The nitroimidazoles misonidazole [1-(2-nitroimidazolyl)-3-methoxypropan-2-ol, MISO) and benznidazole [N-benzyl-(2-nitroimidazolyl) acetamide, BENZO] are able to improve the antitumour selectively of CCNU in mice ('chemosensitisation'), partly through altered CCNU pharmacokinetics (Lee and Workman, 1984). Clinical trials of such combinations are now in progress. The aim of the present study was to determine the effects of MISO and BENZO on CCNU hydroxylation by mixed-function oxidases (MFO) in mice and man.

METHODS

Standard techniques were used for the in vitro metabolism of CCNU by mouse liver microsomes (May et al, 1974). For in vivo studies, drugs were administered ip in mice and orally in man. Concentrations of nitroamidazoles and of CCNU and its monohydroxylated metabolites were determined by reversed-phase HPLC (Workman et al, 1978 and 1984; Lee and Workman, 1983; Lee et al, 1985).

RESULTS AND DISCUSSION

MISO and BENZO both inhibited the ring hydroxylation of

CCNU by mouse hepatic MFO in vitro (Figure 1), with I$_{50}$ values of 5.8 and 0.37mM respectively. Inhibition was of the mixed competitive-non-competitive type. Concentrations which were optimal for chemosensitization in mice (2.5mM MISO and 0.13mM BENZO) produced 30-32% inhibition of metabolism in vitro.

Figure 1. Inhibition by MISO and BENZO of the cyclohexyl ring monohydroxylation of CCNU by mouse liver microsomal MFO in vitro.

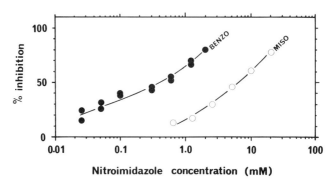

(reproduced from Workman et al, 1986, with permission).

    MISO and BENZO also markedly altered the metabolism of CCNU in vivo. In mice receiving 20mg/kg ip CCNU, the clearance of parent drug was reduced 34% by 2.5mmol/kg MISO and 62% by 0.3 mmol/kg BENZO; concentrations of parent drug at 25 minutes were increased 2-fold and 4-fold respectively.
    In human cancer patients receiving 130mg/m^2 CCNU orally, the parent drug is normally undetectable due to extensive first pass metabolism to the cis- and trans-4-hydroxylated metabolites (Lee et al, 1985). Table 1 confirms that in the absence of BENZO or in patients with peak BENZO concentrations < 20μg/ml parent CCNU was always undetectable (n=13). In contrast, of those patients who achieved BENZO concentrations > 20μg/ml, for which Figure 1 predicts about 30% inhibition of CCNU hydroxylation, only 2/16 failed to show breakthrough of parent CCNU into the plasma. Of those with BENZO concentrations > 26μg/ml (32% inhibition) 12/12 showed CCNU breakthrough.
    We conclude that MISO and BENZO are able to inhibit CCNU hydroxylation by MFO at pharmacological concentrations. Further studies have shown that, as for other imidazole

Table 1.   Relationship between predicted and actual
inhibition of CCNU hydroxylation by BENZO in man.

Patient[1]	BENZO dose[2] (mg/kg)	Plasma BENZO[3] at 4h (μg/ml)	Predicted[4] Inhibition (%)	Peak CCNU[3] (μg/ml)
A-K	0	0	0	0
L	8	10.4	20	0
M	12	20.5	30	0
N	14	26.9	33	0.02
O	14	25.6	32	0
P	17	25.6	32	0.05
Q	20	39.2	38	0.63
E	25	28.3	34	0.31
F	25	48.7	40	0.44
G	25	28.6	34	0.22
H	25	54.3	41	0.17
I	25	22.8	31	0.062
J	25	41.5	39	0.058
K	25	5.7	15	0
R	25	37.9	38	0.23
S	25	32.4	36	0.12
T	40	63.3	43	0.14
U	40	48.3	40	0.21
V	40	27.9	34	0.24

1. Some patients received both CCNU alone and CCNU with
   BENZO on separate occasions.
2. Given orally 4h before an oral dose of 130mg/m^2 CCNU.
3. By HPLC.
4. From Figure 1.

compounds (Wilkinson et al, 1974), both bind as type II
ligands to mouse liver microsomal cytochrome P-450 (Lee et
al, submitted), probably diagnostic of a co-ordination of
the ferric heme with the free imidazole nitrogen.
Inhibition of metabolism leads to marked changes in the
pharmacokinetics of CCNU in mice and man, in some cases
resulting in improved antitumour selectivity (Lee et al,
1985). The in vitro microsomal assay predicted well for
the inhibition of CCNU hydroxylation by BENZO in man.
Nitroimidazoles and related compounds are widely used in a
variety of human diseases. Inhibition of MFO by these

agents is likely to affect the pharmacokinetics and
activity of other co-administered drugs. NItroimidazoles
may also have a role as probes for drug metabolising
enzymes in man.

REFERENCES

Lee, F.Y.F. and Workman, P. (1983). Br. J. Cancer, 47,
     659.
Lee, F.Y.F. and Workman, P. (1984). Br. J. Cancer, 49,
     579.
Lee, F.Y.F., Workman, P., Roberts, J.T. and Bleehen, N.M.
     (1985). Cancer Chemother. Pharmacol, 14, 125.
Lee, F.Y.F., Workman, P. and Cheeseman, K.H. submitted to
     Cancer Res.
May, H.E., Boose, R. and Reed, D.J. (1974). Biochem.
     Biophys. Res. Comm, 57, 426.
Wheeler, G.P., Johnston, J.P., Bourdon, B.J., McCalen,
     G.S., Hill, D.L. and Montgomery, J.A. (1977).
     Biochem. Pharmac, 26, 2331.
Wilkinson, C.F., Hetnarski, K. and Hicks, L.J. (1974).
     Pesticide. Biochem. Physiol, 4, 299.
Workman, P., Marten, T.R., Dale, A.D., Ruane, R.J.,
     Flockhart, I.R. and Bleehen, N.M. (1978). J.
     Chromatog, 145, 507.
Workman, P., White, R.A.S., Walton, M.I., Owen, L.N. and
     Twentyman, P.R. (1984). Br. J. Cancer, 50, 291.
Workman, P., Walton, M.I. and Lee, F.Y.F. (1986).
     Biochem. Pharmac, 35, 117.

6. Extrapolations.

COMPARISON OF MODEL SYSTEMS FOR METABOLISM

Peter Moldeus

Department of Toxicology, Karolinska Institutet, S-104 01
Stockholm, Sweden.

Several model systems are used for studies of drug
metabolism. These include both in vivo and in vitro models
(Figure 1). In this manuscript I have attempted to briefly
describe the various model systems, what they can be used
for, their advantages and limitations.

Figure 1. Model systems for drug metabolism

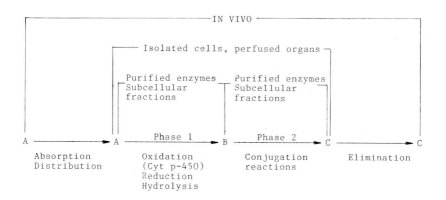

In vivo models are most complex but are the only models
that will give information about all phases of drug
metabolism, i.e. absorption, distribution, phase 1 and
phase 2 metabolism and elimination. Thus they are used for
studies of overall metabolism and metabolite production as
well as for pharmacokinetic studies.

Urine collection and blood sampling are the methods
usually employed but more sophisticated in vivo models are
also used including for instance, bile duct cannulation.

For studies of a drug or other chemicals with unknown metabolism, the in vivo model is usually used initially in order to establish its absorption, distribution and elimination, as well as to identify metabolites formed at various doses. However, when one wants to study specific reactions involved in the metabolism of a drug or study the mechanism of a particular reaction, the in vivo models are not suitable. For these types of studies any of several in vitro systems with varying complexity can be used. The in vitro systems most frequently employed for drug metabolism studies include :

> Isolated purified enzymes
> Subcellular factors
> Tissue homogenates
> Isolated intact cells
>> Freshly isolated
>> Primary cultures
>> Established cell lines
> Perfused organs

In vitro systems from several organs can be used but for studies of drug metabolism the liver is the most commonly used organ. The liver is quantitatively the most important organ and has high activity of most drug metabolising enzymes. Extrahepatic tissues are generally not quantitatively important in the metabolism of most drugs but specific isoenzymes catalysing specific reactions may be present in high concentrations in extrahepatic tissues. There exist, for instance, specific forms of cytochrome P-450 and glutathione transferases in certain extrahepatic tissues. One example of an enzyme that is generally not present within the liver cell is γ-glutamyltranspeptidase which catalyse the metabolism of glutathione conjugates (Meister and Andersson, 1983). This enzyme is present in high concentration in the kidney and is also present in the bile duct and intestine. Thus for studying the further metabolism of a glutathione conjugate to the N-acetylcysteine conjugate (mercapturate), liver in vitro systems should not be used.

Extrahepatic enzymes involved in drug metabolism may also be important for the metabolism of endogenous substrates, like steroids, prostaglandins and fatty acids as well as in the activation of organ specific toxins. Examples of extrahepatic enzymes involved in the metabolic activation or organ specific toxins are prostaglandin synthase and β-lyase. Prostaglandin synthase has been suggested to be involved in the activation of certain kidney and bladder carcinogens such as the aromatic amines benzidine and naphthylamine (Marnett and Eling, 1983).

Prostaglandin synthase has generally high activity in organs with low cytochrome P-450 activity and its role in the metabolic activation in tissues such as the lung and colon of substrates like polycyclic aromatic hydrocarbons may be of significance.

β-Lyase has high activity in the kidney and has been shown to activate certain cysteine conjugates, those from haloalkenes being most prominent (Elfarra and Anders, 1984). Certain cytochrome P-450 isozymes are also present in high concentrations in certain extrahepatic cells. For instance, the activation of 4-ipomeanol in the Clara cells of the lung has been suggested to be catalysed by a certain form of cytochrome P-450 present in high concentrations in those cells and thus being responsible for the rather specific lesion in the lung following 4-ipomeanol exposure (Boyd, 1977).

Isolated purified enzymes are naturally the °purest' model system and the best one to use if one wants to identify and characterise various isoenzymes, study regulation and induction of these isoenzymes and study molecular reaction mechanisms, Furthermore, purified enzymes can be used for preparation of antibodies to be used for studies of activity in less pure systems. For instance, antibodies to an isoenzyme of cytochrome P-450 can be used to identify an activity in a microsomal preparation.

There are, however, certain drawbacks in addition to sometimes intrinsically difficult methodologies, with the use of isolated purified enzymes. For instance, during the purification of membrane-bound enzymes the microenvironment of the enzyme is lost. The activity of purified cytochrome P-450 is thus dependent on addition of a phospholipid fraction. Furthermore, alteration of the amino-acid composition of the enzyme as well as loss of activity of the enzyme towards certain substrates may occur during purification. Moreover, one can generally not determine how much activity a certain isoenzyme contributes to the overall metabolism in the whole cell. Thus extrapolation to the cellular and in vivo situation may be difficult.

The in vitro systems which are probably the most frequently used and which most facile to work with are the subcellular fractions. They are used for subcellular localisation of activity and they can be used for studies of specific reactions and identification of metabolites formed from these reactions with no interference by other reactions. Since optimal cofactor and substrate concentrations can be used, one can study the kinetics of a certain reaction. A subcellular fraction is not as 'pure' as an isolated enzyme but the microenvironment is still intact and for common in vitro metabolism and metabolite identification it is usually an adequate model.

Since, with both isolated purified enzymes and subcellular fractions optimized conditions of cofactors are used and the interaction with other reactions are disregarded, the extrapolation to in vivo may be rather poor.

More suitable systems for such extrapolations are isolated intact cells and perfused organs. With these systems factors that become important include :
- Uptake and intracellular distribution of the substrate.
- Generation of cofactors and cosubstrates.
- Interrelationship between metabolic pathways involved in drug metabolism.
- Competition between endogenous and exogenous substrates.
Uptake and intracellular distribution is usually not a problem since most drug substrates are lipophilic and readily pass through cellular membranes becoming evenly distributed.

The generation of cofactors such as NADPH, NADH, UDPGA (UDP-glucuronic acid) and PAPS (adenosine 3'-phosphate 5'-sulphate phosphate) are necessary to ensure maximal drug metabolising activity. It is thus of vital importance that the cells and organs are viable with sufficient energy production to ensure maximal cofactor synthesis and regeneration. It is also necessary to supply enough substrates for energy production and cofactor biosynthesis. The liver cell normally contains adequate endogenous supply of glycogen to ensure sufficient NADPH generation and ATP synthesis. This may, however, not be true if other organs are used. One reaction that is dependent on the supply of additional exogenous cosubstrate is sulphate conjugation (Moldeus et al, 1979). If, for instance, isolated hepatocytes are incubated in an incubation medium devoid of inorganic sulphate almost no sulphate conjugation occurs. Thus the cell has very limited stores of sulphate to be activated to PAPS. In addition the synthesis of glutathione (GSH) is generally limited by the availability of cytsteine. Thus, under extreme conditions where the utilisation of intracellular GSH is rapid, exogenous cyteine, or cytsteine precursors, should be supplied to the incubation or perfusion medium.

In the intact cell, the interrelationship between metabolic pathways involved in drug metabolism also become important. Competition between different reactions for the same substrate may occur and there is generally a coupling between phase 1 and phase 2 reactions. Consequently, a

substrate that undergoes cytochrome P-450-dependent
hydroxylation will usually not be found in the hydroxylated
form since sulphate conjugation and glucuronidation
generally have higher capacity than the cytochrome P-450
reaction. Thus in this intact cell system the
identification of products of the phase 1 reactions,
particularly involving cytochrome P-450 becomes more
difficult and either enzymatic or acid hydrolytic cleavage
is necessary.

In an intact cell system competition between endogenous
and exogenously added substrates may also become important.
However, since the exogenous substrates are added usually
in relatively high concentrations this is not a major
factor which will influence the metabolism of the exogenous
substrate.

Isolated cells can be used either freshly isolated in
suspension or in primary cultures. Established cell lines
have also been used for drug metabolism studies but since
most of these cell lines have low activity of drug
metabolising enzymes the use of such cells is limited.

Cells isolated from liver (Moldeus et al, 1978) as well
as other organs including intestine (Dawson and Bridges,
1979), lung (Dawson et al, 1982) and kidney (Jones et al,
1979) have been employed in drug metabolism studies. The
preparation of isolated hepatocytes is rather simple and
quite rapid involving perfusion or incubation of the organ
with collagenase. Freshly isolated hepatocytes have
certain advantages over those in primary cultures. These
include the much higher yield of cells and the high
activity of the enzymes involved in drug metabolism. The
major limitation involves the fairly limited lifespan
(approximately 5-7 hours). However, for most studies, even
for studies of mechanism(s) of cytotoxicity, this time of
viability is adequate. One further drawback may be the use
of artifically high oxygen tension during the incubation of
cells in suspension which may alter some drug metabolising
activities. The organ structure is also lost when the
cells are isolated and incubated in suspension. The cell
to cell contact is retained to some extent if the cells are
cultured in monolayers (Bissel et al, 1979). The
hepatocyte primary culture thus has several advantages and
may, for instance, be kept alive for several days thus
permitting long term experiments such as studies on enzyme
regulation and mechanism(s) of cytotoxicity. However, this
system suffers from severe and rapid loss of drug
metabolising enzyme activities. In particular, cytochrome
P-450 decreases rapidly in cultured hepatocytes. This
problem is, to some extent overcome with the use of

appropriate incubation media with the activity of at least most isoenzymes of cytochrome P-450 being maintained over a longer period of time (Steward et al, 1985). A method of culturing hepatocytes which has been even more successful in maintaining high metabolic activity in the hepatocytes is the use of co-cultures. Hepatocytes are cultured together with a rat epithelial cell line (Guillouzo et al, 1985). Using this method hepatocytes cultured for several days have been shown to retain their cytochrome P-450 level and also respond to various inducers. The reason for this effect of the epithelial cells does not seem to be fully understood yet. This method has also been successfully employed in attempts to culture human hepatocytes. This should thus be a very useful method for studying the regulation of human drug metabolising enzymes and mechanisms of hepatotoxicity in man.

Isolated cells are thus a very useful system for studying drug metabolism reactions and much data can be collected from one preparation of cells. As mentioned previously, however, the organ structure is lost and these model systems are less like in vivo than the isolated perfused organ. Several perfused organ models including lung (Mehendale et al, 1981), kidney (Berkersky, 1985) and liver (Thurman and Kauffman, 1980) have been employed for drug metabolising studies, the liver being the most frequently used. In the perfused liver one may thus study the absorption and elimination of a drug and with a cannulated bile duct, study the transport route of a particular metabolite. Pharmacokinetics and first pass elimination of a drug substrate are also readily studied with the isolated perfused liver and the substrate can be continously infused at a constant concentration over a long period of time. Perfusion media resembling plasma can be employed and functional parameters such as pH, oxygen uptake etc, can be continuously monitored. Drug toxicity may also be studied using the isolated perfused organ and leakage of cytosolic enzymes into the perfusion medium, a rather sensitive measure of toxicity, may be monitored. This model system is, on the other hand, more difficult to work with than, for instance, the isolated cells and less information from one experiment can be obtained. Considering all factors, however, the perfused organ is by far the most relevant in vitro system to use if the results obtained are to be correlated to in vivo.

The in vivo metabolism of a drug substrate may still be considerably different from that one may find in an in vitro system. In addition to in vivo effects such as absorption, distribution and protein binding, metabolism in extrahepatic organs may supplement the liver metabolism and certain reactions may occur only in extrahepatic organs. The first pass metabolism through the intestine may, for instance, be of importance as well as metabolism in the lung. Furthermore, a metabolite formed in the liver may be further metabolised in another organ. The enterohepatic re-circulation of certain drugs and conjugates is also not taken into account when the metabolism in an in vitro system is evaluated, neither is the potential role of the intestinal microflora which may indeed be of importance for in the metabolism of certain compounds.

In vitro systems like isolated cells are also used for studies of mechanisms of drug toxicity. Even though these systems have distinct advantages over in vivo models for such investigations, results in these systems may be misleading. A compound may, for instance, be primarily activated in one organ and further activated in the target organ. A possible example of this may be benzene-induced bone marrow toxicity where a primary metabolite of benzene is further activated in the bone marrow cells (Synder et al, 1981). The case of β-lyase-mediated toxicity, where haloalkenes are conjugated to GSH in the liver and further activated in the kidney by γ-glutamyl transpeptidase and β-lyase to a reactive species, has already been discussed.

In conclusion, many different model systems may be used for studies of drug metabolism. Generally, the purpose of a particular study should largely dictate tha choice of model system but results obtained using in vitro systems ought to, as much as possible, be related to in vivo results.

REFERENCES

Bekersky, I. (1985). in "Reviews in Biochemical Toxicology, Vol 7 (Ed. by Hodgson, E., Bend, J.R. and Philpot, R.M). Elsevier North Holland, Amsterdam, p.199

Bissel, P.M., Hammaker, L.E. and Meyer, U.A. (1979). J. Cell. Biol, 59, 722.

Boyd, M.R. (1977). Nature, 2691, 713.

Dawson, J.R., Norbeck, K. and Moldeus, P. (1982). Biochem. Pharmacol, 31, 3549.

Dawson, J.R. and Bridges, J.W. (1979). Biochem. Pharmacol, 28, 3299.

Elfarra, A.A. and Anders, M.W. (1984). Biochem. Pharmacol, 33, 3729.

Guillouzo, A., Clement, B., Begue, J.M. and Guguen-Guillouzo, C. (1985). Biochem. Pharmacol. Suppl. 1, 19.

Jones, D.P., Sundby, G.-B., Ormstad, K. and Orrenius, S.

(1979). Biochem. Pharmacol, 28, 929.

Marnett, L.J. and Eling, T.E. (1983). in "Reviews in Biochemical Toxicology", Vol 5, (Ed. by Hodgson, E., Bend, J.R. and Philpot, R.M). Elsevier, North Holland, Amsterdam, p. 135.

Mehendale, H., Angerine, L.S. and Ohmiya, Y. (1981). Toxicology, 21. 1.

Meister, A. and Anderson, M. (1983). Annual Rev. of Biochem, 52, 711.

Moldeus, P., Hogberg, J. and Orrenius, S. (1978). Methods in Enzymology, 52, 60.

Moldeus, P., Anderson, B. and Gergely, V. (1979). Drug Metab. Disp. 7, 416.

Steward, R.A., Dannan, G.A., Guzelian, P.S. and Guengerich, F.P. (1985). Mol. Pharmacol, 27. 125.

Snyder, R., Lougaore, S.L., Witmer, C.M. and Kocsis, J.J. (1981). in "Reviews in Biochemical Toxicology", Vol 3, (Ed by Hodgson, E., Bend, J.R. and Philpot, R.M). Elsevier, North Holland, Amsterdam, p.123.

Thurman, R.G. and Kauffman, F.C. (1980). Pharmacol. Rev., 31, 229.

COMPARISON OF FETAL AND ADULT DRUG METABOLISING ENZYMES

Karl J. Netter

Department of Pharmacology and Toxicology, University of
Marburg, Lahnberge, D-3550, Marburg, FRG.

It has been known for many decades that the mammalian
fetus lacks the ability to metabolise drugs, or at least
has a very markedly lower activity of oxidising as well as
conjugating enzymes. This obviously has important
consequences for the handling of drugs and other foreign
substances in pregnant individuals. In order to describe
the complex situation quantitatively, it is necessary to
describe the pharmacokinetics in the fetal-placental unit
as well as in the maternal organism.

There have been very many respective efforts as a
consequence of which we are in the position to know fairly
well about the perinatal peculiarities of drug metabolism.
This is treated in a number of reviews which mostly were
published about ten or more years ago, when knowledge about
the mixed function monooxygenase grew explosively not only
for adult tissues but also for fetal tissues and placenta
(Netter, 1971; Dutton and Leakey, 1981; Burke and Orrenius
1982; Bergheim et al, 1973). On the other end of the age
scale, namely with old adult individuals, similar questions
have to be asked with respect to the activity of drug
metabolising enzymes. This has recently been reviewed by
Schmucker (1985).

It is the purpose of this article to discuss the
comparison between fetal and adult drug metabolising
activities.

In order to facilitate comparisons between the
perinatal and the normal adult situation this article will
highlight four different aspects and illustrate them by
selected examples. It must be understood, that this
presentation is not intended to be comprehensive in dealing
with all aspects possible and even less so in dealing with
the complete body of knowledge that is available at
present. With this caveat in mind the present contribution
will treat :
- the areas of comparison
- drug kinetics in pregnancy

  - perinatal activities of drug metabolising systems as
    exemplified by some characteristic drug oxidising
    reactions
  - the question of perinatal inducibility of cytochrome
    P-450
  - perinatal activities of conjugation enzyme systems.

AREAS OF COMPARISON

   Figure 1 has been designed to illustrate the various
points of comparison.

**Figure 1.   A schematic representation of the possible
changes in drug metabolic and kinetic parameters which are
caused by pregnancy.**

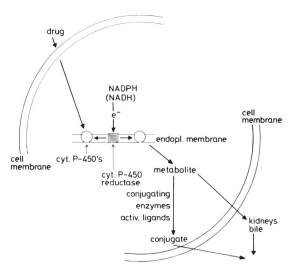

Areas of comparison between adult and fetal drug
metabolising enzymes

Also:
drug metabolism in placenta
pregnancy alters maternal drug kinetics
perinatal inducibility

For further details please consult text.

Firstly, the availability of a drug to the metabolising
cell and its penetration into the cytosol may be an area of
comparison. It is influenced mainly by the fact that the

drug kinetics in the maternal organism are altered during the gestation period. This holds true not only for the maternal organism but also, of course, for the fetus, which is separated from the maternal circulation by the placenta. Secondly, when the metabolisable substance reaches the membraneous monooxygenase system it will interact with an enzyme that is different from the adult stage in various respects: the proportion of the various forms of cytochrome P-450 in the fetus may be different from that in the adult, resulting in an altered metabolic rate. Also the function of the cytochrome P-450 reductase in accepting electrons and reducing cytochrome P-450 may be changed, also resulting in different metabolic rates. In this respect, permutation experiments in reconstituted systems combining either adult cytochrome P-450 with fetal reductase or vice versa should be of great interest. Thirdly, as a consequence of differences in the above two aspects, the metabolite formation during ontogeny may be different. Fourthly, variant activity of conjugating enzyme systems may lead to a different proportion of conjugated metabolites, being excreted into the circulation. Fifthly, an important factor, and also a protective design, must be seen in the fact that the placenta is also able to metabolise drugs, as it contains cytochrome P-450 or at least hemoproteins that catalyse oxidative reactions. Sixthly, in a situation of maternal enzyme induction it is to be examined whether a comparable induction also occurs in the fetal tissues: in other words, inducibility and especially its developmental onset is another area of comparison between fetal and adult drug metabolism. It is also known that kidney function develops perinatally and becomes mainly operative only in the postnatal period, this will have consequences for the excretion of drugs and their metabolites, which, however, will not be dealt with in this article. Neither will there be any emphasis on the developmental changes in bile secretion of foreign compounds.

DRUG KINETICS IN PREGNANCY

Figure 2 shows the drug compartments in pregnancy, Obviously, the feto-maternal unit distinguishes itself from the normal situation by the mere existence of the fetus, the placenta, and the amniotic fluid. These constitute additional compartments which participate in the distribution and, to a smaller extent, to the metabolism of drugs and foreign compounds. The question marks by the metabolism in the fetus and placenta serve to indicate that

Figure 2. The five main compartments for the distribution
and metabolism of foreign compounds during pregnancy.

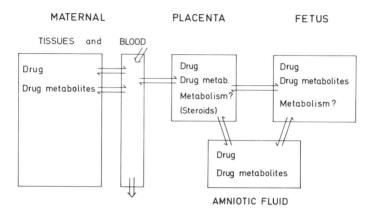

DRUG COMPARTMENTS IN PREGNANCY

here is a qualitative and quantitative difference to the
normal situation. It can be expected that a drug migrates
into the indicated compartments with different distribution
constants, but generally leading to a time lag between the
maxima of drug concentration in the developing
compartments. Also, it must be considered that within the
maternal compartment, the metabolic rate for xenobiotics is
usually decreased which leads to a slower excretion from
the maternal compartment.

Measurements of ampicillin concentrations in maternal
serum, fetal serum, and amniotic fluid by Bray et al. (1966)
illustrate the delayed distribution into the latter two
compartments: these authors have infused 500 mg of
ampicillin in 200 ml 5% glucose within 10 minutes into
pregnant women at term. The determination of ampicillin
levels in maternal serum showed a maximum of about 25μg/ml
immediately after the infusion. This was followed by a
four times lower maximum of about 6μg/ml in the fetal serum
which occurred almost 2 hours later, while in the amniotic
fluid they found about 5μg/mg during a broad maximum
between 4 and 10 hours after administration. This
demonstrates that one must take into account a delayed
distribution into the posterior compartments when making
comparisons about the presence of a given substance in
these regions.

But also, the presence of a foreign compound within the
maternal liver may be subject to drastic influences by

gestation: very recent experiments (Krowke, 1986) show that the concentration of radiolabelled 2,3,7,8-tetrachlorodibenzodioxin (TCDD) in the livers of pregnant mice after application of 25 nmoles/kg is markedly lower than in non-pregnant mice. This phenomenon has been attempted to be explained by various possibilities, such as an induced metabolism due to the strong inducing potency of TCDD, which then must be augmented during pregnancy. Another possibility is a reduction in intestinal absorption or a variation in lipid content or the ability of "TCDD-receptors" to bind the TCDD. At any rate this is an interesting observation, since one usually should expect a decreased metabolism during pregnancy and hence more likely an increased presence of foreign compounds in the maternal organism.

A delayed metabolism during pregnancy is demonstrated by measurements of caffeine concentrations in the saliva of pregnant women during various stages of pregnancy. The half-life of caffeine in four women was generally three times as long during pregnancy than in the same women several weeks post partum, thus serving as their own controls. The same authors have also examined whether caffeine half-life increases gradually with the duration of pregnancy. In fact, it increases from a starting value of 3 hours to a maximum of 10 hours at term, whereby the increase is fairly linear with the duration of pregnancy; the number of women examined at 8 different time points after conception was between 3 and 11. This experiment has a result which is contrary to the above observation on TCDD, namely showing a decrease in metabolic elimination rate during the gestation period, a finding which is more common to most drugs and foreign compounds.

PERINATAL DEVELOPMENT OF OXIDATIVE DRUG METABOLISM

The different rates of oxidative metabolism between adult and neonatal tissues are a further area of comparison. In general, the cytochrome P-450 dependent drug oxidation is very low and almost non-existent during the embryonic and fetal periods and begins to increase postnatally reaching adult levels after several weeks of extra-uterine life. Only some primates and humans possess a considerable fetal activity which amounts to about twenty-five per cent of the adult activity.

Detailed knowledge about the development of drug metabolic activity came through the efforts of Jondorf et al. (1959) roughly simultaneously with the unraveling of the mechanism of the cytochrome P-450 action. These authors

described that in guinea pigs, the oxidation of
monomethylamino-antipyrine is almost non-existant prior to
birth and rises steeply after delivery to about fifty per
cent of the adult level within 10 days and finally arriving
at the maximal level after 4 to 6 weeks. A similar pattern
is true for hexobarbital. These values were obtained as
the amounts of substrates metabolised per gram liver in the
presence of 9000 x g supernatant, a NADPH-generating
system, oxygen and 0.3mM substrate. Again a similar
pattern was also found for the glucuronidation of
phenolphthalein. MacLeod et al.(1972) have studied the
maturational changes in liver parameters in rats; they
obviously found an increase of absolute liver weight with
age, but also an increase in the yield of microsomal
protein per gram wet liver which increases from 17 mg/g at
birth to twice that amount after about a month. This
finding has relevance for quantitative considerations
extrapolated from metabolism data obtained from microsomal
protein. Similarly, the ratio of body weight vs.
aminopyrine-N-demethylation falls from a value of 29 to 1
at the age of one month, when the values are expressed as
per cent of adult. The same authors may be cited here
paradigmatically for many others who have measured the
increase in cytochrome P-450 in the livers of developing
rats with the aid of the reduced carbon monooxide complex;
in male rats there is a steep increase from almost 0 to
about 0.5 nmoles per mg microsomal protein within 3 weeks.
The postnatal increase is less pronounced in female rats
which reach a level of 0.3 nmoles per mg microsomal
protein. Figure 3 illustrates this. At the same time this
figure shows a general pattern which is true not only for
cytochrome P-450 but also for the dependent reactions such
as aminopyrine-N-demethylation and many other drug
metabolic reactions. It is noteworthy that the sex
difference in drug metabolism is most prominent in rats
only, in which females show a lower capacity, while in most
other species there is either no or a very small sex
difference in drug metabolic rates. A similar maturational
increase can also be seen in the activity of cytochrome P-
450 reductase, which shows that both integral parts of the
drug metabolism system develop in harmony. The same is
true for the development of cytochrome b_5 as has been
described by Short and Stith (1973) in pig liver. These
authors also obtained pre-delivery values after 107 days of
gestation which corresponds to about 1 day prior to birth.
They verified also for the swine the same pattern as in the
rat for other metabolic parameters such as NADPH-linked
reductase activity towards cytochrome P-450 and cytochrome

Figure 3.   The normal maturational increase of hepatic cytochrome P-450 in male and female neonatal rats.

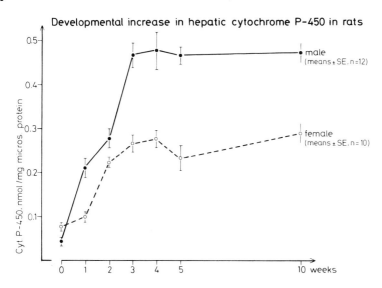

The number of determinations for males and females was 12 and 10, respectively, the bars represent SEM.   Cytochrome P-450 was determined by its carbon monoxide absorption spectrum.   Modified after MacLeod et al.(1972).

c, as well as for ethylmorphine-0-demethylase.   Pelkonen (1973) showed that in humans there is already considerable metabolic activity towards chlorpromazine at an embryonic age of 13 weeks which underlines the above statement that in this respect humans seem to be a certain exception to the general rule that there is practically no fetal metabolism in mammals.   Similar results have been obtained by Dvorchick et al.(1974) who also saw a similar pattern in fetal monkeys.   Furthermore, in rabbits there is also considerable fetal activity, when one compares end-term fetal hepatic activity with that of maternal liver in rabbits.   However, there is great variability for various substrates indicating that certain forms of cytochrome P-450 are differently expressed.   In general, this shows that many end-term fetal and newborn mammals are indeed capable of carrying out a certain amount of oxidative drug metabolism, so that in this respect the dominance of the maternal liver is not absolute.   This is reflected also by observations of Krauer et al.(1973) who found a half-life for the elimination of amobarbital in human newborns of

26±10 hours as compared to that of their mothers with 13±4 hours. Thus, human neonates of one to five days of age have also been shown to be able to metabolise other drugs such as primidone, diphenylhydantoin, caffeine and acetylsalicyclic acid (Horning et al, 1975).

The question of whether various isoenzymes of cytochrome P-450 may show different patterns of developmental increase has been indirectly answered by Kremers et al. (1981) who have characterised various forms of cytochrome P-450 in hepatic cell cultures by their susceptibility to metyrapone and alpha-naphthoflavone as inhibitors. Furthermore, measuring arylhydrocarbon-hydroxylase activity in the homogenates of rat livers from day -4 to +6 they find a steep increase beginning with day one; this is accompanied by a gradual disappearance of alpha-naphthoflavone susceptibility and an equally gradual increase in metyrapone-susceptibility; both changes become apparent already at three days before delivery indicating that in the late fetal stage both these variants of cytochrome P-450 are regulated indepently. Cresteil et al (1986) have described the ontogenesis of various cytochrome P-450 variants in the rat and have found an early expression of the sex difference. In the untreated male animal a different form develops postnatally than in the female: both enzymes have been characterised by antibodies. The same authors have shown that in early postnatal stages cytochrome P-450 can be induced in the newborns whereby phenobarbital produces a selective increase in cytochrome P-450 PB-B while 3-methylcholanthrene selectively increase cytochrome P-450 BNF-B; in both case the untreated controls show practically no increase in these two forms of cytochrome P-450. These findings emphasise the potential value of immunological methods to differentiate between various forms of cytochrome P-450.

ONSET OF INDUCIBILITY

As an outgrowth of the general interest in the phenomenon of enzyme induction early experiments have been undertaken to investigate whether fetal enzyme activity can be induced by applying inducing agents to the mother. Thus Oesch (1975) has shown that transplacental induction of hepatic microsomal benzo-a-pyrene hydroxlase can be achieved in rats by treating the mother with 60mg/kg benzo-a-pyrene intragastrally; under these conditions a steep increase in monooxygenase activity can be seen about two days before delivery, but the epoxide hydrolase remains unaffected. It can be concluded, therefore, that shortly

before the end of the gestation period protein biosynthesis
for cytochromes P-450 can be greatly increased by inducers.
In early pregnancy there is no such effect. The time
course of the development of fetal inducibility has been
further studied by Schubert and Netter (1981) who
predominantly investigated the question of whether
inducibility is facilitated by the act of parturition or
whether there is an internal "clock" which determines the
onset of inducibility. This question was answered by
prolonging the pregnancy in rats beyond day 22 until
maximally day 25. If inducibility would depend on the
previous transition from intrauterine to extrauterine
liver, than there should be no increase in cytochrome P-450
during the prolonged pregnancy in response to inducers such
as phenobarbital. Figure 4 shows that, indeed, the
phenobarbital inducible form also increases very
drastically when the animals are treated with phenobarbital
during interauterine life. However, this is not so when
one used alpha-hexachlorocyclohexane (alpha-HCH). Thus, it
seems that there is a certain prenatal selectivity with
regard to the inducible forms of cytochrome P-450. During
the prolongation of pregnancy by progesterone the molecular
activities for the cytochrome P-450 mediated p-
nitroanisole-demethylation has also been measured under the
influence of both inducers. It is very interesting to
note, that in spite of considerable fluctuations the
molecular activity rises sharply for all three conditions,
that is including the untreated controls, after the 22nd
day of pregnancy. This even more strongly indicates that
shortly before delivery drastic changes in the status of
the catalytic protein occur, and this is independent of the
actual transition from intra- to extrauterine conditions.
At this point it is interesting to note that this is not
entirely true for all transferases, which conjugate foreign
compounds.

In a similar way postnatal inducibility for the hepatic
monooxygenase was found for nuclear membranes suggesting
that the same principles also govern the development of
cytochrome P-450 in a different part of the cell (Romano et
al (1982). However, no experiments about the internal
triggering of inducibility have been performed.

An extensive treatise of the stimulation of onset of
drug metabolising enzymes by glucocorticoids can be found
in the review article by Dutton and Leakey (1981).

GLUCURONYLTRANSFERASES

The biosynthesis of conjugated compounds is a second

Figure 4. Perinatal development of the cytochrome P-450 content and inducibility by phenobarbital (PB) and alpha-hexachlorocyclohexane (alpha-HCH).

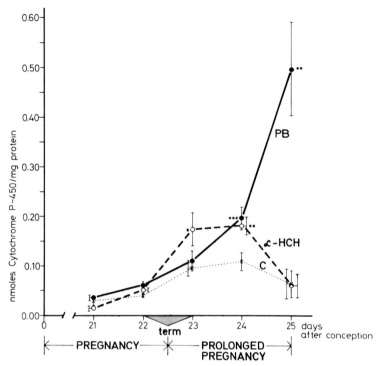

For prolongation of the gestation period pregnant rats were injected with 25 mg/kg progesterone in oil. Normal term was assumed to be day 22 and 23. Animals were always sacrificed at midday. C = controls (untreated)
+ = p < 0.02; ** = p < 0.01; *** = p < 0.002. Fetusses from one litter were pooled and processed. The number of litters varied between 3 and 13.
After Schubert and Netter (1981).

important pathway for the elimination of toxic substances and drugs. Mostly, glucuronic acid is the ligand used for these conjugations, and we shall deal here with the perinatal development of the respective enzyme UDP glucuronyltransferase only. As early as 1966, Dutton observed that the perinatal glucuronyltransferase activity towards different substances varies greatly: when one uses p-nitrophenol as a substrate in newborn rats and in

fetusses the activity during the last days of embryonic
life and the first five days of postnatal life are clearly
higher (up to 200%) than in the maternal liver. On the
other hand when one uses phenolphthalien as a substrate
there is practically no activity during the late fetal
stages and early postnatal period, reaching the equivalent
of maternal activity about five days postnatally. This
observation clearly shows that there must be a family of at
least two enzyme activities with different substrate
specificities. This was later (Wishart and Dutton 1977)
characterised as two families of substrates, which
obviously are accepted by different glucuronyltransferases
(GT_1 and GT_2), which are under different genetic control as
far as their perinatal appearance is concerned. When one
determines the activity of 20 day old fetal liver towards
substrates like 2-aminophenol, 4-methylumbelliferone, 4-
nitrophenol and others, the activity is the same as in
adult male rats. On the other hand, for substrates like
bilirubin, phenolphthalein, morphine, chloramphenicol and
others there is only very little glucuronyltransferase
activity, namely around 10 per cent. The author,
therefore, has classified these two groups of substrates
into "clusters", whereby 2-aminophenol belongs to cluster 1
(with fetal activity) and bilirubin belongs to cluster 2
(without fetal activity). Furthermore, it is quite
remarkable that GT_2 which accepts substrates of cluster 2,
possesses a very much lower activity towards bilirubin, and
activity which develops strictly after birth and continues
to rise to adult levels. GT_1, however, begins to increase
in activity on day 18 of rat pregnancy and rises steeply to
levels higher than adult levels; several days after
delivery this activity will decrease again and approach the
final adult level from a higher perinatal level. In humans
the situation is almost the reverse: in human neonates the
bilirubin UDP glucuronyltransferase activity increases
earlier than that against 2-aminophenol which,
teleologically speaking, is more appropriate in view of the
avoidance of the dangerous icterus neonatorum (Onishi et
al, 1979).

It is appropriate at this point to also investigate the
question of whether the development of glucuronyl-
transferases can be precociously precipitated by prenatal
induction. For this purpose 300μg of dexamethasone were
injected into pregnant rats. This corticoid was chosen
because of its relatively slow inactivation. When doing
so, it could be observed that upon injection on day 14, 15
and 16 of pregnancy the transferase activity of GT_1
(substrate : 2-aminophenol) rose very steeply and reached a

fairly high value even before delivery on day 17. The slope of the increase was the same as that observed for the natural development of the same enzyme beginning on day 18 of pregnancy (Wishart and Dutton, 1977). This experiment shows that the natural triggering of the expression of this protein can be mimicked by dexamethasone. Considering that this effect can be seen as early as about two thirds of the pregnancy it seems that the transferases are more susceptible to exogenous stimulation of onset of activity formation.

CONCLUSIONS

In this article examples have been presented which shall serve to illustrate the following aspects of drug metabolism in normal adults and in the fetus and newborn respectively :

Pregnancy changes maternal drug kinetics usually in the direction to a delayed elimination by metabolic and renal routes. At the same time the addition of new pharmacokinetic compartments leads to a more complex system in which a given foreign compound appears later and at a lower peak concentration in the fetal serum and the amniotic fluid than it can be measured in the maternal serum.

In the same way as other biological functions develop during ontogenesis, the drug metabolic enzyme systems seem to be mainly dormant during the embryonic and fetal stages but rapidly develop into adult-like or even super-adult activities shortly prior and immediately after parturition. This seems to be a general phenomenon which is followed by most drug metabolic activities with some modifications. It is true for drug oxidising enzymes as well as glucuronyltransferases. In the latter group, however, there are remarkable peculiarities for certain enzymes of the transferase family.

Perinatal inducibility seems to be triggered by an endogenous mechanism which is independent of the transgression from intra- to extra-uterine life as such. Conventional enzyme inducers will also induce fetal enzymes, but this becomes possible only shortly before the regular termination of pregnancy and seems to be particularly early in this case of a certain variety of glucuronyltransferase.

REFERENCES

Bergheim, P., Rathgen, G.H. and Netter, K.J. (1973).

Biochem. Pharmacol, 22, 1633.
Bray, R.E., Boe, R.W. and Johnson, W.L. (1966). Am. J. Obst. Gynec, 96, 938.
Burke, M.D. and Orrenius, S. (1982). in "Hepatic cytochrome P-450 monooxygenase system" (Ed. by Schenkman, J.B. and Kupfer, D). Pergamon Press, Oxford, p.47.
Cresteil, T., Beaune, P., Celier, C., Leroux, J.P. and Guengerich, F.P. (1986). J. Pharmacol. Exp. Ther, 236, 269.
Dutton, G.J. (1966). Biochem. Pharmacol, 15, 947.
Dutton, G.J. and Leakey, J.E.A. (1981). Prog.Drug.Res, 25, 189.
Dvorchick, B.H., Stenger, V.G. and Quattropani, S.L. (1974). Drug Metab. Disp, 2, 539.
Horning, M.G., Butler, C.M., Nowlin, J. and Hill, R.M. (1985). Life Sci, 16, 651.
Jondorf, W.R., Maickel, R.P. and Brodie, B.B. (1959). Biochem. Pharmacol, 8, 352.
Knutti, R., Rothweiler, H. and Schlatter, Ch. (1981). Europ. J. Clin. Pharmacol, 21, 121.
Krauer, B., Draffan, G.H., Williams, F.M., Clare, R.A., Dollery, C.T. and Hawkins, D.F. (1973). Clin. Pharmacol. Ther, 14, 442.
Kremers, P., Goujon, F., de Graeve, J., van Cantford, J. and Gielen, J.E. (1981). Europ. J. Biochem, 116, 67.
Krowke, R. (1986). Chemosphere, in press.
MacLeod, S.M., Renton, K.W. and Eade, N.R. (1972). J. Pharmacol. Exp. Ther. 183, 489.
Netter, K.J. (1971). Arch. Gynak, 211, 112.
Oesch, F. (1975). FEBS Letters, 53, 205.
Onishi, S., Kawada, S., Itoh, S., Isobe, K. and Sugiyama, S. (1979). Biochem. J. 184, 705.
Pelkonen, O. (1973). Arch. Int. Pharmacodyn, 202, 281.
Romano, M., Clos, V., Assael, B.M. and Salmona, M. (1982). Chem. Biol. Interact, 42, 225.
Schmucker, D.L. (1985). Pharmacol. Rev. 37, 133.
Schubert, I. and Netter, K.J. (1981). Biochem. Pharmacol, 30, 2901.
Short, C.R. and Stith, R.D. (1973). Biochem. Pharmacol, 22, 1309.
Wishart, G.J. (1978). Biochem. J. 174, 485.
Wishart, G.J. and Dutton, G.J. (1977). Biochem. J. 168, 507.

SPECIES VARIATIONS IN PHARMACOKINETICS

Dennis A. Smith

Department of Drug Metabolism, Fisons plc, Pharmaceutical
Division, Loughborough, Leics. U.K.

The consideration of the relationship between
pharmacokinetic parameters across species is complex.
Undoubtedly guiding rules as to how species handle drugs in
comparison to man would be of enormous importance to the
safety evaluation of future medicines. This paper is
entitled "Pharmacokinetics", a discipline which may be
viewed by some as distinct from compound "Metabolism".
This should not be so and the discipline should be
recognised as a mechanism to quantitate drug disposition
including metabolism in its entirety. Only when
quantitation in terms of rate has been made can comparisons
be meaningfully made. This paper attempts to bridge the
gap between the disciplines. The data, in the literature,
whilst vast, is not usually presented in a form that allows
this to be easily done. In many cases the data has had to
be extrapolated and combined from many sources. To
simplify the considerations here only clearance has been
considered. Clark and Smith (1984) in a review on the
impact of pharmacokinetics on toxicity testing indicate
that clearance is the major variable between species,
rather than such factors as absorption. The approach used
will be to study the clearance of drugs by animals and man
and relate these using simple equations describing drug
clearance. Compounds will be studied both from their
behaviour in animal species relative to man, and on the
basis of their chemistry or specific clearance mechanisms.
The comparisons made do not allow for dose level
differences. Non-linear kinetics could alter some of the
interpretations although effort has been made to use
examples at the lowest dose quoted. The data in rodents
are normally restricted to outbred strains only. The
pharmacokinetic parameters to be considered are systemic
clearance, organ blood flow, organ extraction and intrinsic
clearance. Systemic clearance can be considered to be the
product of organ blood flow and organ intrinsic clearance.
For a drug cleared by a single organ, for instance the

liver, systemic clearance (CL_S) is :

$$CL_S = Q \frac{CL_I}{CL_I + Q} \qquad \cdots\cdots (1)$$

Where Q is the organ blood flow and CL_I the intrinsic clearance of the organ.

$\frac{CL_I}{CL_I + Q}$ represents the extraction (E) of the organ

thus $CL_S = QE$ $\cdots\cdots (2)$

For the purposes of the comparisons these equations will be used to provide a basis. In studying drug clearance across species we must be aware of the nature of the comparison. We can compare systemic clearance to gain an overall view. We can examine more closely and understand differences by consideration of blood flow and intrinsic clearance.

SYTEMIC CLEARANCE ACROSS SPECIES

Figure 1 illustrates the sytemic clearance of a number of drugs in dog, rhesus monkey, rabbit, rat and mouse compared with man. The comparison has been made on a weight normalised basis. It is quite obvious that as a general rule animals clear drugs faster than man, although there are notable exceptions. Inspection of the data may suggest that the largest cluster of drug clearance ratios with man are between 1 to 10 fold greater in dog and 2 to 10 fold greater in rhesus monkey, rabbit and rat. It is hard to determine any trend in the mouse other than considerable scatter. To progress any further in understanding species relationships in pharmacokinetics a closer analysis of the data is necessary. If we first consider the areas in which the majority of drugs lie and the likely trends that could result in clearance values with these ratios, there appears to be an immediate correlation with the clearance ratios and that of Q in equations 1 and 2.

DRUGS OF HIGH HEPATIC EXTRACTION

Cardiac output and hence organ blood flow generally show an inverse relationship to body weight across animal species. Thus in the commonly used laboratory animals shown in Figure 1 the flows are mouse > rabbit > monkey and dog > man. If cardiac output or organ blood flow was a

Figure 1.   Systemic clearance of drugs, normalised for bodyweight, in various animal species, expressed relative to man.

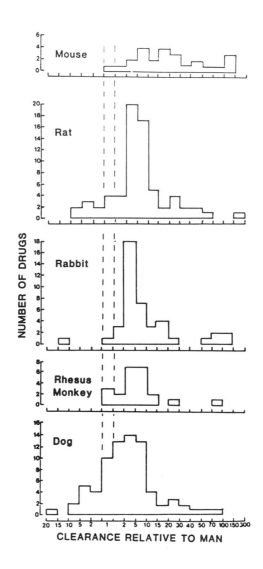

Drugs cleared at identical rates appear as 1. Drugs to the left of this value are cleared at rates lower than man, drugs to the right are cleared at rates greater than man.

major determinant of drug clearance, we would expect a significant number of compounds to be cleared approximately 1-3 fold faster in dog and 4-6 fold faster in the rat. These rates represent the approximate increase in cardiac output or organ blood flow in these species compared with man. Previous inspection of Figure 1 has indicated that many compounds fall close to these values. When the type of drugs falling into this cluster are considered, a significant number of them can be categorised as "high hepatic extraction". With all these drugs hepatic metabolism is very rapid and the sole important clearance pathway. Figure 2 shows the relative rates of systemic clearance in rat and dog for nicardipine, metoprolol, propranolol, domperidone, d-propoxyphene, metoclopramide, lidocaine, lorcainide, fentanyl, bupropion, nifedipine, verapamil, diltiazem and FPL 62129 (a dihydropyridine type Ca^{++} antagonist).

Figure 2. Systemic clearance of high hepatic extraction drugs, normalised for bodyweight, in dog and rat, expressed relative to man.

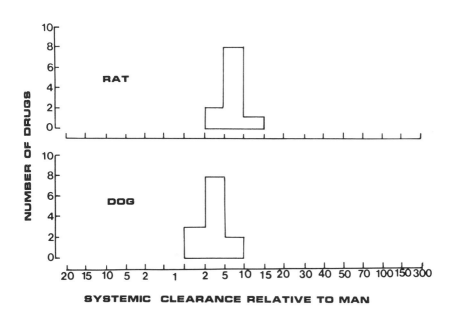

The close correlation is striking although readily explainable by equation 1 since when CL_I (hepatic metabolism) is a large value relative to Q the equation simplifies to

$$CL_S \overset{\sim}{} Q \qquad\qquad \dots\dots (3)$$

The relationship is explored further in Table 1 where
systemic and intrinsic clearance values of high extraction
drugs are considered. Table 1 lists the intrinsic and
systemic clearance values for propranolol, FPL 62129,
metoprolol, domperidone and lidocaine. As might be
expected these drugs show variation in their rate of
metabolism (CL_I) but in all cases the CL_I value is much
larger than liver blood flow. Inspection of the values
shows that the systemic clearance values show little
variation compared to the vast difference in intrinsic
clearance values. For instance FPL 62129 shows similar
intrinsic clearance values in all species, whilst
metoprolol has a much higher value in rat compared to man
and dog. A third situation is presented with propranolol
where both dog and rat values are much greater than man.
Despite these variations the systemic clearance shows the
expected relationship with Q. Figure 3 illustrates the
intrinsic clearance values for most of the drugs in Figure
2. The scatter in intrinsic clearance values compared to
systemic clearance is clear. This variation would be a
major factor in species comparisons if the drugs were
administered orally since the area under the plasma curve
is dependent on CL_I after oral administration. It is
noteworthy that the intrinsic clearance values exceed those
in man, in all cases, for both rat and dog, which could
reflect both liver size and general enzyme content
(cytochrome P-450) increase relative to body weight. It is
more likely in some cases as we will see to represent
specific cytochrome P-450 isoenzyme differences. Further
examination of the relationship between intrinsic clearance
for these drugs between man and rat is made in Table 2.
FPL 62129 and domperidone are representative of the drugs
which show less than a 10 fold difference between man and
rat. Metoprolol, propranolol and lidocaine are representative of the drugs which show large differences in
intrinsic clearance between man and rat. It can be seen
for these three compounds that only one of the routes of
metabolism is responsible for the large change in intrinsic
clearance. Lidocaine and propranolol show disproportionate
rates for their aromatic hydroxylation by the rat, whilst
side chain oxidation, representing both O-dealkylation and
aliphatic hydroxylation is disproportionate for metoprolol.
The data is indicative not of a general increase in enzyme
content but differences in specific isoenzymes. We shall

Table 1. Systemic (S) and intrinsic (I) clearance values (ml min^{-1}kg^{-1}) for five high extraction drugs in man, dog and rat.

DRUG	MAN		DOG		RAT	
	S	I	S	I	S	I
FPL 62129	18	208	48	291	78	261
DOMPERIDONE	13	65	21	100	100	260
PROPRANOLOL	15	50	37	900	74	1800
METOPROLOL	20	60	25	110	120	3200
LIDOCAINE	16	50	40	70	115	1600

Figure 3. Intrinsic clearance of high hepatic extraction drugs, normalised for body weight, in dog and rat, expressed relative to man.

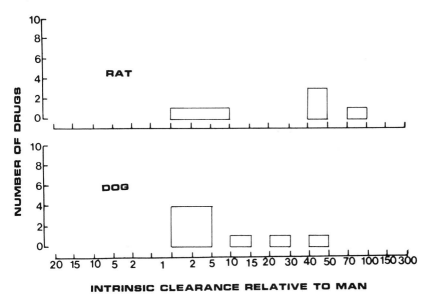

INTRINSIC CLEARANCE RELATIVE TO MAN

return to this in the next section.

Meperidine (pethidine) is an example of a high extraction drug not showing a systemic clearance relationship across species with Q. The systemic clearance in rat (253ml min^{-1}kg^{-1}) is 20 fold greater than man (12ml min^{-1}kg^{-1}) (Dahlstrom et al, 1979; Pond et al, 1981). In

Table 2.   Partial intrinsic clearance values (ml min⁻¹kg⁻¹) for five high extraction drugs in man (M) and rat (R).

DRUG		AROMATISATION	PARTIAL INTRINSIC CLEARANCE			
			N-DEALKYLATION AND AMIDE CLEAVAGE	ALIPHATIC HYDROXYLATION	AROMATIC HYDROXYLATION	CONJUGATION
FPL 62129	M	208				
	R	261				
DOMPERIDONE	M		15		28	
	R		31		146	
METOPROLOL	M		6	45		
	R		32	2912		
LIDOCAINE	M		40		1	
	R		270		1090	
PROPRANOLOL	M		20		20	10
	R		50		1700	50

For β-blocking agents all oxidation products of the oxypropanolamine side chain are termed N-dealkylation man clearance of the drug (mainly N-demethylation, 60%, with some ester hydrolysis, 25%) is hepatic. The rat based on the very high clearance value probably clears the drug by hepatic and extrahepatic mechanisms. Certainly the drug is of high hepatic extraction in the rat but it is tempting to conclude that the much higher excretion of the products of ester hydrolysis in this species are due to non-hepatic esterases. However, there is evidence that meperidine esterase is mainly confined to the liver (Yeh, 1982). One feature of the entire group of drugs is the generalisation that can be made that high extraction of a drug often tends to be a general phenomenon across species even though the principle routes of metabolism may vary. We shall consider in the next section some exceptions to the rule. Consideration of the structure of these drugs extends the view that most high hepatic extraction compounds possess an aromatic portion and are substituted alkyl amines of high lipophilicity. Out of 45 drugs on which human data indicated their hepatic extraction to be > 0.5, 37 possessed these features. Compounds outside of this category included four dihydropyridines, a class of compound that could be termed metabolically labile. It is possible that these features (basicity and lipophilicity) cause concentration of the drug in the hepatocytes and that this feature is of importance in their extraction. More specifically their basicity may have a profound effect on their enzyme binding, however, and extraction would be associated with the ability of the substrate to bind to the enzyme. Such "high affinity" binding obviously fits the concept of high extraction. Compounds that could be included in the above description, but did not show high hepatic extraction, often included a second nitrogen atom in their structure, either as an unsubstituted amine or amide or as part of a ring system such as a pyridine.

DRUGS OF INTERMEDIATE AND LOW EXTRACTION

Figure 4 illustrates the relationship between rat and man for various low and moderate extraction drugs. The drugs are classed as either basic or acidic. Basic drugs shown include theophylline, amphetamine, caffeine, disopyramide, aminopyrine, methadone, amosulolol, camazepam and diazepam, whilst acidic drugs include indoprofen, benoxaprofen, proxicromil, hexobarbitone, diflunisal, flurbiprofen, tolbutamide, phenobarbitone, pentobarbitone, warfarin, naproxen, buprofen and valproic acid. Drugs of low E have CL_I values significantly below blood flow (equation 1). In these cases we can reduce the equation to

$$CL_S \approx CL_I \quad \ldots\ldots\ldots \quad (4)$$

If the systemic clearance is dependent on CL_I then we would expect the systemic clearance to reflect enzyme activity. Most of the drugs shown in Figure 4 are dependent on cytochrome P-450 for clearance. Rat liver contains approximately 2-3 times more cytochrome P-450 than human liver, mainly a reflection of increased liver size relative to body weight. If we mean the rates of in vitro metabolism for many drugs we arrive at a figure that the activity in rat is 10 fold higher than man. Whilst this figure is of doubtful value it does serve as a starting point. Many of the drugs in Figure 4 fall within a 2 to 10 fold increase in clearance relative to man. These include most of the acidic drugs and some of the basic compounds. For instance phenytoin is cleared 7-8 fold faster in rat (man 0.6, rat 4.5ml $min^{-1}kg^{-1}$) and antipyrine shows a similar ratio (man 0.7, rat 6.0ml $min^{-1}kg^{-1}$).

There are compounds in Figure 4 which show large variation across species. The variation is so great that they can be termed high extraction in one species and low extraction in another. The trend is that the smaller species show the higher hepatic extractions. Benzodiazepines are a group of drugs that often show such differences. For instance camazepam, has liver extraction values of rat 0.88 and man 0.07 (Morino, 1985). Examination of equation 1 will indicate very large variation in intrinsic clearance is necessary to cause such a range of extraction values. Intrinsic clearance is over 400 times greater in rat than man, systemic clearance, a product of Q and E is 55 fold greater. Thus in rat systemic clearance depends on Q (equation 3) wherease in man systemic clearance depends on CL_I (equation 4). The metabolism of camazepam is complex but the increase in hepatic extraction across the species correlates with an increased ability to form N_1-desmethyl metabolites. Diazepam also shows high hepatic extraction in rat and not man with systemic clearance in rat over 200 fold greater than in man. Again as seen in other compounds the difference is due to a high intrinsic clearance value for aromatic hydroxylation compared to man.

There are examples of more strongly basic drugs that also show this trend. Amosulalol is an example of such a drug with high hepatic extraction in the rat (E = 0.7) and very low in man. It is possible from the published data (Kamimura et al, 1984; Nakashima et al, 1984; Kamimura et al, 1985) to understand the basis of these differences. Systemic clearance values are 25 fold greater in rat when

Figure 4. Systemic clearance of various low and moderate hepatic extraction drugs, normalised for body weight, in dog and rat, expressed relative to man.

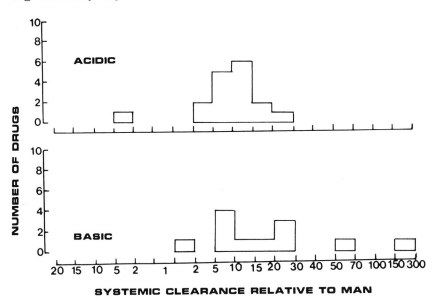

SYSTEMIC CLEARANCE RELATIVE TO MAN

compared to man. The systemic clearance can be divided into renal and metabolic (hepatic) clearance (Table 3). When hepatic clearance is considered on its own and expressed as intrinsic clearance the values are 170 fold greater in rat than man. Making some perhaps ambitious assumptions, it is possible to divide the clearances into partial intrinsic clearances for the various routes. Man can only clear the drug by aromatic hydroxylation, the intrinsic clearance in rat being approximately 10 fold higher. Rat can also clear the drug by N-dealkylation (Table 3) and oxidation of the methyl function very efficiently. The increase in intrinsic clearance and hence increase in E in the rat is due not only to increased rates of metabolism with similar routes (the increase being a relatively modest 10 fold) but an increase in the number of clearance routes available. It is interesting to compare the intrinsic clearance of amosulalol in the rat (250ml $min^{-1}kg^{-1}$) with the intrinsic clearance calculated for some of the "high" hepatic extraction drugs such as nicardipine, metoprolol, propranolol, lidocaine and bupropion, which all have values greater than 1000ml $min^{-1}kg^{-1}$.

Quinidine also shows low hepatic extraction in man and high extraction in the rat. Systemic clearance is 3.9ml

Table 3. Partial systemic and intrinsic clearance values
($ml\ min^{-1}\ kg^{-1}$) for amosulalol.

SYSTEMIC CLEARANCE		HEPATIC INTRINSIC CLEARANCE			
Renal	Hepatic (metabolic)	Total	Aromatic oxidation	N-dealky-lation	Methyl-oxidation
RAT 3.7	53	250	15	37	97
MAN 0.7	1.5	1.5	1.5	-	-

$min^{-1}kg^{-1}$ in man and 76ml min^-kg^{-1} in rat. Intrinsic
hepatic clearance is some 80 fold greater (Rakhit et al,
1984; Harashima et al, 1985; Yu et al, 1982). In man 3-
hydroxylation is the major hepatic clearance pathway
whereas in rat it is O-demethylation. Likewise phenformin
intrinsic hepatic clearance is 3.5ml $min^{-1}kg^{-1}$ in man and
approximately 60ml $min^{-1}kg^{-1}$ in the rat. The hepatic
clearance in both species is by 4-hydroylation (Alkalay et
al, 1979; Oates et al, 1983). Amphetamine (Table 4) is a
drug of moderate extraction showing an 8 fold increase in
systemic drug clearance between man and rat (40ml $min^{-1}kg^{-1}$
compared to 5ml $min^{-1}\ kg^{-1}$). Renal clearance increases
approximately 3 fold between the species (2 and 7ml
$min^{-1}kg^{-1}$). When intrinsic hepatic clearance is considered
side chain oxidation is similar in both species (3ml
$min^{-1}kg^{-1}$) whereas aromatic ring hydroxylation is some 45
fold greater in the rat (45 and 1ml $min^{-1}kg^{-1}$). The
systemic clearance of methadone (Gabrielsson et al, 1985;
Baselt and Bickel, 1973) is 27 fold greater in rat (55ml
$min^{-1}kg^{-1}$) than man 2ml $min^{-1}kg^{-1}$). This is due to an
increase in hepatic extraction. Renal clearance of the
compound only increases 4 fold (0.7 to 2.8ml $min^{-1}kg^{-1}$).
The intrinsic hepatic clearance by this route is 100 fold
greater in rat than man. Early metabolism investigations of
the compound indicated that the major hepatic clearance was
N-demethylation in both species. Recent studies, however,
that have included biliary products, have shown that p-
hydroxymethadone is a major metabolite in the rat (Gerardy
et al, 1986).

Table 4. Partial systemic and intrinsic clearance values (ml.min^{-1} kg^{-1}) for amphetamine.

	SYSTEMIC CLEARANCE		HEPATIC INTRINSIC CLEARANCE		
	Renal	Hepatic (Metabolic)	Total	Aromatic Oxidation	Side chain Oxidation
RAT	7	33	48	45	3
MAN	2	3	4	1	3

It has already been suggested that iso-enzyme differences may be the key to understanding species differences in kinetics. Amphetamine, phenformin, quinidine, methadone and amosulolol demonstrate oxidative metabolism at a distinct distance from a basic amine function. This is directly comparable to metoprolol, propranolol, and perhaps lidocaine. Recently a cytochrome P-450 isoenzyme (P-450 UT-H) has been isolated in rat and man which is at least partly responsible for the hydroxylation of the aliphatic side chain of metoprolol and the ring hydroxylation of propranolol amongst other oxidations including debrisoquine (Guengerich et al, 1986). The active site of this enzyme appears capable of accepting basic molecules of defined proportions. This enzyme is more abundant in rat then man. It or similar isoenzymes would explain the differences in hepatic clearance between rat and man particularly if the rat isoenzyme had a slightly less restricted active site. Evidence that an isoenzyme with a restricted active site is important in the metabolism of these basic compounds by the rat is provided by considering disopyramide (Hinderling and Garrett, 1976; Cook et al, 1982), another drug of low extraction in man but high extraction in the rat. Table 5 lists the clearance in man and rat for the drug. In man clearance is by a combination of renal and metabolic mechanisms. N-dealkyation is the sole major mechanism. In rat clearance is considerably higher due to a disproportionate increase in metabolic clearance. Again the increase is due to the rats ability for aromatic hydroxylation of the compound. The aromatic ring has both amide and pyridine functions that could interfere with the binding of the pheny ring to a "restricted site" cytochrome P-450 and one would expect significant stereospecific metabolism effects with such a compound since it has a chiral centre at the carbon linking the groups. Table 5 shows that aromatic hydroxylation by the rat is very sensitive to such effects.

In conclusion it can be postulated that various cytochrome P-450 isoenzymes contain binding sites for basic functions. Such ionic binding will give the enzyme high affinity for the substrates, high substrate specificity and also high regioselectivity and stereoselectivity of oxidation. The rat enzyme(s) appear to have more tolerance in the active site than man. It is noteworthy that many of the substrates described show large (polymorphic) variation in human metabolism rates.

Table 5. **Partial systemic and intrinsic clearance values** ($mlmin^{-1}kg^{-1}$) **for disopyramide racemate and its enant-iomers.**

SYSTEMIC CLEARANCE				HEPATIC INTRINSIC CLEARANCE	
	Renal	Hepatic (Metabolic)	Total	Aromatic Oxidation	N-dealkylation oxidation
RAT	20	36	78	61	17
MAN	1.8	1.6	1.7	0	1.7
RAT (R-)	17	17	38	13	25
RAT (S+)	22	55	120	110	10

CARBOXYLIC ACIDS IN THE DOG AND MAN

Another area of interest appears in the data in Figure 1. The dog shows a surprising number of compounds which it clears more slowly than man. Analysis of this cluster for trends, indicates that acid group containing drugs particularly carboxylic acid such as NSAI's form a significant proportion of these compounds. However, the fact that a drug contains a carboxylic acid grouping is in itself no determinant, there being several examples of compounds which the dog clears more rapidly than man. Closer examination of data from a number of lipophilic carboxylic acids indicates that man clears this class of compound by two principal mechanisms : acyl glucuronidation and oxidation. For instance proxicromil is cleared by hydroxylation as the sole clearance mechanism; ibuprofen and flurbiprofen are also cleared mainly by hydroxylation although conjugation does occur. Naproxen and fenoprofen are examples of compounds where both mechanisms make significant contributions, whilst benoxaprofen illustrates a compound relying solely on glucuronidation. Indoprofen, somewhat less lipophilic than the other compounds, has a renal component to add to the major acyl glucuronidation process. The contribution that hydroxylation makes to the clearance component will be very structure dependent, for instance the chlorophenyl group of benoxaprofen would be expected to be more resistant to oxidation than the phenyl group of flurbiprofen or the alkyl group of ibuprofen.

When the clearance of these compounds is studied in dog it is immediately apparent that they are all highly resistant to oxidation by this species. For all compounds the dog depends on acyl glucuronidation or taurine conjugation to clear the compounds. In the extreme case where conjugation is prevented by the pKa of the acid group, as with proxicromil, biliary excretion is the sole clearance process (Smith et al, 1985). Where man does not hydroxylate the compounds, for instance benoxaprofen, and depends on conjugation for clearance, the relative clearance in the dog is higher. Where man clears the compound primarily by hydroxylation, as with flurbiprofen, relative clearance by the dog is lower. These trends are illustrated in Figure 5. As a general rule, due to an inability to hydroxylate certain carboxylic acids, the dog shows a relative clearance for these compounds lower than other species. The inability of the dog to oxidise acids, particularly carboxylic acid drugs has been reported for proxicromil (Smith and Neale, 1983), 2-benzylthio-5-trifluoromethyl benzoic acid (Taylor, 1973) 6,8-diethyl-5-hydroxyl-4-oxo-4H-1-benzopyran-2-carboxylic acid (Clark et al, 1982), fenoprofen (Culp, 1971), probenicid (Dayton et al, 1973) bucloxic acid (Gros et al, 1974), flurbiprofen (Risdall et al, 1978), diclofenac (Stierlin and Faigle, 1979), 6,7-dichloro-2-methyl-1-oxo-5-indanyloxy acetic acid (Zacchei et al, 1978), sultosilic acid (Wood et al, 1982) and etodolac (Ferdinandi, 1986). To date little comment has been made on this phenomenon. Once again the ability or inability to oxidise compounds by the cytochrome P-450 system is dependent on a charged group, the binding of which must be highly significant in the orientation of the chemical in the enzyme's active site. Another compound of acidic nature appearing in Figure 5 that the dog cannot oxidise, but is readily oxidised by other species is tolbutamide (Gee et al, 1984). The clearance of this drug is 0.2ml min^{-1}kg^{-1} in man and 0.1ml min^{-1}kg^{-1} in dog. It is interesting that recent work has shown that the cytochrome P-450 enzyme responsible for the hydroxylation of tolbutamide in man is S-mephenytoin 4-hydroxylase (P-450$_{MP}$) (Shimade et al, 1986; Knodell et al, 1986). Comparison of S-mephenytoin clearance in dog and man indicates that man clears the drug (67ml min^{-1}kg^{-1}) much faster than the dog (7ml min^{-1}kg^{-1}) suggesting that the comparable enzyme is absent or defective in the dog (Kupfer and Bircher, 1979; Wedlund et al, 1985). Similarly, the products of oxidation are different with the 4-hydroxy compound produced in man and the 3-hydroxy the major product in dog (Kupfer et al, 1982). Undoubtedly such an absence would explain the striking differences in the stereochemistry of the metabolites of the related compounds such as phenytoin (Maguire et al, 1978; Maguire et al, 1980), when dog and man are compared. As intriguing is if this enzyme, which demonstrates polymorphic behaviour in man, or a similar isoenzyme plays any part in the metabolism of the compounds listed above.

Further evidence for this being so has been recently reported. Tienilic acid is a phenoxyacetic acid derivative which is metabolised in man by oxidation of the thiophene ring to form the 5-hydroxy metabolite (Mansuy et al, 1984). The oxidation of this compound by man has been demonstrated to be catalysed by cytochrome P-450$_{MP}$ (cytochrome P-450-8) leading to the hydroxyl metabolite and also reactive metabolites which bind to the enzyme (Mansuy, 1986). Whilst the hydroxyl metabolite is formed in the rat as well as man, and up to 50% of the dose is excreted as this product in urine, the metabolite is not detected in the dog (Mansuy et al, 1984).

Other oxidation systems also are absent or at low levels in the dog compared to other species and influence the types of compound found in this group. The dog is deficient in the oxidation of phthalazine moieties catalysed by the enzyme aldehyde oxidase. In man this enzyme readily hydroxylates carbazeran (6,7-dimethoxy-1-[4-ethylcarbanoxyloxy]-piperidine). Man has a higher relative clearance than the dog, which relies on O-demethylase as the principal clearance mechanism (Kaye et al, 1984).

It is clear from the above that the enzymologist will play a major role in understanding pharmacokinetic differences across species. Similarly the structure in terms of the conformation and stereochemistry of drugs and their metabolites will be keys to help unlock the puzzle.

Figure 5.   Systemic clearance of various acidic drugs, normalised for body weight, in dog, expressed relative to man.

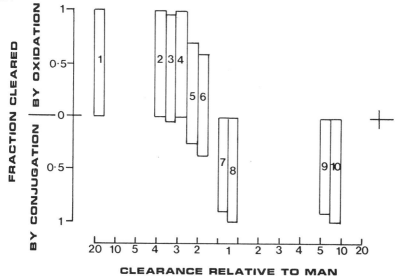

Proxicromil (1), ibuprofen (2), diclofenac (3), tolbutamide (4) are all cleared in man by oxidation whilst flurbiprofen (5) and naproxen (6) are cleared by a combination of oxidation and conjugation. Carprofen (7) diflunisal (8), indoprofen (9) and benoxaprofen (10) are cleared primarily by conjugation.

DRUGS CLEARED BY RENAL PROCESSES

Returning to Figure 1, a number of drugs appearing in the same cluster as those of high hepatic extraction are those cleared predominantly by renal or a combination of renal and biliary clearance. However, if the renally and renal/biliary cleared group of drugs is taken as a whole then considerable scatter appears in the data. Figure 6 illustrates the systemic clearance of nedocromil, probicromil, nadolol, atenolol, sodium cromoglycate, cefotetan, cefmetazole, cefoperazone, moxalactam, cefpiramide and cefazolin in the dog, rabbit, rat and mouse. Cefpiramide is an excellent example of the extremes of the values since the mouse clears the drug 150 fold faster than man. Reported clearance values being 41.5ml $min^{-1}kg^{-1}$ in the mouse and 0.277ml $min^{-1}kg^{-1}$ in man (Sawada et al, 1984).

The importance of drug protein binding in the drug clearance process is widely accepted. Comparison of the binding of drugs to human plasma and that of animal species indicates that mouse, rat and dog tend to have a higher free fraction relative to man (Figure 7). This trend applies particularly to acidic drugs. For instance the free fraction can be 15 to 30 fold greater in the mouse than man. For instance with the cephalosporin cefpiramide (Ma Sui et al, 1982) the free fraction in the mouse (0.56) is 15 fold greater than the free fraction in man (0.037).

Free drug clearance CL_f can be calculated by the equation

$$CL_f = CL_s/fu \qquad \dots\dots\dots (5)$$

where fu is the unbound fraction.

If the same group of drugs is now considered on the basis of their free drug clearance, rather than total drug clearance, a much closer correlation emerges. Figure 8 illustrates the comparison of free drug clearance in dog, rabbit, rat and mouse expressed relative to man. The relationships show a close correlation to organ flows as described for high hepatic extraction drugs. It can perhaps be used to advance the general rule that in the case of renally cleared drugs, correlation can be made with Q and fu. Protein binding effects are not limited to renal clearance processes. For many metabolically cleared drugs they may also be important. In Figure 4 valproic acid shows a 30 fold increase in clearance, between rat and man. Rat has a 7 fold greater free fraction, than man, thus the difference in free drug clearance is only 4 fold (Loscher, 1978). Similarly, the very large ratio for diazepam described earlier reflects to some extent protein binding. However, if CL_I is determined for unbound drug there is still a 65 fold difference (Igari et al, 1983).

CONCLUSIONS

The pharmacokinetics of drugs across a range of species and man has been considered. There is considerable species variation in intrinsic clearance reflecting the complexity of enzymic processes. In general animal species have a higher intrinsic liver clearance than man. The relative values reflect the individual mechanisms (partial intrinsic clearances) that make up the total, probably as a result of specific isoenzymes variation. In circumstances where intrinsic clearance exceeds blood flow (high extraction)

Figure 6.   Systemic clearance of various renally cleared drugs, normalised for bodyweight, in various species, expressed relative to man.

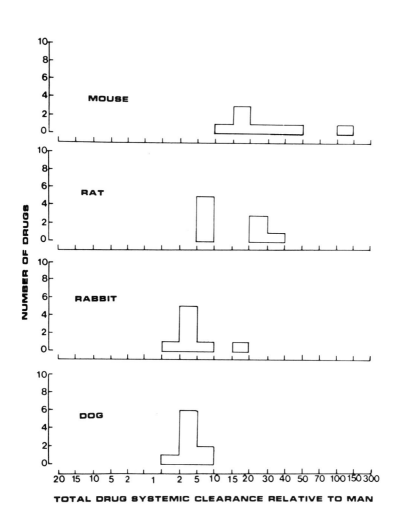

TOTAL DRUG SYSTEMIC CLEARANCE RELATIVE TO MAN

across the species, such differences are of little consequence in determining systemic clearance. In some cases CL_I intrinsic varies across species to such a degree that extraction varies from low to high, in others the drug is low extraction in all cases. To unravel the puzzle,

Figure 7. Protein binding of drugs in dog, rat and mouse
expressed relative to man. Acidic drugs are represented by
the hatched area of the graph, basic drugs by the clear
area.

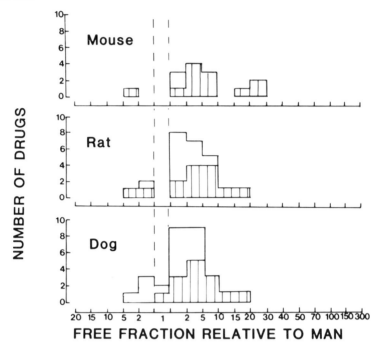

clearance data must be combined with metabolism data. Only
then will the understanding of species differences begin.
Unfortuantely much of the information published is not
suitable for these considerations. Metabolism data is
separated from pharmacokinetics. Often studies on
metabolism and pharmacokinetics are conducted at different
doses, similarly the primary metabolic clearance routes are
often not considered, only the endpoints of metabolite
pathways. If this paper serves to provoke interest in
integrating our experiments and publications then it will
have succeeded.

ACKNOWLEDGEMENTS

The author would like to acknowledge the encouragement
of his colleagues within the Safety Evaluation Group, in
particular Mrs. A. Stevens for the help in preparation and
typing of the manuscript.

Figure 8. Free drug systemic clearance of various cleared drugs, normalised for bodyweight, in various species, expressed relative to man.

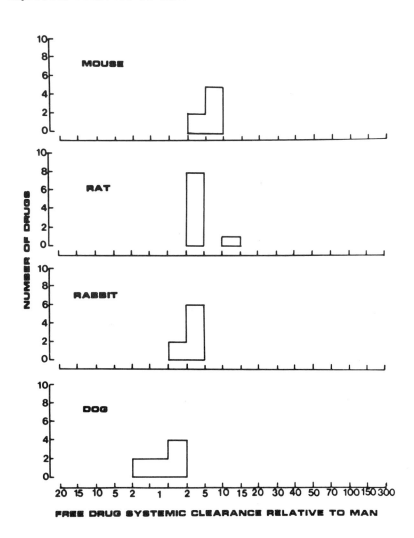

REFERENCES

Alkalay, D., Volk, J., Roth, W., Khemani, L. and Bartlett, F. (1979). J. Pharm. Sic, 68, 156.
Baselt, R.C. and Bickel, M.H. (1973). Biochem. Pharmacol, 22, 3117.
Clark, B., Smith, D.A., Eason, C.T. and Parke, D.V. (1982).

Xenobiotica, 12, 147.

Clark, B. and Smith, D.A. (1984). Crit. Rev. Toxicol, 12, 343.

Cook, C.S., Karim, A., Sollman, P. (1982). Drug. Met. Disp, 10, 116.

Culp, H.W. (1971). Fed. Proc, 30, 564.

Dayton, P.G., Perel, J.M., Cunningham, R.F., Israili, Z.H. and Weiner, I.M. (1973). Drug Met. Disp, 1, 742.

Dahlstrom, B.E., Paalzow, L.K., Lindberg, C. and Bogentoft, C. (1979). Drug Met. Disp, 7, 108.

Ferdinandi, E.S., Sehgal, S.N., Demerson, C.A., Dubuc, J., Zilber, J. Dornik, D. and Cayen, M.N. (1986). Xenobiotica, 16, 153.

Gabrielsson, J.L., Johansson, P., Bondesson, U. and Paalzow, L.K. (1975). J. Pharmacol. Biopharm, 13, 355.

Gee, S.J., Green, C.E. and Tyson, C.A. (1984). Drug Met. Disp, 12, 174.

Gerardy, B.M., Kapusta, D., Dumont, P. and Poupaert, J.H. (1986). Drug Met. Disp, 14, 477.

Gros, P.M., Dari, H.J., Chasseaud, L.F. and Hawkins, D.R. (1974). Arzneim-Forsch, 24, 1385.

Guengerich, F.P., Distelrath, L.M., Reilly, P.E.B., Wolff, T., Shimaga, T., Umbenhauer, D.R. and Martin, M.V. (1986). Xenobiotica, 16, 367.

Harashima, H., Sawada, Y., Sugiyama, Y., Iga, T. and Hanano, M. (1985). J. Pharmacokinet. Biopharm, 13, 425.

Hinderling, P.H. and Garrett, E.R. (1976). J. Pharm. Biopharm, 4, 199.

Igari, Y., Sugiyama, Y., Sawada, Y., Iga, T. and Hanano, M. (1983). J. Pharm. Biopharm, 11, 577.

Kamimura, H., Sasaki, H. and Kawamura, S. (1984). Xenobiotica, 14, 613.

Kamimura, H., Sasaki, H. and Kawamura, S. (1985). Xenobiotica, 15, 413.

Kaye, B., Offerman, J.L., Reid, J.L., Elliott, H.L. and Hillis, W.S. (1984). Xenobiotica, 14, 935.

Knodell, R.G., Hall, S.D., Wilkinson, G.R. and Guengerich, F.P. (1986). Fed. Proc, 44, 320.

Kupfer, A. and Bircher, J. (1979). J. Pharm. Exp, Therap, 209, 190.

Kupfer, A., James, R., Carr, K. and Branch, R. (1982). J. Chrom, 232, 93.

Loscher, W. (1978). J. Pharm. Exp. Therap, 204, 255.

Maguire, J.H., Butler, T.C. and Dudley, K.H. (1978). J. Med. Chem, 21 1294.

Maguire, J.H., Butler, T.C. and Dudley, K.H. (1980). Drug Met. Disp, 8, 325.

Mansuy, D., Dansette, P.M., Foures, C., Jaouen, M., Moinet,

G. and Bayer, N. (1984). Biochem. Pharmacol, 33, 1429.

Mansuy, D. (1987). This volume.

Matsui, H., Yano, K. and Okuda, T. (1982). Atnimicrob. Agents and Chemother, 22, 213.

Morino, A., Nakarmura, A., Nakanishi, K., Tatewaki, N. and Sugiyama, M. (1985). Xenobiotica, 15, 1033.

Nakashima, M., Masaharu, A., Sadao, O., Hashimoto, H., Seki, T., Miyazaki, M. and Takenaka, T. (1984). Clin. Pharm. Ther, 36, 436.

Oates, N.S., Shah, R.R., Idle, J.R. and Smith, R.L. (1983). Clin. Pharm. Ther, 34, 827.

Pond, S.M., Tong, T., Benowitz, N.L., Jacob, P. and Rigod, J. (1981). Clin. Pharm. Ther, 30, 183.

Rakhit, A., Holford, N.H.G., Guentert, T.W., Maloney, K. and Riegelman, S. (1984). J. Pharm. Biopharm, 12. 1.

Risdall, P.C., Adams, S.S., Crampton, E.L. and Marchant, B. (1978). Xenobiotica, 8, 691.

Sawada, Y., Hanano, M., Sugiyama, Y., and Iga, T. (1984). J. Pharmacokinet. Biopharm, 12, 241.

Shimada, T., Misono, M.S. and Guengerich, F.P. (1986). J. Biol. Chem. 261, 909.

Smith, D.A. and Neale, M.G. (1983). Eur. J. Drug Met. and Pharmacokinet, 8, 225.

Smith, D.A., Brown, K. and Neale, M.G> (1985). Drug Met. Disp, 16, 365.

Stierlin, H. and Faigle, J.W. (1979). Xenobiotica, 9, 611.

Taylor, J.A. (1973). Xenobiotica, 3, 151.

Wedlund, P.J., Asfanian, W.S., Jacqz, E., McCallister, C.B., Branch, R.A. and Wilkinson, G.R. (1985). J. Pharm. Exp. Therap, 234, 662.

Wood, S.G., Kirkpatrick, D., Jackson, A.J.S., Hawkins, D.R., Down, W.H., Chasseaud, L.F., Briggs, S.R. and Darragh, A. (1982). Xenobiotica, 12, 165.

Yeh, S.Y. (1982). Drug Met. Disp, 10, 319.

Yu, V.C., Lamirande, E., Horning, M.G. and Pang, K.S. (1982). Drug Met. Disp, 10, 568.

Zacchei, A.G., Wishousky, T.I. and Watson, L.S. (1978). Drug Met. Disp, 6, 313.

EXTRAPOLATION FROM MEASUREMENTS IN VITRO TO DRUG METABOLISM IN VIVO IN MAN

Alan R. Boobis, Stephen Murray, Christopher J. Speirs, Caroline E. Seddon, Gina C. Harries and Donald S. Davies.

Department of Clinical Pharmacology, Royal Postgraduate Medical School, Ducane Road, London. W12 OHS.

INTRODUCTION

The hepatic mixed function oxidase system plays a pivotal role in determining the magnitude and duration of effect of a wide variety of pharmacologically and toxicologically active xenobiotic compounds. Thus, these enzymes may be responsible for terminating the pharmacological effects of a drug such as phenobarbitone or phenytoin, they may activate otherwise innocuous compounds such as paracetamol and aflatoxin B_1 to toxic intermediates, or they may be responsible for or help maintain the pharmacological effects of some drugs such as cyclophosphamide and diazepam, by converting them to active metabolites. Hence, a knowledge of the fate of foreign compounds plays an important role in assessing the potential risk of new and established chemicals in man.

There are major differences in both the routes and rates of metabolism of foreign compounds amongst species. Thus, extrapolation from studies performed in animals to man is difficult and sometimes impossible. One solution is to conduct the studies in man, either directly or with human-derived tissue. In the latter case, the question then arises as to how valid any such in vitro investigations are to the situation in vivo.

GENERAL CONSIDERATIONS

Experiments in man, and with human-derived tissue, are subject to important ethical considerations. Although it is possible to study samples from certain tissues in healthy volunteers, these will be confined to those that can be readily obtained with the minimum of trauma, e.g. peripheral white cells, epidermal cells from the skin and epithelial cells from the buccal mucosa. The more adventurous investigator might be tempted to sample accessible solid tissues such as skeletal muscle and, on at least one occasion in the past (Rubin and Lieber, 1968), the liver itself. However, for the vast majority of investigators, virtually all such sampes will be surplus to tissue removed for diagnostic or palliative reasons. This will include hepatic and pulmonary tissues. There are circumstances where the biopsy samples taken subsequently transpire to be histologically normal, and these can then be used opportunistically to serve as "control samples". In recent years, an additional source of tissue for many groups has been the organ transplant donor, an otherwise healthy individual who has met a traumatic death and who is maintained on life support systems until such time as the removal of the relevant organs or transplantation.

There are several different levels of organisation at which in vitro studies of human drug metabolism can be conducted. These include purified enzyme systems, subcellular fractions, isolated cells in suspension of culture and cultured explants. Practical considerations on the application of each of these techniques will be found elsewhere in this volume.

Both quantitative and qualitative data can be obtained from studies in vitro that should be relevant to the situation in vivo. The effects of genetic, environmental, physiological and pathological factors can be investigated with careful planning and a degree of good fortune. The general purpose of any such study will fall into one of two categories. It may be predictive - what will happen when the investigation is, or in some cases if it could be, performed in vivo; confirmation - are the results in vitro supportive of the data already available from in vivo investigation.

In any such study, it must be borne in mind that there are serious limitations as to how far the in vitro approach can be taken, dependent upon factors such as inter- and intra-cellular architecture, organ-organ interactions, limited supplies of cofactors and nutrients in vivo, physiological control mechanisms, etc. Ultimately, it is almost always necessary to test any extrapolation in vivo. However, with these limitations in mind it should be possible to obtain answers to some of the following questions.

1. WHAT METABOLITE(S) WILL BE PRODUCED IN MAN?

It should be possible to obtain a preliminary answer to this question from studies performed in vitro with subcellular fractions or isolated cells from human liver. However, there are very few reports on any such studies performed in a prospective fashion. This might, in part, be due to the design of early studies of a new drug in man. The compound is very early administered in the radiolabelled form to enable bioavailability to be assessed, and at that time the major metabolites are often identified, based on the results of studies in animals. In addition, the low turnover of some compounds can make identification of metabolites produced in vitro extremely difficult. However, an example of the approach is seen in the metabolic fate of clonidine when incubated with microsomal fractions of human liver. One of the oxidised metabolites, 4-oxoclonidine, identified in that study (Hughes, 1980) was subsequently shown to be produced in vivo (Darda et al, 1978). In view of the complex, multiple, sequential routes of metabolism that occur with very many drugs, the use of isolated hepatocytes, with their full complement of drug metabolising enzymes, will probably be required for adequate metabolic profiling of the majority of compounds.

2. DOES A GIVEN PATHOPHYSIOLOGICAL FACTOR HAVE ANY EFFECT ON DRUG METABOLISM ACTIVITY?

The answer to this question is usually qualitative, or semi-quantitative at best. The development of liver banks containing large numbers of well-characterised samples has enabled the effects of a variety of such factors on drug metabolising activity to be investigated much more closely than in the past (von Bahr et al, 1980; Boobis et al, 1980; Kremers et al, 1981: Meier et al, 1983). The most widely studied of these factors, for obvious reasons, is liver disease. Generally, some measure of overall monooxygenase activity is obtained in vitro and compared with a similar measure in vivo, in almost all cases using different substrates in vivo and in vitro. However, in many instances, this is probably valid, in that the substrates selected are convenient for the type of study, and have been validated as representative for a large number of forms of cytochrome P-450. The substrates used in vitro include aminopyrine (Schoene et al, 1972), ethylmorphine (Farrell et al, 1979), and benzo(a)pyrene (Farrell et al, 1979; Brodie et al, 1981), whereas in vivo the most extensively studied compound is antipyrine (see Vesell, 1979).

As an example of this approach, the effects of severe extrahepatic obstructive jaundice were studied in vitro in liver biopsy samples from such patients (McPherson et al, 1982). Cytochrome P-450 content was substantially reduced (Table 1). In vivo, in the same patients, antipyrine elimination was severely impaired, more than in patients with cirrhosis (Table 1). Thus, the results in vivo confirmed the prediction from the in vitro data that such patients would have severely compromised monooxygenase activity.

Table 1. Effect of liver disease on hepatic cytochrome P-450 content and antipyrine half-life.

PATIENTS	CYTOCHROME P-450 CONTENT (nmol/mg)	ANTIPYRINE t 1/2 (h)
Controls	0.49 + 0.03 (n = 30)	10.4 + 0.4 (n = 12)
Hepatitis/ cirrhosis	0.23 + 0.03 (n = 13)	19.5 + 1.8 [*] (n = 17)
Obstructive jaundice	0.16 + 0.02 (n = 13)	28.3 + 8.0 (n = 16)

[*]   Data from Farrell et al (1979).
Data are modified from Brodie et al (1980) and McPherson et al (1981).

   Other factors that have been, or could be, investigated include race, age, renal disease, endocrine disturbances, malignant disease and sex. There are major differences in the oxidation of a number of substrates between male and female rats (Kato, 1974). It is not clear whether such differences extend to man. Certainly, for some substrates, there are no obvious differences in oxidation between the sexes in vitro (Figure 1). This is reflected in by a lack of any difference between the sexes in the oxidation of a number of drugs, with the exception of the 4-hydroxylation of antipyrine, the clearance of which tended to be greater in females than in males (Figure 2). This is largely in agreement with the findings of Teunessen et al (1982).

3.   IS THE METABOLISM OF A DRUG POLYMORPHIC?

   This question, like many of those listed here, can be

Figure 1. Comparison of hepatic microsomal monooxygenase
activities of biopsy samples from male and female patients.

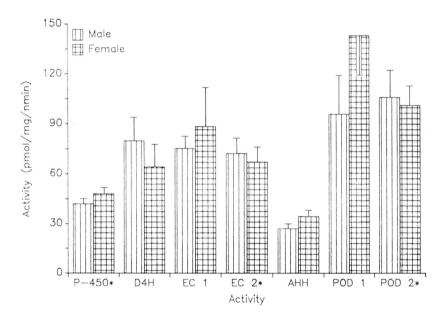

Values are mean±SEM (n > 8). The biopsy samples were all
histologically normal. Activities were determined as
reported elsewhere (Boobis et al, 1980; Boobis et al, 1981;
Kahn et al, 1982). Activities indicated by * have been
reduced by a factor of 10 for ease of plotting.
Abbreviations used are : P-450, cytochrome P-450 (specific
content expressed in pmol/mg); D4H, debrisoquine 4-
hydroxylase; EC 1 and EC 2, the high affinity and low
affinity components respectively of 7-ethoxycoumarin O-
deethylase; AHH, aryl hydrocarbon (benzo(a)pyrene)
hydroxylase; POD 1 and POD 2, the high affinity and low
affinity components respectively of phenacetin O-
deethylase.

answered in vitro only by the opportunistic acquisition of
appropriate liver samples. However, this has been achieved
by a number of groups and the impaired hydroxylation of
debrisoquine and related drugs (Davies et al, 1981; Meier
et al, 1983) and the impaired oxidation of mephenytoin
(Meier et al, 1985) have now been demonstrated in vitro,
thus confirming the involvement of specific isoenzymes of
cytochrome P-450 in such polymorphisms. This has enabled

Figure 2. Comparison of the clearance of drugs to their oxidative metabolites in male and female subjects.

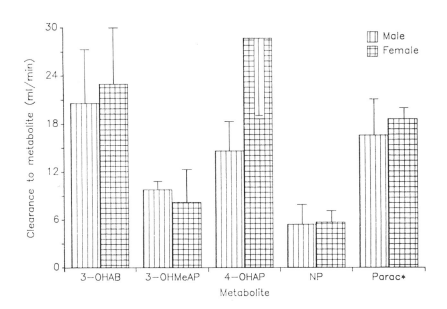

Values are mean±S.D. (n = 3). The method used have been described previously (Boobis et al, 1981; Kahn et al, 1985). The abbreviations used have been described previously (Boobis et al, 1981; Kahn et al, 1985). The abbreviations used are : 3-OHAB, 3-hydroxyamylobarbitone produced from amylobarbitone, 3-OHMeAP, 3-hydroxymethylantipyrine, 4-OHAP, 4-hydroxyantipyrine, NP, norphenazone, all produced from antipyrine; Parac, paracetamol produced from acetanilide.
* Activity has been reduced 20-fold for ease of plotting.

the metabolism of a number of other compounds to be assessed with respect to these polymorphisms, and the prediction that none of the major routes of oxidation of antipyrine would be polymorphic (Davies et al, 1981). This has been substantiated by observations in vivo (Eichelbaum et al, 1983).

An additional means of extrapolating from in vitro studies with respect to possible polymorphic hydroxylation can be achieved by determining the effects of quinidine on the oxidation of the substrate in question. Quinidine is a potent and selective inhibitor of the form of cytochrome P-

450 catalysing the 4-hydroxylation of debrisoquine (Otton et al, 1984). Thus, lack of inhibition by quinidine would strongly suggest that the drug is not oxidised by this form of cytochrome P-450. For example, the O-deethylation of phenacetin was not affected by low concentrations of quinidine (Table 2), and there is now good evidence that this reaction is catalysed by a different isozyme of cytochrome P-450 from that catalysing the 4-hydroxylation of debrisoquine (Kahn et al, 1985; Distlerath et al, 1985). Conversely, inhibition by quinidine would provide evidence that the drug might be polymorphically hydroxylated. For example, the 1'-hydroxylation of bufuralol is inhibited by very similar concentrations of quinidine to those required to inhibit the 4-hydroxylation of debrisoquine (Table 2).

Table 2. IC_{50} values for inhibition of monooxygenase activities by quinine and quinidine.

MONOOXYGENASE ACTIVITY	IC_{50} VALUE (μM)	
	Quinidine	Quinine
Bufuralol 1'-hydroxylase	0.7	> 500
Debrisoquine 4-hydroxylase	0.2	65
Phenacetin O-deethylase	500	120

Data are modified from Speirs et al (in press), where details of the methods used can be obtained.

4.   **WHAT PERCENTAGE OF THE DOSE WILL A GIVEN METABOLITE REPRESENT**

The answer to this question requires the estimation of the relative rates of formation of all competing metabolites. This will depend upon the kinetics of all parallel pathways and the involvement of any downstream reactions. Obviously, the model system used for such extrapolation must be dictated by the routes of metabolism of the compound. For example, soluble enzymes such as aldehyde dehydrogenase may play a major role in the disposition of the substrate and hence inclusion of the cytosolic fraction in the system would be essential.

A simple example of such extrapolation can be illustrated with antipyrine. This compound is metabolised almost exclusively by oxidation by the mixed function oxidases (Brodie et al, 1949). The only major downstream metabolites in vivo are conjugates, which can be hydrolysed to obtain an estimate of total oxidative products formed. From the kinetics of the oxidation of antipyrine to its three main oxidative metabolites, determined with microsomal fractions of human liver (Kahn et al, 1981), it can be predicted that the relative rates of formation of these metabolites in vivo should be 1.50: 1.37: 1.00 for 3-hydroxymethylantipyrine: 4-hydroxyantipyrine: norphenazone. This is in reasonably good agreement with the ratio of these metabolites excreted in urine in vivo which was 1.27: 2.35: 1.00 (Boobis et al, 1981).

5. WHAT IS THE RATE OF FORMATION OF A GIVEN METABOLITE IN VIVO?

Extrapolation from studies in vitro has considerable potential value in answering this question. The kinetics of formation of the metabolite must be determined, and certain essential assumptions concerning microsomal protein yield and total liver weight are necessary. The in vitro parameter of relevance, in the prediction of intrinsic clearance (Cli) to a metabolite, is provided by the ratio of Vmax to (Km+C.f) where C is the concentration of the substrate and f is the unbound fraction of this compound in vitro. This reduces to Vmax/Km when C is very much less than Km, the situation that one usually encounters in vivo when elimination is first order. In vivo, the relevant parameter is the intrinsic clearance to metabolite, Cli (M), which is determined from the following equation, assuming the venous equilibration or well-stirred model (Pang and Rowland, 1977).

$$Cli \ (M) \ = \ (F.M)/(AUCo.f)$$

where M represents the fraction of the dose excreted as the metabolite, F is the fraction of the dose absorbed, AUCo is the area under the plasma concentration - time curve of the parent drug following an oral dose and f is the free fraction of the parent drug. This last parameter is of some importance as the processes responsible for the Cli are dependent upon only the free concentration of the substrate, requiring that this is either known or can be determined, both in vivo and in vitro. Although the former is almost always known, the latter is rarely measured, and may be difficult to determine experimentally. However, accurate prediction of Cli in vivo requires that f is known.

    Studies of this nature have been performed with several
compounds, including antipyrine, paracetamol, bufuralol and
phenacetin. To validate the approach, the kinetics of the
drug should be studied in vivo and in vitro in the same
subjects. This is obviously very difficult in most cases,
and there are only very few instances where such studies
have been performed. It has been possible to investigate
the oxidation of antipyrine in this way (Boobis et al,
1981a). There was very good agreement between the
activities determined in vitro and those observed in vivo
on the same patients (Boobis et al, 1981a).
    Generally, the kinetics of the drug are estimated in a
number of liver samples, often from a liver bank, and
compared with the results of a parallel study performed in
vivo in a number of healthy volunteers. When this approach
was adopted for the oxidation of paracetamol and antipyrine
there was excellent agreement between the results of the in
vivo and in vitro measurements (Table 3). There was
usually less than 2-fold difference between the estimates
of Cli. Neither drug is highly protein bound, so that it
is not necessary to estimate f, the free fraction. One
additional caveat is the quality of the liver. The studies
in vivo are performed in healthy young subjects, whereas
the studies in vitro are performed with liver samples from
patients or organ transplant donors. It is therefore
unlikely that the two studies will be exactly comparable.
    Studies in vitro on the 1'-hydroxylation of bufuralol
serve to illustrate several additional points regarding
this approach. Like many drugs, bufuralol is optically
active so the kinetics of oxidation of both isomers were
determined with human liver samples (Boobis et al, 1985).
At high concentrations of the isomers, oxidation of the
(+)-isomer proceeds at approximately 3-fold the rate of
that of the (-)-isomer. However, when the Km values were
determined, it was apparent that there is a 3-fold
difference in affinities, but in this instance the (-)-
isomer has the better affinity. Thus, the magnitude of Cli
of each isomer by 1'-hydroxylation should be approximately
the same at low substrate concentrations (Table 4). At
higher concentrations one might expect that the (+)-isomer
would be metabolised more rapidly than the (-)-isomer, in
the racemate. However, additional experiments (Boobis et
al, 1985) indicate that the two isomers are substrates for
the same form of cytochrome P-450, and as such will compete
with each other for metabolism. Thus, it can be predicted
that the ratio of (+) to (-)1'hydroxybufuralol in vivo
should be close to 1.00, unless further metabolism is
stereoselective.

Table 3. Comparison of intrinsic clearance of drugs by oxidation estimated in vitro with the values determined in vivo.

REACTION	Km (mM)	Vmax (nmol/mg/ min)	C* (µM)	Cli (in vitro) (ml/min)	Cli (in vivo) (ml/min)
Antipyrine 3-methyl- hydroxylase	9.0	0.60	<0.1	3.72	7.6
Antipyrine 4- hydroxylase	7.3	0.57	<0.1	4.44	14.1
Antipyrine N- demethylase	5.9	0.34	<0.1	3.24	6.0
Paracetamol oxidation	0.95	0.17	<0.2	10.5	26.5

* Estimated maximum concentration of substrate in hepatic cytosol. The methods used have been published elsewhere (Boobis et al, 1981; Seddon et al, in press).

Table 4.   1'Hydroxylation of the isomers of bufuralol.

ISOMER	Vmax (pmol/mg/min)	Km (µM)	Vmax/Km (µl/min/mg)
(+) Bufuralol	153.0	18.7	8.2
(-) Bufuralol	52.0	6.4	8.1

Details of the methods used will be found in Boobis et al, (1985).

7.   DOES ACUTE OR CHRONIC ADMINISTRATION OF A DRUG HAVE ANY EFFECT ON METABOLISM : I.E. IS THERE ANY INDUCTION OR INHIBITION?

The answer to this question may be qualitative, semi-quantitative or quantitative, depending upon the approach adopted. Examples include the inhibitory effect of cimetidine but not of ranitidine in vitro (Knodell et al, 1982) and the inducing properties of phenobarbitone (Remmer et al, 1973), confirming the observations made in vivo. A good example of the ability to extrapolate successfully from in vitro studies of this type to the in vivo situation can be found with the effects of quinidine on the 4-hydroxylation of debrisoquine. Quinidine is an extremely potent and selective inhibitor of this reaction catalysed by microsomal fractions of human liver (Speirs et al, in press). The Ki for quinidine is less than 0.2μM (Otton et al, 1984; Leemann et al, 1986). Although it is not possible to estimate the true hepatic concentration of quinidine, it is known that the peak venous plasma concentration following an oral dose of 300mg is 3μM (Guentert et al, 1979). The hepatic concentration of the drug during absorption must be at least as high as this. Again, it is not possible to estimate the hepatic concentration of debrisoquine directly. However, the peak plasma concentration following an oral dose of 10mg is only 0.09μM (Silas et al, 1978; 1980). As the Km for 4-hydroxylase activity is 125μM (Boobis et al, 1983), it seems very likely that the hepatic concentration following an oral dose of 1mg will be very much less than this. As a consequence, the degree of inhibition of 4-hydroxylase activity will depend only upon the concentration of the inhibitor achieved. Hence, the concentration of quinidine required to produce 70% inhibition, assuming a value for Ki of 0.2μM, would be 0.5μM. If one assumes that the absorption of quinidine is first order, this corresponds to a dose of 50mg. When this dose of quinidine was administered together with 1mg debrisoquine, there was a dramatic increase in the metabolic ratio for debrisoquine in all 8 subjects tested, from a mean value of 1.6 to a mean value of 17.7, implying that there was indeed profound inhibition of the relevant pathway in vivo (Speirs et al, in press).

In a study such as that described above, the experiments can be designed specifically to investigated the variable in question. However, the effects of factors such as cigarette smoking can be compared only in liver samples obtained from smokers and non-smokers, and not on the same samples before and after exposure to the inducing agent. Nevertheless, useful extrapolations can be achieved. For example, it was determined from studies in vitro (Boobis and Davies, 1984) that exposure to anticonvulsant drugs results in the induction of human hepatic epoxide hydrolase. It was thus predicted that the enzymatic hydrolysis of epoxides should be increased in vivo in patients treated chronically with anticonvulsants. This does indeed appear to be the case, at least for the epoxide metabolite of carbemazepine, with increased production of the dihydrodiol metabolite (Eichelbaum et al, 1985).

A further example of extrapolation from measurements in vitro is found in the prediction that some inducing compounds will show selectivity in their effects, as is well known for laboratory animals. For example, the low affinity component of the 0-deethylation of 7-ethoxycoumarin is selectively increased in biopsy samples from patients receiving anticonvulsants, whereas only the high affinity component of this activity is increased in biopsies from cigarette smokers (Table 6). Such differential induction is borne out by the effects of cigarette smoking and rifampicin on the oxidation of phenacetin and antipyrine in vivo (Boobis and Davie, 1984). The 0-deethylation of phenacetin is induced more by cigarette smoking, whereas the oxidation of antipyrine is more affected by rifampicin.

Table 6. Effects of exposure to inducing compounds on the O-deethylation of 7-ethoxycoumarin in vitro.

| SUBJECTS | 7-ETHOXYCOUMARIN O-DEETHYLASE ACTIVITY[*] | |
	High affinity component	Low affinity Component
Non-smokers (16)	60 ± 12	598 ± 79
Smokers (10)	96 ± 17[**]	625 ± 53
Anticonvulsants (non-smoker) (1)	76	1010
Anticonvulsants (smoker) (1)	92	1240

[*] Activities are expressed in pmol/mg/min
[**] $P < 0.05$; smokers versus non-smokers
Activity was determined as previously described (Boobis et al, 1981).

8. IS THE METABOLIC ACTIVATION OF A COMPOUND LIKELY TO POSE ANY RISK TO MAN?

Studies in vitro can provide a valuable interface

between the metabolism and the toxicity of foreign compounds in man. Thus, it is possible to explore the relevance of metabolic activation, particularly where such activation has already been demonstrated to have toxicological significance in animals. In many instances, it is possible only to obtain some estimate of likely, or even possible, hazard from such studies, without any prospect of performing parallel studies *in vivo*. For example, the activation and genotoxicity of aflatoxin B_1 can be readily investigated *in vivo*, with subcellular fractions from human tissues (Plummer et al, 1986), but it will probably never be possible to test directly whether any prediction from such studies is correct, because the compound cannot be administered to man.

In rare circumstances, such comparisons are possible. For example, paracetamol is hepatotoxic only after an overdose. The metabolism and toxicity of paracetamol can be investigated *in vitro* and the results of such studies suggest that man should be relatively resistance to the toxic effects of this compound (Table 7) (Boobis *et al*, in press). The clearance of paracetamol by oxidation can readily be measured in volunteers, and such data show that man is indeed poor at catalysing the conversion of paracetamol to its reactive intermediate (Table 7) (Boobis *et al*, in press). Close scrutiny of the clinical data (Prescott, 1983) would support the suggestion that in most people the dose of paracetamol required to cause liver necrosis is much higher than is believed by some (British National Formulary, 1983).

One further extrapolation from *in vitro* studies remains to be evaluated. A number of heteroaromatic amines, including pyrolysis products of amino acids formed on heating certain foods, are extremely potent mutagens when activated by human liver (Figure 3) (Harries *et al*, in press). Thus, if these compounds are demonstrated to be genotoxic in animals, and there is evidence that at least some of them are (Vuolo and Schuessler, 1985), then this would be cause for concern regarding their role in the aetiology of cancer in man.

CONCLUSIONS

Studies *in vitro* will never replace those *in vivo*. However, they can provide an extremely useful adjunct to such investigations, help to develop testable hypotheses, and confirm suspicions from investigations *in vivo*. There are limitations to the approach, some of them serious, so that is is always necessary to maintain an awareness of the

Figure 3. Relative potency of mutagens in the Ames test with microsomal fractions of human liver as the activating system.

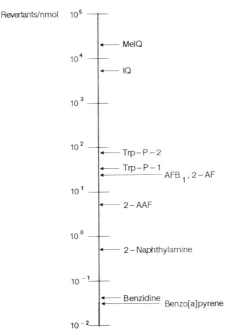

Mutagenicity was determined with S.typhimurium TA98 as previously described (Harries et al, 1986). The abbreviations used are : MeIQ, IQ, Trp-P-1, Trp-P-2, amino acid pyrolysis products; AFB_1, aflatoxin B_1; 2-AF, 2-aminofluorene; 2-AAF, 2-acetylaminofluorene.

confines of the system. Nevertheless, this still provides ample opportunity to utilise an increasingly widely validated approach, which still has considerable potential to be realised in this field.

ACKNOWLEDGEMENTS

The data presented in this chapter are the results, in part, of a program of research into causes of variability of drug oxidation in man, that has been ongoing in our laboratory over the past six years. Many people have been involved in the work, and we wish to extend our thanks and appreciation to them. In particular, we are indebted to M.J. Brodie, G.C. Kahn, E-L Toverud and L.B.G. Tee.

Table 7.   Species differences in the activation and
toxicity of paracetamol.

SPECIES	INTRINSIC CLEARANCE TO GSH ADDUCT IN VITRO (µl/min/mg)	IN VIVO CLEARANCE TO MERCAP- TURATE (ml/min/kg)	TOXICITY IN HEPATOCYTES (EC50, mM)
Rat	0.185	0.378	> 50
Hamster	-	-	3.50
Mouse	2.009	3.418	10.1
Human	0.121	0.205	> 50

Modified from Boobis et al (in press).

We also wish to thank the Professor and staff of the Department of Surgery, Royal Postgraduate Medical School, for their invaluable cooperation in making human liver samples available to us for the use in many of the studies reported here.

We wish to acknowledge the generosity of the pharmaceutical companies who provided many of the substrates and standards that enabled much of the work to be performed.

Finally, but by no means least, we are extremely grateful to those sources of financial support without whom the work could not have been performed. In particular, we would like to acknowledge the support of the Medical Research Council, the Wellcome Trust and the Health and Safety Executive.

REFERENCES

Boobis, A.R. and Davies, D.S. (1984). Xenobiotica, 14, 151.
Boobis, A.R., Brodie, M.J., Kahn, G.C. and Davies, D.S. (1980a). in "Microsomes, Drug Oxidations and Chemical Carcinogenesis", Vol II (Ed. by Coon, M.J., Conney, A.H., Estabrook, R.W., Gelboin, H.V., Gillette, J.R. and O'Brien, P.J). Academic Press, New York, 957.
Boobis, A.R., Brodie, M.J., Kahn, G.C., Fletcher, D.R., Saunders, J.H. and Davies, D.S. (1980b). Br. J. Clin. Pharmac, 9, 11.
Boobis, A.R., Brodie, M.J., Kahn, G.C., Toverud, E.-L.,

Blair, I.A., Murray, S. and Davies, D.S. (1981a). Br. J. Clin. Pharmac, 12, 771.

Boobis, A.R., Kahn, G.C., Whyte, C., Brodie, M.J. and Davies, D.S. (1981b). Biochem. Pharmac, 30, 2451.

Boobis, A.R., Murray, S., Hampden, C.E. and Davies, D.S. (1985). Biochem. Pharmac, 34, 65.

Boobis, A.R., Murray, A., Kahn, G.C., Robertz, G.-M. and Davies, D.S. (1983). Mol. Pharmac, 23, 474.

Boobis, A.R., Tee, L.B.G., Hampden, C.E. and Davies, D.S. (in press). Food Chem. Toxic.

British National Formulary (1983). BMA and Pharmaceutical Society of Great Britain, No. 5, p.29.

Brodie, B.B. Axelrod, J., Soberman, R. and Levy, B.B. (1949). J. Biol. Chem, 179, 25.

Brodie, M.J., Boobis, A.R., Bulpitt, C.J. and Davies, D.S. (1981). Eur. J. Clin. Pharmac, 20, 39.

Danhof, M. and Breimer, D.D. (1979). Br. J. Clin. Pharmac, 8, 529.

Darda, S., Forster, H.J. and Stahle, H. (1978). Arzneim. Forsch, 28, 255.

Davies, D.S., Kahn, G.C., Murray, S., Brodie, M.J. and Boobis, A.R. (1981). Br. J. Clin. Pharmac, 11, 89.

Distlerath, L.M., Reilly, P.E.B., Martin, M.V., Davis, G.C., Wilkinson, G.R. and Guengerich, F.P. (1985). J. Biol. Chem, 260, 9057.

Eichelbaum, M., Bertilsson, L. and Sawe, J. (1983). Br. J. Clin. Pharmac, 15, 317.

Eichelbaum, M., Tomson, T., Tybring, G. and Bertilsonn, L. (1985). Clin. Pharmacokinet, 10, 80.

Farrell, G.C., Cooksley, W.G.E. and Powell, L.W. (1979). Clin. Pharmac. Ther, 26, 483.

Guentert, T.W., Holford, N.H.G., Coates, P.E., Upton, R.A. and Reigelman, S. (1979). Pharmacokinet. Biopharm, 7, 315.

Harries, G.C., Boobis, A.R., Collier, N. and Davies, D.S. (1986). Human Toxic, 5, 21.

Harries, G.C., Boobis, A.R., Sesardic, D., Edwards, R.J. and Davies, D.S. (in press). Food Chem. Toxic.

Hughes, H. (1980). PhD Thesis, University of London.

Inaba, T., Mahon, W.A. and Stone, R.M. (1979). Int. J. Clin. Pharmac. Biopharm, 8, 371.

Kahn, G.C., Boobis, A.R., Blair, I.A., Brodie, M.J. and Davies, D.S. (1981). Anal. Biochem, 113, 292.

Kahn, G.C., Boobis, A.R., Brodie, M.J., Toverud, E.-L., Murrary, S. and Davies, D.S. (1985). Br. J. Clin. Pharmac, 30, 67.

Kahn, G.C., Boobis, A.R., Murray, S., Brodie, M.J. and Davies, D.S. (1982). Br. J. Clin. Pharmac, 13, 637.

Kato, R. (1974). Drug Metab. Rev, 3, 1.

Knodell, R.G., Holtzman, J.L., Crankshaw, D.L., Steele, N.M. and Stanley, L.N. (1982). Gastroenterol, 82, 84.

Kremers, P., Beaune, P., Cresteil, T., De Graeve, J., Columelli, S., Leroux, J.-P. and Gielen, J.E. (1981). Eur. J. Biochem, 118, 599.

Leemann, T., Dayer, P. and Meyer, U.A. (1986). Eur. J. Clin. Pharmac, 29, 739.

McPherson, G.A.D., Benjamin, I.S., Boobis, A.R., Brodie, M.J., Hampden, C. and Blumgart, L.H. (1982). Gut, 23, 734.

Meier, P.J., Mueller, H.K., Dick, B. and Meyer, U.A. (1983).Gastroenterol, 83, 682.

Meier, U.T., Dayer, P., Male, J.-P., Kronbach, T. and Meyer, U.A. (1985). Clin. Pharmac. Ther, 38, 488.

Otton, S.V., Inaba, T. and Kalow, W. (1984). Life Sci, 34, 73.

Pang, K.S. and Rowland, M. (1977). J. Pharmacokinet. Biopharm, 5, 625.

Plummer, S., Boobis, A.R. and Davies, D.S. (1986). Arch. Toxic, 58, 165.

Prescott, L.F. (1983). Drugs, 25, 290.

Remmer, H., Schoene, B. and Fleischmann, R.A. (1973). Drug Metab Dispos. 1, 224.

Rubin, E. and Leiber, C.S. (1968). Science, 162, 690.

Schoene, B., Fleischmann, R.A., Remmer, H. and von Oldershausen, H.F. (1972). Eur. J. Clin. Pharmac, 4, 65.

Seddon, C.E., Boobis, A.R. and Davies, D.S. (in press). Arch. Toxic.

Silas, J.H., Lennard, M.S., Tucker, G.T., Smith, A.J., Malcolm, S.L. and Marten, T.R. (1978). Br. J. Clin. Pharmac, 5, 27.

Silas, J.H., Tucker, G.T., Smith, A.J. and Fieller, N.R.J. (1980). Br. J. Clin. Pharmac, 9, 419.

Speirs, C.J., Murray, S., Boobis, A.R., Seddon, C.E. and Davies, D.S. (in press). Br. J. Clin. Pharmac.

Teunissen, M.W.E., Srivastava, A.K. and Breimer, D.D. (1982). Clin. Pharmac. Ther, 32, 240.

Vesell, E.S. (1979). Clin. Pharmac. Ther, 26, 275.

Von Bahr, C., Groth, C.-G., Jansson, H., Lundgren, G., Lind, M. and Glaumann, H. (1980). Clin. Pharmac. Ther, 27, 711.

Vuolo, L.L. and Schuessler, G.J. (1985). Environ. Mutagen, 7, 577.

7. Biological models for metabolism.

THE USE OF STRUCTURE-ACTIVITY RELATIONSHIPS

David F.V. Lewis[1] , Tim J.B. Gray and Brian G. Lake

BIBRA, Woodmansterne Road, Carshalton, Surrey, SM5 4DS and
[1]Department of Biochemistry, University of Surrey,
Guildford, Surrey, GU2 5XH, England.

INTRODUCTION

It has long been realised that relationships exist between aspects of the chemical structure or physical properties of compounds and their observed effects in biological systems. The study of structure-activity relationships is an attempt to correlate chemical or physical criteria with biological activity. The relationships obtained may be either quantitative or purely qualitative in nature. In this paper we will focus on a few examples of the present and possible future applications of structure-activity relationships in studies of xenobiotic metabolism and toxicology. For more extensive treatments of structure-activity relationships the reader is referred to the excellent publications of Golberg (1983) and ECETOX (1986). Some uses of structure-activity relationships are shown in Table 1 and some examples are discussed below.

Table 1. Some Uses of Structure-Activity Relationships

---

1. Elucidation of the nature of receptor or enzyme binding sites (e.g. determination of critical features of substrates, inhibitors, inducers etc).
2. For an established series the prediction of effects of new members.
3. Determination of the critical features responsible for the effects of a series of compounds.
4. Prediction of metabolic pathways.
5. Prediction of toxicity

CYTOCHROME P-450 STRUCTURAL FEATURES AND INDUCTION

Many studies have shown that multiple forms of cytochrome P-450 exist in the endoplasmic reticulum of liver and other tissues from a variety of species (Guengerich et al, 1982; Ryan et al, 1982). Furthermore, many compounds have been shown to induce rodent hepatic microsomal cytochrome P-450 and whilst there appears to be many types of inducer, two major classes are the drug type (e.g. phenobarbitone) and polycyclic hydrocarbon type (e.g. 20-methylcholanthrene, β-naphthoflavone) enzyme inducers (Nebert et al, 1981; Ryan et al, 1982). The major forms of cytochrome P-450 induced by these two classes of enzyme inducers are known to have different catalytic properties and inhibitor sensitivities. By comparing the molecular geometries of specific substrates, inhibitors and inducers of these two major forms of cytochrome P-450, Lewis et al, (1986) were able to obtain information on the nature of the substrate binding sites of the enzymes. In general, compounds that were substrates, inhibitors or inducers of cytochrome P-448 (i.e. the form induced by polycyclic hydrocarbons) were found to be relatively planar molecules, characterised by a small depth and a large area/depth ratio (Table 2). Conversely, cytochrome P-450 substrates, inhibitors and inducers were relatively bulky, non-planar molecules, characterised by small area/depth ratios and a greater flexibility in molecular conformation. Possibly this type of analysis could be extended to other forms of cytochrome P-450 and hopefully to predict which form(s) of cytochrome P-450 would be likely to be involved in the metabolism of novel compounds.

A number of studies have attempted to derive structure activity relationships for the induction of mixed function odixase enzyme activities (Arcos et al, 1961; Denomme et al, 1986; Fujita et al, 1984; Sage et al, 1985). In early work with a series of polycyclic aromatic hydrocarbons, Arcos et al (1961) attempted to correlate molecular size (measured as the incumbrance area) with induction of azo dye demethylase activity in rat liver. These authors found that in order to induce enzyme activity an optimal molecular size of 85-150 $Å^2$ was required, with compounds having greater or smaller incumbrance areas being essentially inactive. However, this was not an absolute structure activity relationship as several compounds whose incumbrance areas fell within the critical range were also inactive.

It is now known that the mechanisms of induction of cytochrome P-448 by polycyclic hydrocarbon type inducers

Table 2. Relationship between Xenobiotic Molecular Geometry
and Specificity for Cytochrome P-450 or P-448.

CYTOCHROME SPECIFICITY	COMPOUND	AREA/DEPTH RATIO (A)[a]
Cytochrome P-450	Aldrin	10.0
	Ethylmorphine	14.4
	Metyrapone	13.6
	Phenobarbitone	11.2
Cytochrome P-448	Benzo(a)pyrene	38.3
	Dibenz(a,h)anthracene	46.2
	Ellipticine	32.3
	7-Ethoxyresorufin	34.1

[a] For details see Lewis et al, (1986).

involves an interaction with a cytosolic receptor protein
termed the Ah receptor (Nebert et al, 1981). Studies on
the interaction of xenobiotics with the cytosolic Ah
receptor protein have demonstrated that polycyclic
hydrocarbon type inducers exhibit higher binding affinities
than non polycyclic hydrocarbon type inducers (Bandiera et
al, 1982). Furthermore, quantitative structure-activity
relationships (QSARs) have been demonstrated for various
polychlorinated biphenyls and 4'-substituted-2,3,4,5-
tetrachlorobiphenyls between their binding to the cytosolic
receptor of rat liver and induction of enzyme activity
(aryl hydrocarbon hydroxylase and 7-ethoxyresorufin O-
deethylase) in a rat hepatoma cell line (Bandiera et al,
1983; Safe et al, 1985). Molecular geometry, expressed as
area/depth ratio (Lewis et al, 1986), is obviously an
important factor in both receptor binding and enzyme
induction as illustrated in Figure 1 for a series of
polychlorinated biphenyls.

Knowledge of the structural features required for the
binding of halogenated aromatic hydrocarbons to the
cytosolic receptor is important because of the known
relationship between receptor binding, enzyme induction and
toxicity of certain of these compounds. This is
illustrated for 2,3,7,8-tetrachlorodibenzo-p-dioxin (TCDD)
and some related compounds in Table 3 where toxicity
(thymic atrophy) is only a property of compounds which

Table 3. The relationship between thymic atrophy, Ah receptor binding and enzyme induction for some halogenated aromatic hydrocarbons.

Compound	Dose (moles/kg)	C57BL/6J MICE		CHICK EMBRYO
		Relative thymus wt. (% control)	Relative binding affinity	Relative induction of AHH
	3×10^{-7}	39	(100)	(100)
	3×10^{-7}	54	37	67
	1×10^{-6}	97	INACTIVE	INACTIVE
	1×10^{-6}	95		

Data taken from Poland et al (1976) and Poland and Glover (1980).

Figure 1. Relationships between cytosolic receptor binding (A) and enzyme induction (B) with molecular geometries of a series of polychlorinated biphenyls.

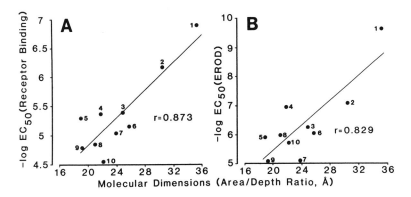

The receptor binding and enzyme induction (7-ethoxyresorufin O-deethylase : EROD) data were taken from Safe et al, (1985) and the molecular geometries were calculated according to Lewis et al, (1986). The polychlorinated biphenyls employed were :
1) 3,3',4,4',5-penta,   2) 3,3',4,4'-tetra,
3) 2,3,4,4',5-penta,   4) 2,3,3',4,4'-penta
5) 2,3,3',4,4',5'-hexa,   6) 2,3,3',4,4',5-hexa,
7) 2,3',4,4',5-penta,   8) 2',3,4,4',5-penta
9) 2,3',4,4',5,5'-hexa   10) 2,3,4,4'-tetra.

interact with the cytosolic receptor and induce enzyme activities.

QUANTITATIVE STRUCTURE-ACTIVITY RELATIONSHIPS (QSARs)

Any QSAR has three components :
i)   The biological activity determined.
ii) The chemical structure descriptors employed (i.e. the data on the physical or chemical properties of the molecules).
iii) The technique used to establish the relationship.
   The biological activity can be almost any measure of effect (e.g. enzyme induction, receptor binding, LD_{50}) and may be derived from both in vivo and in vitro systems. A wide variety of chemical structure descriptors can be employed, some of which are listed in Table 4, ranging from simple criteria such as hydrophobicity (e.g. Hansch values) through to more complex electronic structural

Table 4.   Some chemical structure descriptors.

A. Physico-chemical descriptors

     I.   General - melting and boiling points, pKa values
     II.   Hydrophobicity - partition coefficients, Hansch
            π values
     III.   Electronic - Hammett constant (σ), H-bonding
     IV.   Quantum chemical (including electronic struc-
            tural parameters derived from molecular orbital
            calculations) - atomic charge, dipole moment,
            electron density, frontier orbital electron
            densities, electrophilic and nucleophilic super-
            delocalizabilities.

B. Steric
     -      Molecular volume, shape and surface area, Taft
            steric substituent constant (Es).

C. Structural
     -      Atom and bond fragments, number of atoms or
            rings

---

parameters derived from molecular orbital calculations
(e.g. the MINDO/3 method of Bingham et al, 1975).
     The techniques used to establish the QSAR can range
from simple graphical plots through to computer derived
equations produced by multiple linear regression analysis.
A typical QSAR equation is shown below :

     F (BA)   = ax1 + bx2 + cx3 ....+k

where, F (BA) = a function of the biological activity;
       x1, x2 etc = the chemical structure descriptors;
       a,b etc   = numercial coefficients obtained by
                      regression analysis
       k   = a constant.

     At first sight QSARs appear to be a most valuable tool
for many areas of biological research and product
development. Having established a QSAR for a "training
set" of compounds the relationship derived may be used to
predict the biological activity of additional untested
compounds. This could produce enormous savings in, for

example, the cost of toxicity screening and result in a marked reduction in the use of experimental animals. However, for a number of reasons great caution should be exercised in the use of QSARs. For example, the equations derived will obviously reflect the quality of the biological data employed. This point is particularly important where the biological data is derived from several sources and hence may have been subjected to both methodological and inter-laboratory variations. Obviously the use of poor and inaccurate biological data can in no way be compensated for by sophisticated computer analysis. Similarly, the choise of chemical structure descriptors to derive the QSAR is also important in that they should be appropriate for the biological activity being studied. Furthermore, care should be taken to ensure that the chemical structure descriptors employed in the equation are not inter-related, lest an invalid relationship be obtained. Other factors which may result in spurious relationships include statistical considerations such as the number of compounds used and the number of chemical structure descriptors required for the equation, the delibrate exclusion of outliers from the QSAR and the "clustering" of compounds into distinct groups (see ECETOC, 1986).

PREDICTION OF METABOLIC PATHWAYS

The ability to predict accurately the likely metabolic pathways of novel compounds would clearly be of use in the development of new drugs, pesticides, industrial chemicals etc. One such computer technique to predict metabolism has been developed (Wipke et al, 1983) and as the program is mechanistically based rather than route memory based it is not limited to molecules whose metabolism is known. Possibly the future development of this and other programs will permit the prediction of likely major and minor metabolic pathways and also species differences in metabolism.

PREDICTION OF TOXICITY

One essentially qualitative method employing structure activity considerations to predict toxicity is the "Decision Tree Approach" devised by Cramer et al (1978). This procedure was introduced to attempt to rank food additives and contaminants into different classes based on their probable toxic hazard assessment.

Toxicity may also be estimated on a quantitative basis

by employing QSAR techniques. However, as discussed above, QSARs are best devised employing clearly defined biological endpoints and thus data from in vivo toxicity studies, where many factors (e.g. metabolism, pharmacokinetics) can affect toxicity, may not be suitable. On the other hand useful QSARs have been derived from simpler systems, for example, Konemann (1981) established a QSAR linking aquatic toxicity with partition coefficient for a series of organic compounds of low chemical reactivity.

In our laboratory we have been interested in the usefulness of primary hepatocyte cultures as an in vitro test system (Gray et al, 1983) to screen compounds for potential to produce hepatic peroxisome proliferation in rodents. By measuring the induction of peroxisomal enzyme activities in rat hepatocyte cultures we have been able to derive QSARs linking compound potencies with electronic structural parameters obtained by molecular orbital calculations for both a series of closely related phthalate monoesters (Lake et al, 1986a) and a series of structurally more diverse peroxisome proliferators (Lake et al, 1986b). Hopefully these studies will find application both in the screening of novel compounds and possibly in the elucidation of the mechanism(s) of initiation of peroxisome proliferation in rodent liver.

CONCLUSIONS

The study of structure-activity relationships can be of great use both for the screening of novel compounds and in the elucidation of biochemical mechanisms. Hopefully, as the methods employed continue to develop, more accurate and predictive techniques will evolve. With respect to the application of QSAR techniques in toxicology the future is best summed up in the words of Leon Golberg. "A concerted effort is needed, on the part of all of us, to produce the necessary information - from unpublished sources as well as new systematic approaches - that will permit QSAR studies in toxicology to flourish as never before. Then, and only then, will the application of QSAR assume its rightful place in the hierarchy of hazard evaluation" (Golberg, 1983).

REFERENCES

Arcos, J.C., Conney, A.H. and Buu-Hoi, N.P. (1961). J. Biol. Chem, 236, 1291.
Bandiera, S., Safe, S. and Okey, A.B. (1982). Chem-Biol. Interact, 38, 259.

Bandiera, S., Sawywe, T.W., Campbell, M.A., Fujita, T. and
    Safe, S. (1983). Biochem. Pharmacol, 32, 3803.
Bingham, R.C., Dewar, M.J.S. and Lo, D.H. (1975). J. Am.
    Chem. Soc, 97, 1285.
Cramer, G.M., Ford, R.A. and Hall, R.L. (1978). Food
    Cosmet. Toxicol, 16, 255.
Denomme, M.A., Homonko, K., Fujita, T., Sawyer, T. and
    Safe, S. (1986). Chem-Biol. Interact, 57, 175.
ECETOX (1986). "Structure-activity relationships in
    toxicology and ectoxicology : an assessment" (Ed.
    Tumer, L). ECETOX Monographs No. 8, Brussels.
Fujita, S., Suzuki, M., Peisach, J. and Suzuki, T. (1984).
    Chem. Biol. Interact, 52, 15.
Golberg, L. (1983). in "Structure-activity correlation as a
    predictive tool in toxicology : fundamentals, methods
    and applications" (Ed. Golberg, L). Hemisphere
    Publishing Corporation, Washington.
Gray, T.J.B., Lake, B.G., Beamand, J.A., Foster, J.R. and
    Gangolli, S.D. (1983) Toxicol. Appl. Pharmacol, 67, 15.
Guengerich, F.P., Dannan, G.A., Wright, S.T., Martin, M.V.
    and Kaminsky, L.S. (1982). Xenobiotica, 12, 701.
Konemann, H. (1981). Toxicology, 19, 209.
Lake, B.G., Lewis, D.F.V., Gray, T.J.B., Beamans, J.A.,
    Hodder, K.D., Purchase, R. and Gangolli, S.D. (1986a).
    Arch. Toxicol. Suppl, 9, 386.
Lake, B.G., Lewis, D.F.V., Gray, T.J.B., Hodder, K.D.,
    Beamans, J.A. and Gangolli, S.D. (1986b). Toxicologist,
    6, 113.
Lewis, D.F.V., Ioannides, C. and Parke, D.V. (1986).
    Biochem. Pharmacol, 35, 2179.
Nebert, D.W., Eisen, H.J., Negishi, M., Lang, M.A.,
    Hjelmeland, L.M. and Okey, A.B. (1981). Ann. Rev.
    Pharmacol. Toxicol, 21, 431.
Phillips, J.C., Purchase, R., Watts, P. and Gangolli, S.D.
    (1986). Toxicologist 6, 213.
Phillips, J.C., Purchase, R., Watts, P. and Gangolli, S.D.
    (1987). Food Add. Contam, in press.
Poland, A. and Glover, E. (1980). Mol. Pharmacol, 17, 86.
Poland, A., Glover, E. and Kende, A.S. (1986). J. Biol.
    Chem, 251, 4936.
Ryan, D.E., Thomas, P.E., Reik, L.M. and Levin, W. (1982).
    Xenobiotica, 12, 727.
Safe, S., Bandiera, S., Sawyer, T., Zmudzka, B., Mason, G.,
    Romkes, M., Denomme, M.A., Sparling, J., Okey, A.B. and
    Fujita, T. (1986). Environ. Hlth. Perspec, 61, 21.
Wipke, W.R., Ouchi, G.I. and Chou, J.T. (1983). in
    "Structure-activity correlation as a predictive tool in
    toxicology : fundamentals, methods and applications"

(Ed. Golberg, L). Hemisphere Publishing Corp, Washington, p. 151.

PURIFIED ENZYMES AS BIOLOGICAL MODELS FOR DRUG METABOLISM

G. Gordon Gibson

University of Surrey, Department of Biochemistry, Division
of Pharmacology and Toxicology, Guildford, Surrey, GU2 5XH.
England.

INTRODUCTION

Drug metabolism may be studied at different levels of
biological organisation including the use of whole animals,
organ perfusion systems, tissue slices, cell culture,
tissue homogenates including sub-cellular fractions,
purified enzymes and more recently recombinant DNA
technology and molecular biology. Each of these systems
has its own distinct advantages and disadvantages and the
interested reader is referred to the contribution by Dr.
Peter Moldeus in this volume on the comparison of model
systems for metabolism.

The purpose of this chapter is to focus on the use of
purified enzyme systems in answering particular questions
in drug metabolism and the utility of purified drug
metabolising enzymes will be considered from four
viewpoints. Firstly, to provide information on **FUNDAMENTAL
ASPECTS** of structure activity relationships as seen in the
X-ray crystal structure of a soluble cytochrome P-450 and
the developing area of enzyme engineering using
oligonucleotide-driven site-directed mutagenesis. Secondly, to provide a rational input to **DRUG DESIGN** by
computer simulation of the enzyme active site and, thirdly
to **RATIONALISE** sex and species differences, genetic
polymorphisms and the broad substrate specificity of the
enzymes of drug metabolism. Finally, consideration will be
given to the **DISADVANTAGES** of solely using the above
information, particularly with respect to those factors
that confound even a complete knowledge of the complement
of drug metabolising enzymes in an organism.

FUNDAMENTAL ASPECTS

In order to study the fundamental aspects of the drug-
metabolising enzymes, it is clear that a homogeneous

preparation of the pure enzyme is necessary and this
objective has focussed the minds of protein biochemists
over the past twenty years. This intensive effort has
resulted in the isolation and characterisation of the major
drug metabolising enzymes (Table 1), the structural
features now being validated for many of the enzymes by
recombinant cDNA studies (Nebert, 1985; Phillips et al,
1985; Whitlock, 1986).

Clearly the most definitive structural information on
any enzyme is the X-ray crystal structure and to date this
has been achieved for only one xenobiotic-metabolising
enzyme, the soluble cytochrome P-450$_{cam}$ derived from
Pseudomonas putida (Poulos et al, 1985). Analysis of this
enzyme has yielded a wealth of structural information
including the overall 3-dimensional topography, location
and orientation of the haem prosthetic group, the nature of
the axial haem ligands, the substrate binding site, the
substrate access channel and mechanistic aspects. Although
this structural information is of immense value, it should
be noted that there are many structural and functional
differences between cytochrome P-450$_{cam}$ and the membrane-
bound drug-metabolising cytochrome P-450's and caution must
be exerted in extrapolation between the two systems. There
is therefore a clear need for similar information on the
membranous haemoproteins, although this represents a very
large technical problem in view of the fact that membrane-
bound enzymes are inherently difficult to crystalise for
subsequent analysis. It should also be emphasised that the
3-dimensional configuration of cytochrome P-450 in a
membrane or soluble form may not be identical to that in a
packed crystal.

Purified enzymes have also contributed to an
understanding of how particular amino acid residues in the
enzyme are important in binding either cofactors or the
substrate. A knowledge of the primary amino acid sequence
of a puriied protein then allows protein engineering to be
accomplished by the technique of site directed mutagenesis
with synthetic oligonucleotides (Figure 1). In this
technique, the nucleotide sequence coding for a particular
enzyme can be changed by chemical synthesis of an
oligonucleotide sequence complementary to part of a single-
stranded DNA template that codes for the enzyme. This
oligonucleotide contains a delibrate mismatch (either
single or multiple), an insertion or deletion (Carter,
1986; Walker, 1985). For example, the oligonucleotide may
contain the single mis-match of CGT instead of CAT,
resulting in the ultimate synthesis of a protein that has
an arginine residue instead of a histidine. The catalytic

Table 1. Drug Metabolising Enzymes That Have Been Purified and Characterised

ENZYME	CHARACTERISTICS	REFERENCES
Cytochrome P-450	Exhibits mixed function oxidase, NADPH-oxidase and peroxidase activities; exists as multiple forms	Capdevila et al, 1984 Guengerich, 1982
Microsomal flavin-containing monooxygenase	Also known as Ziegler's enzyme and catalyses N- and S-oxygenation	Ziegler and Poulson, 1978
Prostaglandin synthetase	hydroperoxide component catalyses co-oxidation of drugs during metabolism of PGG2 to PGH2	Hemler et al, 1976; Ohki et al, 1979
Epoxide hydrolase	Catalyses the formation of dihydrodiols from epoxides and exists as multiple forms	Lu and Mawa 1980; Wixtrom and Hammock, 1985
Glucuronyl transferase	Catalyses the conjunction of UDP-glucuronic acid with several functional groups; exists as multiple forms	Burchell, 1981 Zakim et al, 1985
Glutathione S-transferase	Catalyses the condensation of glutathione with electrophilic substrates; multiple forms exist	Boyer and Kenney, 1985 Ketterer, 1986
Sulphotransferase	Catalyses the conjunction of activated inorganic sulphate with phenols, alcohols and hydroxylamines, multiple forms exist.	Jakoby et al, 1984 Singer, 1985

Figure 1.   Site-directed mutagenesis using synthetic
oligonucleotides.

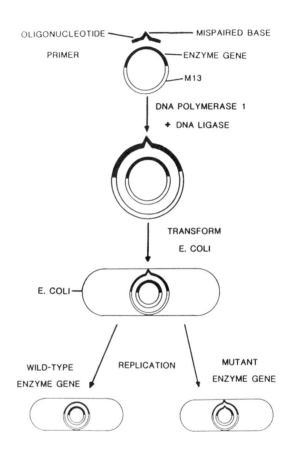

Derived from Walker (1985), with permission.

activities of the native and mutant enzymes are then
compared to evaluate the role of specific amino acid
residues in enzyme function, and this approach has been
taken in the study of β-lactamase (Sigal et al, 1984),
dihydrofolate reductase (Villafranca et al, 1983), lac
permease (Padan et al, 1985) and tyrosyl tRNA synthetase
(Wilkinson et al, 1984).
     A discussion of the site-directed mutagenesis of β-
lactamase highlights the above concepts. This enzyme

hydrolyses the amide bond of penicillins and cepha-
losporins thus inactivating the antibiotic, and therefore
constitutes a mechanism of resistance to this class of
drugs. In the class A family of β -lactamases SER-70 has
been identified as an active site nucleophile, forming an
acyl-enzyme intermediate, important for the catalytic
activity. Using the technique of site-directed
mutagenesis, the SER-70 codon (AGC) was changed to TGC,
resulting in the single substitution of cysteine for serine
(Sigal et al, 1984). The resultant thio-substituted β-
lactamase hydrolyses β-lactam antibiotics with a substrate
specificity that is distinct from the wild type enzyme
(Table 2).

Table 2. **Hydrolysis of β-Lactam Antibiotics by Wild Type
and Mutated β-Lactamase.**

SUBSTRATE	K_m (mM)		k_{cat} (S^{-1})	
	MUTANT	WILD TYPE	MUTANT	WILD TYPE
Benzylpenicillin	0.06	0.05	20	1700
Ampicillin	0.12	0.05	50	2000
Cephaloridine	1.80	1.00	2	1700
Nitrocefin	>2.50	0.11	>400	900

Derived from Sigal et al (1984).

Although the above stategy has not been applied to the
more extensively studied drug metabolising enzymes, the
technology is clearly applicable to this system and the
next few years should see substantial progress in this
area. Of particular value would be the possibility of
increasing/decreasing catalytic activity, altering
substrate specificity and the fusion of enzymes that form a
functional complex (e.g. NADPH-cytochrome P-450 reductase
and cytochrome P-450).

DRUG DESIGN

It has long been the objective of the pharmaceutical
industry to rationally design new drugs and the use of
purified drug metabolising enzymes has an important role to
play in this area of drug research. One very obvious

therapeutic target is the cytochrome P-450 isoenzyme involved in the conversion of androgens to oestrogens, the so-called cytochrome P-450 aromatase. This enzyme is a therapeutic target for anti-cancer drugs, particularly the aromatase inhibitors that are successfully used in the treatment of oestrogen-dependent breast tumours, or other clinical problems associated with oestrogens (Santen et al, 1981). Therefore information on the active site of the aromatase would be of immense value in synthesising specific aromatase inhibitors. This is clearly an achievable target as all the information to date indicates that the aromatase has a different substrate specificity from the other cytochrome P-450 isoenzymes characterised thus far (Tan and Muto, 1986).

The aromatase has been purified to electrophoretic homogeneity from human placenta (Tan and Muto, 1986) and a cloned cDNA has been isolated from a human placental cDNA library in the bacteriophage expression vector λgt11 (Evans et al, 1986). In this latter study, the cDNA clone harbouring the aromatase insert was determined to be 1.8kb in length, sufficiently long to code for the aromatase enzyme. Sequencing of this cDNA will rapidly yield the predicted amino acid sequence of the enzyme and hence facilitate the deduction of the secondary structure by the use of computer-derived graphical modelling. Once this has been achieved, the design of aromatase inhibitors will surely rapidly advance and clearly shows the advantage of this approach over the more traditional structure-activity approaches.

RATIONALISATION OF FACTORS AFFECTING DRUG METABOLISM

Drug biotransformation studies have indicated that many of the enzymes involved have a broad substrate specificity and may exist as multiple forms or isoenzymes. This has been unequivocally established in recent years by the isolation and characterisation of many of these multiple forms (c.f. Table 1 and this volume). Isolation of purified enzymes has allowed the sequencing of these proteins and has shown that sub-families of a given enzyme exist. This has been of advantage in the cytochrome P-450 group of enzymes, where very small differences in amino acid sequences have been noted, resulting in the characterisation of closely-related proteins with different substrate specificities. For example, cytochrome $P-450_b$ and cytochrome $P-450_e$ belong to the pheno-barbital-inducible family and are immunochemically indistinguishable (Vlasuk et al, 1982), primarily because they share 97% sequence homology (Yuan et al, 1983). The primary amino acid sequence differences were observed (in part) in the hypervariable region of genomic exon 7 in residues 344 to 339 as :

P-450$_b$ --- SER - HIS - ARG - LEU - PRO - THR ----
P-450$_e$ --- SER - HIS - ARG - PRO - PRO - SER ----

            334   339

Knowing these differences, synthetic oligonucleotide probes encoding the above different sequences have been synthesised (Omiecinski et al, 1985) and used as probes in hybridisation experiments to determine the differential inductive influence of phenobarbital on their corresponding mRNAs. Clearly then the use of purified enzyme structural information has made a significant impact on the regulation of closely-related isoenzyme forms.

Sex differences in drug metabolism have been documented in experimental animals, particularly the rat (Gustafsson, 1983) and many attempts have been made to rationalise this phenomenon. In view of the existence of multiple forms of drug-metabolising enzymes, it would appear logical that this sexual dimorphism may well be explained in terms of male and female specific isoforms. Protein purification experiments have shown that this is indeed the case, the male rat exhibiting high levels of cytochrome P-450-dependent testosterone 16α-hydroxylase (termed P-450$_{2c}$, 16α or RLM$_5$) (Cheng and Schenkman, 1982; Morgan and MacGeoch, 1985), the enzyme being virtually non-existant in the female. Similarly, a cytochrome P-450 isoenzyme has been purified and characterised from female rat liver and has been shown to be present at a high level in the female, but undetectable in the male (MacGeoch et al, 1984). Thus the purified enzyme data has enabled subsequent analysis of the regulation and expression of these sex-dependent cytochromes P-450 and highlighted the importance of the hypothalamo-pituitary-liver axis in controlling drug metabolism.

Purified enzymes also have an important role to play in rationalising species differences in drug metabolism particularly in the study of human drug metabolism. For example, genetic polymorphisms can make a major contribution to inter-individual variations in drug responsiveness for those drugs whose overall clearance from the body is metabolism-related (Eichelbaum, 1982). Accordingly, an understanding of the human complement of drug metabolising enzymes is of major importance, but there are generally several problems associated with access to large amounts of human tissue for enzyme purification experiments. Therefore an alternative approach has been taken whereby purified enzymes from an appropriate animal model have been obtained, antibodies raised to these enzymes and small samples of human tissue probed with this antibody. A good example of this approach is the characterisation of the human liver cytochrome P-450 isoenzyme responsible for debrisoquine hydroxylation, a reaction that is deficient or substantially reduced in approximately 10% of the Caucasian population. Recent work has reported the purification of a cytochrome P-450 with high debrisoquine hydroxylase activity from the rat and antibodies raised to this enzyme used as a probe in human liver (Distelrath and Guengerich, 1984). This work has shown a significant correlation between human debrisoquine hydroxylase activity and immunoquantitation of the relevant cytochrome P-450 in samples from 44 patients.

The above type of approach has, to date, been used in a retrospective phenotyping mode and the much more intractable problem of prospective typing using purified enzymes or derived antibodies has yet to be successfully applied. In this context it should be pointed out that in vivo assessment of pharmacogenetic polymorphisms clearly presents much less of a problem that the purified enzyme approach (Idle and Smith, 1979).

Purified enzymes and their corresponding antibodies can play several varied and important roles including the rapidly expanding application of molecular biology approaches to drug metabolism studies. For example, cDNA libraries of various tissues can be derived, in one method, by immunoprecipitation of polysomes carrying the required mRNA of interest and therefore constitutes a very useful "clean-up" stage prior to cDNA synthesis by reverse transcriptase. During this clean-up stage, in vitro translations of the semi-purified mRNA's are usually undertaken with subsequent immunoprecipitation of the translated products to ascertain if the message is actually there. Purified enzymes are of great value here to ensure that the immunoprecipitate contains the correct protein corresponding to the appropriate molecular weight of the standard, pure enzyme.

A tremendous stimulus to gene cloning technology has been the ability to screen cDNA libraries for a particular cDNA of interest by using fusion protein vector systems such as bacteriophage λ gt11 (Young and Davis, 1983). This technique depends on an antibody to the enzyme in question and is used to probe clones harbouring the cDNA of interest. Additionally when this procedure has been used successfully to isolate full length cDNA clones, it is of obvious value to ascertain that the correct cDNA has been isolated. This can be achieved in one of several ways including direct comparison of the predicted primary amino acid structure from the cDNA with the authentic sequence obtained by the more traditional method of protein sequencing of the pure protein. The nature of the cDNA can also be ascertained by hybrid arrest or release experiments both of which require pure enzyme for molecular weight validation.

Finally, pure proteins are very useful in constructing the corresponding oligonucleotide probes, which have been successfully used to assess the influence of phenobarbital on cytochrome P-450 mRNA levels in solution hybridisation and Northern blotting experiments (Omiecinski et al, 1985).

DISADVANTAGES OF PURIFIED ENZYMES

The foregoing discussion has centred on the utility of purified enzymes in drug metabolism studies but it should be emphasised that although tremendous advances in our understanding of enzyme structure and function has been gained by such an approach, purified enzymes are only one piece in the jigsaw puzzle. For example, the study of isolated enzyme systems does not take into account several important factors such as the physiological interplay and control exerted between tissues including hormonal factors, supply of oxygen (if necessary for the reaction) and the availability of competition for cofactors.

For membrane-bound drug metabolising enzymes, there are clearly several differences between the membrane environment and the purified enzyme in solution, and these differences may have a profound impact on the catalytic properties of the enzyme. The "latency" of the microsomal UDP-glucuronyltransferases is a good example of this difference where detergents or other membrane disruptants are necessary to fully express activity, whereas they are not necessary when the transferase has been isolated in a soluble, purified form (Dutton, 1980).

Similarly, in the cytochrome P-450 system, the membrane environment plays an important role in controlling both the qualitative and quantitative oxidation of drugs. The organisation and reactivity of cytochrome P-450 in membranes is dependent on the specific organisation with its associated flavo-protein reductase, membrane lipids and cytochrome b_5. All of these latter components can, of course, be isolated and reconstituted into a functional complex, but it is clear there is no guarantee that reconstitution of the above components will accurately mimic the membrane organisation of the complex. A good example of this is that even the simple alteration of the order of addition of the components in a reconstituted system can substantially influence cytochrome P-450 activity (Gorsky and Coon, 1986).

   As shown in Figure 2, information gained from studies on purified enzymes may not be totally representative of the <u>in vivo</u> situation because of the ability of several drug metabolising enzymes to participate in other pathways of intermediary metabolism, not reflected in limited reconstitution experiments.

Figure 2.   Competing Pathways for the Drug Metabolising Enzymes.

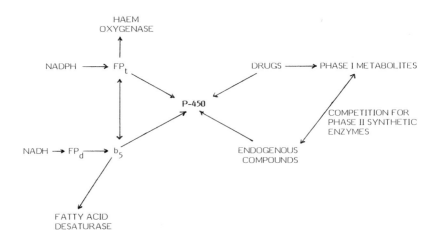

   For example the flow of reducing equivalents through NADPH-cytochrome P-450 reductase to cytochrome P-450 may be diverted during periods of active haem breakdown via haem oxygenase. Similarly, the influence of cytochrome b_5 on cytochrome P-450 reactions may be tempered by the concomitant demand for cytochrome b_5-derived reducing equivalents in fatty acid desaturation.

CONCLUSIONS

The case for purified enzymes in drug metabolism studies is a very substantial one and the science has made tremendous steps forward due to this approach. However, the information gained in these studies must not be considered in isolation and full recognition must be made of the complexities of sub-cellular, tissue and inter-tissue factors that have equally a profound impact on drug metabolism.

REFERENCES

Boyer, T.D. and Kenney, W.C. (1985) in "Biochemical Pharmacology and Toxicology, Volume 1, Methodological Aspects of Drug metabolising Enzymes" (Ed. by D. Zakim and D.A. Vessey), Wiley, New York, p.297.
Burchell, B. (1981). in "Reviews in Biochemical Toxicology" (Hodgson et al, eds), Elsevier, Amsterdam, 1.
Capdevila, J., Saeki, Y. and Falck, J.R. (1984). Xenobiotica, 14, 105.
Carter, P. (1986). Biochem, J, 237, 1.
Cheng, K.C. and Schenkman, J.B. (1982). J. Biol. Chem, 257, 2378.
Distelrath, L.M. and Guengerich, F.P. (1984). Proc. Nat. Acad. Sci (USA), 81, 7348.
Dutton, G.J. (1980). "Glucuronidation of Drugs and Other Compounds", CRC Press, Florida.
Eichelbaum, M. (1982). Clin. Pharmacol, 7, 1.
Evans, C.T., Ledesma, D.B., Schuls, T.Z., Simpson, E.R. and Mendelson, C.R. (1986). Proc. Nat. Acad. Sci (USA), 83, 6387.
Gorsky, L.D. and Coon, M.J. (1986) Drug Metab. Disp, 14, 89.
Guengerich, F.P. (1982). in "Principles and Methods of Toxicology" (Ed. by Hayes, A.W). Raven Press, New York. p.609.
Gustafsson, J.A. (1983). Ann. Rev. Physiol, 45, 51.
Hemler, M.E., Smith, W.L. and Lands, W.E.M. (1976). J. Biol. Chem, 251, 5575.
Idle, J.R. and Smith, R.L. (1979) Drug Metab. Rev, 9, 301.
Jakoby, W.B., Duffel, D.W., Lyon, E.S. and Ramaswamy, S. (1984). in "Progress in Drug Metabolism" (Ed. by Bridges, J.W. and Chasseaud, L.F). Taylor and Francis, London, p.11.
Ketterer, B. (1986). Xenobiotica, 16 957.
Lu, A.Y.H. and Miwa, G.T. (1980). Ann. Rev. Pharmacol, 20,

513.

MacGeoch, C., Morgan, E.T., Halpert, J. and Gustafsson, J.A. (1984). J. Biol. Chem, 259, 15433.

Morgan, E.T. and MacGeoch, C. (1985). Mol. Pharmacol, 27, 471.

Nebert, D.W. (1985). in "Drug Metabolism. Molecular Approaches and Pharmacological Implications" (Ed. by G. Siest), Pergamon Press, Oxford, p..85.

Ohki, S., Ogino, N.,.Yamamoto, S. and Hayaishi, O. (1979). J. Biol. Chem, 254, 829.

Omiecinski, C.J., Waltz, F.G. and Vlasuk, G.P. (1985). J. Biol. Chem. 260, 3247.

Padan, E., Sarkar, H.K., Viitanen, P.V., Poonian, M.S. and Kalback, H.R. (1985). Proc. Nat. Acad. Sci (USA), 82, 6765.

Phillips, A.R., Shephard, E.A., Rabin, B.R., Ashworth, A., Bayney, R.M. and Peeke, S.F. (1985). in "Drug Metabolism. Molecular Approaches and Pharmacological Implications" (Ed. by G. Siest), Pergamon Press, Oxford, p.93.

Poulos, T.L., Finzell, B.C., Gunsalus, I.C., Wagner, G.C. and Kraut, J. (1985). J. Biol. Chem, 260, 16122.

Santen, R.J., Worgul, T.J., Samojlik, E., Interrante, A., Boucher, A.E., Lipton, A., Harvey, H.A., White, D.S., Smart, E., Cox, C. and Wells, S.S. (1981). New England. J. Med. 305, 545.

Sigal, I.S., De Grado, W.F., Thomas, B.J. and Petteway, S.R. (1984). J. Biol. Chem, 259, 5327.

Singer, S.S. (1985). in "Biochemical Pharmacology and Toxicology, Vol 1. Methodological aspects of Drug Metabolising Enzymes" (Ed. D. Zakim and D.A. Vessey), Wiley, New York, p.95.

Tan, L. and Muto, N. (1986). Eur. J. Biochem, 156, 243.

Villafranca, J.E., Howell, E.E., Voet, D.H., Strobel, M.S., Ogden, R.C., Abelsen, J.N. and Kraut, J. (1983). Science, 222, 782.

Vlasuk, G.P., Ghrayeb, J. Ryan, D.E., Reik, L., Thomas, P.E., Levin, W. and Waltz, F.G. (1982) Biochem, 21, 789.

Walker, J.M. (1985). in "Molecular Biology and Biotechnology" (Ed. Walker, J.M. and Gingold, E.B). Royal Society of Chemistry, London, p.325.

Whitlock, J.P. (1986) Ann. Rev. Pharmacol. Toxicol, 26, 333.

Wilkinson, A.J., Fersht, A.R., Blow, D.M., Carter, P. and Winter, G. (1984). Nature, 307, 187.

Wixtrom, R.N. and Hammock, B.D. (1985). in "Biochemical Pharmacology and Toxicology, vol 1. Methodological

Aspects of Drug Metabolising Enzymes" (Ed. by D. Zakim and D.A. Vessey). Wiley, New York, p.1.

Young, R.A. and Davis, R.W. (1983). Science, 222, 778.

Yuan, P.M., Ryan, D.E., Levin, W. and Shively, J.E. (1983.). Proc. Nat. Acad. Sci (USA), 80, 1169.

Zakim, D., Hochman, Y. and Vessey, D.A. (1985). in "Biochemical Pharmacology and Toxicology, vol 1. Methodological Aspects of Drug Metabolising Enzymes" (Ed. D. Zakim and D.A. Vessey). Wiley, New York, p.161.

Ziegler, D.M. and Poulson, L.L. (1978). Method. Enzymol, 52, 142.

INTACT CELLS AS A BIOLOGICAL MODEL FOR METABOLISM

Diane J. Benford

Robens Institute of Industrial and Environmental Health and Safety, University of Surrey, Guildford, Surrey. GU2 5XH. UK.

INTRODUCTION

With the current trend of reducing laboratory animal experimentation for both ethical and financial reasons there is increasing interest in alternative models for studying drug metabolism. Table 1 lists the available models which are also reviewed elsewhere in this volume (Moldeus). As these models increase in distance from man, the amount of data which can be generated from a single preparation is increased. Intact cells are more easily characterised and therefore more reproducible than organ cultures or tissue slices. Compared with the lower models the normal spacial distribution of enzymes and cofactors is maintained, thereby permitting complete metabolic pathways to be followed and producing rates of metabolism which correspond more closely to those observed in the whole organ or animal.

Table 1. Models for drug metabolism studies

1.	Man
2.	Whole animal
3.	Perfused organ
4.	Tissue slices/organ culture
5.	Isolated cells/cultured cells
6.	Subcellular fractions
7.	Purified enzymes
8.	Quantitative structure activity relationships

FACTORS AFFECTING METABOLISM

A frequent criticism of studies in intact cells is the

interlaboratory variation. This is most probably due to inadequate characterisation of the cell preparations or to differences in incubation conditions used. Some viability indices which may be used for hepatocytes are listed in Table 2. The yield quoted here represents 60 to 80% of the maximum, thus lower yields may represent selection of a minority population. Trypan blue exclusion and lactate dehydrogenase (LDH) leakage are the most commonly used but they are relatively insensitive measures of gross damage. Whilst it is not practicable for all these parameters to be routinely determined, they provide useful guidelines for workers new to hepatocyte isolation. With other species and cell types such parameters are much less well documented. However, for interspecies or intertissue comparisons it is essential to have equivalent quality preparations.

Table 2. Viability indices for rat hepatocytes

Yield[a]	$6 - 8 \times 10^7$/g liver
Trypan blue exclusion[a]	>90%
LDH leakage[a]	<10%
Glutathione[a]	50 nmol/10^6 cells
ATP[b]	25 nmol/10^6 cells
02 consumption[b]	25 nmol/min/10^6 cells
Cytochrome P-450[a]	0.3nmol/10^6 cells
7 ethoxycoumarin 0- deethylase[a]	0.2nmol/min/10^6 cells
Gluconeogenesis[c]	17 nmol/min/10^6 cells
Urea synthesis[c]	32 nmol/min/10^6 cells

[a]Typical values obtained in my laboratory with hepatocytes isolated from male Wistar rats (200-250g) by the method described in Benford and Hubbard (1987).

[b]Derived from Cornell (1983). [c]Derived from Goethals et al, 1984).

   Changes in metabolism caused by pretreatment of animals are beyond the scope of this text but incubation conditions may also have considerable effects on rates of metabolism, particularly with conjugating enzymes which are dependent upon an exogenous supply of cofactors or precursors. Glutathione may be depleted during hepatocyte isolation

and, dependent upon incubation conditions, will either be
resynthesised or further depleted (Hogberg and
Kristofferson, 1977). Glutathione itself is not taken up
by hepatocytes and cysteine maybe toxic therefore
methionine must be added to the medium to promote
glutathione synthesis. This is not however true for all
cell types as renal cells can utilise exogenous glutathione
(Orrenius et al, 1983). Sulphation is dependent upon an
exogenous supply of inorganic sulphate (Sundheimer and
Brendel, 1984) and, like glucuronidation, is limited by low
levels of ATP (Wiebkin et al, 1979). The availability of
NADPH may also become limiting for glucuronic acid
synthesis and conjugation (and to a lesser extent for
cytochrome P450 dependent oxidation) in hepatocytes from
fasted animals. This is avoided by addition of lactate or
glucose to the medium (Smith and Orrenius, 1984). Tissue
culture media are often used to circumvent these problems
but the majority of these contain phenol red which, as a
substrate for glucuronyltransferase may also be a
competitive inhibitor.

Another factor which may alter rates of metabolism is
the serum or albumin added to maintain cell viability which
may bind certain substrates. Most substrates are obviously
relatively lipophilic and can only be introduced into the
cell suspension in an organic solvent. High solvent
concentrations may be toxic to the cells and will inhibit
or activate various enzymes and should therefore be
restricted to 0.5% or less. The oxygen tension is also
critical. Carbogen (5% CO_2 : 95% O_2) is often used to
maintain cell viability but this may promote lipid
peroxidation in untreated cells and decrease rates of
reductive metabolism (Stacey et al, 1982). Conversely
insufficient oxygen will result in cell death and/or
decreased rates of oxidation.

Despite the above problems with metabolism studies in
intact cells it has been demonstrated that they metabolise
at rates which correspond more closely to the whole organ
or animal than do subcellular fractions (Billings et al,
1977). Subcellular fractions often give higher activities
because conditions are optimised for a particular enzyme.
Whilst this is desirable for studies on that enzyme it does
not necessarily reflect the conditions that pertain in the
whole cell whether in isolation or in situ. Thus
saturating levels of substrate and cofactors are used which
may not be attained in vivo. High concentrations of many
model substrates such as biphenyl and 7-ethoxycoumarin are
toxic to hepatocytes necessitating the use of sub-
saturating levels.

METABOLISM STUDIES IN LIVER CELLS

Extensive reviews have been published of metabolism studies in isolated hepatocytes (Fry 1982a; Moldeus et al, 1983; Smith and Orrenius, 1984) and will not be repeated here. In addition to studies of metabolic pathways and the effects of reactive metabolites within hepatocytes, these cells have also been used as an exogenous metabolising system for toxicity or carcinogenicity studies in bacteria or cell cultures which contain little or no endogenous drug metabolising capacity (Bridges and Hubbard, 1980; Fry, 1982b; Bridges et al, 1983). With certain classes of compound such as nitrosamines (Jones et al, 1981) and benzo(a)anthracenes (Platt et al, 1986), hepatocyte-mediated mutagenicity assays correlate more closely with in vivo carcinogenicity than do homogenate-mediated assays. However hepatocytes are not always superior to subcellular fractions for this purpose as highly reactive metabolites may not leave the hepatocyte.

Arguably the most valuable use of intact cells is for the study of interspecies comparisons, invariably with extrapolation to man as the ultimate aim. Methods for isolation of human hepatocytes by perfusion of a wedge of liver are now well-established (see Guillouzo et al, this volume). However few laboratories have access to regular supplies of normal liver and it is essential therefore to perfect methods of cryopreservation in order to maximise the use of available material. In agreement with Guillouzo (this volume), studies in my laboratory have shown that attachment rate is preferable to trypan blue exclusion as a measure of the quality of cryopreserved and thawed hepatocytes. We have also confirmed the report of Gomez-Lechon et al (1984) that fast freezing rates are superior to the more conventional $1^{\circ}C/min$ (Lawrence and Benford, unpublished results).

Although metabolism data generated in isolated hepatocytes will normally relate to the total metabolism of a compound in vivo it may not explain specific effects of certain hepatotoxins. Hepatocytes from different regions of the liver lobule vary considerably in their content of drug metabolising enzymes and in their sensitivity to toxic compounds. Table 3 shows the relative activities of periportal and centrilobular hepatocytes. Cytochrome P450, epoxide hydrolase and glutathione transferase activities are all greater in the centrilobular region whereas glutathione content and sulphotransferase activity are lower. This may contribute to the greater susceptibility of centrilobular hepatocytes to hepatotoxins such as

paracetamol and bromobenzene. The use of selected
populations of hepatocytes may therefore facilitate
elucidation of toxic metabolite formation and effects.
Subpopulations of hepatocytes may be separated by
digitonin-collagenase perfusion (Lindros and Penttila,
1985), density gradient centrifugation (Tonda and Hirata,
1983) or centrifugal elutriation (Willson et al, 1985).

Table 3. Heterogeneity of Hepatocytes.

	PERIPORTAL	CENTRILOBULAR
Size	1	1.09
O_2 (in vivo)	↑	↓
P-450	1	1.6
P-450 reductase	1	2
Epoxide hydrolase	1	1.3
Glutathione transferase	↓	↑
Glutathione	↑	↓
UDP Glucuronyl transferase	1	1
Sulphotransferase	↑	↓

The relative distribution of enzyme activities are
compared and not the relative proportions within a region
(from Baron and Kawabata, 1983).

        Similarly, the liver sinusoidal cells are often ignored
but contain levels of drug metabolising enzymes which
although much lower than in hepatocytes, may explain
certain hepatotoxic effects (Lafranconi et al, 1986).

METABOLISM STUDIES IN CELLS FROM EXTRAHEPATIC TISSUES

        The drug metabolising enzymes of many extrahepatic
tissues are concentrated in a minority cell type(s). Thus
the use of whole tissue, whether as isolated organ, tissue
slices or homogenised and subfractionated tissue, results
in dilution of the enzyme activity. The contribution of
extrahepatic cells to total metabolism of a compound may be
small but first pass effects at the site of entry to the
body, or toxic metabolite mediated effects (see Cohen and
Moss, this volume) may be considerable. Table 4 lists the
major extrahepatic cell types which contain appreciable

levels of drug metabolising enzymes with references for
their isolation.

**Table 4. Isolation procedures for extrahepatic metabo-
lising cells.**

TISSUE	CELL TYPE	REFERENCE
Lung	Clara cell, alveolar type II cell, alveolar macrophage	Devereux & Fouts, 1982; Domin et al, 1986
Trachea	Ciliated epithelial cells	Massey & Fouts, 1985
Small Intestine	Mucosal epithelial cells	Shirkey & Schiller, 1980
Colon	Epithelial cells	Burger et al, 1985
Kidney	Proximal tubule segments	Endon, 1983
Skin	Sebaceous cells, differentiated keratinocytes	Coomes et al, 1983, 1984

The majority of studies with extrahepatic cells have been
designed to detect enzyme activity and consequently
homogenates of isolated and purified cell preparations have
been used for the enzyme assays rather than intact cells.
Whilst this approach simplifies the methods and provides
much information on particular enzyme systems, the use of
intact cells would also be valuable for the reasons
detailed above. In addition lower levels of activity can
be detected in intact cells because they remain viable for
much longer periods than cell homogenates or fractions.
However as isolation of pure preparations of extrahepatic
cells is generally more technically complex and produces
much lower yields than with hepatocytes their routine use
is impractical unless great improvements in preparation and
storage methods are made.

METABOLISM STUDIES IN CULTURED CELLS

Total cytochrome P-450 declines rapidly in rat
hepatocytes between 8 and 24 hours in culture. Depending
on the culture conditions this may be followed by an
increase of highly active isozyme(s) similar to those
induced by polycyclic aromatic hydrocarbons. Many attempts
have been made to maintain cytochrome P-450, including
addition of hormones (Dickins and Peterson, 1980), addition
of metyrapone and omission of cyst(e)ine (Lake and Paine,
1982) or co-culture with rat liver epithelial cells (Begue
et al, 1984). Whilst these methods maintain the total
cytochromes P-450 content (determined by the reduced-carbon
monoxide difference spectrum) measurement of specific
isoenzymes reveals that the relative populations are
altered. Thus present methods for culturing rat
hepatocytes are not suitable for studying rates and routes
of metabolism when it is essential that these relate to the
in vivo levels. Isolated hepatocytes are more suited to
this purpose and the viable lifetime of 4 to 5 hours is
generally sufficient.

However cultured hepatocytes can be used for studies of
enzyme regulation and metabolite-mediated toxicity. The
changes in enzyme populations are largely quantitative not
qualitative, therefore toxicity of most chemicals requiring
metabolic activation will still be observed because
cultured hepatocytes may be exposed to a compound for much
longer periods than either freshly isolated cells or the
liver in situ. The cytochrome P-450 population of cultured
human hepatocytes appears to be much more stable than that
of rat (Guillouzo et al, 1985, and this volume). Because
the longer incubation periods possible in culture allow
detection of lower levels of activity human hepatocytes in
culture may prove superior to freshly isolated suspensions
as a model for metabolism.

Similarly, with extrahepatic tissues cytochrome P-450
is probably more stable over short periods of culture.
Explant cultures or epithelial cell outgrowths have been
used for studying metabolism of carcinogens in many human
tissues (Harris et al, 1982; Autrup et al, 1985; Harris,
1987).

CONCLUSIONS

Intact cells are possibly the best model for metabolism
when attempting to extrapolate results to the whole animal
or to man. The lack of requirement for added cofactors
results in rates and routes of metabolism which correspond

more closely with those observed in vivo than subcellular fractions produce, and complete metabolic pathways can be studied. Techniques are generally less complex and much more data can be generated from a single preparation than with isolated organs. However viability of intact cells should be strictly monitored throughout use and incubation conditions should be carefully selected.

REFERENCES

Autrup, H., Seremet, T., Arenholt, D., Dragsted, L. and Jepsen, A. (1985). Carcinogenesis, 6, 1761.

Baron, J. and Kawabata, T.T. (1983). in "Biological Basis of Detoxication" (Eds. J. Caldwell and W.B. Jakoby). Academic Press, New York, P.105.

Begue, J.M., Guguen-Guillouzo, C., Pasdeloup, N. and Guillouzo, A. (1984). Hepatology, 4, 839.

Benford, D.J. and Hubbard, S.A. (1987). in "Biochemical Toxicology : A Practical Approach" (Eds. K. Snell and B.M. Mullock). IRL Press, Oxford, p.57.

Billings, R.E., McMahon, R.E., Ashmore, J. and Wagle, S.R. (1977). Drug Met. Disp, 5, 518.

Brides, J.W. and Hubbard, S.A. (1980). in "The Predictive Value of Short-term Screening Tests in Carcinogenicity Evaluation" (Eds. G.M. Williams, et al). Elsevier, Amsterdam, p.69.

Bridges, J.W., Benford, D.J. and Hubbard, S.A. (1983). in "Animals in Scientific Research : An Effective Substitute for Man?" (Ed. P. Turner). MacMillan Press, London, p.47.

Burger, H.J., Hauber, G., Schlote, W. and Schwenk, M. (1985). Am. J. Physiol, 248, C271.

Coomes, M.W., Norling, A.H., Pohl, R.J., Muller, D. and Fouts, J.R. (1983). J. Pharmacol. Exp. Ther, 225, 770.

Coomes, M.W., Sparks, R.W. and Fouts, J.R. (1984). J. Invest. Dermatol, 82, 598.

Cornell, N.W. (1983). in "Isolation, Characterisation and Use of Hepatocytes" (Eds. R.A. Harris and N.W. Cornell). Elsevier, Amsterdam, p.11.

Devereux, T.R. and Fouts, J.R. (1982). Meth. Enzymol, 77, 147.

Domin, B.A., Devereux, T.R. and Philpot, R.M. (1986). Mol. Pharmacol, 30, 296.

Dickins, M. and Peterson, R.E. (1980). Biochem. Pharmacol, 29, 1231.

Endon, H. (1983). Jap. J. Pharmacol, 33, 423.

Fry, J.R. (1982a). in "Reviews on Drug Metabolism and Drug Interactions" (Eds. A.H. Beckett and J.W. Gorrod).

Freund Publishing House Ltd, Tel Aviv.

Fry, J.R. (1982b). Toxicol, 25, 1.

Goethals, F., Krack, G., Deboyser, D., Vossen, P. and
   Roberfroid, M. (1984). Fund. Appl. Toxicol, 4, 441.

Gomez-Lechon, M.J., Lopez, P. and Castell, J.V. (1984). In
   Vitro, 20, 826.

Guillouzo, A., Beaune, P., Gascoin, M.N., Begue, J.M.,
   Campion, J.P., Guengerich, F.P. and Guguen-Guillouzo,
   C. (1985). Biochem. Pharmacol, 34, 2991.

Harris, C.C., Trump, B.F., Graftstrom, R. and Autrup, H.
   (1982). J. Cell. Biochem, 18, 285.

Harris, C.C. (1987). Cancer Res. 47, 137.

Hogberg, J. and Kristoferson, A. (1977). Eur. J. Biochem,
   74, 77.

Jones, C.A., Marlino, P.J., Lijinsky, W. and Huberman, E.
   (1981). Carcinogenesis, 2, 1075.

Lafranconi, W.M., Glatt, H.R. and Oesch, F. (1986).
   Toxicol. Appl. Pharmacol, 84, 500.

Lake, B.G. and Paine, A.J. (1982). Biochem. Pharmacol, 31,
   2141.

Lindros, K.O. and Penttila, K.E. (1985). Biochem. J. 228,
   757.

Massey, T.E. and Fouts, J.R. (1985). J. Cell Biol. Toxicol.
   1, 297.

Moldeus, P., Jernstrom, B. and Dawson, J.R. (1983).
   "Reviews in Biochemical Toxicology" Vol 5 (Eds. E.
   Hodgson, J.R. Bend and R.M. Philpot). Elsevier,
   Amsterdam, p.239.

Orrenius, S., Ormstad, K., Thor, H. and Jewell, S.A.
   (1983). Fedn. Proc. 42, 3711.

Platt, K.L., Utesch, D., Gemperlein-Mertes, 1., Glatt, H.R.
   and Oesch, F. (1986). Fd. Chem. Toxic, 24, 721.

Shirkey, R.J. and Schiller, C.M. (1980). J. Appl. Biochem,
   2, 196.

Smith, M.T. and Orrenius, S. (1984). in "Drug Metabolism
   and Drug Toxicity" (Eds. J.R. Mitchell and M.G.
   Horning). Raven Press, New York, p.71.

Stacey, N.H., Ottenwalder, H. and Kappus, H. (1982).
   Toxicol. Appl. Pharmacol, 62, 421.

Sundheimer, D.W. and Brendel, K. (1984). Life Sci, 34, 23.

Tonda, K. and Hirata, M. (1983). Chem. Biol. Interact, 47,
   277.

Wiebkin, P., Parker, G.L., Fry, J.R. and Bridges, J.W.
   (1979). Biochem. Pharmacol, 28, 3315.

Willson, R.A., Liem, W.H., Miyai, K. and Muller-Eberhard,
   U. (1985). Biochem. Pharmacol, 34, 1463.

DIAZEPAM METABOLISM IN CULTURED HEPATOCYTES FROM RAT, RABBIT, DOG, GUINEA-PIG AND MAN.

Richard J. Chenery[1], Andrew Ayrton[1], Harriet G. Oldham[1], Penelope Standring[1], Sarah J. Norman[1], Thomas Seddon[1] and Robert Kirby[2]

[1]Smith Kline and French Research Ltd, The Frythe, Welwyn, Herts, UK and [2]Transplantation Department, The Queen Elizabeth Hospital, Queen Elizabeth Medical Centre, Birmingham, UK.

Diazepam is widely used clinically with well-characterised species differences in both rates and routes of metabolism (Ruelius et al, 1965; Schwartz et al, 1965; Andrews and Griffiths, 1984). Diazepam is completely absorbed after oral administration and completely metabolised by demethylation and hydroxylation to produce nordiazepam, temazepam and oxazepam in man. However, in some laboratory species the 4'-hydroxylation pathway of metabolism is known to be important, producing a complex range of metabolites. Moreover, discrepancies exist between the metabolites known to be produced in vivo and the ability of the in vitro microsomal systems to reflect these activities (Andrews and Griffiths, 1984). We have, in this study, characterised both the rate and routes of diazepam metabolism in hepatocyte preparations from rat, dog, guinea-pig, rabbit and man in order to help evaluate the utility of the hepatocyte system in investigating species differences in drug metabolism.

The disappearance of diazepam from the culture medium was rapid in rat, dog and guinea-pig hepatocytes but slow in human hepatocytes (Table 1) and this is in agreement with in vivo studies where it is known that diazepam is metabolised rapidly in laboratory species, but in man, hepatic extraction is estimated to be low resulting in a long half-life for diazepam (Guentert, 1985). Marked variations were also observed in the intrinsic clearance of nordiazepam, temazepam and oxazepam, and this variation was consistent with the metabolite profile produced from diazepam in each species (Table 2), indicating that the metabolite profile could be attributed to a combination of the rate at which a metabolite was formed and the rate at which it was removed from the medium by further metabolism

Table 1. The Intrinsic Clearance of Diazepam, Nordiazepam, Temazepam and Oxazepam in Rat, Dog, Guinea-Pig, Rabbit and Human Hepatocytes.

| | Intrinsic Clearance $(ml.hr^{-1}.mg\ protein^{-1})$ | | | |
	Diazepam	Nordiazepam	Temazepam	Oxazepam
Rat	1.40	1.47	1.27	1.08
Dog	1.08	0.00	1.15	0.38
Guinea-pig	1.08	0.37	1.10	0.44
Rabbit	0.45	0.15	0.44	0.14
Human	0.32	0.09	>0.05	0.16

Hepatocytes were prepared and then introduced into culture. After 2hr in culture the parent benzodiazepine (diazepam, nordiazepam, temazepam or oxazepam) dissolved in WME at 15 µM was added and the disappearance of substrate measured every 15 min over a 2 hour time course. Benzodiazepine concentration was determined by HPLC.

The demethylation of diazepam to nordiazepam predominated in dog, guinea-pig and human hepatocytes and the steady accumulation of nordiazepam in dog and human hepatocytes was a consequence of minimal further metabolism of nordiazepam in these systems. In contrast, rabbit hepatocytes produced 4'-hydroxydiazepam as the predominant metabolite, and this metabolite was extensively glucuronidated. In rat hepatocyte cultures the recovery of metabolites corresponding to authentic standards was low, even after hydrolysis with β-glucuronidase, suggesting extensive further metabolism of most primary metabolites. These in vitro data are in good agreement with the known species differences in metabolite production from diazepam in vivo. Thus, demethylation to nordiazepam and 3-hydroxylation to temazepam are the major pathways of diazepam metabolism in man. In contrast, in the rat and the rabbit the formation of 4'-hydroxy metabolites is predominant. In the dog, diazepam is rapidly demethylated to nordiazepam which is removed from the circulation only very slowly by 3-hydroxylation to oxazepam.

In conclusion, the data presented in this study and from other studies indicate that isolated or cultured hepatocytes offer an excellent system to study qualitative and quantitative species differences in drug metabolism.

Table 2. The Metabolite Profile of Diazepam in Hepatocytes
from Rat, Dog, Guinea-Pig, Rabbit and Human Liver.

	Concentration (% of initial diazepam)									
	Rat		Dog		G-Pig		Rabbit		Human[*]	
	-	+	-	+	-	+	-	+	-	+
Diazepam	20	23	36	36	8	5	46	46	62	62
Nordiazepam	12	12	48	48	54	53	17	17	25	25
Temazepam	4	4	4	3	-	-	-	-	11	11
Oxazepam	-	-	4	4	4	8	-	-	-	-
4'-OH Diazepam	5	14	-	-	-	8	3	38	-	-
4'-OH Nordiazepam	-	-	-	-	-	5	-	-	-	-
TOTAL	41	53	92	91	66	79	66	101	98	98

Hepatocytes were prepared and then introduced into culture.
Hepatocytes from rat, dog, guinea-pig and rabbit were
allowed to attach for 2hr before addition of diazepam (15
µM). The metabolite profile was determined at 120 minutes
before (-) and after (+) treatment with bacterial β-glucuronidase. [*]The metabolite profile with human hepatocytes
was determined in cells cultured for 36hr and then
incubated with 50µM diazepam for 24 hr.

Clearly, many further studies will be required to fully
establish the relationships between metabolism in vivo and
metabolism in the hepatocyte system.

REFERENCES

Andrews, S.M. and Griffiths, L.A. (1984). Xenobiotica, 14,
    751.
Guentert, T.W. (1984). In "Progress in Drug Metabolism"
    (Ed. Bridges, J.W. and Chasseaud, L.F). Taylor and
    Francis, London, p.241.
Ruelius, H.W., Lee, J.M. and Alburn, H.E. (1965). Arch.
    Biochem. Biophys, 111, 376.
Schwartz, M.A., Koechlin, B.A., Postma, E., Palmer, S. and
    Krol, G. (1965). J. Pharmacol. Exptl. Ther, 149, 423.

XENOBIOTIC BIOTRANSFORMATION ENZYMES ARE PRESENT IN RAT LIVER KUPFFER AND ENDOTHELIAL CELLS

Pablo Steinberg, W. Mark Lafranconi, Thomas Friedberg and Franz Oesch.

Institute of Toxicology, University of Mainz, Obere Zahlbacher Str. 67, D - 6500 Mainz, Federal Republic of Germany.

INTRODUCTION

The mammalian liver is composed of several different cell types. Parenchymal cells, which constitute about 90 per cent of the total cell mass, only represent about 65 per cent of the total cell number (Daoust, 1958). The rest corresponds to nonparenchymal cells, mainly sinusoidal cells, but also haemopoietic, bile duct and blood vessel wall cells. Four types of sinusoidal cells have been described: endothelial, Kupffer, fat-storing and pit cells. They only account for about 6 per cent of the total liver volume but contribute considerably to the total number of liver cells (about 30 per cent) (Fabrikant, 1968; Greengard et al, 1972). Further, endothelial, Kupffer and fat-storing cells constitute about 54, 29 and 17 per cent of sinusoidal cells respectively (Munthe-Kaas et al, 1976; Blouin et al, 1977; Blomhoff et al, 1984).

When a xenobiotic enters the hepatic circulation the first cells it encounters are the Kupffer and endothelial cells, which form the sinusoidal lining of the liver. While much has been written about the xenobiotic metabolising capacity of parenchymal cells, there is not much informaiton about the presence of drug metabolising enzymes in nonparenchymal cells. In order to characterise the distribution and inducibility of drug metabolising enzymes within different cell populations of the rat liver, the activities of aminopyrine-N-demethylase, ethoxyresorufin O-deethylase, epoxide hydrolase and glutathione transferase in isolated liver parenchymal, Kupffer and endothelial cells from control, phenobarbital-, 3-methylcholanthrene- and Aroclor 1254- pretreated rats have been measured.

MATERIALS AND METHODS

All chemicals were purchased from commercial sources and were of the highest grade available. Male Sprague-Dawley rats (200-250g body weight) were treated with either corn oil (controls), phenobarbital, 3-methylcholanthrene or Aroclor 1254 as described by Wolf and Oesch (1983).

Based on previous reports in the literature (de Leeuw et al, 1982; Brouwer et al, 1984), parenchymal and sinusoidal lining cells were isolated from different animals in order to obtain higher yields of the latter. The two sinusoidal lining cell types (Kupffer and endothelial cells) were isolated from the same livers. Parenchymal cells were isolated by a collagenase perfusion method (Glatt et al, 1981). Nonparenchymal cell suspensions were prepared as described by Knook and coworkers (Praaning-van Dalen and Knook, 1982; Brouwer et al, 1984) by using pronase E, an enzyme which selectively destroys parenchymal cells. The nonparenchymal cell suspensions were further separated into endothelial and Kupffer cells by centrifugal elutriation (Brouwer et al, 1984). Ten isolations of Kupffer and endothelial cells from control, phenobarbital-, 3-methylcholanthrene- and Aroclor 1254- pretreated rats were performed; the cells were frozen in liquid nitrogen and stored at -70°C until used. For the enzyme assays the ten samples of Kupffer and endothelial cells from each group were split into 5 pairs (n = 5).

Cell viability was estimated from the capacity of the cells to exclude 0.25% trypan blue and from the cellular ultrastructure as observed by electron microscopy. Cell counts were performed with a haemocytometer. Kupffer cells, endothelial cells and lymphocytes present in the different cell fractions were distinguished from each other by light microscopy after they had been stained for peroxidase and non-specific esterase: in the rat, peroxidase is found exclusively in Kupffer cells (Wisse, 1974) while, although esterase is present in all liver cells, lymphocytes do not possess this enzyme (Wisse and Knook, 1979). Fat-storing cells were identified by fluorescence microscopy (Blomhoff et al, 1984). The percentages of lymphocytes, Kupffer, endothelial and fat-storing cells were afterwards confirmed by transmission electron microscopy as previously described (Knook et al, 1982).

The enzyme assays were carried out in cell homogenates obtained by sonicating the thawed cells and in all cases the amount of product was linear with both time and protein concentration. Aminopyrine N-demethylase activity was measured by determining formaldehyde production as described by Mazel (1971). Ethoxyresorufin O-deethylase was measured fluorimetrically according to the method of Burke and Mayer (1974). Epoxide hydroxylase activity was determined radiometrically with (^{3}H)-benzo(a)pyrene 4,5-oxide (Schmassmann et al, 1976). Glutathione transferase activity was measured spectrophotometrically according to the method of Habig et al (1974), using 1-chloro-2,4-dinitrobenzene as substrate. Protein determinations were performed as described by Lowry et al (1951). Statistics were done by Dunnett's test for multiple comparisons with a control (Dunnett, 1964).

RESULTS AND DISCUSSION

The yield, viability, purity and protein content of isolated parenchymal, Kupffer and endothelial cells from control rats are given in Table 1. The total yield of isolated parenchymal cells following collagenase digestion of the liver was $264 \pm 35 \times 10^6$ cells per rat liver (n=4), which included $2 \pm 1\%$ endothelial cells, $3 \pm 2\%$ Kupffer cells and $5 \pm 4\%$ fat-storing cells. Non-parenchymal liver cells were prepared from the total liver cell suspension by incubation with pronase E. The non-parenchymal cell suspension used for the separation of Kupffer and endothelial cells by centrifugal elutriation contained $210 \pm 60 \times 10^6$ cells per rat liver (n=10; $59 \pm 3\%$ endothelial cells, $31 \pm 3\%$ Kupffer cells and $8 \pm 2\%$ fat-storing cells). The recovery of Kupffer and endothelial cells following elutriation was $90 \pm 4\%$ and $87 \pm 3\%$ lymphocytes and $4 \pm 2\%$ Kupffer cells. The Kupffer cell preparations were found to contain $10 \pm 4\%$ endothelial cells, $3 \pm 2\%$ fat-storing cells and $0.2 \pm 0.1\%$ parenchymal cells.

Pretreatment of the animals with phenobarbital, 3-methylcholanthrene or Aroclor 1254 did not effect the yield, viability and purity of the isolated parenchymal, endothelial and Kupffer cells. Aroclor 1254 significantly increased the protein concentrations of parenchymal, Kupffer and endothelial cells by about 80%, 30% and 25% respectively; phenobarbital and 3-methylcholanthrene only increased the protein concentration in the parenchymal cell population by about 25% and 15% respectively. The methods of cell isolation provided Kupffer and endothelial cell populations that were essentially free from whole parenchymal cells and parenchymal cell debris. This was essential because of the generally high specific activity of parenchymal cell enzymes and the relatively low

Table 1. Characteristics of the isolated liver cell
populations from control rats

CELL TYPE	NUMBER OF RATS	YIELD x 10^6/ rat liver	VIABILITY %	PURITY %	PROTEIN μg/ 10^6 cells
Parenchymal	4	264+35	85+7	90+3	1478+156
Kupffer	10	25+6	93+2	86+4	109+25
Endothelial	10	59+10	95+3	88+4	69+18

Values represent mean + SD.

activities expected in the sinusoidal lining cells.
    The activities of aminopyrine N-demethylase,
ethoxyresorufin O-deethylase, epoxide hydrolase and
glutathione transferase were determined in the different
rat liver cell populations. These data are shown in Table
2. Measurable activities of the four enzymes were detected
in parenchymal cells as well as in Kupffer and endothelial
cells. In all cases, the parenchymal cells possessed
greater enzyme activities than did the sinusoidal lining
cells. In preprations from control animals, ethoxyresorufin O-deethylase and epoxide hydrolase activities
were on the average 5-fold higher in parenchymal cells than
in Kupffer or endothelial cells. The differences were
smaller in the case of aminopyrine N-demethylase (3- to 5-
fold) and glutathione transferase (2.3- to 3.5-fold)
activities. Although not statistically significant,
epoxide hydrolase and glutathione transferase activities
were higher in endothelial cells than in Kupffer cells.
    Pretreatment of the animals with phenobarbital led to
an increase in aminopyrine N-demethylase, epoxide hydrolase
and glutathione transferase activities in all three cell
types; aminopyrine N-demethylase activity was enhanced to a
greater extent (4.5-, 9-and 13-fold in parenchymal, Kupffer
and endothelial cells respectively) than epoxide hydrolase
and glutathione transferase activities (1.6- to 2.6-fold in
the three cell populations).
    The administration of 3-methylcholanthrene increased
ethoxyresorufin O-dethylase, epoxide hydrolase and
glutathione transferase activities in parenchymal as well
as Kupffer and endothelial cells. The most dramatic

Table 2. Drug metabolising enzyme activities in isolated parenchymal, Kupffer and endothelial cells from control, phenobarbital-, 3-methylcholanthrene- and Aroclor 1254- pretreated rats[a].

ENZYME ASSAY	CELL TYPE	CONTROL	PHENOBARBITAL	3-METHYL-CHOLANTHRENE	AROCLOR 1254
Ethoxy-resorufin[b] O-deethylase	Parenchymal	54±12	67±8	1317±159*	1478±287*
	Kupffer	10±6	8±3	89±10*	95±13*
	Endothelial	10±4	11±5*	67±5*	72±11*
Aminopyrine N-demethylase[c]	Parenchymal	15±3	76±9*	15±4	67±14*
	Kupffer	3±2	39±6*	2±1	31±4*
	Endothelial	5±2	44±6*	8±3	27±8*
Epoxide hydrolase[b]	Parenchymal	3368±479	5385±614*	4479±560*	5100±716*
	Kupffer	592±138	1562±267*	944±187*	1637±203*
	Endothelial	829±145	1621±194*	1107±118*	1716±220*
Glutathione Transferase[c]	Parenchymal	1054±138	1796±278*	1520±190*	1870±359*
	Kupffer	301±72	681±155*	597±123*	578±101*
	Endothelial	460±119	709±93*	652±132*	784±122*

[a] All enzyme assays were carried out in broken cell preparations. Values are means $\pm$ SD of 4 rats per treatment in the case of parenchymal cells, while ten samples of Kupffer and endothelial cells from each group were split into 5 pairs (n=5).
[b] Activity is expressed as pmol product formed/min/mg protein
[c] Activity is expressed as nmol product formed/min/mg protein
* Indicates significantly different from the corresponding control value 'p $<$ 0.05, Dunnett's test).

increase in enzyme activity was observed in the case of ethoxyresorufin O-deethylase (24-, 9- and 7-fold in parenchymal, Kupffer and endothelial cells respectively), while epoxide hydrolase and glutathione transferase activities were increased 1.3- to 2-fold in the three cell types. Aroclor 1254 enhanced all investigated enzyme activities in parenchymal, Kupffer and endothelial cells. The increase of ethoxyresorufin O-deethylase activity was greater in parenchymal (27-fold) than in sinusoidal lining cells (7- to 9-fold). On the other hand, Kupffer and endothelial cells displayed greater increases in aminopyrine N-demethylase and epoxide hydrolase activities than parenchymal cells. An average 1.8-fold increase in glutathione transferase activity was observed in parenchymal as well as sinusoidal lining cells.

The cytochrome P-450 assays were selected according to their specificity for particular forms of the enzymes: the ethoxyresorufin O-deethylase assay is specific for the forms of cytochrome P-450 which are inducible by 3-methylcholanthrene (Burke and Mayer, 1974) while the aminopyrine N-demethylase assay appears to be relatively specific for those forms of cytochrome P-450 that are inducible by phenobarbital (Mazel, 1971). As the 3-methylcholanthrene- and the phenobarbital-inducible forms of cytochrome P-450 are quantitatively very important forms, the two assays provide some estimate of the overall cytochrome P-450 enzymatic activity in parenchymal, Kupffer and endothelial cells. Parenchymal as well as Kupffer and endothelial cells possess oxidative (aminopyrine N-demethylase and ethoxyresorufin O-deethylase) and post-oxidative (epoxide hydrolase and glutathione transferase) enzyme activities, one striking feature is that Kupffer and endothelial cells have extremely low oxidative enzyme activities and relatively high post-oxidative enzyme activities. Hence sinusoidal lining cells might have a lower ability to oxidize xenobiotics to reactive electrophiles and a greater ability to conjugate or hydrolyse those products that may be formed. Oxidative and post-oxidative enzyme activities were enhanced in all three cell types by phenobarbital, 3-methylcholanthrene or Aroclor 1254; however, the effect of the inducers on epoxide and glutathione transferase activities was low by comparison to the efect on aminopyrine N-demethylase and ethoxyresorufin O-deethylase activities.

ACKNOWLEDGEMENTS

This work was supported by the Deutsche

Forschungsgemeinschaft (SFB 302) and the Alexander von Humboldt Foundation (P.S., W.M.L.).

REFERENCES

Blomhoff, R., Holte, K., Naess, L. and Berg, T. (1984). Exp. Cell. Res, 150, 185.

Blouin, A., Bolender, R.P. and Weibel, E.R. (1977). J. Cell. Biol. 72, 441.

Brouwer, A., Barelds, R.J., de Zanger, R. and Knook, D.L. (1984). in "Centrifugation, a practical approach", 2nd edition (Ed Rickwood, D). IRL Press, Oxford and Washington, D.C. p.183.

Burke, M.D. and Mayer, R.T. (1974). Drug Metab. Disp, 2, 583.

Daoust, R. (1958). in "Liver funtions, Publication 4 (Ed. Brauer, R.W.). American Institute of Biological Science, Washington, D.C. p.3.

de Leeuw, A.M., Barelds, R.J., de Zanger, R. and Knook, D.L. (1982). Cell Tissue Res. 223, 201.

Dunnett, C.W. (1964). Biometrics, 6, 482.

Fabrikant, J.I. (1968). J. Cell. Biol, 36, 551.

Glatt, H.R., Billings, R., Platt, K.L. and Oesch, F. (1981). Cancer Res, 41, 270.

Greengard, O., Federman, M. and Knox, W.E. (1972). J. Cell. Biol, 52, 261.

Habig, W.H., Pabst, M.J. and Jakoby, W.B. (1974). J. Biol. Chem, 249, 7130.

Knook, D.L., Seffelaar, A.M. and de Leeuw, A.M. (1982). Exp. Cell Res, 139, 468.

Lowry, O.H., Rosebrough, J., Farr, A.L. and Randall, R.J. (1951). J. Biol. Chem, 193, 265.

Mazel, P. (1971). in "Fundamentals of Drug Metabolism and Drug Disposition" (Eds. LaDu, B.N., Mandel, H.G. and Way, E.L.). Williams and Williams, Baltimore, p. 546.

Munthe-Kaas, A.C., Berg, T. and Seljelid, R. (1976). Exp. Cell Res, 99, 146.

Praaning-van Dalen, D.P. and Knnok, D.L. (1982). FEBS Lett, 141, 229.

Schmassmann, U., Glatt, H.R. and Oesch, F. (1976). Anal. Biochem, 74, 94.

Wisse, E. (1974). J. Ultrastruct. Res, 46, 393.

Wisse, E. and Knook, D.L. (1979). in "Progress in Liver Disease", Vol VI (Eds. Popper, H. and Schaffner, F). Grune and Stratton, New York, p.153.

Wolf, C.R. and Oesch, F. (1983). Biochem. Biophys. Res. Comm, 111, 504.

THE STEREOSELECTIVE FORMATION OF BENZO(A)PYRENE DIHYDRODIOLS BY PURIFIED RAT LIVER CYTOCHROMES P-450

Michael Hall[1], Deborah K. Parker[1], Maro Christou[2], Colin R. Jefcoate[2] and Philip L. Grover[1].

[1]Chester Beatty Laboratories, Institute of Cancer Research, Royal Cancer Hospital, Fulham Road, London. SW3 6JB. UK, [2]Department of Pharmacology, University of Wisconsin Medical School, Madison, W1 53706, USA.

Benzo(a)pyrene (BP) is a member of the polycyclic aromatic hydrocarbons (PAH), a group of compounds widely distributed in the environment and known to possess carcinogenic potential. This potential is expressed by their activation in animal tissues to an "ultimate carcinogenic" form which is capable of binding to cellular macromolecules including DNA. In the case of BP the ultimate carcinogen is the (+)-anti-BP-7,8-dihydrodiol 9,10-epoxide, derived from the precursor (-)-BP-7R, 8R-dihydrodiol (Conney, 1982; Cooper et al, 1983). The metabolic activation of PAH via a diol-epoxide is catalysed by the sequential action of cytochromes P-450 and epoxide hydrolase in a regio-and stereoselective manner, the proportion of parent hydrocarbon finally appearing in the form of its ultimate carcinogen being a reflection of the specificities and relative levels within the tissue of the enzymes involved and, in particular, the cytochrome P-450 profile. Pretreatment of animals with various xenobiotics will lead to changes both in the regio- and stereoselective metabolism of PAH within tissues (Conney, 1982; Yang et al, 1985) and also in the cytochrome P-450 profile (Ryan et al, 1982). Cytochrome P-450 isozymes purified from differently-induced rat liver microsomes have previously been shown to exhibit different regioselectivities with respect to BP metabolism (Wilson et al, 1984). In the present study an investigation was made of the stereoselective metabolism of BP to its 4,5-, 7,8-, and 9,10-dihydrodiols by three forms of purified rat liver cytochrome P-450, viz a constitutive form, P-450a, a form induced by phenobarbital (PB), P-450b, and a form induced by 3-methylcholanthrene (3-MC), P-450c.
Microsomes were prepared from the livers of uninduced,

PB-induced and 3-MC-induced male Sprague-Dawley rats by
differential centrifugation, and cytochromes P-450a,b and c
were isolated from these preparation (Wilson et al, 1984).
[^{3}H]BP was incubated with these purified isozymes in a
reconstituted system, and also with uninduced (control) rat
liver microsomes in the presence or absence of added
epoxide hydrolase (Wilson et al, 1984). Resulting [^{3}H]BP
metabolites were extracted, separated on reverse phase
h.p.l.c. and quantitated by liquid scintillation counting
as previously described for DMBA (Christou et al, 1984).
Enantiomers of the separated [^{3}H]BP-4,5-, -7,8-, and -9,10-
dihydrodiols were resolved by normal phase h.p.l.c. on
Pirkle columns packed with a chiral stationary phase of
(R)-N-(3,5-dinitrobenzoyl)phenylglycine either ionically or
covalently bonded to γ-aminopropyl silanised silica. The
resolved enantiomers were quantitated from the amount of
radioactivity that coeluted with added authentic reference
materials.

Data obtained for the regioselective metabolism of BP
to its dihydrodiol derivatives by uninduced microsomes and
the three isolated P-450 isozymes are given in Table 1.
Some differences are apparent here compared with data
previously presented by Wilson et al (1984), most obviously
the relative amounts of BP-9,10-dihydrodiol produced by
cytochromes P-450a and c. However, the marked preference
of the BP-induced isozyme P-450b for metabolism of BP in
the K-region to form the 4,5-dihydrodiol (Table 1) is in
agreement with this earlier work.

**Table 1. Regioselectivity of BP dihydrodiol formation by
purified cytochromes P-450.**

ENZYME SOURCE	AMOUNT OF BP DIHYDRODIOL EXTRACTED[a]		
	4,5-	7,8-	9,10-
Control rat liver microsomes + EH	9.5	3.4	9.2
P-450a	20.0	15.3	16.7
P-450b	100.0	<0.5	<0.5
P-450c	13.7	11.0	3.5

[a]Expressed as (pmol/mg microsomal protein/min) for control
rat liver microsomes and as (pmol/nmol.P-450/min) for
purified cytochromes P-450.

Table 2 presents the data obtained for the stereoselective formation of the dihydrodiols by the various enzyme preparations. Each dihydrodiol was extracted with an optical purity > 80%, with the enantiomer possessing R,R absolute configuration predominating in each case. However, there do appear to be subtle differences between the stereoselectivities of the preparations. For instance, cytochrome P-450a, although a constitutive isozyme form, demonstrated a higher stereoselectivity of BP dihydrodiol formation that did the uninduced microsomal preparation. In addition, the PB-inducible form of cytochrome P-450, P-450b, appeared to show a lower degree of stereoselectivity in the formation of all three BP dihydrodiols than either P-450a or P-450c. Jerina et al, (1984) have attempted to map the steric requirements of the catalytic binding site of cytochrome P-450c by consideration of the absolute configuration of metabolites formed by this enzyme. Based upon the differences in the stereoselective formation of naphthalene and anthracene 1,2-oxides by cytochromes P-450b and P-450c, it was suggested (van Bladeren et al, 1985) that the binding sites of these two isozymes were markedly different. A comparison of the data obtained for cytochromes P-450b and c in the present work (Table 2), although less dramatic than that presented by van Bladeren et al (1985), could be taken as supporting evidence for this contention.

The more striking differences between the three cytochrome P-450 isozymes investigated here, however, is in their regioselectivity of BP metabolism (compare data in Tables 1 and 2). This would imply that the binding sites of the various isozymes differ in the orientation in which they are capable of accommodating the BP molecule, with P-450b possibly having a more closely-defined structure than isozymes P-450a or c, but that the alignment of the bound molecule to the haem iron is similar in all the isozymes thus resulting in >90% of the R,R enantiomer of each dihydrodiol. Hence it seems likely that the regioselectivities of isolated cytochrome P-450 isozymes may be more important than their stereoselectivities when considering the susceptibility of tissues to PAH-induced carcinogenesis.

REFERENCES

Christou, M., Wilson, N.M. and Jefccate, C.R. (1984). Carcinogenesis, 5, 1239.
Conney, A.H. (1982). Cancer Res, 42, 4875.
Cooper, C.S., Grover, P.L. and Sims, P. (1983). Progress in

Table 2.   Stereoselectivity of BP dihydrodiol formation by purified cytochromes P-450.

ENZYME SOURCE	BP DIHYDRODIOL ENANTIOMER RATIO		
	4S,5S:4R,5R	7S,8S:7R,8R	9S,10S:9R,10R
Control rat liver microsomes	2:98	5:95	2:98
Control rat liver microsomes + EH	2:98	5:95	2:98
P-450a	2:98	<1:>99	1:99
P-450b	5:95	10:90	5:95
P-450c	1:99	1:99	4:96

Drug Metabolism, vol 7 (Eds. Bridges, J.W. and Chasseaud, L.F), John Wiley and Sons Ltd, London, P. 295.

Jerina, D.M., Sayer, J.M., Yagi, H., van Bladeren, P.J., Thakker, D.R., Levin, W., Chang, R.L., Wood, A.W. and Conney, A.H. (1984). in "Microsomes and Drug Oxidations", (Eds. Boobis, A.R., Caldwell, J., De Matteis, F. and Elcombe, C.R). Taylor and Francis, London, p.310.

Ryan, D.E., Thomas, P.E., Reik, L.M. and Levin, W. (1982). Xenobiotica, 12, 727.

Van Bladeren, P.J., Sayer, J.M., Ryan, D.E., Thomas, P.E., Levin, W. and Jerina, D.M. (1985). J. Biol. Chem, 260, 10226.

Wilson, N.M., Christou, M., Turner, C.R., Wrighton, S.A. and Jefcoate, C.R. (1984). Carcinogenesis, 5, 1475.

Yang, S.K., Mushtaq, M. and Chiu, P.-L (1985). in "Polycyclic Hydrocarbons and Carcinogenesis", ACS Symposium Series No., 283 (Ed. Harvey, R.G). American Chemical Society, Washington, D.C. p.19.

GALACTOSAMINE/ENDOTOXIN-INDUCED HEPATITIS IN MICE : A MODEL FOR PEPTIDO-LEUKOTRIENE MEDIATED TOXICITY

Albrecht Wendel and Gisa Tiegs

Physiologisch-Chemisches Institut der Universitat, Hoppe-Seyler-Str. 1, D - 7400 Tubingen, West Germany.

INTRODUCTION

In rats, in vivo administration of endotoxin (E) leads to an immediate increase of the secretion of leukotriene-immunoreactive material into the bile (Hagmann et al, 1984). It is also known that galactosamine (GalN)-induced hepatitis in mice, rats and rabbits is potentiated by simultaneous administration of endotoxin. On the other hand, inhibitors of leukotriene synthesis or receptor antagonists were shown to prevent GalN/E-induced lethality in mice (Hagmann et al, 1984).

Recently we reported that the new anti-inflammatory seleno-organic compound ebselen (PZ51, Nattermann, Cologne) inhibited rat leukocyte 5-lipoxygenase activity with an IC_{50} of 20μM (Safayhi et al, 1985). In order to study the effects of this drug in vivo we set up a mouse model of acute hepatotoxicity using GalN/E and compared the results obtained with alternative models of drug-induced liver injury in the mouse. Special interest was directed towards the role of hepatic glutathione. For numerous drugs and xenobiotics, it is documented that glutathione depletion leads to enhanced susceptibility of animals to hepatotoxicity. We were interested in differentiating the effects of the hydroxylated leukotrienes from those of the peptidoleukotrienes derived from glutathione by manipulating the liver glutathione content in vivo.

METHODS

The basic principles of the mouse liver hepatotoxicity model are shown in Figure 1. Details are given as described by Wendel and Tiegs (1986).

RESULTS

1. Endotoxin-induced hepatitis in GalN-sensitised mice was

Figure 1.   Experimental design of GalN/E-induced liver injury in male NMRI mice.

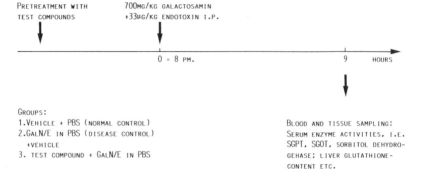

Figure 2. Metabolism of eicosanoids and its inhibition in vivo.

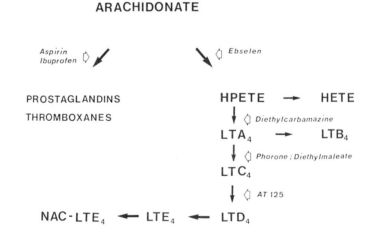

significantly prevented by in vivo inhibitors of leukotriene synthesis, while compounds interfering with prostanoid production were ineffective (Table 1 and Figure 2).

2.   Severe depletion of the hepatic glutathione content by phorone or diethylmaleate pretreatment prevented GalN/E hepatitis as well as lethality (Table 2). In contrast, a

mere glutathione synthesis block leading to moderate depletion had no significant effect.

3. When the further processing of LTC_4 was blocked by inhibiting glutamyl transpeptidase with AT 125, an apparent protection from GalN/E hepatitis was observed (Table 2).

4. Oral pretreatment of mice with 600mg/kg ebselen (c.f. Table 1), offered essentially no protection against liver injuries induced by 400 mg/kg paracetamol, or 520 mg/kg bromobenzene, or 3.2 g/kg carbon tetrachloride, or 60 mg/kg allyl alcohol (data not shown).

Table 1. **Influence of different in vivo inhibitors of arachidonic acid metabolism on endotoxin induced hepatitis in galactosamine-sensitised mice.**

TREATMENT	SGPT	n
none	70+30	8
disease control	10440+8640	49
200µg/kg dexamethasone [a,c]	100+60***	8
220mg/kg aspirin [a,b]	8010+8000	8
45 mg/kg ibuprofen [a,b]	7160+7800	10
78 mg/kg diethylcarbamazine [a,c]	290+180***	10
600mg/kg ebselen [b]	140+100***	12
60 mg/kg ebselen [b]	730+890***	21
6 mg/kg ebselen [b]	1300+2200***	21

*** $p < 0.001$; SGPT: U/liter; a) doses correspond to 50% inhibition of carageenan paw oedema; b) orally; c) intraperitoneally. Analogous data for SGOT and sorbitol dehydrogenase activities.

CONCLUSIONS

1. In mice, GalN/E hepatitis seems to be a suitable in vivo model for screening compounds interfering with arachidonate metabolism selectivity on the leukotriene branch.

2. In contrast to the effect on a large variety of hepatotoxins metabolized by the microsomal MFO, hepatic glutathione depletion protects mice from GalN/E liver injury. We interpret this by the inability of the organ to form leukotrienes in the depleted state.

Table 2. Influence of liver glutathione status of <u>starved</u> mice on GalN/E hepatitis.

Treatment	SGOT	liver glutathione[a]	Mortality[b]
Vehicle control	70+30	18+2	0/8
disease control	2210+1850	22+3	15/16
phorone + GalN/E	50+30**	1+0.1	0/8
DEM + GalN/E	90+30**	1.5+0.4	0/8
BSO + GalN/E	3170+2730	11.4+4.4	6/8
AT 125 + GalN/E	175+170***	62+8[c]	0/16

**p<.01, [a] at the time GalN/E was given; [b]within nine hours; [c]fed mice. Analogous data for SGOT and SDH activities, glutathione : nmol per mg protein.

DEPLETION : 250 mg/kg phorone (diiso-propylidene acetone) i.p. 90 min prior to GalN/E (see Figure 2).
400 mg/kg diethyl maleate (DEM) in oil i.p. three times every 20 min within the first hour prior to GalN/E.
SYNTHESIS BLOCK : 880 mg/kg buthionine sulfoximine (BSO) i.p. 8 hours prior to GalN/E.
CATABOLISM BLOCK: 50 mg/kg at 125 (= acivicin), intravenously 60 min prior to GalN/E.

3. Our results suggest that neither LTB_4 not LTC_4 but rather a metabolite of the peptidoleukotrienes might be responsible for mediating GalN/E induced hepatotoxicity.

ACKNOWLEDGEMENT

Supported by the Deutsche Forschungsgemeinschaft, Grant We 686/10-1.

REFERENCES

Hagmann, W., Denzlinger, C. and Keppler, R. (1984). <u>Circ. Shock</u> 14, 233.
Safahyhi, H., Teigs, G. and Wendel, A. (1985). <u>Biochem. Pharmacol,</u> 34, 2691.
Wendel, A. and Tiegs, G. (1986). <u>Biochem. Pharmacol,</u> 35, in press.

RECONSTITUTION OF THE LIVER DRUG OXIDATION SYSTEM IN A SOLUBLE MONOMERIC STATE

G.I. Bachmanova, E.D. Skotselyas, I.P. Kanaeva, E.V. Petrachenko, D.R. Davydov, S.A. Gordeev, V.A. Karyakin, G.P. Kuznetsova, E.N. Korneva and A.I. Archakov.

Institute of Physico-Chemical Medicine, M. Pirogovskaya 1, Moscow, 119828, USSR.

INTRODUCTION

The microsomal monooxygenase system may be reconstituted from isolated cytochrome P-450 and NADPH-specific flavoprotein (FP) in the presence of detergents and phospholipids (Dean and Gray, 1982; Kominami et al, 1984; Miwa and Lu 1984). It has earlier been shown in our laboratory that in the presence of Emulgen 913 (E), mixed equimolar complexes of P-450 and FP with molecular weights of 700 kD are formed which can oxidase benzphetamine (BP) and dimethylaniline (Kanaeva et al, 1985). However, there remains the problem of whether the monooxygenase system can be reconstituted from FP and P-450 monomers in solution. We have therefore made an attempt to reconstitute the liver microsomal monooxygenase system from haemo- and flavoprotein monomers.

MATERIALS AND METHODS

Isolation of P-450 (LM2) and FP, determination of protein molecular weights and rate of BP N-demethylation were performed as described previously (Kanaeva et al, 1985). LM2 and FP monomers were obtained after 2-hour incubation at $4^\circ C$ of 2.5µM LM2 and 2.5µM FP in 100 mM K-phosphate buffer, pH 7.5 containing 0.25 g/l of E. The kinetics of NADPH-dependent LM2 reduction were determined by a stopped flow technique with further processing of kinetic curves on a Silex computer (Davydov et al, 1985).

RESULTS AND DISCUSSION

It has been shown by gel filtration that, in the absence of E, FP and LM2 oligomers consist of 20 and 14 subunits, respectively (Kanaeva et al, 1985). At an E concentration of 0.05 g/l a mixed complex (700 kD) was formed, FP and LM2 stoichiometry being 5:5. Protein monomers were obtained at an E concentration of 0.25 g/l after a 2-hour incubation at 4°C. The FP molecular weight was equal to 135 kD and that of LM2 was 70 kD as some E is associated with proteins.

In the absence of E, LM2 reduction and BP oxidation were not observed, while in presence of E (0.05 g/l for complex and 0.25 g/l for monomers), these reactions proceeded. The higher initial rates of LM2 reduction and BP oxidation were observed in the system containing the protein complex (Table 1). As the soluble reconstituted systems under investigation contain enzymes in aggregate states, it is necessary to take into consideration the effective concentrations of components when calculating kinetic parameters of the reactions catalysed by these systems. Therefore on the formation of 700 kD complex containing 5 molecules of each FP and LM2 at the initial 1 µM protein concentrations, the concentration of complex equals 2.10^{-7}M and that of LM2 in the complex is 7.10^{-3}M. The concentration of the proteins in monomeric state is equal to 10^{-6}M. Shown in Table 1 are rate constants of LM2 reduction and BP oxidation calculated in terms of the effective concentrations of the proteins. In this case the reactions prove to proceed more efficiently in the monomeric system. In the complexes electron transfer reactions proceed within a non-dissociating system, which makes it different from the monomeric and, apparently, microsomal ones. Thus, the data obtained show the possibility of reconstitution of the membranous microsomal monooxygenase system in solution from proteins existing in monomeric state in the presence of detergent. More detailed investigated of the monomeric reconstituted system has shown that NADPH-dependent reduction of LM2 is an exponential monophasic reaction (Figure 1, a.b) in contrast to that taking place in microsomes and proteoliposomes (Davydov et al, 1985). The monomeric system exhibits reductase activity at a 1:1 ratio of FP and LM2 (Figure 1c). The pseudo-first order in the absence of substrate is $5.4.10^{-3}s^{-1}$, the dissociation constant is $0.22.10^{-6}$M. It means that the electron transfer reaction between FP and LM2 occurs in full accordance with the mass action law for bimolecular reaction.

REFERENCES

Davydov, D.R., Karyakin, A.V., Binas, B., Kurganov, B.I. and Archakov, A.I. (1985). Eur. J. Biochem, 150, 115.

Figure 1. NADPH-dependent reduction of LM2 in reconstituted monomeric system.

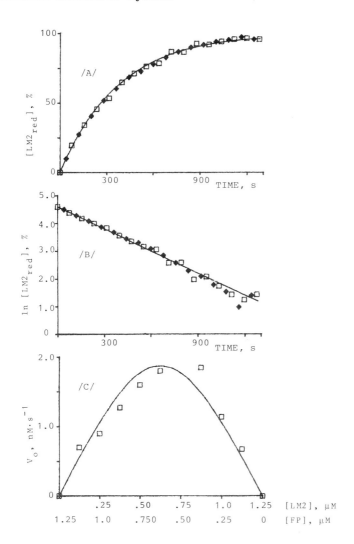

A,B : Kinetics of the reaction in linear and
semilogarithmic coordinates in different cases of reaction
initiation. Conditions : 0.1M K-phosphate buffer, pH 7.5;
0.25 g/l of Emulgen; 1mM NADPH; 0.5μM LM2 and 0.5μM FP:
anaerobiosis; CO. T = 25°C. The content of each syringe
was : □ - (LM2) + (NADPH+FP); ◆ - (NADPH) + (FP + LM2).
C : Dependence of initial reduction rate on FP and LM2
concentrations.

Bachmanova et al.

Table 1. Kinetic parameters of LM2 reduction and BP N-demethylation in reconstituted systems.

SYSTEMS	V_o, $M.s^{-1}$		k''_{app}, $M^{-1}s^{-1}$	
	Redn.	Demethn.	Redn.	Demethn.
AGGREGATES 1μM FP+1μM LM2 +<0.01 g/l Emulgen	0	0	0	0
COMPLEXES 1μM FP+1μM LM2 +0.05 g/l Emulgen	1.6×10^{-6}	0.23×10^{-6}	0.12×10^{4}	1.7×10^{2}
MONOMERS 1μM FP+1μM LM2 +0.25 g/l Emulgen	0.6×10^{-6}	0.06×10^{-6}	0.62×10^{6}	5.8×10^{4}

V_o - initial reaction rate of BP demethylation and LM2 reduction in the presence of 0.5 mM BP. T = 37°C.

k''_{app} - apparent second order rate constant of reactions calculated with effective protein concentrations considered:

for complexes
$$k''_{app} = \frac{V_o}{[FP + LM2]_c \cdot [LM2]_{ic}},$$
where $[FP + LM2]_c$ is complex concentration and $[LM2]_{ic}$ is concentration of LM2 in complex;

for monomers $k''_{app} = \dfrac{V_o}{[FP] \cdot [LM2]}$

Dean, W.L. and Gray, R.D. (1982). J. Biol. Chem, 257, 14679.

Kanaeva, I.P., Skotselyas, E.D., Kuznetsova, G.P., Antonova, G.N., Bachmanova, G.I. and Archakov, A.I. (1985). Biochemistry, USSR, 80, 1382.

Kominami, S., Hara, H., Ogishima, T. and Takemory, S. (1984). J. Biol. Chem, 259, 2991.

Miwa, G.T. and Lu, A.Y.H. (1984). Arch. Biochem. Biophys, 234, 161.

8. Biological techniques and drug metabolism

PRESERVATION OF HUMAN LIVER CELLS AND THEIR FUNCTION

Andre Guillouzo, Christophe Chesne, Damrong Ratanasavanh,
Jean-Pierre Campion and Christine Guguen-Guillouzo.

Unite de Recherches Hepatologiques U 49 de l'Inserm,
Hopital de Pontchaillou, 35033 Rennes Cedex - France.

INTRODUCTION

Qualitative and quantitative interspecies differences
are common among various liver functions, including drug
metabolism, of which a number of studies have reported
differences in both the rates and the routes, particularly
when comparisons involved experimental animals and man.
Therefore, there was an increasing need to perform
experiments directly on human hepatocytes. This cell type,
which represents about two-thirds of the total hepatic cell
population, expresses most of the liver functions,
including uptake from the blood of nutrient components and
their subsequent metabolismn, storage and distribution to
blood and bile as well as biotransformation of endogenous
and exogenous compounds.

Early attempts to cultivate human liver cells were
performed by explantation of minced-small tissue fragments.
Adult tissue samples constantly yielded few hepatocytes and
overgrowth of a minority of primitive cells usually
resembling myofibroblasts occurred and were able to be
subcultivated. Fetal liver samples also yielded an
heterogenous cell population but the percentage of
hepatocytes was much higher than in explant cultures of
adult liver and their survival was longer (Guguen-Guillouzo
et al, 1986).

A major progress in obtaining viable hepatocytes was
made by the introduction of collagenase as a dissociating
enzyme and for adult human liver by the adaption of the
two-step collagenase perfusion method to the dissociation
of either a portion of the whole liver or biopsies (Clement
et al, 1984; Guguen-Guillouzo et al, 1982; Reese and Byard,
1981; Strom et al, 1982).

Freshly isolated hepatocytes do not survive for more
than a few hours in suspension. To survive longer they
must attach to a support. In which conditions they may

continue to express their specific functions is of major
importance. It has been shown that rodent hepatocytes are
very unstable in culture and that they rapidly lose their
most differentiated functions (Bissell and Guzelian, 1980;
Guguen-Guillouzo and Guillouzo, 1983; Sirica and Pitot,
1980). Only specific, well defined conditions have been
found to temporarily delay dramatic phenotypic alterations
in these cells (Rojkind et al, 1981; Guguen-Guillouzo et
al, 1983).

Other major problems exist with human hepatocytes,
namely their limited availability and individual variation
in metabolic functions. In order to work with cells from
several donors it is essential to store them for long
periods. This leads to the need for a reproducible method
of hepatocyte cryopreservation.

This review will briefly summarise the protocol for
isolation of adult human ·hepatocytes and then will focus on
the preservation of the cells either by culture or by
freezing. Preservation of fetal human parenchymal cells
will not be considered.

ISOLATION OF ADULT HUMAN HEPATOCYTES

Both portions of the whole liver and biopsies of
various sizes can be dissociated. Whole livers are
obtained from kidney donors, biopsies by resection either
from patients undergoing partial hepatectomy or from kidney
donors. Liver samples must be perfused within 45-60
minutes after resection except if the samples have been
washed and chilled using a buffer usually employed for the
preservation of the organ before transplantation. In this
case several hours can separate liver removal from the
perfusion. The flow rates of perfusates must be adapted to
the size of the organ portion to be perfused. Thus, a
limited area of the left lobe representing 5 to 10% of the
whole liver can be dissociated as previously described
(Guguen-Guillouzo et al, 1982). In outline, a polyethylene
catheter is introduced deeply in the anterior branch of the
left lobe and liver is first washed with a calcium-free
Hepes buffered solution pH7.6, at 75 ml/min at 37°C for 20
min then with the same buffer containing 0.05% collagenase
and 5mM $CaCl_2$ at a flow rate of 50ml/min for 20 min. At
the end of the perfusion, the well-perfused part of the
liver is transferred to L15 Leibovitz medium containing
0.2% bovine serum albumin.

Similar flow rates are selected for perfusing large
liver biopsies weighing 100g or more, through the largest
vascular orifice. Biopsies weighing only 5-10g are

perfused with 100ml of calcium-free Hepes buffer at 16-18ml/min then with 100ml of the enzymatic solution at a flow rate of 8-10 ml/min. Cell aggregates can be further dissociated by incubation for 20 min in the Hepes buffered collagenase solution at 37°C with gentle stirring. The buffer with or without collagenase is heated at 40-41°C to reach the liver at 37°C. The solutions are neither oxygenated nor recirculated.

Cell suspensions are filtered on gauze and allowed to sediment for 20 min to eliminate cell debris and non-parenchymal cells. They are then washed three times by low-speed centrifugation. The cell yield depends on the size of the well-perfused part of the liver. Large biopsies often yield more than 10^9 parenchymal cells, small biopies 20 to 60 x 10^6 cells. Viability ranges between 70 and 90% (Figure 1).

Figure 1. Phase-contrast micrograph or freshly isolated adult human hepatocytes. Bar : 20μm.

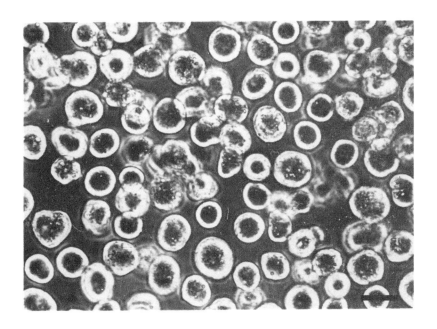

PRESERVATION OF HUMAN HEPATOCYTES WITHOUT FREEZING

In suspension, freshly isolated hepatocytes do not survive for more than a few hours. In addition it must be kept in mind that they memorise signals to which they are

responding in vivo. Several factors may be responsible for
variations in cellular functions (Table 1). Thus, Houssin
et al (1983) have measured some functional activities of
freshly isolated hepatocytes from two kidney donors. One
patient received glucose by perfusion while the other did
not during the 30h between trauma and kidney removal. In
the latter case, glycogen and ATP content as well as
lactate + pyruvate production were much lower. Recently we
found a cytochrome P-450 content of twice the normal value,
in hepatocytes obtained from a 25 year old woman who died
five days after massive consumption of barbiturates
(Guillouzo et al, 1985). In addition, within a few hours
hepatocytes cannot perform all their functional capacities,
i.e. conjugate some drugs or respond to inducers.

**Table 1.   Factors influencing functional capacity of
freshly isolated hepatocytes.**

Genetic polymorphisms
Nutritional status of the donor
Premedication
Liver disease
Time separating liver resection from the dissociation
  process
Cell viability after liver dissociation

Therefore, hepatocyte cultures theoretically represent
the only in vitro model for long-term studies in a well-
defined environment. We have tested various culture
conditions and found that both cell survival and
maintenance of specific functions can vary greatly
depending upon the conditions used.
When seeded at the density of about $0.5 - 0.8 \times 10^6$
cells per ml of medium in conventional culture conditions
(i.e. in polystyrene flasks in a nutrient medium containing
fetal calf serum) about 60% of adult human hepatocytes
attach to the plastic within a few hours, aggregate and
form monolayers of granular epithelial cells (Figure 2a).
When the cells are attached, and every day thereafter, the
medium containing hydrocortisone hemisuccinate is renewed.
The first medium renewal is usually performed ater 4-6
hours but must be delayed to 10 hours or more when plating
efficiency and spreading are low. As a rule, human
hepatocytes attach and spread more slowly than do rat

Figure 2.   Phase-contrast micrographs of cultured adult
human hepatocytes.

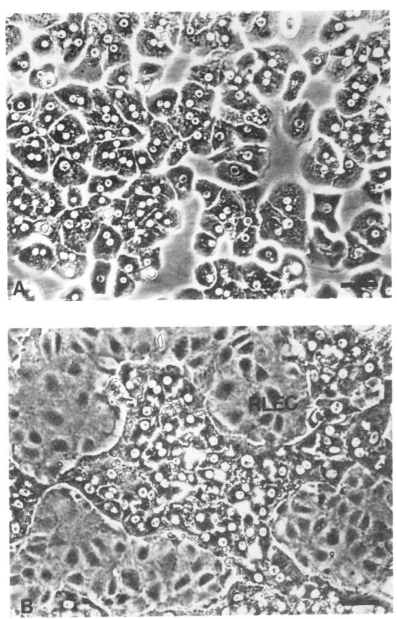

A : 2-day pure culture; B : 12-day co-culture with rat
liver epithelial cells (RLEC). Bar : 40μm.

hepatocytes. This difference probably results from longer
treatment of human hepatocytes with collagenase and time
separating liver resection or removal from the beginning of
perfusion.

In conventional culture conditions, human hepatocytes
survive for 2 or 3 weeks. During the first week, they
exhibit a fine structure similar to that found in in vivo
cells and express specific functions at high levels.
However quantitative variations occur probably due to the
new environment which is dramatically different from that
existing in vivo. Thus, the albumin secretion rate is
stimulated for 5-6 days before dropping (Clement et al,
1984). Total cytochrome P-450 content progressively
declines although it still represents about 50% of its
initial value after 7-8 days. However, it is increased
after 3 daily additions of 3.2mM sodium phenobarbital and
no major changes appear to occur in the isozymic pattern.
Indeed two isozymes (cytochrome P-450-5 and P-450-8) which
correspond to the two major families of cytochrome P-450
are well expressed for several days (Guillouzo et al, 1985)
and the heterogenous cell distribution observed in vivo is
retained in culture (Ratanasavahn et al, 1986). Other
enzymes, such as epoxide hydrolase and NADPH-cytochrome c
reductase are still well maintained (Ratanasavanh et al,
1986).

That drug metabolising enzymes remain active for
several days is well demonstrated by identification of the
metabolites of various drugs formed after a 24h incubation
(Begue et al, 1983; Guillouzo et al, 1986). As summarised
in Table 2 the major pathways are demonstrated for at least
4 days in pure human hepatocyte cultures. These findings
clearly demonstrate that in primary culture human
hepatocytes are more stable than rat hepatocytes,
particularly with respect to the cytochrome P-450 dependent
monooxygenase system (Guillouzo, 1986).

Recently, we have used short-term primary cultures of
adult hepatocytes from rat, rabbit and man to study species
differences in drug metabolism. Ketotifen was selected as
a model substrate because its metabolic pathways are well
known and different in man and several animal species. The
major in vivo pathways were demonstrated in vitro, namely
oxidation in rat hepatocytes, oxidation, glucuronidation
and sulphation in rabbit hepatocytes, reduction and
glucuronidation in human hepatocytes (Le Bigot et al,
1986).

Among the various conditions proposed to enhance
survival of rodent hepatocytes with maintenance of specific
functions the most promising one seems to be co-culture

Table 2.   Metabolic pathways of Ketotifen, Pindolol and Fluperlapine in man and in cultured adult human hepatocytes.

Drug	Metabolic Pathways	In Vivo	In Vitro	Reference
Ketotifen	Reduction	+	+	Begue et al 1983
	Glucuron-idation	+	+	Le Bigot et al
Pindolol	Oxidation	+	+	Guillouzo, Begue,
	Sulphation	+	+	Maurer & Koch
	Glucuron-idation	+	+	(unpublished results)
Fluperla-pine	N-oxidation	+	+	Guillouzo, Begue,
	N-demethylation	+	+	Maurer and Koch
	Sulphation	+	+	(unpublished
	Glucuroni-dation	+	+	results)

Metabolites from the three drugs (Sandoz) were determined in urine and in culture media after a 24h incubation with ^{14}C-drugs. All pathways indicated as present in vitro were identified at least during the first 4 days of culture.

with rat liver epithelial cells (Figure 2b). Indeed, rat hepatocytes were found to survive for several weeks in co-culture and to express specific functions at higher levels and for longer periods than in pure culture (Guguen-Guillouzo et al, 1983). Direct contacts between the two cell types are required; they do not involve intercellular junctions but rather specific membrane protein(s) (Guguen-Guillouzo, 1986). Corticosteroids but not serum must be added to the nutrient medium. The co-culture system has been successfully applied to human hepatocytes. As with rat hepatocytes, these cells interact with rat liver epithelial cells and in these conditions they may survive for several months (Clement et al, 1984). Both secretion of plasma proteins and drug metabolism capacity are better maintained than in pure culture. Thus, whereas glucuronidation of ketotifen is no longer detected by day 6, it is still active ater 3 weeks in co-culture (Begue et al, 1983). Drug metabolising enzymes may respond to inducers. A 2-fold increase in the cytochrome P-450 concentration was measured after 3 daily additions of 3.2mM sodium phenobarbital in 9·days adult human hepatocyte co-cultures.

Long-term studies on cultured human hepatocytes remain scarce. There is no well conducted study related to genetic polymorphism. Important differences in drug metabolisms have been reported during the first 24h of culture (Moore and Gould, 1984; Tee et al, 1985) but whether they were related to genetic polymorphism or to one of other factors listed in Table 1 was not elucidated. Clearly a large number of different hepatocyte populations would have to be investigated to clarify this major problem.

PRESERVATION OF HUMAN HEPATOCYTES AFTER FREEZING

Because of the irregular availability of human liver samples and the large numbers of cells obtained from a single perfusion, a method for storing hepatocytes is needed. Cryopreservation appears to be the only conceivable method. A successful freezing protocol must yield stocks of cells that can be restored to full activity. Most cryopreservation protocols have been devised for rat hepatocytes and they have stressed the importance of the cryoprotectant and its concentration, the cooling rate and the conditions of thawing (Table 3). Only one differs markedly, Gomez-Lechon et al (1984) have reported that the cooling rate is critical and must be fast. However, to our knowledge, these findings have not yet been confirmed. Freezing of one human liver cell suspension has also been reported (Moore and Gould, 1984). All the results underline that cell viability is decreased and metabolic activities are impaired after freezing (Table 3). Cell viability was usually determined by the trypan blue exclusion test, which cannot be considered as a good functional test. Moreover, the cells were used either just after thawing or within 1-2 days, therefore before damage repair. During the last months we have reconsidered freezing protocols in order to find conditions which allow hepatocytes to attach to a support and to repair their damage in culture. This study was performed on rat hepatocytes and will be published elsewhere (Chesne et al, manuscript in preparation). In outline, hepatocytes were suspended in the nutrient medium containing 10% fetal calf serum and augmented with DMSO (10%), glycerol (1%) and 1,2-propanediol (1%). The freezing rate was $1^{O}C/min$ in a Minicool LC40 (distributed by CFFPO, Sassenage France).

Table 3. Freezing conditions and functional capacity of cryopreserved hepatocytes.

SPECIES	CRYO-PROTECTANT	COOLING RATE °C/MIN	VIABILITY (%)	ATTACH-MENT (%)	COMMENTS	REFERENCES
Rat	10% DMSO	2-7	80-85	ND	Gluconeogenesis impaired	Le Cam et al (1976)
Rat	12% DMSO	1-2	60-70	28	Metabolic activities impaired	Nutt et al (1980) Fuller et al (1982)
Rat	10% DMSO	1	80	-	Metabolic activation of cyclophosphamide preserved	Karlber and Lindahl-Kiessling (1981)
Rat	10% DMSO	1	70-80	-	Ectopic transplantation	Kusano et al (1981)
Rat	20% DMSO	1	80	66	Microsomal associated functions decreased after 24h	Novicki et al (1982)
Rat	10% DMSO	2-39	78	59	Metabolic activities much better preserved in fast frozen cells after 24h	Gomez-Lechon et al (1984)
Human	10% DMSO	1	78	-	Benzopyrene metabolism reduced after 24h	Moore and Gould (1984)
Rat	10% DMSO	1-2	42	37	Faster decrease of the cytochrome P-450 content after 20h	Jackson et al (1985)
Rat	10% DMSO 1% Glycerol 1,2 propanediol	1	66	40	Long-term survival in co-culture with maintenance of albumin secretion and paracetamol	Chesne et al (in preparation)
Human	"	1	75	35	Long term survival in co-culture with maintenance of active albumin secretion	Chesne et al (in preparation)

After the temperature was reduced to $-50^{\circ}C$ the ampoules were placed in liquid nitrogen. Ater rapid thawing, the cells were set up either as conventional culture or as co-culture. The percentage of attached cells represent about 40% compared to that obtained with unfrozen cells. Cryopreserved cells attached and spread more slowly and functional activities were temporarily impaired. Functional activities were restored much better in co-culture than in pure culture indicating that this system is more suitable. In co-culture frozen hepatocytes were able to survive for several weeks, to secrete plasma proteins and to metabolise paracetamol at rates similar to those found with unfrozen cells. Two human hepatocyte populations were also investigated and the results were similar to those observed with rat hepatocytes. The cells also had lower plating efficiency than did unfrozen heptocytes. However, both fine structure and biochemical activities were improved particularly in co-culture after a few days. In co-culture frozen human hepatocytes exhibited a well-preserved fine structure (Figure 3) and albumin production was high. All our experiments lead to the conclusions that : 1) cell viability after cryopreservation must be defined on a functional basis and attachment to a support seems to be a good criterion; 2) the percentage of attached cells after cryopreservation may greatly depend on some of the factors listed in Table 1; 3) several hours are required for damage repair. Therefore we believe that the co-culture system which allows hepatocytes to survive for several weeks, is appropriate for studies on cryopreserved human hepatocytes. Since, only functionally active cells survive this makes possible comparisons between cultures from various donors.

ACKNOWLEDGEMENTS

We thank Mrs. M. Rissel for preparing the micrographs and A. Vannier for typing the manuscript.

REFERENCES

Begue, J.M., Le Bigot, J.F., Guguen-Guillouzo, C., Kiechel, J.R. and Guillouzo, A. (1983). Biochem. Pharmacol, 32, 1643.

Bissell, D.M. and Guzelian, P.S. (1980). Ann. NY Acad. Sci, 349. 77.

Clement, B., Guguen-Guillouzo, C., Campion, J.P., Glaise, D., Bourel, M. and Guillouzo, A. (1984). Hepatology, 4, 373.

Figure 3. Electron micrographs of cultured adult human hepatocytes after cryopreservation.

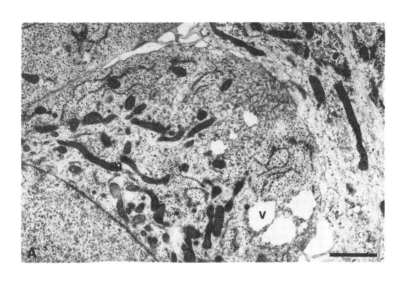

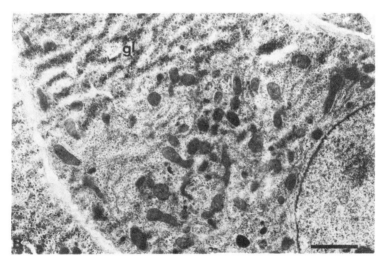

A : 10-day pure culture; B : 10-day co-culture. While in pure culture, hepatocytes contained vacuoles (v) and elongated mitochondria (m), in co-culture, they exhibit a typical fine structure with large amounts of glycogen particles (gl). Hepatocytes were stored for 1 month in liquid nitrogen. Bar : 1µm.

Fuller, B.J., Grout, B.W. and Woods, R.J. (1982). Cryobiology, 19, 493.

Gomez-Lechon, M.J., Lopez, P. and Castell, J.V. (1984). In Vitro, 20, 826.

Guguen-Guillouzo, C. (1986). In "Isolated and Cultured Hepatocytes" (Eds. Guillouzo, A. and Guguen-Guillouzo, C). J. Libbey, London and INSERM Paris, p. 259.

Guguen-Guillouzo, C. and Guillouzo, A. (1983). Mol. Cell. Biochem, 53/54, 35.

Guguen-Guillouzo, C., Bourel, M. and Guillouzo, A. (1986). In "Progress in Liver Disease" (Eds. Popper H. and Schaffner, F). Grune and Stratton, Orlando, Vol VIII, p.33.

Guguen-Guillouzo, C., Campion, J.P., Brissot, P., Glaise, D., Launois, B., Bourel, M. and Guillouzo, A. (1982). Cell. biol. Int. Rep. 6, 625.

Guguen-Guillouzo, C., Clement, B., Baffet, G., Beaumont, C., Morel-Chany, E., Glaise, D. and Guillouzo, A. (1983). Exp. Cell Res, 143, 47.

Guillouzo, A. (1986). In "Isolated and Cultured Hepatocytes" (Eds. Guillouzo, A. and Guguen-Guillouzo, C). J. Libbey London and INSERM Paris, p.313.

Guillouzo, A., Beaune, P., Gascoin, M.N., Begue, J.M., Campion, J.P., Guengerich, F.P. and Guguen-Guillouzo, C. (1985). Biochem. Pharmacol, 34, 2991.

Guillouzo, A., Begue, J.M., Maurer, G. and Koch, P. (1986). Submitted for publication.

Houssin, D., Capron, M., Celier, C., Cresteil, T., Demaugre, F. and Beaune, P. (1983). Life Sci, 33, 1805.

Jackson, .B.A., Davies, J.E. and Chipman, J.K. (1985). Biochem. Pharmacol, 34, 3389.

Karlber, I. and Lindahl-Kiessling, K. (1981). Mut. Res. 85, 441.

Kusano, M., Ebata, H., Onishi, T., Saito, T. and Mito, M. (1981). Transplant. Proc, 13, 848.

Le Bigot, J.F., Begue, J.M., Kiechel, J.R. and Guillouzo, A. (1986). Life Sci, in press.

Le Cam, A., Guillouzo, A. and Freychet, P. (1976). Exp. Cell. Res, 98, 382.

Moore, C.J. and Gould, M.N. (1984) Carcinogenesis, 5, 1577.

Novicki, D.L., Irons, G.P., Strom, S.P., Jirtle, R. and Michalopoulos, G, (1982). In Vitro, 18, 382.

Nutt, L.H., Attenburrow, V.D. and Fuller, B.J. (1980). Cryo-Lett, 1, 513.

Ratanasavanh, D., Beaune, P., Baffet, G., Rissel, M., Kremers, P., Guengerich, F.P. and Guillouzo, A. (1986). J. Histochem. Cytochem, 34, 527.

Reese, G.A. and Byard, J.R. (1981). In Vitro, 17, 935.

Rojkind, M., Gatmaitan, Z., Mackensen, S., Giambrone, M.A., Ponce, P. and Reid, L. (1981). J. Cell. Biol, 87, 255.

Sirica, A.E. and Pitot, H. (1980). Pharmacol. Rev, 31, 205.

Strom, S.C., Jirtle, R.L., Jones, R.S., Novicki, D.L., Rosenberg, M.R., Novotny, A., Irons, G., McLain, J.R. and Michalopoulos, G.M. (1982). J. Natl. Cancer Inst. 68, 771.

Tee, L.B., Seddon, T., Boobis, A.R. and Davies, D.S. (1985). Brit. J. Clin. Pharmacol, 19, 279.

DNA CLONING : TECHNOLOGY AND APPLICATIONS TO DRUG METABOLISM

Ian R. Phillips[1] Elizabeth A. Shephard[2] and Alan Ashworth[2]

[1]Department of Biochemistry, St. Bartholomew's Hospital Medical College, University of London, Charterhouse Square, London. EC1M 6BQ. UK and [2]Department of Biochemistry, University College London, Gower Street, London. WC1E 6BT, UK.

INTRODUCTION

A fundamental goal of research on drug metabolism is to understand the molecular mechanisms that enable organisms to metabolise the extremely wide range of both naturally occurring and synthetic substances that are used as therapeutic drugs. Such metabolic versatility can largely be ascribed to: (1) the multiplicity of cytochromes P-450; (ii) the relatively low substrate specificity of many of these proteins; and (iii) the ability of organisms selectively to induce the appropriate member of the cytochrome P-450 super-family of proteins required to metabolise a particular drug. Another important question in drug metabolism concerns the molecular basis of inherited individual human variations in the metabolism of many drugs. The application of recombinant DNA technology has already led to a dramatic increase in our understanding of many of these topics. The use of this technology to investigate these and other aspects of drug metabolism will undoubtedly increase in the future. In this paper we describe methods for the synthesis and isolation of cloned DNA sequences and then consider how such cloned DNAs can be used in research on drug metabolism.

WHAT IS DNA CLONING?

In contrast to proteins, individual DNA molecules, being composed of only four different nucleotides, are extremely difficult to purify by standard biochemical methods. We have to resort, instead, to a biological technique known as "DNA cloning". The basis of this technique is the transformation of a population of bacteria with a mixture of DNA molecules, under conditions where each bacterium takes up only a single molecule of foreign DNA. The DNAs can then be "isolated" from each other by separating the bacteria into individual colonies i.e. "clones". In effect, DNA cloning is merely a means of isolating and amplifying specific genes. DNA cloning became possible only after many fundamental discoveries and technical advances, These include methods for: (i) generating suitable DNA molecules; (ii) cutting and joining DNA molecules at specific sites; (iii) propagating foreign DNAs in bacteria and (iv) screening bacteria for the DNA of interest.

CONSTRUCTION OF A cDNA LIBRARY

Figure 1 illustrates a standard procedure for constructing a cDNA library. Total RNA is extracted from the appropriate tissue and poly $(A)^+$-containing mRNA is isolated by oligo (dT)-cellulose affinity chromatography. Using oligo(dT) as a primer the enzyme RNA-dependent DNA polymerase (often referred to as reverse transcriptase) can synthesise a complementary DNA (or cDNA) copy of the mRNA. The mRNA template is then removed by alkaline digestion and a second DNA strand is synthesised either by reverse transcriptase or the Klenow fragment of E. coli DNA polymerase. The hairpin loop is removed by digestion with the single-strand specific nuclease S1, leaving a double stranded cDNA. The population of cDNA molecules reflects the abundance of mRNA species in the original preparation. If foreign DNAs were introduced directly into bacteria they would almost certainly be degraded. Even if they survived intact, being incapable of replicating themselves, the DNA molecules would be "diluted" as the bacteria divided. To ensure the survival and propagation of cDNAs in bacteria they are inserted into a suitable vector such as the plasmid pAT153. This contains an origin of replication, enabling it to replicate independently in bacteria, and two genes coding for drug resistence factors.

Bacterial enzymes known as restriction endonucleases cut double-stranded DNA molecules at specific sites (usually four or six base pairs long). Many of these enzymes make staggered cuts that create short four-base single-stranded complementary tails on the ends of each fragment. A fragment of DNA produced by digestion with such a restriction endonuclease can anneal by complementary base pairing to any other DNA fragment generated by the same enzyme. The fragments can then be covalently joined by the enzyme T4 DNA ligase. In this way it is possible to

Figure 1. A standard procedure for the construction of a cDNA library (see text for details).

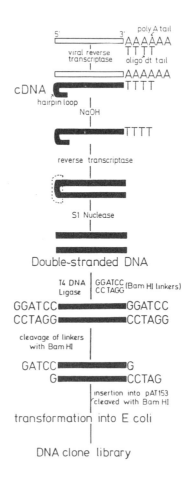

join DNA molecules from different sources thus creating a hybrid or "recombinant" DNA molecule.

The plasmid pAT153 contains a single recognition site for the restriction endonuclease Bam HI. Recognition sites for Bam HI can be artificially generated at the end of the cDNAs by attaching small synthetic oligonucleotides (known as "linkers") that contains the appropriate sequence. Digestion of the linker-cDNA molecules with Bam HI will create DNA fragments capable of annealing with Bam HI-cut pAT153 to generate recombinant, or hybrid, plasmids.

Treatment of the bacterium E.coli with Ca^{2+} ions followed by a brief "heat-shock" renders their membranes permeable to DNA. In this state the bacteria are "competent" to take up a recombinant plasmid. This process, known as "transformation" is relatively inefficient. However, the use of vectors carrying genes for antibiotic resistance provides a means of selecting the bacteria containing a recombinant plasmid. The insertion of foreign DNA into the Bam HI site of pAT 153 inactivates the tetracycline-resistance gene, leaving the ampicillin-resistance gene functional. Thus, bacteria that have taken up the plasmid can be selected by growth in a medium containing ampicillin. The sensitivity of the ampicillin-resistent bacteria to tetracycline will confirm the successful insertion of a cDNA into the plasmid.

The transformed bacteria, which constitute a "cDNA library" are grown as individual colonies on nitrocellulose filters. All cells in a colony are derived from a single bacterium and thus represent a bacterial "clone". The conditions used for transformation ensure that each bacterium takes up no more than one recombinant plasmid. Thus every cell in a colony will harbour an identical plasmid, whereas other colonies will contain plasmids carrying different cDNA inserts. Therefore, by cloning the bacteria we have, in effect, produced clones of foreign DNA. This process is referred to as "molecular cloning".

Before constructing a cDNA library it may be useful to ascertain the abundance of the mRNA of interest. This can be done by the following procedure. Total RNAs or polyribosomes are translated in an in vitro system such as a rabbit reticulocyte or wheat germ lysate containing a radiolabelled amino acid such as $[^{35}S]$methionine. The translation products are then immunoprecipitated with an antibody to the protein of interest and the immunoprecipitate is electrophoresed through an SDS/polyacrylamide gel. Precipitated radiolabelled antigen can be identified by fluorography, cut out of the gel and its radioactivity determined. The representation of a cDNA in a library can be increased by enriching the corresponding mRNA before synthesising cDNA. This can be achieved through size fractionation of the mRNA by density gradient centrifugation or gel electrophoresis. But, unless the mRNA is of an unusual size this approach will not result in a very substantial enrichment. A greater degree of enrichment can be obtained by using a specific antibody to immunoprecipitate polyribosomes that are actively synthesizing the corresponding antigen and thus contain the corresponding mRNA. However, unless the mRNA

is of extremely low abundance, the ability to construct
large libraries and to screen them at high colony densities
obviates the need for enrichment of mRNAs.

SCREENING A cDNA LIBRARY

Having constructed a cDNA library, containing perhaps
millions of independent clones, we are faced with the
"needle in the haystack" problem of identifying bacterial
colonies containing a specific cDNA.

The basis of many screening procedures is a technique
known as colony hybridisation. Baterial colonies are
replica-plated onto nitrocellulose filters. One set of
replica filters is retained as master filters. The
bacteria on the other set of filters are lysed and their
DNA is denatured and fixed to the filter. The filter is
then incubated with a ^{32}P radiolabelled single-stranded DNA
complementary in sequence to the mRNA of interest. The DNA
will bind to its complementary sequence by base-pairing.
The colonies that contain this sequence can be identified
by radioautography and picked from the corresponding master
filter. This procedure would, of course be applicable only
for isolating cDNAs of highly abundant mRNAs (e.g. globin
in reticulocytes) or highly enriched mRNAs. A modification
of the technique, referred to as "differential colony
hybridisation" allows the identification of cDNA clones
coding for mRNAs present in different abundance in two
similar RNA populations. This technique is particularly
useful for mRNAs of enzymes involved in drug metabolism
because many of them are inducible. The utility of the
method is illustrated by the isolation of a cloned cDNA
coding for a phenobarbital-inducible cytochrome P-450
(Phillips et al, 1983). A cDNA library was constructed
representative of total mRNA from the livers of
phenobarbital treated rats. The library was plated in
triplicate on nitrocellulose filters. Each set of filters
was incubated with ^{32}-P-labelled single-stranded cDNAs
complementary to the entire population of liver mRNAs from
phenobarbital-treated, ß-napthoflavone-treated or untreated
rats. Because of variations in mRNA abundance bacterial
colonies that contain a plasmid coding for a phenobarbital-
inducible mRNA will give a more intense hybridisation
signal with "PB" cDNAs than with "NF" or "control" cDNAs.
We have used a similar approach to isolate cloned cDNAs
coding for ß-naphthoflavone-inducible cytochromes P-450
(Phillips et al, 1985a).

If the sequence of a protein is known it is possible to
identify its cDNA by screening a library with radiolabelled

synthetic oligonucleotides complementary in sequence to the corresponding mRNA. In practice a stretch of amino acid residues with low codon redundancy is chosen. A pool of short oligonucleotides (approx. 17 bases), representing all possible mRNAs coding for this stretch of amino acids, is synthesised. Alternatively, a single longer oligonucleotide (approx. 30 bases), synthesised on the basis of codon usage, can be used to screen the library under conditions that allow some mismatching of base-pairs.

Another powerful screening method involves the use of a specific antibody to detect bacteria synthesising the corresponding antigen. An advantage of this technique is that is requires no knowledge of the sequence of the protein. To ensure that the foreign DNA is efficiently expressed by the bacteria the cDNA is inserted adjacent to a strong prokaryotic transcriptional promotor in a so-called "expression vector" such as λgt11 (Young and Davis, 1983). For screening purposes the bacterial proteins, rather than the DNA, are fixed to a nitrocellulose filter. The filter is incubated with the appropriate antibody and the position of the bound antibody is visualised immunochemically by means of a second antibody-enzyme complex. We have recently used this method to isolate cDNAs coding for cytochrome P-450 reductase, cytochrome b5, cytochrome b5 reductase, some species of cytochrome P-450, serum albumin and fatty acid binding protein.

The identity of an isolated cDNA clone can be checked by a technique known as hybrid-selected translation. Plasmid DNA is isolated from the bacteria, denatured and fixed to a small piece of nitrocellulose filter. The filter is incubated with a population of poly $(A)^+$ RNA that contains the appropriate mRNA species. The mRNA selectively bound by the cDNA is eluted and translated in a cell-free system containing (^{35}S)-methionine. The translation product of the selected mRNA is visualised by SDS/polyacrylamide gel electrophoresis followed by fluorography (Phillips et al, 1983). The identity of the protein can be confirmed by immunoprecipitation of the translation product with an appropriate antibody.

APPLICATION OF CLONED DNAs TO PROBLEMS RELEVANT TO DRUG METABOLISM

Over the past five years cloned DNA sequences coding for many cytochromes P-450 and other proteins involved in Phase I and Phase II of drug metabolism have been isolated. The utility of cloned DNAs for research on drug metabolism will be illustrated by reference to experiments on cytochromes P-450.

STRUCTURE AND EVOLUTION OF CYTOCHROMES P-450 AND THEIR GENES

One of the most fundamental properties of a protein is its amino acid sequence. Despite the introduction of automated methods for protein sequencing this can be determined more rapidly via sequencing of cloned DNA. To date over 25 distinct cytochromes P-450 have been identified. The homology of their amino acid sequences ranges from ∼20% to ∼97%. On the basis of sequence homology members of the cytochrome P-450 superfamily of proteins have been assigned to individual families (homology ∼50%) and sub-families (homology ∼70%) (Nebert et al, 1986). So far eight different families have been identified, some of which contain only one known member whereas others have more than ten. From a knowledge of the primary structure of a cytochrome P-450, predictions can be made concerning its secondary structure and its topology within membranes of the endoplasmic reticulum (Haniu et al, 1986).

By comparing the sequences of orthologous proteins of different species we can estimate their rate of evolution. Cytochromes P-450 appear to have evolved relatively rapidly, with the time taken for a 1% change in sequence (known as the unit evolutionary period) being only 2-2.5 million years. Despite this rapid rate of evolution regions have been identified that are conserved among all known cytochromes P-450 (Gotoh et al, 1983) and hence are likely to be involved in common functions of these proteins. An important application of cloned DNAs is their use as molecular hybridisation probes for the corresponding mRNA and gene(s). The technique of Southern blot hybridisation enables us to detect fragments of DNA whose sequence is identical or very similar to that of a cloned DNA. After digestion of genomic DNA by a restriction endonuclease the DNA fragments are resolved on the basis of size by electrophoresis through an agarose gel. The DNA is transferred from the gel to a nitrocellulose filter and incubated with a radiolabelled cloned DNA. The fragments of genomic DNA homologous to the cloned sequence are revealed by radioautography.

An analogous technique referred to as Northern blotting involving the size fractionation of RNA molecules by electrophoresis through an agarose gel under denaturing conditions permits us to detect, size and quantify specific mRNAs. Southern and Northern blotting provide the basis for many applications of recombinant DNA technology.

Analysis of genomic DNA by Southern blotting reveals that some cytochromes P-450 are encoded by multigene families whereas others have only one gene (Ashworth et al, 1984). Genes coding for several cytochromes P-450 have been isolated by screening libraries of genomic DNA with the corresponding cloned cDNA. The internal organisation of the genes has been determined through a combination of hybridization experiments and DNA sequencing. Genes coding for members of different P-450 families differ in size, in the number and position of their intervening sequences and in their chromosomal localisation. Analysis of the genomic DNA can also provide an insight into the evolution of cytochrome P-450 gene families. It appears that the major phenobarbital-inducible P-450 was established as a multigene family before the adaptive radiation of mammals about 85 million years ago. The gene family was expanded in rodents and rabbits about 60 million years ago, and in rats there has been a further amplification within the last 20 million years (Phillips et al, 1985a). In contrast the major 3-methylcholanthrene inducible P-450 and an isosafrole-inducible P-450 known as P-450c and P-450d, respectively have been conserved throughout rodent and rabbit evolution as single genes (Nebert et al, 1985).

CONTROL OF GENE EXPRESSION

The ability of an organism to metabolise drugs is influenced by its genetic composition, physiological factors such as age and sex, and environmental factors such as diet and exposure to foreign chemicals including drugs themselves. To a large extent the effect of these factors is mediated via changes in the amounts of the proteins (particularly cytochromes P-450) that are responsible for drug metabolism. Clearly the elucidation of the mechanisms involved in controlling the synthesis of these proteins will have important implications for our understanding of drug metabolism. The isolation of appropriate cloned DNAs has made it possible to address this question directly. Our own group, for example, has used a cloned cDNA coding for the major phenobarbital-inducible cytochrome P-450 (PB P-450) to investigate the mechanism of induction of this protein by phenobarbital. A key question is the level at which the induction is controlled. The results of these experiments are summarised in Table 1. The induction of the protein is mediated by a 20-fold increase in its 2100 nuclectide-long mRNA. In turn, this can be almost entirely accounted for by an increase in the rate of transcription

Table 1.   Mechanism of induction of PB P-450 by phenobarbital.

	FOLD INDUCTION BY PHENOBARBITAL
Total Cytochrome P-450	2-3
PB P-450	43
PB P-450 mRNA (translatable)	22
PB P-450 mRNA (cytoplasmic)	20
PB P-450 mRNA (nuclear)	20
Transcription of PB P-450 gene(s)	16

of the gene(s) coding for PB P-450 (Pike et al, 1985).
Thus to induce PB P-450 in liver microsomal membranes
phenobarbital must act, either directly, or indirectly, at
the level of the genome. Analysis by Southern blotting
revealed that phenobarbital caused no amplification or
rearrangement of PB P-450 genes. The induction of other
cytochromes P-450 by compounds such such as 3-
methylcholanthrene is also mediated at the level of gene
transcription (Gonzalez et al, 1984). Recently, workers
have begun to investigate the developmental stage-specific
and tissue-specific regulation of cytochrome P-450 gene
expression. An interesting aspect of this work is the use
of synthetic oligonucleotides to distinguish mRNAs coding
for two closely related members of the phenobarbital-
inducible cytochrome P-450 gene family (Omiecinski, 1986).
    Having established that the induction of cytochromes P-
450 is largely controlled at the level of gene
transcription it is important to determine the DNA
sequences involved in regulating the expression of these
genes. The approach taken is to fuse various sections of a
cytochrome P-450 gene to a gene coding for a readily
identifiable enzyme such as chloramphenicol
acetyltransferase (CAT). The ability of the cytochrome P-
450 gene sequences to respond to an inducer by increasing
the synthesis of CAT, is then tested following transfection
of the gene constructs into a suitable eukaryotic cell
line. This method has identified both positive and
negative cis-acting DNA sequences and enhancer-like
elements in 3-methylcholanthrene inducible cytochrome P-450
genes (Jones et al, 1985). One of the next steps will be
the identification of trans-acting protein factors that

regulate gene expression by interacting with these DNA sequences.

PB P-450 mRNA is also induced, albeit it to a lesser extent than by phenobarbital, by foreign compounds such as dexamethasone, pregnenolone-16α-carbonitrile and isosafrole, all of which are known to induce other cytochrome P-450 isozymes (Ryan et al, 1980; Schuetz et al, 1984). We have also found that PB P-450 mRNA is induced by naturally occurring terpenoids such as camphor and pinene. In contrast β -naphthoflavone, although an inducer of certain cytochromes P-450, actually decreases the amount of PB mRNA (Shephard et al, 1982; Phillips et al, 1983). Thus it is evident that a specific isozyme can be induced by several structurally different compounds; certain foreign compounds can also induce more than one species of cytochrome P-450; and some inducers of cytochromes P-450 can simultaneously decrease the amounts of other cytochromes P-450. The lack of specificity in the induction of cytochromes P-450, together with the low substrate specificity exhibited by many of these proteins, are undoubtedly important factors contributing towards the ability of organisms to detoxify such an extremely wide range of naturally occurring and synthetic hydrophobic foreign compounds.

MOLECULAR PHARMACOGENETICS

Individual human variations are well known in the metabolism of several therapeutic drugs, and there is evidence that similar variations exist in the activation of chemical carcinogens. This metabolic variability may be due, in part, to genetically determined factors relating to the structure or expression of cytochrome P-450 isozymes. The isolation and characterisation of cloned DNAs coding for human cytochromes P-450 will greatly facilitate the elucidation of the structure of these proteins and is essential for investigating the molecular basis of genetically determined variations in the metabolism of foreign compounds. Our approach (and that of other groups) has been to use cloned DNAs coding for cytochrome P-450 of animals to isolate, from a human liver cDNA library, cloned sequences coding for the corresponding proteins of man (Phillips et al, 1985b). This has the advantage of bypassing completely the need to purify and characterise human cytochrome P-450 proteins. Recently, others have isolated human cytochrome P-450 cDNA clones by screening a human liver expression library with antibodies raised to purified human proteins that are associated with known polymorphisms in drug metabolism (Umbenhaer et al, 1986). Cloned DNAs coding for human cytochromes P-450 will be used to investigate the molecular genetic basis of inherited variations in drug metabolism. If correlations can be established between individual haplotypes and inherited variations in the metabolism of foreign compounds it may be possible to design genetic tests to identify those at high risk from treatment with particular drugs, and individuals prone to developing certain chemically-induced cancers.

PROTEIN ENGINEERING OF CYTOCHROMES P-450

Two important questions concerning the mechanism of action of cytochromes P-450 are (i) how are single species of cytochrome P-450 able to bind and metabolise many structurally different compounds, and (ii) how can these proteins catalyse some extraordinarily difficult chemical transformations?

Although considerable progress has been made in the past two decades on the catalytic cycle of the cytochrome P-450 mediated mono-oxygenase, virtually nothing is known about the location, within cytochromes P-450, of regions involved in important functions such as catalysis, haem-binding and interaction with other proteins of the mono-oxygenase. Recently it has been shown that, after transformation with a DNA sequene coding for a mammalian cytochrome P-450 under the control of a strong yeast promotor, yeast cells are capable of expressing the foreign gene and accumulating high levels of functional protein product (Oeda et al, 1985).

This system together with techniques of site-directed mutagenesis, presents the opportunity of testing the effect on protein function of altering specific amino acid residues, and hence provides a powerful means of investigating the mechanism of action of cytochromes P-450. Indeed, through the use of this technology, it may be possible, in the future, to produce cytochromes P-450 possessing novel functions of potential use in the synthesis of new drugs.

ACKNOWLEDGEMENTS

Work in our own laboratories has been supported by the Medical Research Council and the Cancer Research Campaign.

REFERENCES

Ashworth, A., Shephard, E.A., Rabin, B.R. and Phillips,

I.R. (1984). Biochem. Soc. Trans, 12, 669.
Gonzalez, F.J., Tukey, R.H. and Nebert, D.W. (1984). Molec. Pharmacol, 26, 117.
Gotoh, O., Tagashira, Y., Iizuka, T. and Fujii-Kuriyama, Y. (1983). J. Biochem, 93, 807.
Haniu, M., Ryan, D.E., Levin, W. and Shively, J.E. (1986). Arch. Biochem. Biophys, 244, 323.
Jones, P.B.C., Galeazzi, D.R., Fisher, J.M. and Whitlock, J.P. Jr (1985). Science 227, 1499.
Nebert, D.W. and Gonalez, F.J. (1985). TIPS 6, 160.
Nebert, D.W., Kimura, S. and Gonzalez, F.J. (1985). in "Microsomes and Drug Oxidations" (Ed. Boobis, A.R., Caldwell, J. De Matteis, F. and Elcombe, C.R). Taylor and Francis, London and Philadelphia, P.145.
Nebert, D.W., Adesnik, M., Johnson, E., Kemper, B., Phillips, I.R. and Waterman, M.R. (1986). DNA in press.
Oeda, K., Sakaki, T. and Ohkawa, H. (1985). DNA 4, 203.
Omiecinski, C.J. (1986). Nucl. Acids Res, 14, 1525.
Phillips, I.R., Shephard, E.A., Ashworth, A. and Rabin, B.R. (1983). Gene, 24, 41.
Phillips, I.R., Shephard, E.A., Rabin, B.R., Ashworth, A. and Pike, S.F. (1985a). in "Microsomes and Drug oxidations" (Ed. by Boobis, A.R., Caldwell, J., DeMatteis, F. and Elcombe, C.R). Taylor and Francis, London and Philadelphia, p. 118.
Phillips, I.R., Shephard, E.A., Ashworth, A. and Rabin, B.R. (1985b). Proc. Natl. Acad. Sci, USA, 82, 983.
Pike, S.F., Shephard, E.A., Rabin, B.R. and Phillips, I.R. (1985). Biochem. Pharmacol, 34, 2489.
Ryan, D.E., Thomas, P.E. and Levin, W. (1980). J. Biol. Chem. 225, 7941.
Schuetz, E.G., Wrighton, S.A., Barwick, J.L. and Guzelian, P.S. (1984). J. Biol. Chem, 259, 1999.
Shephard, E.A., Phillips, I.R., Pike, S.F., Ashworth, A. and Rabin, B.R. (1982). FEBS LETT, 150, 375.
Sogawa, K., Gotoh, O., Kawajiri, K. and Fujii-Kuriyama, Y. (1984). Proc. Natl. Acad. Sci, USA 81, 5066.
Suwa, Y., Mizukami, Y., Sogawa, K. and Fujii-Kuriyama, Y. (1985). J. Biol. Chem, 260, 7980.
Umbenhaer, D.R., Lloyd, R.S. and Guengerich, F.P. (1986). Fed. Proc, 45, 1854.
Young, R.A. and Davis, R.W. (1983). Proc. Natl. Acad. Sci, USA 80,, 1194.

THE INTERFERON MEDIATED LOSS OF CYTOCHROME P-452

Kenneth W. Renton[1], Shabbir M. Moochhala[1], G. Gordon Gibson[2] and Ryszard J. Makowski[2]

[1]Department of Pharmacology, Dalhousie University, Halifax, N.S. Canada, [2] Department of Biochemistry, University of Surrey, Guildford, Surrey, England.

In both animals and man, cytochrome P-450 in the liver is depressed during viral infections and following the administration of interferon or interferon inducing agents (Renton and Mannering, 1976; Renton 1983). Initially evidence that interferon depressed drug biotransformation was obtained using mouse strains which had varying abilities to produce interferon (Singh and Renton, 1981) but more recently the utilisation of highly purified cloned interferons has provided unequivocal proof that interferon can be directly involved in the depression of drug biotransformation (Singh et al, 1982; Parkinson et al, 1982). In our laboratory we have demonstrated that the incorporation of labelled amino acids into cytochrome P-450-rich fractions isolated from liver microsomes was depressed by interferon and suggested that the synthesis of the apo-protein of cytochrome P-450 was impaired (Singh and Renton 1984). In more recent studies it has been suggested that interferon stimulates the synthesis of xanthine oxidase in the liver and that the free radicals produced by this enzyme destroy cytochrome P-450 within the membrane (Ghezzi et al, 1985; Deloria et al, 1985). This paper provides evidence to suport our initial idea that the loss of cytochrome P-450 involves a diminished synthesis of the hemoprotein.

Different isozymes of cytochrome P-450 were depressed to varying degrees by the interferon inducer poly rI.rC in rats treated with a variety of inducing agents. Cytochrome P-452 as measured by lauric acid hydroxylation was depressed by 60% and was the isoenzyme most affected. Synthesis of this isoenzyme was thereore utilised to investigate the effects of poly rI.rC on the cell free synthesis of cytochrome P-450.

Rats were treated with clofibrate (400 mg/kg for 3 days) to induce the levels of cytochrome P-452 in hepatic microsomes (Tamburini et al, 1984). RNA was then isolated from these induced animals 24 hours after the administration of poly rI.rC or saline using the method of Cox (1968). Total amounts of RNA isolated from both groups of animals were identical. The RNA was then translated in an in vitro cell free translation system (Bethesda Research Labs; Gaithesburg, Maryland, USA) and the incorporation of ^{35}S-methionine into protein determined (Pelham and Jackson 1976). The amount of label incorporated into TCA precipitable material was identical in both groups of animals (Table 1), indicating that the total translational capacity of the liver in poly rI.rC treated rats was identical to that in saline treated animals.

Table 1. The effects of poly rI.rC on the synthesis of cytochrome P-452 in a cell free translation system.

TREATMENT	TOTAL INCORPORATION IN TRANSLATION MIXTURE (cpm x 10^5/incubation mix)	SPECIFIC INCORPORATION INTO CYTOCHROME P-452 (cpm/µg RNA)
Control	2.63 ± 0.65	108 ± 26
Poly rI.rC	3.17 ± 0.47	55 ± 8 [*]

[*]Significantly different from control; P < 0.05; n=4
All animals received clofibrate (400 mg/kg for 3 days) and then poly rI.rC (10 mg/kg) or saline for twenty four hours before livers were homogenised and RNA isolated. Incorporation was measured as the amount of ^{35}S-methionine incorporated. Total incorporation was determined from the TCA-precipitable fraction of the translation incubation mixture. Specific incorporation was determined from the labelled material which bound to a specific anti-P-452 antibody and which was removed from the incubation mixture with an S. Aureus preparation.

Translation mixtures were then incubated with a specific antibody raised to purified cytochrome P-452 (Tamburini et al, 1984) and the immunoglobulin-cytochrome P-450 complex was adsorbed to a S. Aureus preparation. The

Figure 1. SDS-polyacrylamide gel electrophoresis of the protein which binds to anti-P-452 antibody following the in vitro translation of RNA isolated from clofibrate induced rats treated with poly rI.rC or saline. The major bands of radioactivity occurred at a molecular weight of approximately 53 kD.

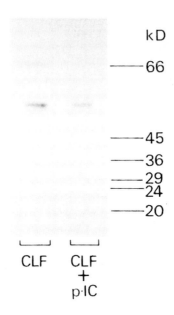

amount of ^{35}S-methionine incorporated into the protein binding to this antibody was only 51% of controls in the translation mixture containing RNA obtained from poly rI.rC treated rats (Table 1). SDS electrophoresis and autoradiography of the immune-adsorbed material indicated that a major band of incorporation occurred at a molecular weight of approximately 53 kD indicating that the translation product isolated was cytochrome P-452 (Figure 1). This band at 53kD was considerably less intense in the poly rI.rC treated animals compared to controls. This data clearly indicates that the interferon inducer depressed the capacity of the liver to translate the apo-protein of cytochrome P-452. Recent experiments in our laboratory also indicate that cytochrome P-447 (induced by β-naphtho-flavone), synthesis is impaired in similar manner.

These experiments provide evidence that interferon or interferon inducers are likely to depress cytochrome P-450 levels in the liver by diminishing the synthesis of the apo-protein.

ACKNOWLEDGEMENT

This work was supported by the Medical Research Councils of Canada and UK.

REFERENCES

Cox, R.A. (1968). Meth Enzymol, 12, 20.
Deloria, L., Gooderham, N. and Mannering, G.J. (1985). Biochem. Biophys. Res. Commun, 131, 109.
Ghezzi, P., Bianchi, M., Gianera, L., Landolfo, S. and Sajmona, M. (1985). Cancer Res, 45, 3444.
Parkinson, A., Lasker, J., Kramer, M.J., Huang, M.T., Thomas, P.E., Ryan, D.E., Reik, L.M., Norman, R.L., Levin, W. and Conney, A.H. (1982). Drug Metab. Dispos, 10, 579.
Pelham, H. and Jackson, R.J. (1976). Europ. J. Biochem, 67, 247.
Renton, K.W. (1983). in "Biological Basis of Detoxication". (Ed. by Caldwell, J. and Jakoby, W.B. Academic Press, New York, p.307.
Renton, K.W. and Mannering, G.J. (1976). Biochem. Biophys. Res. Commun, 73, 343.
Singh, G. and Renton, K.W. (1981). Mol. Pharmacol, 20, 681.
Singh, G. and Renton, K.W. (1984). Can. J. Physiol. Pharmacol, 62, 379.
Singh, G., Renton, K.W. and Stebbing, N. (1982). Biochem. Biophys. Res. Commun, 106, 1256.
Tamburini, P., Masson, H.A., Bains, S.K., Makowski, R.J., Morris, B. and Gibson, G.G. (1984). Eur. J. Biochem. 139, 235.

THE SUICIDAL REDUCTIVE ACTIVATION OF CARBON TETRACHLORIDE BY PROTOHAEM

Maurizio Manno[1,3], Laurence J. King[1] and Francesco De Matteis[2]

[1]Department of Biochemistry, Division of Pharmacology and Toxicology, University of Surrey, Guildford, Surrey, GU2 5XH, [2]MRC Laboratories, Toxicology Unit, Biochemical Pharmacology Section, Woodmansterne Road, Carshalton, Surrey, SM5 4EF. [3]Present address: Istituto di Medicina del Lavoro, Universita degli Studi di Padova, Via Facciolati 71, 35127 Padova, Italy.

INTRODUCTION

During the reductive metabolism of carbon tetrachloride (CCl_4) by NADPH-reduced microsomes, cytochrome P-450, the enzyme responsible for CCl_4 activation, is rapidly inactivated and in the process equimolar amounts of protohaem, the prosthetic group of cytochrome P-450, are also lost (de Groot and Haas, 1981). The CCl_4-dependent loss of haem is due to an irreversible change of the tetrapyrrolic ring (Manno et al, 1986). In these experiments the loss of cytochrome P-450 and haem were both significantly prevented by carbon monoxide (CO), suggesting that the destruction of cytochrome P-450 is a suicidal process where haem is both the site of CCl_4 activation and the target of its reactive metabolites.

The evidence presented here indicates that anaerobic haem itself may reductively activate CCl_4, and also undergo suicidal degradation. We have made use of this non-enzymatic model to study the mechanism of haem destruction by CCl_4 and a reverse phase ion pairing h.p.l.c technique has been developed to investigate the products of haem degradation.

MATERIAL AND METHODS

Chemicals and Biochemicals : [^{14}C]-CCl_4 was purchased from New England Nuclear Research Products (Boston, Mass, USA). Methaemalbumin (MHA), a water soluble complex of haem with human albumin (Sigma), was prepared by the method of Tenhunen et al (1968) using either unlabelled or ^{14}C-

labelled haem.

Assays : haem was measured by the pyridine/haemochrome assay (Paul et al, 1953) and by the oxalic acid method (Morrison, 1965). All incubations were in 0.1M phosphate buffer, pH 7.4, made anaerobic by bubbling with nitrogen and the addition of an oxygen-scavenging system comprising 600 U/ml catalase, 12.5 U/ml glucose oxidase and 60 mM D-glucose.

The H.P.L.C. Technique : A reverse phase ion pairing gradient elution method was developed for separation of haem products from haem. Pigments were extracted from the incubation mixture with two volumes of 80% methanol containing 20mM tetrabutylammonium hydroxide buffered with phosphate (TBA). Extracts were injected and eluted by mixtures of the two following solvents : A) 35% methanol in water, containing 2.5mM TBA, B) 95% methanol containing 1mM TBA. After one minute elution with 100% A, a 13 min linear gradient to 58.3% A in the A + B mixture was followed by a second linear gradient reaching 100% B in the following 7 min. This concentration was kept constant for the remaining 9 min. Separation was carried out on a column of 30cm x 3.9mm of internal diameter, packed with μ Bondapak C18 10μm particles (Waters) and fitted with a guard column of 3cm x 3.9mm packed with 30-38 μm particles (Whatman).

RESULTS AND DISCUSSION

A rapid loss (84% in 5 min) of haem was observed during the anaerobic incubation at $22^{\circ}C$ of 1.6 μM MHA with 1 mM CCl_4 and 2.9 mM sodium dithionite. The loss of haem in this non-enzymatic system was accompanied by an equimolar loss of its protoprophyrin IX moiety and was almost totally prevented by CO. When protoporphyrin IX itself was incubated with CCl_4/dithionite, no loss was observed. These results indicate that, in this non-enzymatic model, like for microsomal incubations, a) haem undergoes drastic modification of the tetrapyrrolic ring, b) a reduced free haem iron is necessary for CCl_4 activation.

When [^{14}C]-MHA was incubated anaerobically for 5 min without any addition (control) or with CCl_4/dithionite and the radioactivity was extracted in methanol/TBA, the recovery of radioactivity was in both cases quantitative, indicating that volatile products of haem were not formed as a result of CCl_4-dependent haem destruction. On injection of these extracts into the h.p.l.c. system, total radioactivity recovered was the same for control and CCl_4/dithionite incubations (94 and 93% respectively). Both the absorbance at 400nm and the radioactivity associated with the haem peak markedly decreased after treatment, but 40-50% of the injected radioactivity was found in several new non-haem fractions eluted immediately before or after haem. These new fractions showed, however, negligible absorbance at 400nm and no fluoresence.

When [^{14}C]-CCl$_4$ was incubated with MHA and sodium dithionite, approximately 20% of the injected radioactivity was found in those h.p.l.c fractions known, from the experiments with ^{14}C-labelled haem, to contain haem or haem products. When the CCl$_4$-dependent loss of haem and the amount of CCl$_4$ bound to haem products were compared, a one to one stoichiometry was found between haem loss and [^{14}C]-CCl$_4$-derived adduct formation, suggesting that one molecule of CCl$_4$ binds covalently to one molecule of haem.

CONCLUSIONS

1. A non-enzymatic model for the cytochrome P-450-dependent reductive activation of CCl$_4$ has been investigated by using methaemalbumin as a "suicidal" activator.
2. As with cytochrome P-450, the loss of haem caused by CCl$_4$ in this non-enzymatic model was accompanied by equimolar loss of its protoporphyrin IX ring and was prevented by carbon monoxide. Several unidentified products were partially separated from haem by a reverse phase iron pairing h.p.l.c. system and shown to contain radioactivity from prelabelled haem and also from ^{14}C-labelled CCl$_4$. In addition, the amount of CCl$_4$-derived radioactivity bound to haem products was calculated to be equimolar to the amount of haem lost.
3. We conclude that the destruction of haem caused by CCL$_4$ in both the cytochrome and the non-enzymatic system is a typical suicidal inactivation reaction, where the same molecule of haem responsible for the activation of CCl$_4$ may undergo destruction by a CCl$_4$ reactive intermediate.

ACKNOWLEDGEMENT

This work has been partly supported within the framework of the CNR Applied Project 'Medicina Preventiva e Riabilitativa', grant number 85.00811.56. M.M. is grateful to the British Council for a Research Fellowship.

REFERENCES

de Groot, H. and Haas, W. (1981). Biochem. Pharmacol, 30, 2343.

Manno, M., de Matteis, F. and King, L.J. (1986). Human Toxicol, 5, 118.
Morrison, G.R. (1965). Anal. Chem, 37, 1194.
Paul, K.G., Theorell, H. and Akeson, A. (1953). Acta. Chem. Scand, 7, 1284.
Tenhunen, R., Marver, H.S. and Schmid, R. (1968). Proc. Natl. Acad. Sci, USA, 61, 748.

THE IN VITRO METABOLISM OF AMINO AZAHETEROCYCLES

J.W. Gorrod

Chelsea Department of Pharmacy, King's College London (KQC), Manresa Road, London, SW3 6LX, UK.

Aromatic aminoazaheterocycles are a group of molecules of diverse structure possessing a wide range of pharmacological properties. Some are used in clinical medicine whilst others are mutagens and carcinogens. Biological oxidation of the constituent nuclear nitrogen leads to the formation of innocuous N-oxides, whereas oxidation of the exo amino groups produces toxic hydroxylamines (Gorrod 1979; Gorrod 1985). For a number of years work in this laboratory has been focussed on elucidating the nature of nitrogen atoms vulnerable to biological oxidation, the nature of the enzymes involved and the factors influencing substrate specificity of these enzymes.

To this end we have established that a number of 3-substituted pyridines are oxidised by a hepatic microsomal P-450 dependent system (Cowan et al, 1978; Gorrod and Damani 1979a and b). These observations were extended to include both 2 and 4-substituted pyridines (Wareing, 1983) and included isomeric aminopyridines. At that time no definite evidence for metabolic oxidation of either the nuclear or exo nitrogens of amino pyridines could be obtained. The in vitro metabolism of these latter substrates have recently been re-examined using sensitive HPLC techniques and chemically converting any unstable hydroxylamine formed to the corresponding nitro compound. Preliminary metabolic studies, using microsomal preparations from the dog, show that all the isomeric aminopyridines are N-oxidised, producing the nuclear N-oxide, but in addition the 3-isomer gave the hydroxylamine. This initial observation is interesting since 3-aminopyridine is mutagenic in the presence of norharman, unlike the 2 and 4-isomers (Sugimura et al, 1982).

Further investigations, using 2-aminopyridine as substrate, showed that 2-nitropyridine was produced as a metabolite (the hydroxylamine probably being an intermediate) when rabbit hepatic preparations were used.

Surprisingly, no metabolites were observed using microsomal preparations from hamster.

It is of interest that whilst pyridines and substituted pyridines are susceptible to N-oxidation by a variety of species in vitro, pyrazine, pyrimidine and pyridazine are at best very poor substrates for this process. This is probably related to the availability of the lone pair of electrons rather than the electron density of the whole nitrogen atom. Albert (1968) has calculated the electron densities of the constituent nitrogen of pyridine to be -0.097 and those of pyrimidine to be -0.095. Recently Webb (1986) has re-calculated the charge densities on the two molecules and found total N-electron densities of -0.26 and -0.28. This would not seem to be a difference great enough to account for their different susceptibilities to biological and chemical oxidation (Katritsky and Lagowski, 1971). Webb has also calculated the nitrogen lone pair densities for the two molecules and found a value of 1.54 lone pair electrons for pyridine and only 1.29 for pyrimidine, this is much more in line with the reactivity of the molecules towards oxidants. It will be interesting to extend these calculations to pyrazine, pyridazine and symmetrical triazine and establish the influence of substituent amino groups on this parameter.

We have concurrently been investigating the metabolic N-oxidation of 5- and 6-substituted 2,4-diaminopyrimidines. This group of compounds includes trimethoprim, metoprine and pyrimethamine. Considerable evidence is available on the in vivo N-oxidation of these compounds (See Gorrod, 1985 for references) but to date no in vitro data has been reported. Liver microsomal studies with pyrimethamine in our laboratory has demonstrated the metabolic formation of both isomeric 1- and 3-N-oxides with several animal species (Table 1).

Table 1. **In vitro hepatic microsomal metabolism of pyrimethamine by different animal species.**

SPECIES	3-N-OXIDE	1-N-OXIDE
	n moles formed/mg protein	
Rat	21.0	1.0
Hamster	31.5	3.7
Mouse	45.0	3.4
Guinea Pig	10.5	0

The results for pyrimethamine show that the 3-N-oxide is formed in greater amount in all the species studied. The 1-N-oxide only accounts for 5-10% of the total N-oxides in rat, hamster and mouse and was not produced by guinea pig hepatic preparations. In the case of the 2,4-diaminopyrimidines substituted in the six position with the diethylamino or piperidino moiety only the 3-N-oxide could be detected in any species. The failure of pyrimethamine to form the 1-N-oxide in guinea pig hepatic preparations is indicative that more than one enzyme is involved in N-oxidation of this substrate by the other species.

By using various inducing agents and inhibitors, the biological N-oxidation of pyrimethamine, 2,4-diamino-6-diethylaminopyrimidine and 2,4-diamino-6-piperidinopyrimidine has been shown to be mediated via cytochrome P-450 dependent pathways. This is illustrated in Tables 2 and 3.

Table 2.   The effect of inhibitors and inducers on rat liver N-oxidation of pyrimethamine.

INHIBITOR OR INDUCER	PERCENTAGE N-OXIDES FORMED[1]	
	3-N-OXIDE	I-N-OXIDE
Control	100	100
SKF 525 10^{-5}M	45	50
" " 10^{-3}M	33	25
$CO:O_2$ (2:1)	38	0
" (5:1)	34	0
Phenobarbitone[2]	621	4555
β-Naphthoflavone[3]	96	166

[1]Compared with control experiments carried out under identical conditions.
[2]Animals were treated with phenobarbitone (80mg/kg ip) on each of three days prior to sacrifice.
[3]Animals were treated with i.p. injections of β-naphthoflavone (80mg/Kg) on each of two days prior to sacrifice.

A further example of the metabolism of an aminoazaheterocycle is 9-benzyl-6-aminopurine (9BA) which

Table 3. The effect of inhibitors and inducers on rat liver microsomal 2,4-diamino-pyrimidine-3-N-oxidase activity

SUBSTRATE	INHIBITOR OR INDUCER	CONCN	3-N-OXIDE FORMED[1]
2,4-Diamino-6-piperidino-pyrimidine	Control	-	11.8 (100%)
	SKF 525-A	10^{-4}M	5.4 (46%)
	"	10^{-3}M	2.7 (23%)
	n-octylamine HCl	10^{-4}M	8.11 (69%)
	"	10^{-3}M	5.58 (47%)
"	Control	-	10.82 (100%)
	phenobarbitone[3]	-	24.46 (226%)
	β-naphthoflavone[3]	-	12.88 (119%)
2,4-Diamino-6-diethylamino-pyrimidine	Control	-	6.76 (100%)
	SKF 525-A	10^{-4}M	3.38 (50%)
	"	10^{-3}M	1.35 (20%)
	n-octylamine HCl	10^{-4}M	4.39 (65%)
	"	10^{-3}M	3.04 (45%)
"	Control	-	13.18 (100%)
	phenobarbitone[3]	-	24.46 (186%)
	β-naphthoflavone[3]	-	13.50 (102%)

[1]n moles/mg protein [2]Percentage of activity in control experiments carried out under identical conditions [3]Pre-treatments as described in Table 2.

is an analogue of Aprinocid. Preliminary in vitro studies of 9BA using liver microsomes of various animal species showed that debenzylation of 9BA was the main metabolic pathway. On the basis of HPLC analysis we observed that 9-benzyladenine-1-N-oxide (9BANO) was formed using hamster hepatic preparations. However, neither 9BANO nor 9B6HP were detected using rabbit or rat liver.

The formation of 2-aminopyridine-N-oxide and 2-hydroxylaminopyridine from 2-aminopyridine by rabbit microsomes raises questions as to the enzymology of the processes. From the above experiments it appears that nuclear N-oxidation of amino aromatic azaheterocycles is mediated by a phenobarbitone inducible form of cytochrome P-450. Even in the case of substrate having two nuclear nitrogens vulnerable to biological N-oxidation, the evidence indicates that both are oxidised via a phenobarbitone inducible form (Table 3). This situation is clearly different from that observed during the N-oxidation of the exo-amino group of 3-amino-1-methyl-5H-pyrido-[4,3b]-indole (Trp-P-2), the corresponding dimethyl compound (Trp-P-1) (Yamazoe et al, 1980; Hashimoto et al, 1980a); 2-amino-6-methylpyrido [1,2a:3,2d]imidazole (Glu-P-1) (Hashimoto et al, 1980b); 2-amino-3-methylimidazole [4,5f]-quinoline (IQ), (Okamoto et al, 1981). Yamazoe et al (1984) showed that the high spin form of P-448 (P-448IIa) from rat liver was better than the low spin form, (P-448IId) at N-oxidising both Glu-P-1 and IQ, as measured by the number of Salmonella revertants produced under standard incubation conditions. Trp-P-2 was well oxidised by both forms of cytochrome P-448.

As it is usually considered that all forms of cytochrome P-450 oxidise substrates by a common mechanism it is difficult to envisage one that will produce two species of N-oxidation products from a single substrate. It could be that different cytochromes bind the substrate in different orientations in order to achieve different end products. These differences may be explicable in terms of the amine-imine tautomerism hypothesis (Gorrod 1985) in which it is proposed that certain aminoazaheterocycles are bound to cytochrome to produce an imine tautomer which then becomes an alternative substrate leading to the formation of an hydroxylamine.

Further experiments will be necessary to elucidate the enzymic mechanisms by which a single substrate can produce multiple N-oxidation products and characterise the factors both chemical and biological, which influence each pathway. As N-oxidation products have diverse toxicological and pharmacological properties, knowledge of the factors which influence their formation is clearly important.

ACKNOWLEDGEMENTS

The data cited in this communication have been obtained by Ms N. Iles and Ms K. El-Ghomari, Mr. P.J. Watkins, Mr

S.P. Lam and Dr S. Noorazar and will be published in full elsewhere.

REFERENCES

Albert, A.A. (1968). "Heterocyclic Chemistry", 2nd edition, The Athlone Press, London, UK. p.64.

Cowan, D.A., Damani, L.A. and Gorrod, J.W. (1978). Biomedical Mass Spectrometry, 5, 551.

Gorrod, J.W. (1979). in "Drug Toxicity" (ed. Gorrod, J.W). Taylor and Francis, Basingstoke, UK. p.1.

Gorrod, J.W. (1985). in "Biological Oxidation of Nitrogen in Organic Molecules" (Ed. Gorrod, J.W., Damani, L.A). Ellis Horword Ltd, Chichester, UK. p.219.

Gorrod, J.W. and Damani, L.A. (1979a). Xenobiotica, 9, 209.

Gorrod, J.W. and Damani, L.A. (1979b). Xenobiotica, 9, 219.

Hashimoto, Y., Shudo, K. and Okamato, T. (1980a). Biochem. Biophys. Res. Comm, 96, 355.

Hashimoto, Y., Shudo, K. and Okamato, T. (1980b). Biochem. Biophys. Res. Comm, 92, 971.

Katritsky, A.R. and Lagowski, J.M. (1971). Chemistry of the Heterocyclic N-oxides. Academic Press, London, UK.

Okamoto, T., Shudo, K., Hashimoto, Y., Kosuge, T., Sugimura, T. and Nishimura, S. (1981). Chem. Pharm. Bull, 29, 590.

Sugimura, T., Nagao, M. and Wakabayashi, K. (1982). in "Biological Reactive Intermediates II part B" (eds. Snyder, R., Parke, D.V., Kocsis, J.J., Jollow, D.J., Gibson, G.G. and Witner, C.M). Plenum Press, New York, USA. p.1011.

Wareing, M.P.A. (1983). PhD Thesis, University of London.

Webb, G.A. (1986). Personal Communication.

Yamazoe, Y., Ishii, K., Kamataki, T., Kato, T. and Sugimara, T. (1980). Chem. Biol. Interact, 30, 125.

Yamazoe, Y., Shimada, M., Maeda, K., Kamataki, T. and Kato, R. (1984). Xenobiotica, 14, 549.

INTERACTION OF POTENTIAL QUINONE CYTOSTATIC DRUGS WITH DNA

Nicolaas J. de Mol[1], Irma L. Groothuis-Pielage[1], Klaas Lusthof[1] and Jean Decuyper[1,2]

Departments of (1) Pharmaceutical Chemistry and (2) Analytical Pharmacy, State University of Utrecht, Catharijnesingel 60, 3511 GH Utrecht, The Netherlands.

INTRODUCTION

A number of naturally occuring antibiotics with anti-tumour activity possess a quinone moiety. According to the concept of bioreductive alkylation, reduction of these drugs increases their biological activities (Kappus, 1986 and references therein). Our research of the DNA interactions of a series of aziridinyl benzoquinones (Figure 1) is part of a multi-disciplinary project in the Netherlands in which a series of new benzoquinones are synthesized (Twente University of Technology, CT Department) and pharmacologically screened (REPGO-TNO, Rijswijk).

Figure 1. Aziridinyl Quinones

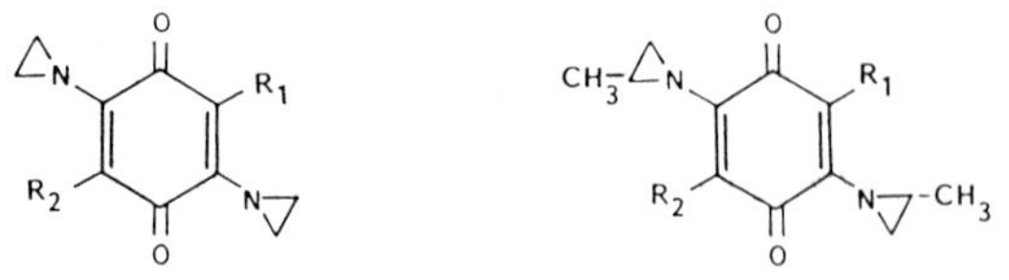

Compound	R_1	R_2
TW013	H	H
TW025	Br	C_2H_5
TW026	N◁	F
TW032	CH_3	C_2H_5
TW039	CH_3	$(CH_2)_2$-O-CO-NH_2
Trenimon	N◁	H
Carboquone	CH_3	$COHCH_3$-CH_2-O-CO-NH_2
AZQ(Diaziquone)	$R_1 = R_2 = NH$-CO-O-C_2H_5	

Compound	R_1	R_2
Me-TW039	CH_3	$(CH_2)_2$-O-CO-NH_2
TW053	CH_3	Br
TW073	$R_1 = R_2 = NH$-CO-O-C_2H_5	

462

The electrochemical reduction mechanism of the quinones is studied by the Department of Analytical Pharmacy, State University of Utrecht. Reduction of the electron-deficient quinone nucleus to the electron-rich hydroquinone may facilitate ring opening of the aziridinyl rings by increasing the PK value of the aziridinyl nitrogen. The opened aziridinyl ring is a potential alkylating species for which DNA is a likely target. It is thought that the reductive activation is predominant in hypoxic media like tumour cells in solid tumours (Kennedy et al, 1980). As alkylation of DNA is considered to be a crucial step in the antitumour activity of the aziridinyl quinones we started an investigation into the effects of these compounds on DNA.

EFFECTS OF AZIRIDINYL BENZOQUINONES IN A BACTERIAL DNA REPAIR TEST

The effects of several aziridinyl benzoquinones on DNA were investigated using a bacterial DNA repair test. As shown in Table 1, exposure of DNA repair deficient bacteria (E.coli K12 (uvr B^-/recA$^-$/lac$^+$) to aziridinyl benzoquinones leads to an inactivation of these bacteria. In our experimental conditions, no effect was recorded on DNA repair proficient bacteria (E.coli K12 (uvr$^\pm$/rec$^\pm$/lac$^-$). An endogenous reductive activation of aziridinyl-benzoquinones can be suspected because, on the first hand, polarographic analysis has allowed us to demonstrate that these bacteria were able to reduce the aziridinyl-benzoquinone and, on the other hand, addition of methylnaphthoquinone, a reductase inhibitor, during the exposure of bacteria to aziridinyl benzoquinone, decreased the effect.

From these results, it appears that DNA is the target for aziridinyl-benzoquinone effect because in the DNA repair test used, effects are assumed to be closely related to DNA damage. The very low activity of methylaziridinyl compounds (Me-TW039, TW053 and TW073) could be due to steric hindrance decreasing the interactions with DNA.

Beside DNA alkylation, DNA damage could also be induced by reactive oxygen species which are known to be produced during redox cycling of quinone compounds (Kappus, 1986). We have thus examined the effect of catalase and of superoxide dismutase in the DNA repair test. Catalase was without effect, but superoxide dismutase reduced the efficiency of the drugs. This indicates that the superoxide anion, or related species, may also be involved in the induction of DNA damage .

Table 1. Activity of a series of aziridinylquinones in a DNA repair test.

COMPOUND	ACTIVITY IN DNA REPAIR DEFICIENT E.COLI K-12* +s.d.(RELATIVE TO TWO39)	ACTIVITY IN L_{1210} CLONO-GENIC ASSAY (ID_{75}** IN ng/ml)
TWO73	0.03 + 0.01	-
TWO53	0.04 + 0.01	-
Me-TWO39	0.07 + 0.02	-
Carboquone	0.22 + 0.02	28.9
TWO32	0.49 + 0.05	692
TWO25	0.51 + 0.05·	0.34
TWO39	1	3.8
TWO13	2.65 + 0.20	3.9
TWO26	3.76 + 0.25	1.2

The quinones are activated by bacterial reductase. Also included is the activity in the L_{1210} clonogenic assay.

*Under our experimental conditions no inactivation of the colony-formimg ability of the DNA repair proficient strain is observed. **ID_{75} is the concentration needed for reduction of the number of colonies to 75%

In order to investigate further the interaction between DNA and reduced aziridinyl benzoquinones, in vitro experiments were carried out.

DNA EFFECTS OF TWO39 REDUCED BY NaBH₄

Covalent binding of TWO39 reduced by $NaBH_4$ on DNA was determined by UV spectroscopy. As shown in Figure 2, an absorbance around 350nm can be recorded in DNA after reaction with $NaBH_4$ reduced TWO39 and removal of unbound TWO39. This indicates the presence of covalent adducts of TWO39 with open aziridinyl ring. The amount of TWO39 covalent adducts increases linearly when the reaction is carried out with increasing TWO39 concentrations.

We investigated the cross-linking ability of TWO39 after $NaBH_4$ reduction by studying the melting behaviour of DNA. The melting temperature (T_m) of DNA increases with increasing number of adducts. This could indicate that

Figure 2. UV spectrum of calf thymus DNA which has been reacted with TWO39 reduced by NaBH$_4$.

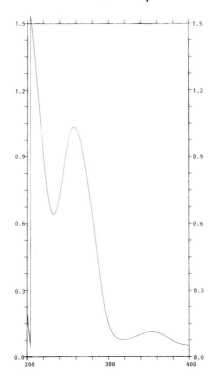

Reaction conditions were: 0.93 µg/µlDNA (2.9mMnucleotide), 1.4mM TWO39, 14 mM NaBH$_4$ and 100mM acetatebuffer pH 5.3

interstrand cross-links are formed. The ring opening, which is essential for alkylation, is acid catalyzed (Akhtar et al., 1975), thus we studied the pH dependence of DNA-adduct formation, by NaBH$_4$ reduced TWO39, with UV detection of the adducts. It can be observed from Figure 3 that the amount of adduct decreases if the reaction has been performed at higher pH. The experimental values seem to fit very closely with a curve giving the amount of an acid in the protonated form with pK_a = 5.24. This value could correspond to the pK_a of the aziridinyl ring of TWO39 in the hydroquinone form. Beside the alkylating properties of aziridinylhydroquinones it can be expected that these compounds are also able to promote the generation of DNA breakage, particularly by way of reactive oxygen species. We used the superhelical pBr 322 plasmid DNA in order to

monitor strand breaks with NaBH$_4$ reduced TW039. After
reduction, a conversion of superhelical circular DNA into
circular relaxed DNA is observed. This indicates the
induction of single strand breaks. Here also lower pH
value increases the amount of single strand breaks.
Further experiments are needed in order to determine the
reactive species implicated in this reaction. Transfection
experiments will be performed to study direct effects on
DNA.

We will further study the DNA effects of aziridinyl
quinones with various ways of reduction: electrochemically
and enzmically. To study DNA effects on the molecular
level we will use in vitro replication and sequencing
techniques.

**Figure 3. Absorbance at 350 nm of calf thymus DNA which
has been reacted with TW039 reduced by NaBH$_4$ as a function
of pH.**

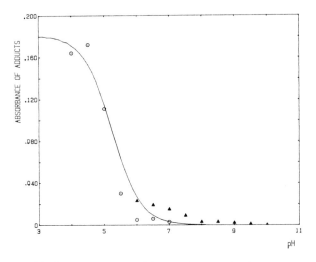

Reaction conditions were: 0.93µg/µl DNA (2.9 mM nucleotide),
1.4mM TW039, 14mM NaBH$_4$, 100mM acetatebuffer (O) or
trisacetate buffer (▲).

ACKNOWLEDGEMENTS

We are indebted to Prof. Reinhoudt and Dr. Verboom of the
Twente University of Technology for synthesis of the TW
compounds. We thank Dr. Baas, Institute for Molecular
Biology, University of Utrecht, for support in the

preparation of pBr 322. and Drs. Driebergen, Department of Analytical Pharmacy, University of Utrecht for helpful discussion. We thank Dr. Mohn, University of Leiden for providing us with the bacterial strains for the DNA repair test.

REFERENCES

Akhtar, M.H.,Begleiter, A., Johnson, D., Lown, J.W., McLaughlin, L., and S.-K. Sim (1975), Can. J. Chem.53, 2891.

Kappus, H. (1986), Biochem. Pharmacol. 35, 1.

Kennedy, K.A., Rockwell, S., and Sartorelli, A.C., (1980), Cancer. Res. 40, 2356.

INFLUENCE OF CYTOCHROME b_5 ON ELECTRON FLOW FROM NADPH-CYTOCHROME c(P-450) REDUCTASE TO CYTOCHROME P-450

Ines Golly and Peter Hlavica

Walter Straub-Institut fur Pharmakologie und Toxikologie der Universitat, Nussbaumstrasse 26, D-8000 Munchen 2, Federal Republic of Germany

INTRODUCTION

Cytochrome b_5 is well known to donate the second electron to oxyferrous cytochrome P-450 in certain types of drug oxidations (White and Coon, 1980). Apart from its functions as an electron carrier, cytochrome b_5 appears to modulate monooxygenase activity via protein-protein interaction (Hlavica, 1984; Morgan and Coon, 1984). The present report centres on the regulative role of cytochrome b_5 in electron transfer from NADPH-cytochrome c(P-450) reductase to cytochrome P-450.

MATERIALS AND METHODS

Preparation of microsomal fraction from the livers of phenobarbital-treated rabbits, purification of cytochromes $P-450LM_2$ and b_5 and NADH/NADPH-dependent reductase, incorporation of the hemoproteins into microsomal membranes or phospholipid, and measurement of NADPH-cytochrome P-450 reductase and NADPH oxidase activity was performed as described previously (Golly and Hlavica, 1985). Suicidal inactivation of cytochrome $P-450LM_2$ by chloramphenicol (CAP) was achieved by pre-incubation of the microsomal fractions with 1mM antibiotic for 2 h at $37^{\circ}C$; this was followed by purification of the modified haemoprotein.

The kinetics of cytochrome P-450 reduction were assessed by stopped-flow technique. The reaction mixtures contained: 2 µM cytochrome $P-450LM_2$ (either native or CAP-modified), 0.2 µM NADPH-cytochrome P-450 reductase (or 0.5 µM NADH-cytochrome b_5 reductase plus 1 µM cytochrome b_5), 1 mM hexobarbital, and 0.33 mM NADPH (or NADH) in 0.15M phosphate buffer, pH 7.4; the mixtures were gassed with CO for 5 min.

RESULTS AND DISCUSSION

Incorporation into rabbit liver microsomal fractions of detergent-solubilized cytochrome b$_5$ causes a decrease both in the maximum velocity of NADPH-supported cytochrome P-450 reduction and the affinity of the system for the reductant (Figure 1B). This is unlikely to result from the ability of cytochrome b$_5$ to serve as an alternative electron acceptor shunting reducing equivalents away from cytochrome P-450, since NADPH utilization is markedly inhibited (Figure 1A). Similarly, deceleration of cytochrome P-450 reduction is not the consequence of cytochrome b$_5$-induced impairment of the electron-transferring capacity of NADPH-cytochrome c P-450 reduction (data not shown). Cytochrome b$_5$ also does not influence the process of anchoring of reductase to cytochrome P-450 LM$_2$ (Golly and Hlavica, 1985).

Figure 1. Influence of extra-bound cytochromes b$_5$ and Mn(III)-b$_5$ on NADPH activation in the presence of hexobarbital, as measured in terms of NADPH oxidation (A) or cytochrome P-450 reduction (B).

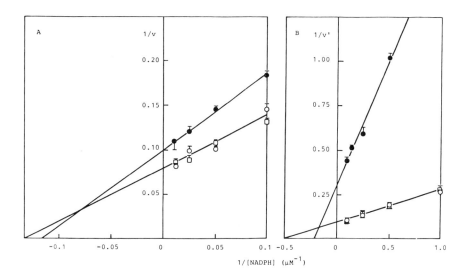

o, controls; cytochromes b$_5$ (●) and Mn (III)-b$_5$ (□) added to give a molar ratio to P-450 of 1.7:1 and 0.9:1, respectively.

Cytochrome b_5 is thus proposed to perturb in some way electron transfer from the reductase flavins to the haem iron of cytochrome P-450; however, changes in the redox potential of the haemoprotein do not appear to be involved (Guengerich, 1983). Most interestingly, there is a remarkable modulation in the kinetic characteristics of microsomal cytochrome P-450 reduction as the molar ratio of cytochrome b_5 to cytochrome P-450 is raised: the amplitude of the slow phase gradually increases at the expense of the relative contribution of the fast phase (Figure 2). This

Figure 2. Influence of extra-bound cytochrome b_5 on the kinetics of microsomal cytochrome P-450 reduction in the presence of hexobarbital.

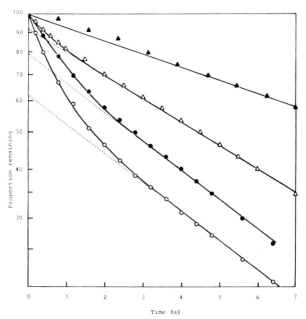

o, control; **●**, control heated for 30 min at 37°C; cytochrome b_5 added to yield a molar ratio to P-450 of 0.9:1 (Δ) and 1.4:1 (▲), respectively.

is not due to dispersal by cytochrome b_5 of the cytochrome P-450 clusters within the membranes: sedimentation equilibrium experiments reveal that the number of cytochrome P-450 molecules per individual b_5/P-450 aggregate remains fairly constant (data not shown). The phenomenon thus possibly arises from disturbed interaction of phospholipid with the haem moiety of cytochrome P-450 (Figure 3); the lipid component is well known to regulate electron flow between reductase and haemoprotein (Ingelman-

Figure 3. Influence of cytochrome b$_5$ on the interaction of dilauroyl phosphatidylcholine (DLPC) with cytochrome P-450 LM$_2$.

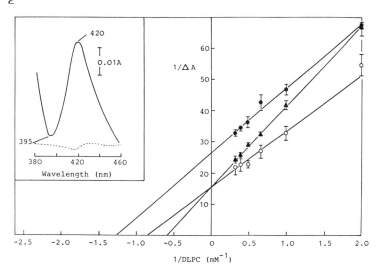

The incubation mixtures contained 15μM P-450 LM$_2$ and the amounts of DLPC indicated (o); in some experiments, 18 μM cytochrome b$_5$ (●) or 18μM Triton X-100 (▲) was added. Inset: reverse type I spectrum produced by the addition of DLPC to P-450LM$_2$.

Sundberg et al., 1983). An alternative possibility is that cytochrome b$_5$ interfers directly with the electron transport from flavo- to haemoprotein. This view receives support from studies with CAP-modified cytochrome P-450 LM$_2$: the labelled pigment is less effective than the native one in accepting electrons both from the reductase and cytochrome b$_5$ (Figure 4). These findings suggest that the haem region of cytochrome b$_5$ and the reductase flavins indeed compete for a common site on the cytochrome P-450 molecule, that regulates electron transfer from these structures to the haem iron of the monoxygenase. Further work is in progress to elucidate the mechanisms involved.

REFERENCES

Golly, I and Hlavica, P. (1985) in "Cytochrome P-450, Biochemistry, Biophysics and Induction" (Eds. Vereczkey, L. and Magar, K.), Akademiai Kiado, Budapest, p. 177
Guengerich, F. P. (1983) Biochemistry 22, 2811

Figure 4. **Kinetics of reduction of native (o) or CAP-modified (●) cytochrome P-45(LM$_2$.**

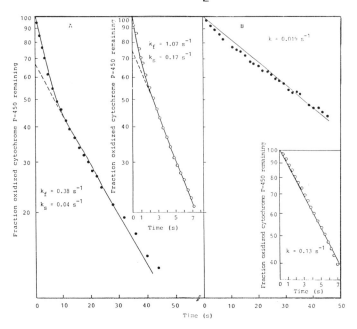

Systems tested: (A) NADPH-cytochrome c(P-450) reductase/P-450LM$_2$; (b) NADH-cytochrome b$_5$ reductase/b$_5$/P-450LM$_2$.

Hlavica, P. (1984) Arch. Biochem. Biophys. 228, 600.

Ingelman-Sundberg, M., Blank J., Smettan, G. and Ruckpaul, K. (1983) Eur. J. Biochem. 134, 157.

Morgan, E.T. and Coon, M. J. (1984) Drug Metab. Dispos. 12, 358.

White, R.E. and Coon, M. J. (1980) Ann. Rev. Biochem. 49, 315.

MULTIPLICITY OF CYTOCHROME P-450 ACTIVITIES: STOICHIOMETRICAL APPROACH

Alexander I. Archakov and Andrei A. Zhukov

Department of Biochemistry, Medico-Biological Faculty
2nd Moscow Medical Institute, Ostrovityanova 1, Moscow, USSR

Of numerous activities exhibited by different haemoproteins, cytochrome P-450 has been shown capable of acting as a monooxygenase, peroxidase (both H_2O_2 and organic peroxide-dependent), electron carrier and oxidase. While catalysing monooxygenation of organic substrates is commonly considered the main physiological function of the enzyme, these reactions are always accompanied by the release of free superoxide anions, hydrogen peroxide and water in oxidase reactions (Nordblom and Coon,1976; Ullrich and Kuthan, 1980, Zhukov and Archakov, 1982; Gorsky et al.,1984), which distorts the classic "monooxygenase" stoichiometry. The first two of the above three reduced oxygen species formed in P-450-catalyzed oxidase reactions are rather reactive and can interact with various macromolecules to modify them, while water formation (at least at first glance) appears to be harmless. This is why it is of importance to develop a methodological approach that could allow one to follow separately the formation of O_2-, H_2O_2 and H_2O during P-450-dependent NADPH oxidation in microsomes. The approach to be described consists in measuring the stoichiometry of O_2 consumption, NADPH and organic substrate oxidation, O_2- and H_2O_2 formation in P-450-catalysed reactions.

Microsomes were isolated from the liver of phenobarbital-pretreated rabbits. NADPH oxidation was followed by the decrease in absorbance at 340nm. The oxygen consumption rate was determined polarographically. The rates of benzphetamine and dimethylaniline N-demethylation were measured by the accumulation of formaldehyde (Nash, 1953). H_2O_2 was determined by the thiocyanate method (Thurman et al., 1972). To determine the rate of O_2- formation the superoxide dismutase-sensitive rate of reduction of succinylated cytochrome c was calculated. The rate of O_2^- formation was estimated using xanthine/xanthine oxidase system for calibration.

RESULTS AND DISCUSSION

One of the questions that can be settled by measuring stoichiometry is that of whether H_2O_2 can be formed through direct 2-electron reduction of P-450-bound dioxygen or the only way of its generation is the dismutation of previously released superoxide radicals. Indeed, with the latter alternative being the case, the ratio of the rates of O_2^- and H_2O_2 formation must equal 2 according to the stoichiometry of O_2^- dismutation:

$$2O_2^- + 2H^+ = H_2O_2 + O_2 \qquad (1)$$

while smaller ratios should indicate that a portion of H_2O_2 is formed directly, the smaller being the ratio, the greater the portion.

Another interesting problem which can be solved using this approach is that of the fate of NADPH and O_2 unaccounted for by organic substrate oxidation and H_2O_2 formation, it is not clear which of the two alternative mechanisms is involved:

$$NADPH + H^+ + RH + O_2 = NADP^+ + ROH + H_2O \qquad (2)$$
$$2NADPH + 2H^+ + O_2 = 2NADP^+ + 2H_2O \qquad (3)$$

Again, one can see that the answer can be found by measuring the ratio of "unaccounted" NADPH and O_2. The values of 2 and 1 would point to the oxidase and monooxygenase pathway, respectively.

We measured the stoichiometry of NADPH oxidation both in the absence and in the presence of various P-450 substrates (Table 1). The ratio of O_2^- to H_2O_2 formed was about unity in all cases thus indicating that about half the H_2O_2 is formed directly, while another half results from O_2^- dismutation.

As for the ratio of unaccounted NADPH and O_2 it is indicative of the oxidase mechanism involving complete 4-electron reduction of the dioxygen molecule. It is of interest that perfluorodecalin used as a chemically inert component of artificial blood (Geyer, 1975; Maugh, 1979) also interacts with microsomes to stimulate the oxidase reaction of water formation. This illustrates the fact that chemical inertness is not necessarily equal to the biological one. Figure 1 presents the possible ways of electron transfer to oxygen catalyzed by P-450. The overall catalytic process is seen to consist of four cycles including a monooxygenase and three oxidase ones, the latter involving direct 1-, 2- and 4-electron reduction of the dioxygen molecule. The 1- and 2-electron oxidase reactions result in the formation of reactive oxygen species (O_2^- and H_2O_2), which can lead to the inactivation of cytochrome P-450 and other macromolecules (Karuzina and Archakov, 1985; Laura <u>et al</u>., 1983).

Table 1. Stoichiometry of **NADPH oxidation in liver microsomes**

SUBSTRATE ADDED	NADPH (a)	O_2 (b)	P (c)	O_2^- (d)	H_2O_2 (e)	$\dfrac{a-c-e}{b-c-e}$	$\dfrac{d}{e}$
None	25	18	0	9	11	2.0	0.8
Benzphetamine	123	108	72	29	24.3	2.3	1.2
Dimethylaniline	73	52	17	–	13.3	2.0	–
Perfluorohexane	61	34	0	10.2	10.1	2.1	1.0
Perfluorodecalin	42	24	0	–	9	2.2	–

Figure 1. Cytochrome P-450 activities.

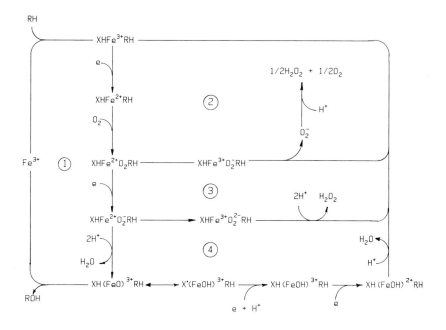

RH stands for an organic substrate; XH is an electron donating group in the P-450 molecule.

Detailed presentation of the related material is to be
found elsewhere (Zhukov and Archakov, 1985).

REFERENCES

Geyer, R.P. (1975) Federat. Proc., 34, 1499.
Gorsky, L.D., Koop, D.S. and Coon, M.J. (1984) J. Biol.
   Chem., 259, 6812.
Karuzina, I.I. and Archakov, A. I. (1985) Biokhimiya, 50,
   1805 (Russ.).
Laura, F., Oliver, C.N., Coon, M.J. and Stadtman, E.R.
   (1983) Proc. Natl. Acad. Sci. USA, 80,1521.
Maugh, T.H. (1979) Science, 206,205
Nash, T. (1953) Biochem. J., 55, 416.
Nordblom, J. D. and Coon, M.J. (1977) Arch. Biochem.
   Biophys., 171, 385
Thurman, R.G. Ley, H.G. and Scholz, R. (1972) Eur. J.
      Biochem., 25, 420.
Ullrich, V. and Kuthan, H. (1980) in "Biochemistry,
   Biophysics, and Regulation of Cytochrome P-450" (Ed. by
   Gustafsson, J.-A., Carlstedt-Duke, J., Mode A. and
   Rafter, J.), Elsevier, Amsterdam, p267.
Zhukov, A.A. and Archakov, A.I. (1982) Biochem. Biophys.
   Res. Commun., 109, 813
Zhukov, A.A. and Archakov, A.I. (1985) Biokhimya, 50, 1983
   (Russ).

9. Metabolism and kinetics in safety evaluation.

METABOLISM AND TOXICOKINETICS STUDIES IN THE SAFETY EVALUATION OF DRUGS AND OTHER CHEMICALS

Dennis V. Parke

Department of Biochemistry, University of Surrey, Guildford
Surrey, GU2 5XH

INTRODUCTION

The safety evaluation of drugs and other chemicals has evolved rapidly over the past half century, from a purely empirical procedure to a highly complex, experimentally-determined and scientifically-based assessment. The procedures vary from one government agency to another, and from one industrial company to the next, but essentially fall into one of the four approaches listed in Table 1, namely, the 'Empirical' procedure- now largely abandoned, 'Current Good Practice' - widely used by most drug regulatory agencies, 'Ideal' - a more economic and desirable system advocated in the U.S.S.R. which relates safety evaluation to the extent of usage, and 'QSAR' - the system used for evaluating new industrial chemicals by the US Environmental Protection Agency, that initially replaces animal studies by chemical/toxicity structure-activity relationships. One of the most regrettable features of many safety evaluation procedures is that statistics are often used as a substitute for sound science, with empirical studies being given token respectability by validation with statistical procedures, instead of using experimental procedures established on the sound scientific basis of metabolism studies, toxicokinetics, and a knowledge of the molecular mechanisms of the chemical toxicity.

Chemical toxicity is not solely the property of the chemical concerned, but it is the consequence of three independent factors, namely, (i) the intrinsic properties of the chemical (its lipophilicity, molecular structure, and electronic conformations) (ii) the biological characteristics of the living organism (species, genetics, age, sex) exposed to the chemical, and (iii) the total environment of that living organism (nutrition, exposure to other chemicals, radiation, etc.). Although chemical toxicity may result from many different mechanisms, some of which are shown in Table 2, these all point to the

TABLE 1 Alternative Approaches to Safety Evaluation of Chemicals

Empirical	Current Good Practice	Ideal	QSAR
Lethality and morphological studies, mostly on rodents, with emphasis on statistics. Little or no concern with mechanisms, metabolism or toxicokinetics.	Limited but adequate animal studies. Species and doses chosen from metabolic and toxicokinetic studies.	Progressive development of safety evaluation from QSAR and in vitro tests to 2-generation studies, neuro-toxicology and behavioural toxicology, related to scale of production and nature of usage.	Physico-chemical parameters, and log P. Structure/activity relationships with chemicals of known toxicity, metabolism and toxicokinetics.
	Human risk assessments made on scientific basis from animal experiments and human studies, including mechanisms of toxicity and comparative receptor studies.	Choice of animal species, doses and human risk assessment based on mechanisms, and comparative metabolism, toxicokinetic and receptor studies.	Chemical is discarded if toxic, and re-designed instead of conducting animal toxicity studies.
		(USSR, Sanockij, 1975)	(US Environmental Protection Agency)

Table 2   Some Mechanisms of Chemical Toxicity

---

1. Direct interaction with cell constituents, enzyme inhibition - e.g. cyanide.
2. Lethal synthesis, inhibition of ATP synthesis - e.g. fluoroacetamide.
3. Metabolism to reactive intermediates, arylation of DNA - e.g. benzo(a)pyrene.
4. Oxidation of thiol enzymes and glutathione - e.g. quinones.
5. Redox cycling and generation of reactive oxygen - e.g. paraquat.
6. Radical formation, lipid peroxidation, membrane damage - e.g. carbon tetrachloride.
7. Neoantigen formation, immunological injury - e.g. dinitrofluorobenzene.

---

involvement of a common factor, namely, that chemical toxicity is the consequence of inadequate detoxication. Some of the reasons for this are as follows:

1. saturation of detoxication pathways , e.g. paracetamol is toxic only at high dosage, when the detoxicating glucuronide and sulphate conjugations have been overwhelmed, and the alternative metabolic pathway of oxidative metabolism leads to the formation of quinoneimes, depleting glutathione and resulting in redox cycling, covalent binding and tissue necrosis (Hinson, 1983); bromobenzene is a similar example and is toxic only when liver glutathione has been depleted (Pessayre, et al, 1979).
2. impairment of conjugation as occurs in starvation (Pessayre et al., 1979; Tong et al., 1986) and in studies with isolated cell systems, where the detoxicating glutathione, UDP-glucuronic acid, etc, are not regenerated as occurs in in vivo (Boobis et al., 1986) (this is a limitation to studying chemical toxicity in isolated systems).
3. the presence of impurities which inhibit detoxication mechanisms, e.g., impurities present in the pesticides malathion and phenthoate inhibit the carboxylesterase enzymes which normally detoxicate these insecticides (Lee and Fukuto, 1982). This results in a marked increase in the toxicity of the pesticide in mammalian species.

4. chemical structure, since the structure of many chemicals determines molecular site of the Phase 1 oxygenations and the nature of the oxygenase which metabolises the chemical. Oxygenation in conformationally-hindered positions of the chemical molecule inhibits subsequent conjugation and detoxication, resulting in the formation of reactive intermediates and chemical toxicity. This occurs with large, planar, highly lipophilic moleculae, e.g. benzo(a)pyrene, which are preferentially metabolised by the cytochrome P-448 (Lewis et al, 1986).

5. species differences, eg, malathion is toxic to insects but non-toxic to mammals, due to different pathways of metabolism - insects oxidatively metabolise the pesticide to malaoxon, a potent inhibitor of acetylcholinesterase, whereas mammals detoxicate the chemical by hydrolysis to malathion diacid, a pathway catalysed by carboxylesterases.

6. genetic differences, eg. the peripheral neurotoxicity and hepatotoxicity of perhexiline in those individuals who exhibit genetic impairment of the cytochrome P-450 which results in the oxidative deactivation of this drug (Gould et al, 1986).

A drug or chemical may therefore be metabolised to yield metabolites which are then conjugated, resulting in detoxication, or may be activated to reactive intermediates, each of these enzymic reactions proceeding at rates characteristic of the chemical in question and of the animal concerned (see Figure 1). Furthermore, the drug itself, or possibly a metabolite, reacts with the "pharmacological receptor" to elicit the pharmacological activity and, similarly, the drug or metabolites also may react with other receptors to evoke toxic activity. Hence, the pharmacological and toxicological activities of drugs and chemicals will depend on the tissue concentrations of the receptors, the tissue concentration of the drug or metabolite, and the affinities of the receptors for these chemicals.

From these considerations, it is readily apparent that the essential factors which determine the relative toxicity of chemicals in different animal species, and in different human individuals, are largely dependent on the activities and tissue concentration(s) of the enzymes and coenzymes concerned with detoxication , which are reflected in:

(i) the routes of metabolic detoxication and/or activation of the chemical,

(ii) the rates of its metabolism and clearance from the body,

Figure 1. Scheme for Metabolism of Drugs by Detoxication and Activation, their Toxicokinetics and Receptor Activities

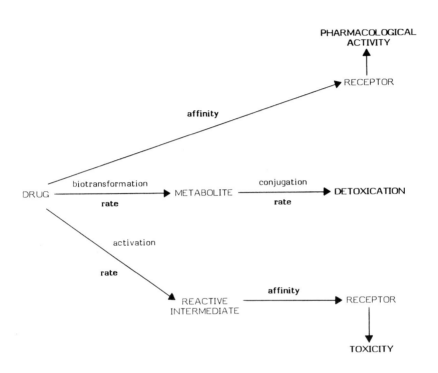

(iii)   the molecular mechanism(s) of toxicity, and
(iv)   the affinities of the chemical and/or its metabolites for the various receptors involved in the pharmacological/toxicological activities.

As toxicity is thus dependent on the pathways of metabolism and on the rates at which these different processes occur, metabolism and pharmacokinetic studies are central to the whole procedure of safety evaluation, and are indispensible in the selection of appropriate animal species for the experimental toxicity studies. Metabolism and pharmacokinetic studies are also essential in the selection of appropriate doses to be administered to these animal models, and in scientific interpretation of the animal toxicity data for human risk assessment. Where the mechanism(s) of toxicity has been elucidated and the receptor(s) identified, a knowledge of the relative tissue concentrations of these receptors and their affinities for

the chemicals concerned, in both animals and man, is highly
valuable in interpreting the significance of the animal
toxicity data. Without the scientific application of
metabolic, toxicokinetic, mechanistic, and receptor studies
to the safety evaluation of drugs and chemicals, toxicity
testing in animal models becomes an expensive but largely
pointless ritual, since the significance of the animal
toxicity data for potential human hazard is uninterpretable,

THE ROLE OF METABOLISM STUDIES

The metabolism of drugs and chemicals may lead to two
major consequences, namely, (i) the detoxication of the
chemical and its enhanced clearance from the body, or (ii)
the activation of the chemical to reactive intermediates,
forming electrophiles which may covalently bind to
essential intracellular macromolecules or result in the
production of highly reactive oxygen radicals by redox
cycling, etc, thereby resulting in toxicity (Guengerich and
Liebler, 1985; Mason, 1985). Recent studies have indicated
that, due to essential diffences in the spatial
conformations and the natures of the active sites of the
microsomal mixed-function oxidase cytochromes, metabolism
by the cytochromes P-450 generally results in oxygenations
that lead to subsequent conjugation and, hence, to
detoxication. In contrast, the cytochrome P-448 family of
enzymes generally inserts oxygen into hindered positions of
a chemical molecule, which are not readily susceptible to
subsequent conjugation, and hence results in activation of
the molecule with the formation of reactive indtermediates
(Lewis et al, 1986).

The selection of appropriate animal species as models
for man, based on the similarity of the major routes of
metabolism of the chemical, is most essential, since
empirical selection of the animal species based on short
life-span, low-cost, ready availablity, knowledge of
background pathology, can lead to costly errors when these
animals do not metabolise the drug or chemical in a manner
similar to man. For example, carbenoxolone, a terpenoid
ester that was the first effective anti-peptic ulcer
treatment, and is now used as an anti-viral agent, was
first evaluated for safety using rats, mice and rabbits.
However, the drug, is metabolised in man, ferret and dog by
conjugation with glucuronic acid, which is then almost
entirely excreted via the bile into the faeces, whereas, in
rat, mouse and other rodents and lagomorphs, it is
metabolised in the gastrointestinal tract by bacterial
hydrolysis to enoxolone and succinic acid, with the

subsequent excretion of succinate in the urine and
enoxolone glucuronide in the bile (Iveson et al, 1971).
Because it is an old drug, developed in the late 1950s, it
was one of the earliest casualties of the empirical choice
of animal species in safety evaluation studies, and initial
safety evaluation procedures had to be repeated in the more
appropriate species of ferret, dog and monkeys (see Figure
2).

**Figure 2. Species Differences in the Pathways of
Metabolism of Carbenoxolone**

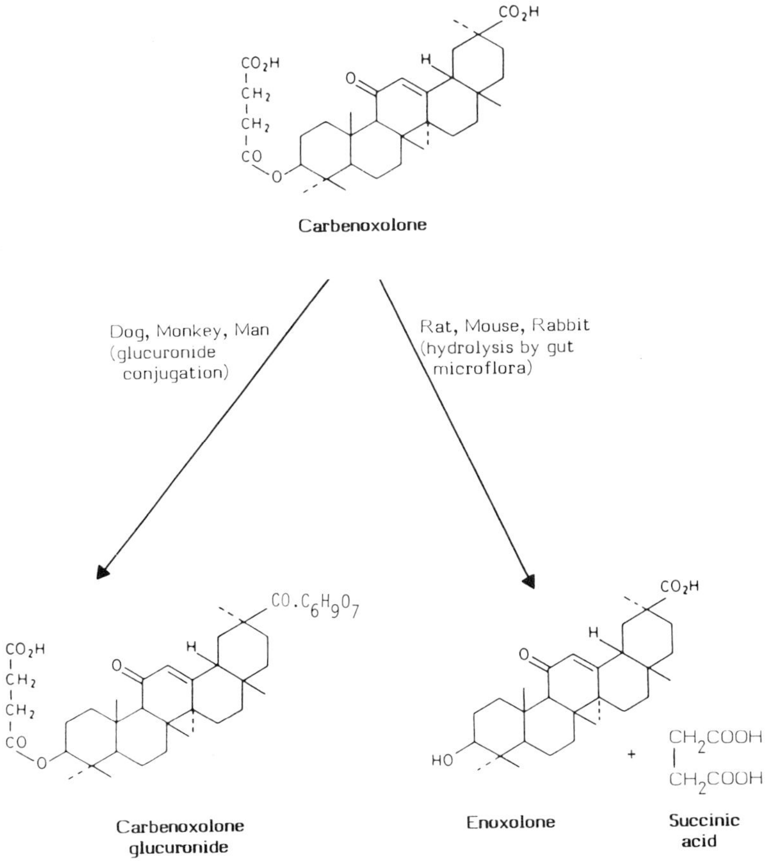

Carbenoxolone

Dog, Monkey, Man
(glucuronide
conjugation)

Rat, Mouse, Rabbit
(hydrolysis by gut
microflora)

Carbenoxolone
glucuronide

Enoxolone

Succinic
acid

Similarly, the non-steroidal anti-inflammatory drug,
feprazone, an analogue of phenylbutazone, is metabolised by
different pathways in man, dog and rat. In the rat it is

hydroxylated to 4'-hydroxyfeprazone and dihydroxyfeprazone, in dog it is metabolised to 4'-hydroxyfeprazone and also forms a cyclic metabolite resulting from epoxidation of the isoprenyl double bond, but in human subjects oxidative metabolism is minimal, and the major metabolite is a C-glucuronide (Gaetani et al, 1979).

THE ROLE OF TOXICOKINETICS

The importance of comparative toxicokinetics in animals and man, for the selection of suitable animal species and the choice of appropriate doses in safety evaluation studies, is now well appreciated. Nevertheless, greater collaboration between the pharmacokineticist and the toxicologist, would result in much more meaningful toxicology studies and the saving of considerable time and expense. Pharmacokineticists are too seldom consulted concerning the choice of animal species and dose levels when chronic toxicity and carcinogenicity studies are being planned. The consequences of such practice are seen in the case of the oral chromone, anti-asthmatic drug candidate, FPL 52757, which was found to be hepatotoxic, but only in dog and man. Toxicology studies in all other species showed no adverse effects, and metabolism studies in a variety of species did not indicate any significant differences between animals and man. It was only when metabolism, toxicokinetics, and receptor studies were considered altogether, that it was obvious that the dog was the only appropriate animal model for evaluating the safety of the drug for human use (Clark et al, 1982; Clarke et al., 1985). Because only dog and man exhibit impaired oxidative metabolism of the drug, the consequent slow clearance, and toxicity due to detergent activity of the parent drug on the hepatocyte membranes, the dog is the only species which adequately reproduces the toxic effects seen in man.(see Table 3).

Similarly, the species-different rates of oxidative metabolism of chloroform to the reactive intermediate, carbonyl chloride, probably the toxic metabolite responsible for the carcinogenicity of chloroform in the mouse, indicates that this occurs most readily in small animals (see Table 4) (Brown, et al, 1974). From the work of Walker (1980) and others, it is now readily appreciated that the rates of oxidative metabolism of drugs and toxic chemicals are inversely related to the body weight of the animal species concerned. As may be seen from Table 4, mice oxidatively metabolise chloroform (first to $^{14}COCl_2$ then to $^{14}CO_2$) to the extent of approximately 80% of the

Table 3. Relationship of Toxicity of a Chromone Anti-
Asthma Drug to its Systemic Clearance.

Species	Dose (mg/kg)	Clearance (mg/kg/h)	Hepatotoxicity
Rat	10	138	none (400 mg/kg per day)
Rabbit	10	44	none (100 mg/kg per day)
Squirrel Monkey	10	59	none (300 mg/kg per day)
Dog	1	20	
	5	12	
	10	13	
	50	1	extensive centrilobular necrosis and fatalities after 6 doses at 40 mg/kg per day)
Man	1	15	raisedplasma amino-transferase levels

Clark et al, 1982; Clarke et al, 1985)

Table 4 Species Differences in the rates of Oxidative
Metabolism of Chloroform and its Dependence on Body Weight

Species	Body Wt.(g)	% Dose Excreted in 2 Days as:		
		$^{14}CO_2$	$^{14}CHCL_3$ unchanged	Total Recovered
Mouse CBA	20-30	76+5	7+2	83
C57	20-30	79	5	84
CF/LP	20-30	76	6	82
Rat (Sprague-Dawley)	200-300	66+4	20+5	86
Monkey (Squirrel)	500-1000	18+2	79+3	97

Dose of chloroform was 60mg/kg (from Brown et al, 1974)

dose; the rat, at ten times the bodyweight of the mouse, oxidatively metabolises 65% of dose, and the squirrel monkey at some 20 to 50 times the mouse body weight, oxidatively metabolises only some 20% of dose. It is obvious that the amount of chloroform that would be oxidatively metabolised by man would be extremely small (ca. 1% dose) and that most would be exhaled unchanged. Thus, the likelihood of chloroform constituting a significant risk of cancer in man is remote, and an appreciation of the mechanism of toxicity and the species differences in the pharmacokinetics of chloroform, might have precluded the naive assumption that chloroform has significant carcinogenic potential in human.

Often on increasing the dose of a drug or chemical, the toxicokinetic parameters may undergo change, due to saturation of metabolic pathways, saturation of a route of excretion, etc, indicating non-linear kinetics. It is therefore important to take this into consideration when selecting the doses for chronic toxicity studies. In general, the low dose would be chosen as the pharmacokinetic equivalent of the human dose, or a simple multiple of this; the middle dose should, if possible, be chosen at the maximum dose within the range of linearity of the toxicokinetics; and only the highest dose should be chosen in the non-linear toxicokinetic range, i.e. on the other side of the 'metabolic break-point' (Feron and Kroes, 1986). A comprehensive account of the impact of non-linear toxicokinetics on chemical toxicity, and the importance of determining the rates of metabolic detoxication at different doses before undertaking chronic toxicity studies, is given in a review, with specific reference to the industrial chemical dioxane, by Dietz et al, (1982).

Similarly, the toxicokinetics of a drug or chemical may change with repeated dosage, due to enzyme induction, enzyme inhibition, enterohepatic recirculation, drug accumulation, etc. It is therefore essential to determine the kinetics of a chemical after repeated dosage, say for 1 month, in the animal species selected for chronic toxicity studies, before undertaking such studies, so as to avoid excessively high doses which would precipitate marked toxicity not experienced at normal dosage of the drug, or to anticipate higher dosage likely to be required because of enzyme induction.

Man is genetically highly heterogeneous, and the safety evaluation of chemicals in studies with genetically homogeneous experimental animal models can reveal only the major forms of toxicity. No animal experiments can be completely satisfactory for the safety evaluation of drugs and chemicals for human use, and final validation in human populations, by clinical pharmacology/toxicology and human pharmacokinetic studies, is an essential aspect of the safety evaluation procedure for new drugs. Genetic differences in the activities of the drug-metabolising enzymes in human populations, resulting in genetically-dependent toxicity due to impaired detoxication and drug accumulation have long been known in respect of the rates of drug acetylations (e.g. isoniazid) (Evans et al, 1960) and the hydrolysis of esters (eg, suxamethonium) (Price-Evans, 1965). However, the toxicity of sulphapyridine and other sulphonamide drugs appears to involve more than differences in acetylator status, and the immunologically-mediated adverse effects of these drugs (e.g. Stevenson-Johnson syndrome) seems to be mediated by the genetically-dependent formation of a lymphotoxic, oxygenated, reactive intermediate (Shear et al, 1986). Indeed, several genetic differences have been observed in the activities of the various human cytochromes P-450, resulting in differences in the rates of oxidative metabolism, detoxication and clearance of a number of drugs including debrisoquine, desmethylimipramine, sparteine and nortryptiline (Guengerich et al, 1986), and genetic variability in the pharmacokinetics of certain β-adrenoceptor antagonists, such as metoprolol, has been shown to be dependent on the extent of oxidative metabolism (Tucker et al, 1986).

In the case of drugs and chemicals that are diastereoisomeric mixtures (eg, perhexiline, mephenytoin, bufuralol, and the synthetic pyrethroid insecticides), one particular isomer may be metabolised in a different manner, or at a different rate, from the other isomers, resulting in accumulation and toxicity which are dependent on the isomeric composition of the chemical. In some instances, the metabolism in man of the different stereoisomers may be genetically dependent, and the hepatotoxicity of perhexiline has been attributed to genetic differences in the oxidative metabolism of the drug and to pharmacokinetic differences of the various diastereoisomers (Gould et al, 1986).

Clinical pharmacokinetic studies of new drugs in substantial populations of patients, including the elderly who frequently exhibit impaired oxidative drug metabolism and renal excretion (Triggs, 1986), have long been considered desirable. In view of the now recognised. problems of genetic polymorphism in the metabolic detoxication and clearance of drugs, and the possibilities of enzyme induction (e.g. diphenylhydantoin) and inhibition (e.g. cimetidine), such studies become highly essential.

Unfortunately, repeat-dose, clinical pharmaco-kinetic studies in patients are still an aspect of drug safety evaluation which is often neglected, sometimes with disastrous results (e.g. benoxaprofen).

MECHANISMS OF TOXICITY AND RECEPTORS

The design of animal chronic toxicity studies, without some prior knowledge of the mechanism of toxicity of the chemical under consideration, is scientifically unsound, as the mechansism may obviously vary markedly from chemical to chemical and from species to species. Furthermore, the mechanism of toxicity cannot be considered in isolation of knowledge concerning the routes and rates of metabolism of the chemical, as these processes are essential to detoxication.

Elucidation of the mechanism(s) of toxicity, frequently allows a specific receptor to be identified. These may be membrane or cytosolic receptors (e.g., the steroid receptors), enzymes (eg, the cholinesterases, cytochrome oxidase or cytochrome P-450 or P-448), or biological redox buffers or detoxication/chemical defence enzymes (eg, glutathione, glutathione peroxidase) (see Table 5). When the receptors have been identified, it is possible to carry out comparative receptor studies in vitro, e.g., by studying the inhibition of individual cholinesterases of human erythrocytes by organophosphorus pesticides and comparing the effects with those of the erythrocyte enzymes of experimental animals (Chemnitius et al, 1983), or by determining the comparative tissue concentrations and affinities of steroid receptors for anti-steroid drugs, such as tamoxifen (Rose et al, 1985) or gestodene (Iqbal et al, 1986). In this way, excellent predictions of the potential human toxicity of many pesticides and steroid-inhibiting drugs, have been calculated from animal toxicity studies and comparative receptor experiments.

Many chemicals with proven carcinogenicity (e.g. benzo(a)pyrene) and with other toxicity (e.g., 2,3,7,8-tetrachlorodibenzodioxin) have been shown to have high affinity for a cytosolic receptor that results in the specific induction of the cytochromes P-448. This receptor also binds epidermal growth factor (Karenlampi et al, 1983), and regulates the same m-RNAs which are regulated by a number of oncogenes (Matrisian et al., 1985). Moreover, these chemicals are selectively metabolised by the cytochromes P-448, so it was perhaps not surpising to find that the spatial conformation of the active site of the enzyme, cytochrome P-448, is very similar to that of the

Table 5   Some Receptors Mediating Toxicity

RECEPTOR	TYPICAL SUBSTRATE/INHIBITOR

Steroid	
androgen	dihydrotestosterone, bifluranol
oestrogen	oestradiol, tamoxifen
progestogen	progesterone, gestodene
mineralocorticoid	aldosterone
Cholinesterase	
acetylcholinesterase	acetylcholine, parathion
Others	
opiate	morphine, naloxene
glutathione	bromobenzene
cytochrome P-450	acetylenic compounds
DNA	beno(a)pyrene diol epoxide

---

cytosolic receptor (Lewis et al, 1986). Computerised
molecular graphics of substrates, inhibitors and inducing
agents of the microsomal cytochromes, have indicated that
substrates and inducing agents of the cytochromes P-450 are
globular molecules with molecular dimensions in which
area/depth^2 approaches unity, whereas, in contrast, the
substrates, inhibitors and inducers of the cytochromes P-
448 are large planar molecules with area/depth ^{2} of greater
than 5 (see Table 6 and Figure 3) (Lewis, et al, 1986). An
evaluation of the affinity of drugs and chemicals for this
cytosolic receptor is now finding wide application in
safety evaluation studies both by determining their
induction of cytochrome P-448 (Iwasaki et al, 1986) and by
computergraphic studies (Parke et al, 1986).
    The design of drugs, pesticides and other chemicals is
frequently based on the principle of selective toxicity,
namely, species differences in the toxicity of the
chemical, its metabolic detoxication, or its activation.
    In evaluating the potential toxicity of these chemicals
in man, these differences in metabolism, toxicokinetics,
mechanisms of toxicity and receptor studies are central to
any scientific approach to safety evaluation. The paradox
is that the very philosophy of 'selective toxicity' on
which the design of so many drugs, pesticides and food

Figure 3. Computer-calculated Molecular Dimensions of
Substrates of the Cytochromes P-450 and P-448

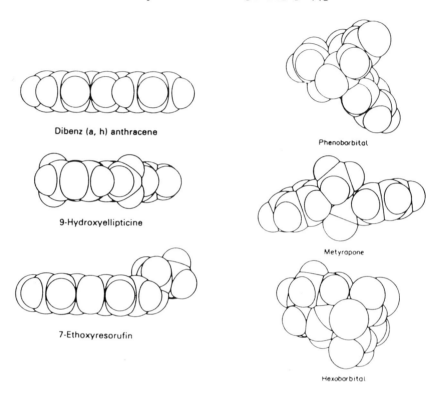

Dibenz (a, h) anthracene

9-Hydroxyellipticine

7-Ethoxyresorufin

Phenobarbital

Metyrapone

Hexobarbital

Cytochrome P-450: hexobarbital (substrate), metyrapone
(inhibitor) and phenobarbital (inducing agent). Cytochrome
P-448: 7-ethoxyresorufin (substrate), 9-hydroxyellipticine
(inhibitor) and dibenz(a,h)anthracene (inducing agent)
(see Lewis et al, 1986).

additives is based, becomes the major obstacle to
determining the safety of these chemicals for man by the
use of toxicity studies in experimental animal models.

REFERENCES

Boobis, A.R., Tee, L.B.G., Hampden, C.E. and Davies, D.S
    (1986) Food Chem. Toxicol, 24, 731.
Brown, D.M., Langley, P.F., Smith, D. and Taylor, D.V
    (1974) Xenobiotica, 4, 151.

Table 6. The Molecular Dimensions of Carcinogens and Toxic Chemicals and Their Activation by Cytochrome P-448

Chemical	Molecular Dimension (area/depth2)	Prefered Cytochrome	Toxicity
Dibenz(a,h)anthracene	14.4	448	carcinogen
Benzo(a)pyrene	12.0	448	carcinogen
Dimethylaminoazobenzen	9.7	448	carcinogen
9-Hydroxyellipticine	7.0	448	cytotoxin + carcinogen
2-Acetamidophenol	5.0	448	carcinogen
Paracetamol	4.8	448	hepatotoxin at highdose
Aflatoxin	3.2	448/450	hepatotoxin hepatocarcinogen
Metyrapone	2.0	450	adrenal suppression non-carcinogen
DDT	1.9	450	cholinesterase inhibition, non-carcinogen
Phenobarbitone	1.1	450	hypnotic, non-carcinogen

Chemnitius, J.-M., Haselmeyer, K.-H and Zech, R. (1983) Biochem. Pharmacol, 32, 1693.

Clark, B., Smith, D.A., Eason, C.T., and Parke, D.V (1982) Xenobiotica, 12, 147.

Clarke, A.J., Clarke, B., Eason, C.T. and Parke, D.V (1985) Regulat. Toxicol. Pharmacol. 5, 109.

Dietz, F.K., Stott, W.T. and Ramsey, J.C. (1982) Drug Metab. Rev, 13, 963.

Evans, D.A.P., Manley, K.A., McKusick, V.C. (1960) Br. Med. J. ii, 485.

Feron, V.J. and Kroes, R. (1986) J. Appl. Toxicol. 6, 307

Gaetani, M., Yamaguchi, H., Vidi, A., Hashimoto, Y. and Donetti,A. (1979)Pharmacol. Res.Commun. 11, 719.

Gould, B.J., Amoah, A.G.B. and Parke, D.V. (1986) Xenobiotica 16, 367.

Guengerich, F.P., Distlerath, L.M. Reilly, P.E.B., Wolff,

T., Shimada, T., Umbenhauer, D.R. and Martin, M.V. (1986) Xenobiotica 16, 367.

Guengerich, F.P. and Liebler, D.C. (1985) C.R.C. Crit. Rev. Toxicol. 14, 259.

Hinson, J.A. (1983) Environ. Hlth. Perspect. 49, 71.

Ioannides, C., Lum, P.Y. and Parke, D.V. (1984) Xenobiotica 14, 119.

Iqbal, M.J., Colletta, S.D., Houmayoun-Valyani and Baum, M. (1986) Br. J. Cancer. 54, 447.

Iwasaki, K., Lum, P.Y., Ioannides, C. and Parke, D.V. (1986) Biochem. Pharmacol. 35, 3879.

Iveson, P., Lindup, W.E., Parke, D.V. and Williams, R.T. (1971) Xenobiotica 1, 79.

Karenlampi, S.O., Eisen, H.J., Hankinson, O. and Nebert, D.W. (1983) J. Biol. Chem. 258, 10378.

Lee, S.G.K. and Fukuto, T.R (1982) J. Toxicol. Environ. Hlth. 10, 717.

Lewis, D.F.V., Ioannides, C. and Parke, D.V. (1986) Biochem. Pharmacol 35, 2179.

Mason, R.P. (1985) Environ. Hlth. Perspect 64, 1.

Matrisian, L.M., Glaichenhaus, N., Gesnel, M.-C. and Breathnach, R. (1985) EMBO J. 4, 1435.

Parke, D.V., Ioannides, C. and Lewis, D.V.F. (1986) FEST Supplement, TIPS, 14.

Pessayre, D., Dolder, A. and Artigou, J.-V. (1979) Gastroenterology, 77, 264.

Price-Evans, D.A. (1965) Ann. N. Y. Acad. Sci. 123, 178.

Rose, C., Thorpe, S.M, Andersen, K.W., Pedersen, B.V., Mouridsen, H.T., Blichert-toft, M and Rasmussen, B.B. (1985) Lancet i, 16.

Sanockij, I.V. (1975) In: "Methods used in the U.S.S.R. for establishing biologically safe levels of toxic substances", Geneva, WHO, p9.

Shear, N.H., Spielberg, S.P., Grant, D.M., Tang, B.K. and Kalow, W. (1986) Ann. Int. Med. 105, 179.

Tong, S., Masson, H.A., Iannides, C., Bechtel, W.D. and Parke, D.V. (1986) Xenobiotica 16, 595.

Triggs, E.J. (1986)In Development of Drugs and Modern Medicine". (Eds J.W. Gorrod, G.G. Gibson and M.Mitchard) Ellis Horwood, Chichester. p 451.

Tucker, G.T., Lennard, M.S., Jackson, P.R. and Woods, H.F. (1986) In: "Development of Drugs and Modern Medicine," (Eds. J.W. Gorrod, G.G. Gibson and M. Mitchard.) Ellis Horwood, Chichester. p. 462.

Walker, C.H. (1980) In: "Progress in Drug Metabolism", Vol. 5,(Eds. J.W. Bridges and L.F. Chasseaud). Wiley: Chichester. p. 113.

RELATION OF DRUG METABOLISM TO DRUG DESIGN

Johann W. Faigle

Research and Development Department, Pharmaceuticals Division, CIBA-GEIGY Limited, Basle, Switzerland.

INTRODUCTION

In this article, the term metabolism will be used in a broad sense as defined by Di Carlo (1982) :

"Xenobiotic metabolism is the sum of processes affecting the fate of foreign substances in the organism"

Accordingly, the following discussions will consider both the chemical reactions and the transport processes of drugs in the body, although emphasis will be placed on the former.

Rational drug design means the application of previously recognized correlations of biological activity with physicochemical properties. The final aim of drug design should not be to increase activity. It should rather be to reach a better ratio between activity and toxicity of a drug, i.e. to increase its selectivity.

Since the interactions of drugs with living organisms are complex, the drug designer often focusses on intrinsic activity only. This activity can be measured in simple biological systems, such as enzyme preparation or isolated organs. In doing so, however, he neglects the kinetic processes governing the concentration of the active substances in the target tissue in vivo. He normally also neglects the possible appearance of active or reactive metabolites.

Optimal intrinsic activity does not imply optimal metabolic properties. The groups of substituents in a drug molecule which determine the biological effects have little or nothing to do with those parts which determine its fate in the body. Therefore, rational drug design must take the metabolic aspects of drug action into account as well.

Numerous concepts and methods do exist which make use of metabolic knowledge in the design and development of new drugs. In the present account, an attempt will be made to discuss these approaches from a practical point of view. Their chances and limitations will be illustrated by selected, actual examples.

However, it is not intended to give a complete review of the published literature in the field. A great number of excellent articles on individual topics is available, and the reader will be referred to the most recent ones in the text.

THE ERRATIC APPROACH

In routine biotransformation studies one often detects biologically active metabolites. An active metabolite may favourably differ from the parent compound regarding its activity profile or its pharmacokinetic characteristics. So it may become a drug candidate in its own right. Several important drugs in our armamentarium have actually resulted, more or less by chance, from such an unsystematic and erratic approach.

In a strict sense, this approach would not even fit into the above definition, according to which drug design is a predictive and systematic process. Nevertheless, the erratic approach shall be included here, since its impact on drug development is still important. For review articles on active metabolites and their relevance see Drayer (1982). Oelschlager (1982), Dostert and Strolin-Benedetti (1984) and Garattini (1985).

A classic example is desipramine (Figure 1). It has become an established antidepressant following its detection as a metabolite formed by oxidative N-dealkylation of imipramine (Herrmann and Pulver, 1960). Desipramine is a selective blocker of nor-adrenaline uptake, whereas imipramine blocks the uptake of both serotonin and noradrenaline. The biotransformation of desipramine is less complex that that of the parent drug (Gram and Christiansen, 1975). The latter is converted to other primary metabolites (cf. Figure 1); they include pharmacologically active ones, such as the products of N-oxidation and C-hydroxylation. Apart from a different neurobiochemical profile, therefore, desipramine offers favourable metabolic properties.

Biotransformation of diazepam leads to three active compounds, i.e. temazepam, nordazepam and oxazepam (Figure 2). All of them have been developed as independent, tranquillizing drugs. The metabolic reactions involved are N-demethylation and C-hydroxylation (Mandelli et al, 1978), both being catalysed by microsomal mono-oxygenases. Such reactions are known to be sensitive towards enzyme

Figure 1. Active metabolites as independent drugs : Desipramine resulting from N-demethylation of imipramine.

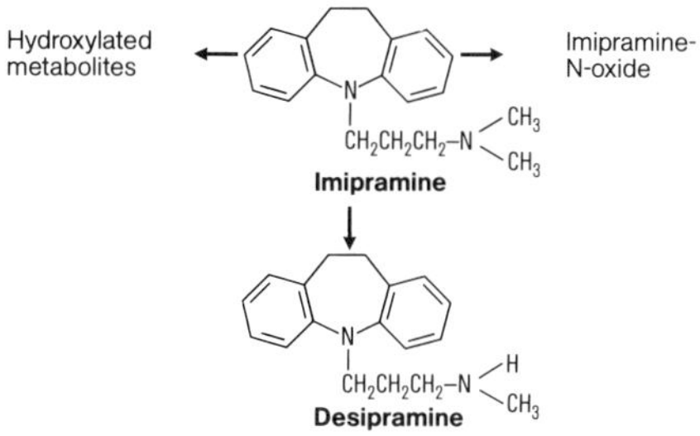

(From Herrmann and Pulver, 1960).

induction or inhibition caused by other xenobiotics. Among the three metabolites, oxazepam has presumably found the widest acceptance. Its biotransformation proceeds in one step by direct O-glucuronidation, which is less sensitive than oxidative pathways. The half-life of oxazepam is shorter than that of diazepam. Again, the metabolite differs from the parent drug in several aspects, which may be therapeutically important.

Figure 2. Active metabolites as independent drugs : Temazepam, nordazepam and oxazepam resulting from C-hydroxylation and N-demethylation of diazepam.

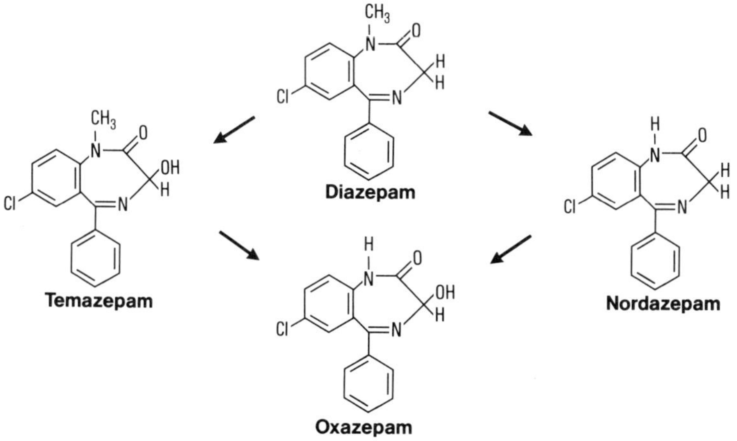

(From Mandelli et al, 1978).

Although the erratic approach may appear outdated at first sight, it should still be pursued in modern drug research and development. However, the main goal should not necessarily be to obtain a second pharmacon in addition to an existing one. It should rather be to develop an active metabolite instead of the initially foreseen parent compound. In doing so, it would often be possible to end up with a product showing less pharmacokinetic variability, less complex biotransformation and better therapeutic performance.

When employing this approach in industrial drug development, the time factor has to be considered. The entire process from the synthesis of a new chemical entity to its approval as a drug lasts 10 to 15 years. Roughly one third of this period is needed for preclinical work (Davies et al, 1986). Therefore, metabolism studies in man can only be initiated after considerable investments have been made already. At that stage it is impossible to replace the trial drug by an active metabolite, without undue delay of development and increase in cost.

It is essential that potentially active metabolites be recognised as early as possible. Suitable animal models or, better, in vitro models with human organ preparations, such as liver homogenates, offer a way out (Maurer, 1983). In addition, attempts should be made to predict biotransformation based on historic knowledge. Therefore, putative metabolites can be synthesised and tested for biological activity at a very early stage. Computer assisted metabolism prediction (CAMP) has already proved useful in some cases (von Wartberg et al, 1984). When this tool is further refined, it will eventually allow reliable forecasting of the structures of metabolites of any compound in any species. Thus, the erratic approach may turn into a more systematic one.

THE THEORETICAL APPROACH

Most of the drugs used today have been created by the traditional, empirical way : Several thousand substances have to be synthesised and screened for biological activities in animal models. Only a few of them can be made available for clinical trials, and only one may become a new drug. Ideally, however, it should be possible to design a drug solely by the theoretical approach, i.e. by prediction of its pharmacodynamic, toxic and metabolic properties before synthesis. This kind of ab ovo design is still a dream, because of our ignorance about structure-activity and structure-metabolism relationships. Yet, a

few promising concepts have come up which allow
optimization of certain metabolic characteristics starting
from a lead compound. One may divide these concepts into
qualitative and quantitative ones. Figure 3 summarises the
main features of three well established qualitative
concepts. They have been proposed for the design of
prodrugs, "hard" drugs and "soft" drugs. In all three
cases, the design aims at predictable, predetermined ways
of drug transformation or excretion. Quantitative
pharmacokinetic aspects have normally to be neglected.
These concepts have been successfully applied in many
cases. Their theoretical background will be discussed
below, and a few typical examples will be given in the next
section.

Figure 3. Drug design concepts based on metabolism : Ideal
properties of prodrugs, "hard" drugs and "soft" drugs.

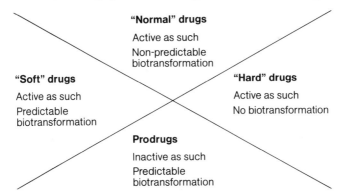

"Normal" drugs
Active as such
Non-predictable
biotransformation

"Soft" drugs
Active as such
Predictable
biotransformation

"Hard" drugs
Active as such
No biotransformation

Prodrugs
Inactive as such
Predictable
biotransformation

A prodrug is an intentionally-formed derivative of an
active substance. Prodrugs can be used to enhance
absorption, to mask side-effects, to extend duration of
action, or to allow site-specific delivery. Ideally, the
prodrug itself is inactive; as soon as its goal is
achieved, it should be quantitatively converted to the
active agent in vivo by an enzymatic or non-enzymatic
process (Notari, 1981; Wermuth, 1983; Stella et al, 1985).
    Carrier-linked prodrugs contain the active molecule
covalently bound to a transport moiety, which is normally
lipophilic. This moiety should be non-toxic and should be
rapidly excreted after its hydrolytic release in the body.
In principle, many types of reversible prodrug linkages
would exist. They include esters, amides, carbamates and
glycosides, among others. In practice however, the ester
linkage is the most widely used one. In vivo, it is
cleaved by esterases present mainly in liver and blood.

The bioprecursors represent a different class of prodrugs (Wermuth, 1983). They result from a molecular modification of the active substances, but they do not contain a carrier group. In vivo they are reconverted to the active substance, e.g. by enzymatic oxidation or reduction.

The aim of the "hard" drug concept is to design active molecules which resist biotransformation and are excreted unchanged (Figure 3). This concept of metabolic stabilisation has been put forward by Ariens and his group (Ariens and Simonis, 1982, and references therein). The term "hard" drugs has been proposed by others (Bodor, 1984). Metabolic stabilisation would imply a longer persistence of the drug in the body and less waste of the active agent. The appearance of potentially toxic, electrophilic, alkylating intermediates of biotransformation would be avoided. The same is true for the unintended formation of pharmacologically active metabolites. Inter- and intra-subject variability of drug response, and the risk of drug-drug interactions would be reduced. Compared to conventional drugs, therefore, "hard" drugs should render therapy safer and simpler.

Metabolic stabilisation can be achieved by shielding vulnerable positions of an active molecule, for instance, or by replacing vulnerable substituents by stable ones. Substitution of hydrogen by halogen may serve as an example. However, it is difficult to design the ideal "hard", non-metabolisable drug, and still maintain optimal properties regarding absorption and excretion (Bodor, 1984).

The "soft" drug concept provides another way to safer therapeutic agents (Figure 3). A "soft" drug is pharmacologically active as such; it undergoes a predictable and controllable conversion into non-toxic, inactive metabolites, after having exerted its therapeutic effects (Bodor, 1984 and references therein). The ideal "soft" drug should be designed such that it is inactivated by one metabolic step, preferentially by hydrolysis. Again, potentially hazardous, reactive intermediates resulting primarily from oxidative biotransformation are avoided. Thus, the therapeutic benefits to be expected from "soft" drugs are similar to those described for "hard" drugs.

In practice, a metabolically sensitive group or bond is built in a non-critical position of a lead molecule. For instance, part of an n-alkyl side-chain is replaced by an ester group to yield an isosteric "soft" analogue. The ester is easily cleaved in vivo by esterases. Further structrual modifications may be needed to reach the optimal rate of deactivation. However, often it will not be possible to fully suppress additional, undesirable routes of biotransformation.

The above three concepts are based on qualitative structure-metabolism relationships; they still demand a large amount of empericism and intuition. A truly rational design of new drugs would necessitate that the relevant descriptors of the biological activities in vivo can be related quantitatively to the relevant descriptors of molecular structures (Figure 4). This straightforward approach is not possible today, owing to the complex situation in the living organism. Therefore, analyses of quantitative structure-activity relationships (QSAR) have concentrated on intrinsic activity (cf. Introduction). Additionally, analyses of quantitative structure-pharmacokinetic relationships (QSPR) have been attempted, to take the metabolic fate of drugs into account (Rowland, 1983; Seydel, 1984; Schaper and Seydel, 1985; Mayer and van de Waterbeemd, 1985).

Figure 4. Quantitative structure-activity relationships. Descriptors of molecular structures, of biological activities and of metabolic properties of drugs.

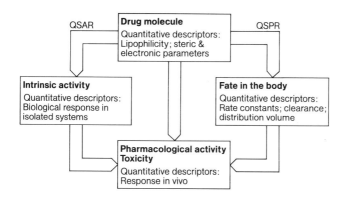

These authors refer to numerous practical examples describing an observed change in a pharmacokinetic parameter as a function of lipophilicity. The kinetic parameters considered include the rate constants of absorption and elimination, the distribution volume, the protein binding constants and the clearance. Other descriptors of molecular structure than lipophilicity have rarely been used. Such analyses have provided a better understanding of kinetic processes within certain classes of compounds. They may also have helped to optimise the metabolic characteristics in some cases, but their impact on the design of new drugs and new leads still appears insignificant.

A better success rate can only be expected when it is possible to analyse each step in drug action by an individual, quantitative method (Mayer and van de Waterbeemd, 1985). Such a multiple approach can be written as :

$$\text{overall QSAR} = f \ (\text{QSAR}_i, \text{QSPR}_j, \text{QSBR}_k, \text{QSTR}_l)$$

where i,j,k,l = 1 to n. QSBR and QSTR would describe the quantitative structure-biotransformation and structure-toxicity relationships. Quite obviously, tremendous efforts will have to be made, before we can think of such a solution.

THE PRAGMATIC APPROACH

Drug design by the pragmatic approach relies on the predictive means available today. It especially tries to make use of the three qualitative concepts presented above from a theoretical point of view (Figure 3). It must be kept in mind, however, that the objectives of these concepts are puristic and absolute. Often it is not possible to fully comply with them, and one must allow for compromises. The following examples will illustrate the pragmatic approach.

Figure 5 shows the structural formula of CGS 14831, which is a potent inhibitor of the angiotensin converting enzyme (ACE) system (Schaller et al, 1985). Its development as an antihypertensive has been hampered by insufficient absorption from the gastrointestinal tract. Being an amino acid with two carboxyl functions, CGS 14831 possesses strongly polar properties detrimental to rapid diffusion through lipoid membranes. The prodrug CGS 14824 A, an inactive mono-ethyl ester, is absorbed in man to the extent of > 40% of dose. A small fraction of the absorbed prodrug is eliminated by direct metabolic conjugation, and is thus lost for the pharmacological effect. Yet, the main part is hydrolysed to the active agent CGS 14831, presumably by hepatic esterases (Waldmeier et al, 1986). At present, CGS 14824A is undergoing clinical trials with promising initial results.

The non-steroidal, anti-inflammatory agent sulindac also meets some essential criteria of a prodrug (Figure 6).

Figure 5. Enhancement of absorption by use of a prodrug : Comparison of CGS 14831, an ACE inhibitor, with its inactive prodrug CGS 824A (Waldmeier et al, 1986).

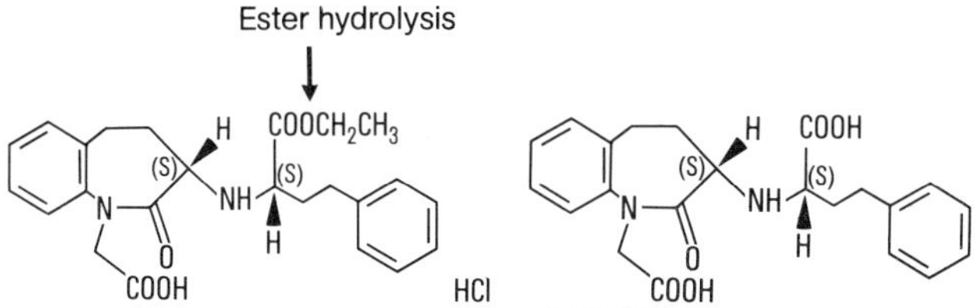

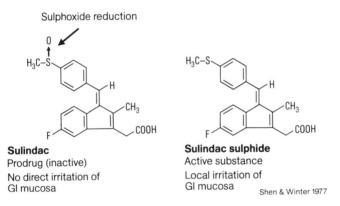

Ester hydrolysis

CGS 14824 A

Prodrug (inactive)
Absorption ⩾ 40 % of dose

CGS 14831

Active substance
Absorption < 5 % of dose

Figure 6. Diminution of toxicity by use of a prodrug : Comparison of sunlindac sulphide, an anti-inflammatory agent, with its inactive prodrug sulindac (Shen and Winter, 1977).

Sulphoxide reduction

Sulindac
Prodrug (inactive)
No direct irritation of
GI mucosa

Sulindac sulphide
Active substance
Local irritation of
GI mucosa

Shen & Winter 1977

Unlike the classical prodrugs, it does not contain a cleavable carrier group in its molecule. It is a sulphoxide, and may be assigned to the subclass of bioprecursors (cf. Wermuth, 1983). Sulindac is metabolised by reversible reduction to the sulphide and by irreversible oxidation to the sulphone. The sulphide strongly inhibits prostaglandin synthetase, while the two other compounds do not (Shen and Winter, 1977). This inhibition seems responsible for both the intestinal irritation and the anti-inflammatory effects observed after oral doses of sulindac sulphide. By administration of sulindac as an inactive precursor, the local effects on the gastro-intestinal mucosa are reduced, but the therapeutic efficacy is largely maintained.

Comparison of the two anti-diabetic drugs tolbutamide and chlorpropamide illustrates the consequences of metabolic stabilisation, in accordance with the "hard" drug concept (Figure 7). Tolbutamide is eliminated from the body mainly by oxidation of the aromatic methyl group to a carboxyl function. In man, it has a comparatively short half-life of about 6 hours (Beyer and Jensen, 1974). In the molecule of chlorpropamide, the vulnerable group (H₃C-) is replaced by a stable one (Cl-). The elimination half-life is in fact prolonged to 33 hours (Taylor, 1972). In spite of this metabolic stabilisation, however, chlorpropamide is not a "hard" drug. Only a small fraction of the dose is excreted unchanged by the kidneys. The main part is removed by alternative biotransformations, particularly hydroxylation in the alkyl side-chain.

Figure 7.   Metabolic stabilisation by replacement of a vulnerable group : Comparisons of two anti-diabetics drugs, tolbutamide and chlorpropamide (Taylor, 1972; Beyer and Jensen, 1974).

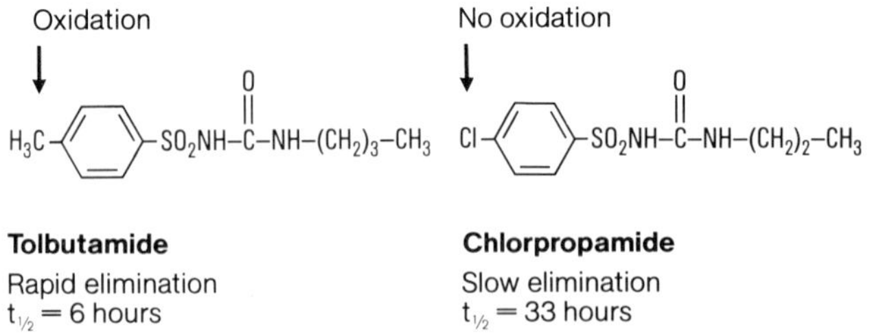

Oxidation

No oxidation

$H_3C-\langle\rangle-SO_2NH-\overset{\overset{O}{\parallel}}{C}-NH-(CH_2)_3-CH_3$ $Cl-\langle\rangle-SO_2NH-\overset{\overset{O}{\parallel}}{C}-NH-(CH_2)_2-CH_3$

Tolbutamide

Rapid elimination
$t_{1/2}$ = 6 hours

Chlorpropamide

Slow elimination
$t_{1/2}$ = 33 hours

The prostacyclin analogue iloprost is a powerful platelet aggregation inhibitor and vasodilator. It is orally active in man, but its short half-life of 20-30 minutes is a serious drawbrack (Skuballa et a;. 1986). Elimination proceeds mainly by β-oxidation of the upper side-chain (Figure 8). Replacement of the vulnerable methylene group by an oxygen atom, accompanied by some other structural modifications, has led to compound ZK96 480. In the rat model, the hypotensive action of this agent lasts two to three times longer than that of iloprost, and the effective dose is more than five times lower. Thus, metabolic stabilisation has clearly been achieved, but it is unknown whether ZK 96480 is eliminated unchanged or by enzymatic attack at other sites of the molecule.

Atracurium, a neuromuscular blocking agent, can be considered as a result of "soft" drug design. The molecule possesses two types of sensitive parts, i.e.

Figure 8. Metabolic stabilisation by replacement of a vulnerable group : Comparison of two platelet aggregation inhibitors and vasodilators, iloprost and ZK96480 (Skuballa et al, 1986).

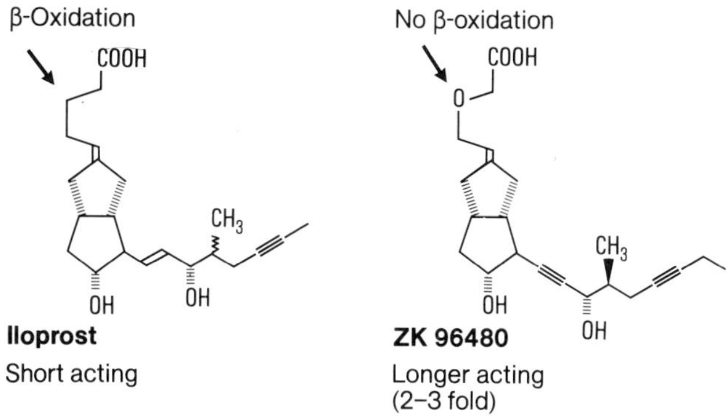

β-Oxidation

COOH

Iloprost
Short acting

No β-oxidation

COOH

ZK 96480
Longer acting
(2–3 fold)

quaternary N-functions and ester groups (Figure 9). In vivo under physiological conditions of pH and temperature, a non-enzymatic Hofmann elimination takes place at the quaternary N-functions. Moreover, the ester groups undergo hydrolysis, which is catalysed by esterases in plasma (Neill et al, 1983). Therefore, atracurium is inactivated by two-non-oxidative processes that are not dependent on liver and kidney function. This certainly contributes to a safe and simple use of the drug in patients. In their advertisements in medical journals, the producers of atracurium actually emphasise the beneficial metabolic properties of their drug.

Figure 9. Avoidance of oxidative biotransformation : Reactions governing the elimination of atracurium, a neuro-muscular blocking agent (Neill et al, 1983).

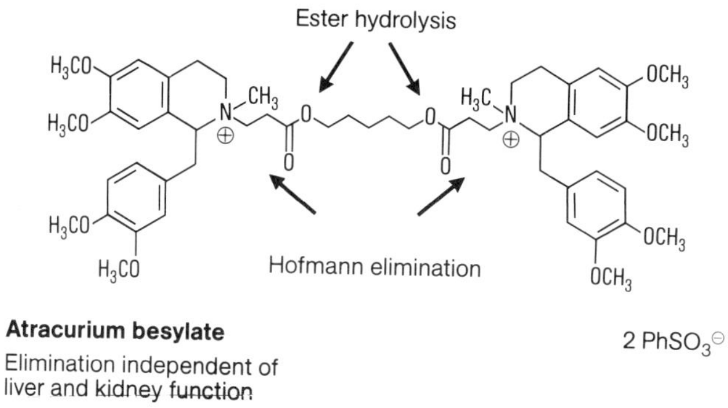

Ester hydrolysis

Hofmann elimination

Atracurium besylate
Elimination independent of
liver and kidney function

$2 \text{ PhSO}_3^{\ominus}$

Carbamazepine is an important, first-line drug for the treatment of epilepsy. Its elimination from the organism in mainly governed by oxidative processes, i.e. epoxidation in the azepine ring, and hydroxylation and methoxylation in the benzene rings (Figure 10). These metabolic processes are inducible by carbamazepine itself or by other anti-epileptic drugs (Faigle and Feldman, 1982). Furthermore, they may be adversely influenced by concomitantly administered enzyme inhibitors.

Figure 10. Oxidative vs. non-oxidative biotransformation : Reactions governing the elimination of two related anti-epileptic drugs, carbamazepine and oxcarbazepine (Faigle and Feldmann, 1982; Schutz et al, 1986).

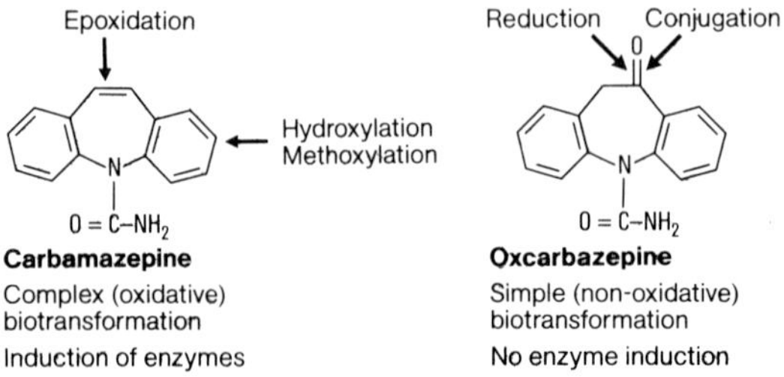

Oxcarbazepine is an anti-epileptic trial drug closely related to carbamazepine. The molecule contains a carbonyl group as a "metabolic handle", which gives rise to a much simpler biotransformation. In the human body, this ketone is enzymatically reduced to a secondary alcohol, which is also pharmacologically active. The latter is largely inactivated by 0-glucuronidation. Oxidative pathways play a subordinate role only (Schutz et al, 1986). In this respect, oxcarbazepine can be taken as a "soft" analogue of carbamazepine. It has potential advantages over the established drug, especially regarding the pharmacokinetic variability brought about by enzyme induction and inhibition. The clinical results available so far are in agreement with these assumptions.

The examples illustrating the pragmatic approach are self-explanatory and do not need further comments, except for one : When applying qualitative metabolic concepts to drug design, use should also be made of quantitative methods like QSPR, whenever sufficient data are available.

CONCLUSIONS

Metabolic findings and predictions do have an important

impact on the design and development of new and better therapeutic agents.

In the course of industrial drug research and development, the medicinal chemist and his counterpart in drug metabolism should consider the metabolic aspects as early as possible. Experimental input should also be obtained at an early stage with suitable in vitro and animal models.

Use should be made of theoretical concepts, such as the prodrug, the "hard" drug and the "soft" drug concept. Within the series of active compounds, they allow one to optimize the metabolic characteristics or to render drug therapy simpler and safer. Avoidance of oxidative bio-transformation is an essential feature of these concepts.

A fully rational design of new drugs would have to be based on quantitative relationships between the relevant descriptors of structure on the one hand, and the relevant descriptors of biological activity and metabolism on the other. Such an integrated approach is not possible with the knowledge and means available today. For partial aspects of drug design, however, analysis of quantitative relationships may already be of great help.

REFERENCES

Ariens, E.J. and Simonis, A.M. (1982). in "Strategy in Drug Research" (Ed. Keverling Buisman, J.A). Elsevier Amsterdam, p.165.

Beyer, W.F. and Jensen, E.H. (1974). in "Analytical Profiles of Drug Substances", Vol. 3 (Ed. Florey, K). Academic Press, New York, p.513.

Bodor, N. (1984). Medicinal Res. Rev, 4, 449.

Davies, I.B., Grind, I.M., Pottage, A. and Turner, P. (1986). J. Roy. Soc. Med, 79, 96.

Di Carlo, F.J. (1982). Drug Metab. Rev, 13, 1.

Dostert, P. and Strolin-Benedetti, M. (1984). Actualites de Chimie Therapeutique, 11e, Serie, 237.

Drayer, D.E. (1982). Drugs, 24, 519.

Faigle, J.W. and Feldmann, K.F. (1982). in "Antiepileptic Drugs" (Ed. Woodbury, D.M., Penry, J.K. and Pippenger, C.E). Raven Press, New York, p.483.

Garattini, S. (1985). Clin. Pharmacokinet, 10, 216.

Gram, L.F. and Christiansen, J. (1975). Clin. Pharmacol. Therap 17, 555.

Herrmann, B. and Pulver, R. (1960). Arch. Internat. Pharmacodyn. Therap, 126, 454.

Mandelli, M., Tognoni, G. and Garattini, S. (1978). Clin. Pharmacokinet, 3, 72.

Maurer, G. (1983). in "Drug Metabolism and Drug Design : Quo Vadis?" (Ed. Briot, M., Cautreels, W. and Roncucci, R). Centre de Recherches CLIN MIDY, Montpellier, p.103.

Mayer, J.M. and van de Waterbeemd, H. (1985). Environ. Health. Perspec, 61, 295.

Neill, E.A.M., Chapple, D.J. and Thompson, C.W. (1983). Brit. J. Anaesthesia, 55, 23S.

Notari, R.E. (1981). Pharmacol. Therap, 14, 25.

Oelschlager, H. (1982). in "Strategy in Drug Research" (Ed. Keverling Buisman, J.A). Elsevier, Amsterdam, p.203.

Rowland, M. (1983). in "Quantitative Approaches to Drug Design" (Ed. Dearden, J.C). Elsevier Amsterdam, p.155.

Schaller, M.D., Nussberger, J., Waeber, B., Bussien, J.P., Turini, G.A., Brunner, H. and Brunner, H.R. (1985). Eur. J. Clin. Pharmacol, 28, 267.

Schaper, K.-J. and Seydel, J.K. (1985). in "QSAR and Strategies in the Design of Bioactive Compounds" (Ed. Seydek, J.K). VCH Verlagsgescellschaft, Weinheim, p.173.

Schutz, H., Feldmann, K.F., Faigle, J.W., Kriemler, H.-P and Winkler, T. (1986). Xenobiotica (in press).

Seydel, J.K. (1984). Methods and Findings in Experimental and Clinical Pharmacology, 6, 571.

Shen, T.Y. and Winter, C.A. (1977). in "Advances in Drug Research ". Vol. 12 (Ed. Harper, N.J. and Simmonds, A.B). Academic Press, London, p.89.

Skuballa, W., Schillinger, E., Sturzebecher, C.-St. and Vorbruggen, H. (1986). J. Med. Chem. 29, 313.

Stella, V.J., Charman, W.M.N. and Naringrekar, V.H. (1985). Drugs, 29, 455.

Taylor, J.A. (1972). Clin. Pharmacol. Therap, 13, 710.

Von Wartburg, B.R., Voges, R. and Sieber, W. (1984). in "Abstracts of the 9th European Workshop on Drug Metabolism", Pont-a-Mousson, p.6.

Waldmeier, F., Faigle, J.W. and Schmid, K. (1986). "Abstracts of the 10th European Drug Metabolism Workshop", Guildford, p.45.

Wermuth, C.G. (1983). in "Drug Metabolism and Drug Design: Quo Vadis" (Ed. Briot, M., Cautreels, W. and Roncucci, R). Centre de Recherches CLIN MIDY, Montpellier, p.253.

SIGNIFICANCE OF MEASURING BLOOD LEVELS OF DRUGS

Silvio Garattini

Istituto di Ricerche Farmacologiche "Mario Negri", Via
Eritrea, 62 - 20157, Milano, Italy.

INTRODUCTION

About 30 years ago, advances in modern analytical
technology, making it possible to measure relatively small
concentrations of chemicals in biological materials, added
a new dimension to pharmacology.

It became possible to discuss pharmacological problems
not only in terms of doses but in terms of concentrations
in blood and in tissues, thus relating levels of drugs to
pharmacological or toxicological effects. This approach
was obviously extended to man in view of the relatively
easy availability of samples of biological fluids, i.e.
blood and urine and though much less frequently, of biopsy
specimens from different tissues. Mathematical models have
also provided a means of exploring the relations between
drug concentrations in blood and tissues over a set time
course.

The initial approach was relatively simplistic and the
aim was to use blood levels of drugs as a parameter to
individual therapy; it was generally believed that
adjusting the blood concentration of drugs at an optimal
level would prove useful in overcoming variability in the
pharmacological and therapeutical effects of drugs in
individual patients.

In these three last decades we have learned that the
problem is not so simple and that many factors interfere in
the relationship between blood levels and effects of drugs.
This review aims at illustrating some of these factors,
using examples taken from research work carried out in this
laboratory.

AN ALMOST IDEAL SITUATION

Several examples of good relationships between blood
levels and pharmacological effects are available in the
literature. Usually it is necessary to have drugs which

are not metabolized and equilibrate their blood and tissue
concentrations well. An example is reported in Figure 1,
depicting the relationship between plasma and striatal
levels of apomorphine (Figure 1a) in rats given several
doses (0.6-5mg/kg i.p) at a set time (Bianchi et al, 1986).
The high correlation (r = 0.944) of these two parameters
means it is possible to use blood concentrations for
establishing correlations with a pharmacological effect of
apomorphine, the stereotyped behaviour (Figure 1b) which is
usually attributed to the direct agonistic activity of
apomorphine on post-synaptic dopamine receptors (Anden et
al, 1967; Ernst 1967). In this case there is also a good
statistical correlation (r = 0.855) although it is evident
from the graph that individual rats may have equal blood
levels of drugs but different quantitative responses
(stereotyped score) to apomorphine.

The relationship may be even better when sharper end
points are considered. For instance in inbred mice
(CD_2F_1/CrlBR) the oral LD_{50} (1746 mg/kg) of caffeine was 5
times the i.v. LD_{50} (319 mg/kg) while the concentrations of
caffeine at these doses in brain and in blood were
comparable for the two routes. This supports the
importance of establishing tissue concentrations, more than
doses, as a useful parameter. These results suggest a
possible threshold brain concentration for the lethal
effect of caffeine, around 1 μ mol/g (190μg/g) regardless of
the route of administration (Bonati et al, 1985).

These examples are however relatively rare and they
represent more the exception than the rule.

DOSES VERSUS BLOOD LEVELS

The dose is an "exogenous" unit. As soon as a dose is
administered to a living organism it becomes a
concentration (an amount expressed per unit of blood volume
or tissue weight). In some cases there may be a good
proportion between the administered dose and the blood
concentration; Figure 2 shows for instance that the
administration of oral theobromine to rats over a dose
range of 100 times results in a corresponding increase of
the blood levels (Bonati et al, 1984a). However as also
shown in Figure 2 this is not always the case: caffeine,
another methylxanthine, shows a disproportionate increase
in blood levels over the same range of doses (Latini et al,
1978) and even steeper is the relationship between doses
and brain levels in the case of 1-fenfluramine (Caccia,
unpublished results).

The fact that raising the doses does not cause a

Figure 1. Relationship between plasma and striatal levels
of apomorphine after administration of apomorphine (0.6-
5mg/kg i.p) to rats (A).   Relationship between plasma
apomorphine levels and stereotypy (B). For details see
Bianchi et al, 1986.

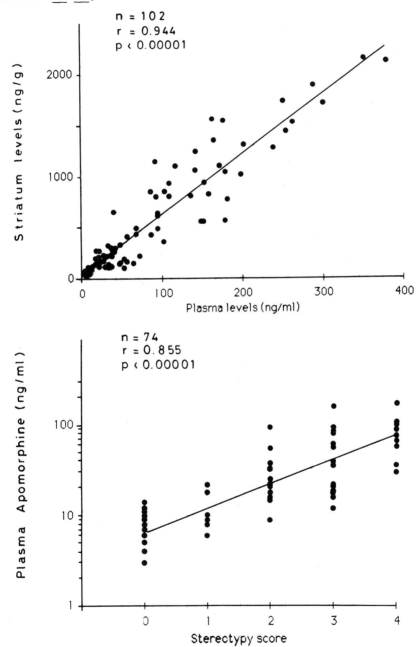

Figure 2.   Relations between blood AUC (caffeine and
theobromine) and brain AUC (1-fenfluramine) and the
administered dose to rats.

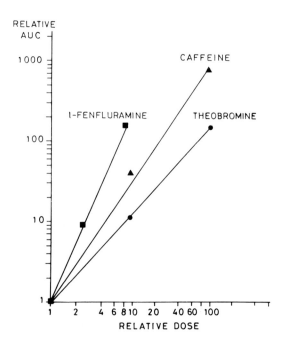

similar increase in blood levels may depend on several
reasons including limited capacity of the body to
metabolize or excrete a given chemical.

   This situation, usually referred to as dose-dependent
pharmacokinetics, is unfortunately influenced by several
factors including animal species, making any extrapolation
across species difficult. With caffeine, dose-dependent
kinetics for pharmacological doses are only observed in
rats; in fact, on raising the dose of caffeine from 1 to 10
mg/kg orally the increase in blood levels (expressed as
area under the curve - AUC - which represents the area
covered by the concentration versus time) is about 46 for
rats but between 12 and 16 for mice, rabbits, monkeys and
man (Bonati et al, 1984b).

   In other cases the dose-dependence kinetics is not
predictable by measuring blood levels but it can be seen in
tissues. For instance on raising the oral dose of
amiodarone in rats by 3 times (from 25 to 75mg x 3 weeks)
plasma levels increased by about 3 times but the liver

levels increased by 10 times and lung levels by about 13 times (Latini et al, 1986).

Since dose-dependent pharmacokinetics may be peculiar for given individuals and tissues, adjustment of the dose to reach optimal blood concentrations may become a very difficult matter.

BLOOD LEVELS VERSUS TISSUE LEVELS

It is often difficult to predict the relation between blood levels and concentrations of a drug in a tissue relevant for the drug's effect; there may be no relation between changes in blood versus tissue concentrations. A first example can be taken from clinical studies with an antiarrhythmic drug, amiodarone. This drug was given for therapeutic purposes for a short or long time to two groups of patients undergoing surgery. The short-term treatment was 12.2 ± 2.2 days (n = 9) and the long-term treatment was 23.1 ± 4.9 months (n = 12) with daily amiodarone doses of 4.7 ± 0.6 and 3.4 ± 0.4 mg/kg respectively. About 30h after the last dose, patients underwent heart surgery and it was possible to measure amiodarone in biopses of atrial tissue as well as in plasma. Table 1 reports the results. Plasma amiodarone was comparable in the two groups while the atrial levels were almost 2.5 times higher in the long-term treatment than in the short treatment group (Barbieri et al, 1986). Since amiodarone accumulates in cardiac tissue with a ratio of about 30 it is very difficult to predict from plasma levels the concentration present in the heart, the organ where amiodarone exerts its effect. Therefore an apparent lack of change in plasma levels does not guarantee that no changes have occurred in tissues.

The profile of distribution in a single tissue may differ widely from one tissue to another and it is usually unpredictable unless direct measurements have been made. Therefore in these cases blood levels cannot be directly extrapolated to any one tissue. Figure 3 presents a profile of tissue concentrations of adriamycin in a patient with breast tumour. 48h after a dose of 75 mg/m^2 of adriamycin, an antitumour drug, there are striking differences, even 40 times, between for instance the concentrations of adriamycin in fat and lymph nodes (Tossi et al, in preparation).

In other cases the blood levels have no importance because they are not measurable at times when the pharmacological effects are still present. The following example is pertinent; tertatolol is a typical β-adrenergic blocker which, like other analogues, reduces heart rate in

Table 1.   Amiodarone (Am) concentrations in surgical
patients treated with the drug for variable lengths of
time, <12 days (S) and >23 months (L).

GROUP	PLASMA	ATRIUM	FAT
S	0.46+0.07 (0.08-0.74)	13.2+2.5 (4.2-29.0)	33.7+11.7 (2.2-79.1)
	n.s. [1]	*	**
L	0.55+0.08 (0.16-1.18)	30.2+5.6 (11.5-75.0)	140.2+22.6 (70.0-305.3)

Figures are means + S.E.M. Ranges are in parentheses under
the mean.
[1]Levels of significance, Student's t test; n.s. p>0.05
*   p<0.01 ** p<0.001

Figure 3.   Levels of adriamycin (ADR) in breast, tumour,
lymph nodes (linph) and other tissues 48h after a dose of
75 mg/m^2 of adriamycin.

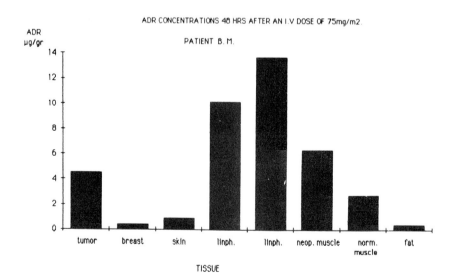

ADR CONCENTRATIONS 48 HRS AFTER AN I.V DOSE OF 75mg/m2.

PATIENT B.M.

animals and in man.   In a study in volunteers (De Blasi et
al, 1986) it was found that tertatolol had a long duration
of action (more than 48h) after a single dose (5mg).   As
depicted in Figure 4 the bradicardiac effect was still
present when tertatolol was no longer measurable in plasma
(sensitivity of the method < 2 ng/ml).

Figure 4.   Effects of tertatolol (5mg) in normal volunteers
(n = 6).

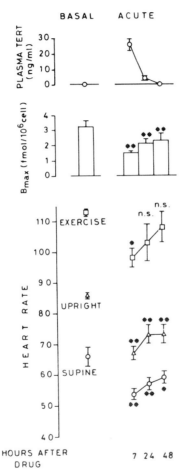

From top to bottom the panels show : plasma tertatolol
levels 7,24 and 48h after administration; density of β -
adrenergic receptors (B_{max}) of lymphocytes; heart rate
after exercise, upright and supine positions.   For details
see De Blasi et al (1986).

   Measurements of β-adreneric receptors in lymphocytes
(which correlate with measurements in cardiac tissue)
indicate that tertatolol reduces the density of these
receptors (B_{max}); other studies show there is a significant
correlation between the decrease in B_{max} and the reduction
of heart rate under different conditions (see Figure 5).
No correlation was apparent between heart rate and the
affinity constant of β-adreneric receptors (data not
shown). These findings suggest that blood levels are not
valid indicators of the effect of tertatolol because the
important factor is the reduction of the density of β-
adrenergic receptors induced by the drug (De Blasi et al,
1986).

Figure 5. Relations between decrease of heart rate and
decrease of lymphocyte B_{max} induced by tertatolol in normal
volunteers (De Blasi et al, 1986).

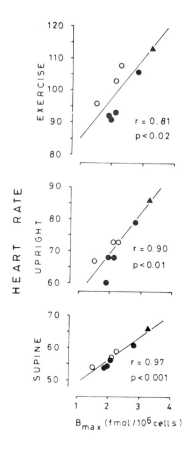

PRESYSTEMIC VERSUS SYSTEMIC BLOOD LEVELS

Usually drugs are assayed in venous blood representative of the systemic circulation but it may be more important - particularly when a drug is given orally - to measure the concentration in the portal circulation (presystemic). Aspirin can be taken as a typical example. As is well known, this drug inhibits platelet aggregation because it blocks cyclooxygenase which is important for synthesis of prostaglandins, among them thromboxane which is a potent platelet aggregating agent (Moncada and Vane, 1979). The effect of aspirin is long-lasting in platelets because it originates from irreversible acetylation of cyclooxygenase (Roth et al, 1975). In a typical experiment in volunteers an oral dose of 320mg of aspirin resulted in some subjects in a measurable level of systemic aspirin, while in others no aspirin was detectable. This difference is not due to problems of drug absorptions because in both groups there were measurable levels of salycilate, the major metabolite of aspirin which does not block cyclooxygenase. Yet the two groups of volunteers showed an over 95% decrease of thromboxane and marked inability of the platelets to aggregate (Cerletti et al, 1985).

A number of studies have shown that blockade of cyclooxygenases in platelets occurs in the portal circulation before aspirin is metabolised in the liver (first-pass metabolism) (Ali et al, 1980; Siebert et al, 1983). Therefore in this case the level of aspirin measured in the general circulation is irrelevant in determining its antiaggregatin effect because the main measurement is the one in the portal circulation where aspirin actually acts. This finding also explains why an oral dose of aspirin inhibits the cyclooxygenase (level of prostacyclin) in the mesenteric vessels more than in systemic vessels. A scheme of these experimental findings is presented in Figure 6 (Cerletti et al, 1986).

BLOOD LEVELS OF THE PARENT DRUG AND METABOLITES

Measurement of a drug in blood is not always meaningful because drugs are frequently transformed in the body into other chemical species (metabolites) which may have pharmacological effects that account for all or part of the effect of the parent drug (or interfere with it), see for review (Garattini 1985).

Benzodiazepines are typical examples of drugs which are metabolised to form active metabolites (Garattini et al, 1973a). For instance when diazepam is given to mice its

Figure 6.   Scheme of "first pass" metabolism of oral
aspirin and its effect on cyclooxygenase of platelets,
vessel walls and peripheral organs (De Blasi et al, 1986).

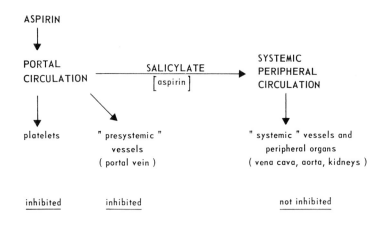

pnarmacological errect (e.g. anticonvulsant) is long-
lasting because it is sustained firstly by diazepam in the
brain, then by N-desmethyldiazepam and by oxazepam
(Garattini et al, 1973a). This situation does not occur in
rats where diazepam's anticonvulsant effect is relatively
short-lasting (Garattini et al, 1973a).
     In the case of trazodone, an antidepressant agent, an
active metabolite is formed: m-chlorophenylpiperazine, a
serotoninergic agonist (Cervo et al, 1981). The levels of
this metabolite are higher in brain than in plasma (Caccia
et al, 1985a).
     In some cases it may be difficult to measure the
metabolite(s) in blood because they rapidly enter tissues
and never accumulate in blood. Antrafenine, an analgesic
agent, is metabolised with the formation of m-trifluoro-
methyl-phenylpiperazine. After the administration of 25
mg/kg oral antrafenine this metabolite is undetectable in
plasma but is present in the brain at a concentration of
100 ng/g (Caccia et al, 1985b). Enpiprazole, a potential
antidepressant agent, is metabolised to o-
chlorophenylpiperazine. Even after the administration of
100 mg/kg of enpiprazole orally, this metabolite is
undetectable in plasma but is present in the brain at the
concentration of 1.3µg/g (Caccia et al, 1985b). It is
evident from these two cases that it would be difficult to
relate plasma levels of the parent compound to
pharmacoloical effect because the active metabolites are

detectable only in brain.

The metabolites do not always show the activity of the parent compound because in some instances they have different effects. Recent studies have indicated that N-desmethyldiazepam, the metabolite of diazepam in man (Garattini et al, 1973b), differs from the parent compound because it shows partial agonistic activity. It has been calculated that the intrinsic potency of N-desmethyldiazepam (taking the value of 1 for diazepam) on leptazol convulsion is equal to 0.43 in rats (Mennini et al, 1986) and 0.37 in mice (Frey and Loscher, 1982). Since the ratio between diazepam and N-desmethyldiazepam in individual patients may vary widely (Garattini et al, 1973b), this could help explain the variability in the degree of sedation exerted by diazepam and other benzodiazepines which are metabolised with the formation of N-desmethyldiazepam (Caccia and Garattini, 1984).

Buspirone is an anxiolytic agent (Goldberg and Finnerty, 1979) which acts with a mechanism different from benzodiazepines (Garattini et al, 1982). Buspirone is metabolised in the body with the formation of 1-pyrimydil-piperazine (PmP), a metabolite which accumulates in the brain (Caccia et al, 1982). As reported in Table 2, buspirone and PmP show completely different effects on brain monoamine receptors; buspirone is particularly effective on striatal dopamine receptors (D_2) and hippocampal $5HT_1$ receptors and on the subtype $5HT_{1A}$ in the cortex while PmP is particularly effective on 2-adreno-ceptors in the cortex (Garattini and Mennini, 1986).

Table 2. **Different effects exerted by buspirone and its metabolite 1-pirimydil-piperazine (PmP) on a number of monoamine receptors.**

RECEPTOR	LIGAND	BUSPIRONE IC_{50} (μM)	PmP
$5HT_1$	^{3}H-5HT[a]	1.2	4.7
$5HT_2$	^{3}H-SPIPERONE[a]	2.2	>10.0
$5HT_{1A}$	^{3}H-BOHDPAT[a]	0.03	3.0
D_2	^{3}H-SPIPERONE[b]	0.6	>10.0
α_2-adren	^{3}H-clonidinea	13.0	0.02

a Experiments using rat cortex
b Experiments using striatum

It would be difficult and even misleading to try to explain some of buspirone's pharmacological effects without knowing about the presence and effect of PmP. Buspirone's action on the inhibition of apomorphine stereotype is likely to be explained by the effect of the drug itself on D_2 receptors, an effect that is not related to the action of PmP (inactive on D_2 receptors); however the antagonistic effect of buspirone on clonidine inhibition of intestinal motility (ED_{50} = 7.16 mg/kg i.p) is entirely by PmP (ED_{50} = 0.49 mg/kg i.p) because of its action on α_2-adrenoceptors (ligand ^{3}H-clonidine or ^{3}H-yohimbine) on which buspirone is essentially inactive (Garattini and Mennini, 1986). A similar explanation is offered for the inhibitory effect of buspirone on the potentiation of hexobarbital sleeping time or on the lowering of MOPEG.SO$_4$ (the brain metabolite of NA) induced by clonidine (Bianchi and Garattini, 1986).

In some cases the metabolite may even antagonise the parent compound's effect. This is the case of salicylate, the major metabolite of aspirin which, at appropriate concentrations, blocks both the platelet antiaggregation (Dejana et al, 1981) and the irreversible cyclooxygenase inhibition (Cerletti et al, 1982) induced by aspirin. It is clear that in this case too the explanation of the effects of aspirin on platelet aggregation and perhaps its other pharmacoloical and toxicological effects, may depend more on the ratio of plasma salicylate: aspirin than on the plasma levels of aspirin (see also the previous considerations on the importance of presystemic blood levels of aspirin). In fact as reported in Table 3, an intravenous dose (40 mg) of aspirin inhibits thromboxane formation more in the presence of a low than a high level of plasma salicylate (Cerletti et al, 1984).

BLOOD LEVELS IN NORMAL AND PATHOLOGICAL CONDITIONS

The presence of pathology during the use of drugs in experimental studies and in clinical conditions complicates the question of the relationship between blood levels and effects. Liver disease may impair drug metabolism; obesity may affect drug distribution to target organs; low plasma albumins may increase the relative amount of the unbound drug fraction; a tumour may change blood drug levels or renal insufficiency may affect blood levels of drugs that are excreted mostly in the urine.

In this last case blood level measurement may be very important for readjusting the doses in relation to the degree of renal impairment. An example is given by pharmacokinetic studies on teicoplanin, a new, wide

Table 3. Antagonistic effect of salycilate (SAL) on the inhibition of platelet thromboxane (TXB$_2$) synthesis induced by aspirin (ASA) in normal volunteers[a].

VOLUNTEER	DOSE OF SAL mg	SAL (C40)	ASA (Co)	RATIO SAL/ASA	TxB2 % INHIBITION
		PLASMA LEVELS (μg/ml)			
GT	250	22.2	8.1	2.8	90
AL	250	19.8	6.4	3.1	93
CO	250	16.8	4.3	3.9	68
ED	1000	85.6	6.8	12.6	51
MB	1000	80.1	8.3	9.7	25
MW	1000	63.3	12.5	5.1	58

[a]Derived from Cerletti et al, 1984.
ASA (40 mg i.v) at the time of salicylate determination

spectrum antibiotic (Parenti et al, 1978). As reported in Figure 7, serum and renal clearances of teicoplanin are directly related to the creatinine clearance (Bonati et al, 1986a). This information is helpful in formulating guidelines for the proper use of this antibiotic as summarised in Table 4. Obviously the problem is much more complicated in cases where the metabolite(s) are excreted in urine depending on their activity (inactive, contributing different effect or antagonist) in relation to the parent drug.

BLOOD LEVELS AND DRUG INTERACTIONS

The extensive literature on drug interactions has shown that several such interactions can be detected by measuring blood drug levels. Independently from the clinical significance of drug interactions, for which there are abundant reviews, drug interactions are mentioned here in relation to pharmacological studies which are frequently aimed at clarifying the mechanisms of drug action. In general, measurements of drug levels in blood, and in some cases, tissues, are essential to establish whether there is

Figure 7. Relationships between total serum teicoplanin
clearance and creatinine clearance (a), and teicoplainin
renal clearance vs. creatinine clearance (b) after a 3
mg/kg i.v. dose in subjects with different renal function.

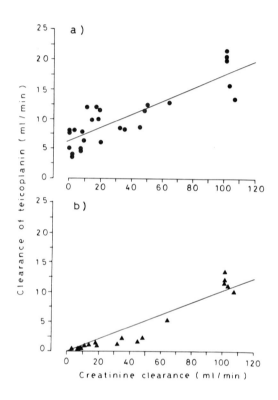

synergism or antagonism between two drugs on a metabolic or
"mechanistic" basis.

    Denzimol is a new anticonvulsant agent (Nardi et al,
1981) which potentiates the action of other anticonvulsants
such as benzodiazepine. However the mechanism of synergism
between denzimol and diazepam may differ considerably,
depending on the dose utilised. Relatively small doses of
denzimol (1.5 mg/kg i.p) increase the density of
benzodiazepine GABA receptors (Mennini et al, 1984) making
the system hypersensitive to the action of diazepam as an
anticonvulsant. At higher doses (5 mg/kg) the effect of
denzimol involves changes of the diazepam metabolism
(Caccia et al, 1986) as indicated in Figure 8 which reports
the blood levels of diazepam given alone or in combination
with denzimol. Pharmacokinetic analysis of these findings

Table 4. Guidelines for modification of teicoplanin dosage regimen in uremic patients[a].

MODIFICATION OF DOSAGE REGIMEN	DEGREE OF RENAL INSUFFICIENCY[b]		
	NORMAL	MILD-MODERATE	SEVERE[c]
Variable maintenance dose, constant dosage interval			
Dose (fraction of normal)[a]	1	1/2	1/3
Dosage interval (multiple of normal)	1	1	1
Variable dosage interval, constant maintenance dose			
Dose (fraction of normal)	1	1	1
Dosage interval (multiple of normal)	1	2	3

[a]Loading dose is always 400 mg i.v. regardless of degree of renal function. [b]Renal function was defined by creatinine clearance as follows: normal = > 80ml/min; mild-moderate = 30-80 ml/min; severe = < 10ml/min. [c]Patients requiring hemodialysis or peritoneal dialysis should not receive additional doses to compensate drug cleared since the amount cleared by these procedures is very limited. Derived from Bonati et al, 1986a and b.

shows that the plasma clearance of diazepam is 34.3 ± 4.8 ml/min kg-1 and 19.8 ± 4.6 when given alone or with denzimol respectively. Accordingly, brain levels of diazepam are higher in combination with denzimol than after diazepam alone (Caccia et al, 1986).

DO EQUAL BLOOD LEVELS MEAN EQUAL EFFECTS

The meaning of blood levels have been discussed on the assumption that in different subjects equal levels of drugs (and/or their metabolites) may result in a similar effect. However this assumption is misleading because the action of a drug does not depend only on its concentration but also on the "sensitivity" of the system - an enzyme or a receptor - on which the drug acts. Table 5 summarises the

Figure 8. Mean plasma concentration-time curves of diazepam after intravenous injection (1 mg.kg^{-1}) to control and denzimol (5 mg.kg^{-1} p.o) treated rats.

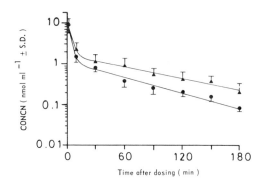

Data are the means ± s.d. for six control (●) and five denzimol (▲)-treated rats.

sensitivity of a small series of human ovarian carcinoma cells exposed to adriamycin (Morasca et al, 1983). It would be clearly impossible to establish an optimal blood concentration of adriamycin considering that the concentrations needed to kill 50% of cancer cells range from 0.16 to >40 µg/ml.

Table 5. In vitro sensitivity of human ovarian carcinoma cells after 24h incubation with adriamycin.

PATIENT	ED_{50} (µg/ml)
1	40
2	0.16
3	>40
4	0.16
5	1
6	10
7	10
8	1

The reason for this different sensitivity is exemplified in Figure 9 which shows that the absolute concentration of

adriamycin is irrelevant, the important thing being the
cancer cells' capacity to bind adriamycin covalently to
macromolecules including DNA (Pantarotto et al, 1986).
This may permit a distinction between sensitive cells
showing macromolecule binding proportional to the uptake,
and resistant cells showing no binding even in the presence
of active adriamycin uptake.

The examples of important individual variability of
targets for drug action could be multiplied ad libitum.
Table 6 shows that the density of β-adrenergic receptors of
human blood lymphocytes may differ by a factor of about 4
in a small number of subjects while the constant of
affinity may change by a factor of more than 2. Even more
variable is basal free fatty acid (FFA) release by human
subcutaneous adipocytes ranging from 0.03 to 1.00 µEqt/g/h
(Table 7). The basal level is not related to the
mobilising effect of noradrenaline which may increase FFA
release by about 6 to about 47 times.

Figure 9. Intracellular kinetics of adriamycin in "in
vitro" sensitive and resistant human lymphoid cells.

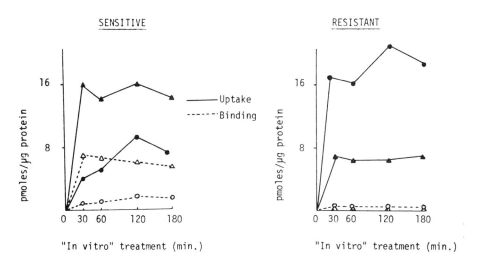

The target tissue's response rather than blood levels
is more important in determining a drug's effect in
arrhythmic patients. As shown in Figure 10, responders or
non-responders to flecainide do not differ in terms of
plasma levels. Similarly the levels of amiodarone and of
its active metabolite desethylamiodarone are not different

Table 6. Individual variability of density and affinity of
β-adrenoceptors in intact human lymphocytes.

β -adrenergic receptors in intact human lymphocytes

SUBJECT	B_{max} (sites/cells)	K_D (nM)
A	813	0.75
B	813	0.78
C	910	0.64
E	1915	0.41
F	1933	0.54
G	2174	0.71
H	3036	0.71
I	3469	0.95

β-adrenoceptors were measured using ^{3}H-CGP 12,177 as
radioligand.

Table 7. Basal lipolysis (release of free-fatty acids =
FFA) of human subcutaneous adipocytes and variability of
response to in vitro added noradrenaline (NA).

SUBJECT	FFA RELEASE (µEq/g/h) FROM HUMAN SUBCUTANEOUS ADIPOCYTES		FACTOR OF INCREASE
	BASAL	NA (10^{-6}M)	
1	0.73	4.9	5.9
2	0.79	5.0	6.3
3	1.00	6.4	6.4
4	0.95	6.8	7.1
5	0.23	2.6	11.3
6	0.37	6.7	18.1
7	0.18	6.9	38.3
8	0.23	9.7	42.1
9	0.03	1.4	46.6

in sensitive and resistant patients (A.D.E.G, 1986).
      All these examples indicate that equal blood levels are
not synonymous with equal drug activity because of the
variability of the target system, thus adding complexity to
the problem.

BLOOD LEVELS AND THERAPEUTIC WINDOWS

      Despite the difficulties mentioned above in utilising
blood levels of drugs for predicting pharmacological
effects and optimising therapy in individual patients, in a
number of cases it has proved possible to establish ranges
of blood levels (therapeutic windows) which statistically
may represent a useful departure point for adopting dose
regimens. Table 8 summarises these "therapeutic windows"
for some drugs.

**Table 8. Plasma concentrations ranges within which
therapeutic effects can be expected for widely used drugs.**

Drug	Therapeutic level (mg/L)
Anti-infective agents	
Amikacin	15-25
Gentamicin	4-10
Tobramicin	4-10
Anticonvulsants	
Valproic acid	50-150
Carbamazepine	4-12
Ethosuximide	40-100
Phenytoin	10-201
Phenobarbitone	72-120 (adult)
	37-73 (child)
Primidone	5-12
Cardiovascular agents	
Quinidine	1-5
Digoxin	0.8-2.4µ/L
Disopyramide	2-75
Various	
Lithium	0.7-1.5 mEq/L
Theophylline	5-20

How useful these indications are in current therapeutic
practice, outside specialised clinical research centers, is

Figure 10.   Plasma levels of flecainide (A) and amiodarone
(B) in responders (R) and non responders (NR).

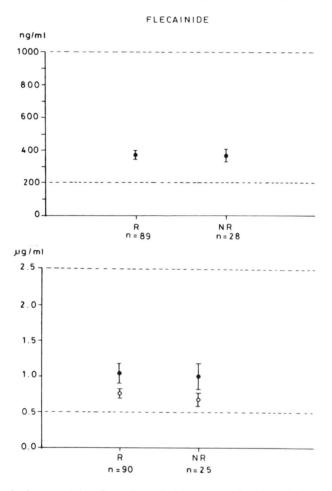

For amiodarone the levels of the parent drug (●) and of its
metabolite desethylamiodarone (O) are reported.

very difficult to state because of a lack of data.   A
study was therefore made recording the requests for drug
assays in 18 large Italian hospitals.   The results,
summarised in Table 9, indicate that with the exception of
digoxin for which there is a large demand, blood level
monitoring is rarely requested even for drugs that are
widely used (Traina et al, 1986; Bonati et al, 1986b).
    The results for digoxin were analysed at two successive

Table 9. Requests for serum drug measurements in eighteen
Italian hospitals during 1984.

DRUG	NO. OF REQUESTS	
	RANGE	MEDIAN
Anti-infective agents		
Amikacin	24-48	36
Gentamicin	16-28	22
Tobramicin	16	-
Anticonvulsants		
Valproic acid	8-516	100
Carbamazepine	12-380	160
Ethosuximide	4-32	12
Phenytoin	8-312	96
Phenobarbitone	24-1344	280
Primidone	8-76	30
Cardiovascular agents		
Quinidine	4-596	8
Digoxin	44-16096	650
Disopyramide	160	-
Various		
Lithium	8-232	108
Salicylates	8-212	28
Theophylline	56-988	164

determinations to establish to what extent they were useful
in improving therapeutic outcome. The advantage of
monitoring blood levels was not evident, but this could
probably be improved with more adequate knowledge of
pharmacokinetic principles (Traina et al, 1986; Bonati et
al, 1986b).

CONCLUDING REMARKS

Thirty years of studies concerning drug kinetics and
metabolism have resulted in some loss of the initial
optimism because the problem of relating blood levels to
pharmacological and therapeutic activity of drugs appears
much more complex than expected. A tentative scheme
identifying some of the factors which complicate relations
between blood levels and drug effects is presented in
Figure 11. Drug and metabolism levels must be considered
in the light of target sensitivity, bearing in mind that a

Figure 11. Some factors which make it difficult to extrapolate pharmacological effects from measurements of drug blood levels.

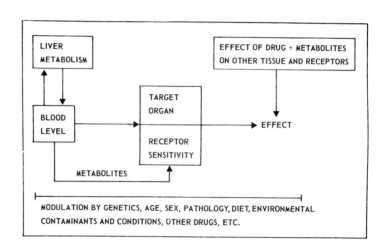

number of variables interfere with the final result.

It is difficult at present to establish general rules because each drug represents a special case that must be studied and understood in all its peculiarities. Perhaps in selected cases the possibility of measuring not only the drug (and active metabolites) blood levels but also the sensitivity of the target may make for greater accuracy in our predictions. The next decade may well bring interesting developments of this approach.

REFERENCES

A.D.E.G. - Antiarrhythmic Drug Evaluation Group-Milan, Italy. (1986). Acta. Pharmacol. Toxicol. Suppl. V. in press.

Ali, M., McDonald, J.W., Thiessen, J.J. and Coates, P.E. (1980). Stroke, 11, 9.

Anden, N.-E., Rubenson, A., Fuxe, K. and Hokfelt, T. (1967). J. Pharm. Pharmacol, 19, 627.

Barbieri, E., Conti, F., Zampieri, P., Trevi, G.P., Zardini, P., D'Aranno, V. and Latini, R. (1986). J. Am. Coll. Cardiol, in press.

Bianchi, G. and Garattini, S. (1986). Br. J. Pharmacol, submitted for publication.

Bianchi, G., Landi, M. and Garattini, S. (1986). Eur. J. Pharmacol, submitted for publication.

Bonati, M., Jiritano, L., Bortolotti, A., Gaspari, F., Filippeschi, S., Puidgemont, A. and Garattini, S. (1985). Toxicol. Let, 29, 25.
Bonati, M., Latini, R., Sadurska, B., Riva, E., Galletti, F., Borzelleca, J.F., Tarka, S.M., Arnaud, M.J. and Garattini, S. (1984a). Toxicology, 30, 327.
Bonati,M., Latini, R., Tognoni, G., Young, J.F. and Garattini, S. (1984b). Drug Metab. Rev, 15, 1355.
Bonati, M., Traina, G.L., Villa, G., Salvadeo, A., Gentile, M.G., Fellin, G., Rosina, R., Covenaghi, L. and Buniva, G. (1986a). Clin. Pharmacokinet, in press.
Bonati, M., Traina, G.L., Colombo, T. and Tognoni, G. (1986b). Lancet, 1, 623.
Caccia, S., Conforti, L. and Conti, I. (1986). J. Pharm. Pharmacol, 38, 469.
Caccia, S., Fong, M.H., Garattini, S. and Notarnicola, A. (1985a). Biochem. Pharmacol, 34, 393.
Caccia, S., Fong, M.H. and Urso, R. (1985b). J. Pharm. Pharmacol, 37, 567.
Caccia, S. and Garattini, S. (1984). in "Handbook of Experimental Pharmacology", Vol 74 (Ed. by Frey, H.H. and Janz, D). Springer-Verlag, Berlin, p.574.
Caccia, S., Garattini, S., Mancinelli, A. and Muglia, M. (1982). J. Chromatogr. 252, 310.
Cerletti, C., Bonati, M., Del Maschio, A., Galletti, F., Dejana, E., Tognoni, G. and de Gaetano, G. (1984). J. Lab. Clin. Med, 103, 869.
Cerletti, C., Gambino, M.C., Bucchi, F., Rajtar, G., Riva, E. and de Gaetano, G. (1986). Agents Actions, submitted for publication.
Cerletti, C., Latini, R., Dejana, E., Tognoni, G., Garattini, S. and de Gaetano, G. (1985). Biochem. Pharmacol, 34, 1839.
Cerletti, C., Livio, M. and de Gaetano, G. (1982). Biochim. Biophys. Acta, 714, 122.
Cervo, L., Ballabio, M., Caccia, S. and Samanin, R. (1981). J. Pharm. Pharmacol, 33, 813.
De Blasi, A., Lipartiti, M. and Garattini, S. (1986). Am. J. Nephrol, in press.
Dejana, E., Cerletti, C., De Castellarnau, C., Livio, M., Galletti, F., Latini, R. and de Gaetano, G. (1981). J. Clin. Invest, 68, 1108.
Ernst, A.M. (1967). Psychopharmacologia, 10, 316.
Frey, H.H. and Loscher, W. (1982). Pharmacology, 25, 154.
Garattini, S. (1985). Clin. Pharmacokinet, 10, 216.
Garattini, S., Caccia, S. and Mennini, T. (1982). J. Clin. Psychiatry, 43, 19.
Garattini, S., Marcucci, F, Morselli, P.L. and Mussini, E.

(1973b). in "Biological Effects of Drugs in Relation to their Plasma Concentrations" (Ed. by Davies, D.S., Prichard, B.N.C). Macmillan Press, London. p.211.

Garattini, S. and Mennini, T. (1986). in "Neuropharmacology 11", Humana Press, Clifton, NJ. in press.

Garattini, S., Mussini, E., Marcucci, F. and Guaitani, A. (1973a). in "The Benzodiazepines" (Ed. by Garattini, S., Mussini, E., Randall, L.O). Raven Press, NY. p.75.

Goldberg, H.L. and Finnerty, R.J. (1979). Am. J. Psychiatry, 136, 1184.

Latini, R., Bizzi, A., Cini, M., Veneroni, E., Marchi, S. and Riva, E. (1986). J. Pharmacokin. Biopharm, submitted for publication.

Latini, R., Bonati, M., Castelli, D. and Garattini, S. (1978). Toxicol. Lett, 2, 267.

Mennini, T., Gobbi, M. and Garattini, S. (1986). Biochem. Pharmacol, submitted for publication.

Mennini, T., Gobbi, M. and Testa, R. (1984). Life Sci, 35, 1811.

Moncado, S. and Vane, J.R. (1979). Pharmacol. Rev. 30, 293.

Morasca, L., Erba, E., Vaghi, M., Ghelardoni, C., Mangioni, C., Sessa, C., Landoni, F. and Garattini, S. (1983). Br. J. Cancer, 48, 61.

Nardi, D., Tajana, A., Leonardi, A., Pennini, R., Portioli, F., Magistretti, M.J. and Subissi, A. (1981). J. Med. Chem, 24, 727.

Pantarotto, C., Sanfilippo, O., Del Monte, M., Bastone, A., Coltro Campi, C. and Silvestrini, R. (1986). Proc. Am. Ass. Cancer Res, 27, 423.

Parenti, F., Beretta, G., Berti, M. and Arioli, V. (1978). J. Antibiot (Tokyo), 31, 276.

Roth, G.J., Stanford, N. and Majerus, P.W. (1975). Proc. Natl. Acad. Sci, (USA), 72, 3073.

Siebert, D.J., Bochner, F., Imhoff, D.M., Watts, S., Lloyd, J.V., Field, J. and Gabb, B.W. (1983). Clin. Pharmacol. Ther, 33, 367.

Traina, G.L., Colombo, F., Del Favero, A., Patoia, L., Gaspari, F., Bonati, M. and Tognoni, G. (1986). Acta. Pharmacol. Toxicol. suppl.V, in press.

SINGLE VERSUS CHRONIC DOSING IN THE SAFETY EVALUATION OF XENOBIOTICS: PHARMACOKINETIC CONSIDERATIONS

M. Danhof

Center for Bio-Pharmaceutical Sciences, Division of
Pharmacology, University of Leiden, P.O. Box 9503, 2300 RA
Leiden, The Netherlands.

INTRODUCTION

The purpose of safety evaluation is to make an
assessment of the potential toxic effect that a compound
may have. In order to make such an assessment, it seems
essential that the compound under investigation is
administered in such a way that sufficiently high
concentrations in a target tissue are obtained to detect
such toxic effects, but also that these concentrations are
maintained at this level for a sufficiently long period of
time. This means that the concentration versus time
profile ("exposure") of the parent compound and/or
metabolites may be expected to be of crucial importance in
the safety evaluation.

Generally the concentration versus time profile of a
compound in vivo is determined by a), the pharmacokinetic
properties of the compound under study and b), the dosing
regimen.

These two factors determine in the first place, the
concentration versus time profile in the blood. However
the concentrations in the target tissue(s) are also
ultimately dependent on these factors since these are
generally closely related to and always dependent on the
concentrations in the blood. Furthermore, the
concentration versus time profile of (exposure to) any
toxic metabolites is also determined by the concentration
of the parent compound.

In this paper a description will be given of the
various concentration versus time profiles that are
obtained upon different dosing regimens. Also, an overview
will be presented of the various factors determining these
concentration versus time profiles. It will be emphasised
that in the safety evaluation of xenobiotics, detailed
knowledge of the pharmacokinetic properties of the compound
under investigation is required, since this allows the
design of dosing regimens resulting in concentration versus

time profiles that are relevant with regard to the assessment of potential toxic effects.

CONCENTRATION VERSUS TIME PROFILE AND PHARMACOKINETICS FOLLOWING SINGLE DOSE ADMINISTRATION

The concentration versus time profiles and pharmacokinetics of drugs following different modes of administration have been described in various textbooks (Rowland and Tozer, 1980). Generally the concentration versus time profile of a compound can be described using the simple pharmacokinetic model depicted in Figure 1.

Figure 1. Schematic representation of the fate of a foreign compound in the body.

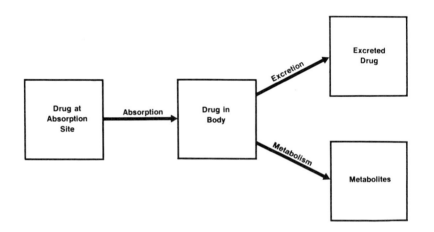

The processes of absorption, renal excretion and hepatic metabolism are indicated with arrows and the compartments with boxes (Rowland and Tozer, 1980; reproduced with permission).

In this model the different boxes represent compartments which can be differentiated into so-called transfer and chemical compartments. In this particular pharmacokinetic model the compound is administered at the site of absorption (i.e. oral administration, intraperitoneal injection, subcutaneous injection) from where it is absorbed into the body. Subsequently the drug is eliminated either in the unchanged form by the kidney or by metabolism in the liver. In the pharmacokinetic model, drug at the site of absorption, drug in the body and drug excreted are clearly in different places. These places may be referred to as a location or transfer compartment. In contrast, metabolism involves a chemical conversion and the metabolite is therefore a chemical compartment.

From the model it can, on the basis of mass balance considerations, easily be visualised that the amount of drug in the body, and thus its concentration, is determined by the simultaneously occurring processes of absorption and elimination resulting in a profile that is represented in Figure 2.

Figure 2. Time course of drug in each of the compartments shown in Figure 1.

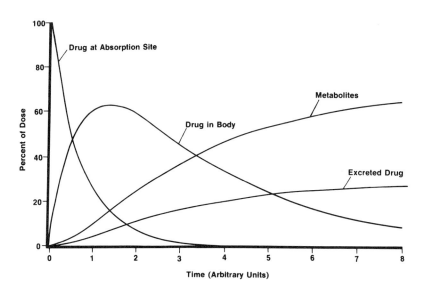

The amount in each compartment is expressed as fraction of the dose administered (Rowland and Tozer, 1980; reproduced with permission)

The concentration versus time profile of a compound in the body can be characterized by the following pharmacokinetic parameters:
a. the rate and extent of absorption (minus the amount of drug lost as result of a possible "first-pass" effect),
b. the volume of distribution (V), which is defined as the ratio between the amount of drug in the body and the plasma concentration at a given point in time and
c. the clearance of the compound, as a measure for the rate

of elimination (CL).

The value of the volume of distribution of a given compound
is dependent mainly on its physicochemical properties (i.e.
lipophilicity). The value of the clearance is determined
by a number of physiological processes according to the
equation:

$$CL = \frac{Q \times f_u \times CL_{int}}{Q + f_u \times CL_{int}} \qquad (1)$$

in which Q is the blood flow to the organ of elimination,
f_u is the fraction unbound to protein and CL_{int} is the
intrinsic organ clearance. For a compound which is
eliminated by metabolism CL_{int} is related directly to
enzyme kinetic parameters according to the following
equation:

$$CL_{int} = \frac{V_{max}}{K_m + C} \qquad (2)$$

For a drug which is eliminated in the unchanged form by the
kidney, CL_{int} can generally be directly related to the
glomerular filtration rate. Thus, the physiological
parameters of blood flow to organs of elimination, fraction
unbound to protein, intrinsic and organ clearance, and the
physicochemical properties of the drug studied are the
determinants of the pharmacokinetic parameters, clearance,
volume of distribution and rate and extent of absorption.
In turn, the values of these pharmacokinetic parameters
determine the height of the concentrations as well as the
rate at which these concentrations change upon a given
dosing regimen.

**CONCENTRATION VERSUS TIME PROFILE AND PHARMACOKINETICS UPON
CHRONIC DOSING**

As far as chronic dosing is concerned two different
modes of administration can be distinguished:
a. continuous infusion, whereby the drug is administered at
a zero order rate and
b. repetitive dosing, whereby bolus doses of the compound
are   administered at regular intervals.
These two modes of administration result in markedly

different concentration versus time profiles. Upon continuous infusion there is from the beginning of the infusion a gradual increase in concentration, which then reaches a constant value; the so-called steady-state concentration. The value of the steady-state concentration, upon infusion of the drug at a certain rate is solely determined by the clearance of the drug according to the following equation:

$$C_{ss} = \frac{R_{inf}}{CL} \qquad (3)$$

in which C_{ss} is the steady-state concentration, R_{inf} is the infusion rate, and CL is the clearance. The time to reach the plateau is determined by the elimination half-life of the drug, with the understanding that a concentration within 90% of the ultimate steady-state concentration is reached after a duration of the infusion of 3 to 4 times the elimination half-life.

Upon repetitive dosing, a concentration profile similar to that during infusion is observed, with the understanding that the steady-state concentrations will be constant, but fluctuate between maximal and minimal values around the average steady-state concentration (Figure 3).

In principal, upon repetitive dosing two different concentration versus time profiles can be obtained, depending on the ratio between the elimination half-life and the dosing interval. In the case when the dosing interval is much longer than the elimination half-life, the previous dose has almost completely been eliminated from the body when the following dose is administered, thus resulting in an "intermittent" concentration versus time profile (curve B in Figure 3). However, when the dosing interval is smaller then the elimination half-life, a significiant accumulation of the drug in the body will occur (curve A in Figure 3).

The average steady-state plasma concentration that is reached upon a certain repetitive dosing regimen is determined by the clearance of the compound according to the following equation:

$$C_{av} = \frac{F \times D}{\tau} \times \frac{1}{Cl} \qquad (4)$$

in which C_{av} is the average steady-state plasma concentration, F is the bioavailability, D is the

maintenance dose and τ is the dosing interval and Cl is the
clearance.

Figure 3. Time course of drug in the body upon repetitive
dosing.

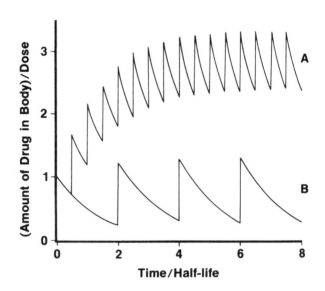

Curve A: bolus dose administered twice every half-life;
Curve B: same bolus dose administered once every two half-
lives (Rowland and Tozer, 1980; reproduced with
permission).

The degree of accumulation that occurs upon repetitive
dosing is generally expressed as the so-called accumulation
ratio which is defined as the ratio between the average
amount of drug in the body at the plateau and the amount
absorbed from each dose. The value of the accumulation
ratio is determined by the elimination half-life of the
compound and the dosing interval according to the equation:

$$R_{ac} = \frac{1.44 \times t_{1/2}}{\tau} \qquad (5)$$

in which R_{ac} is the accumulation ratio, $t_{1/2}$ is the
elimination half-life and τ is the dosing interval.

Thus alterations in the ratio between the elimination
half-life and the dosing interval result in changes in the

degree of accumulation (Figure 4A). In addition however, this also affects the ratio between the minimal and maximal plasma concentrations, with the understanding that this difference increases when the elimination half-life is short compared to the dosing interval (Figure 4B).

Figure 4. Schematic representation of the effects of alterations in the ratio between elimination half-life and dosing interval on the degree of accumulation and difference between maximal and minimal concentrations at plateau.

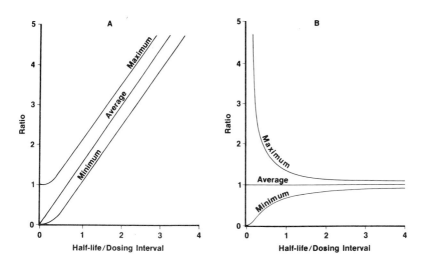

A: More frequent administration results in a greater degree of drug accumulation. B: Less frequent administration results in larger relative differences between maximum and minimum concentrations (Rowland and Tozer, 1980; reproduced with permission).

IMPLICATIONS OF SPECIES DIFFERENCES IN PHARMACOKINETICS

The existence of wide species differences in the pharmacokinetics of various compounds may have important implications for safety evaluation (Nau et al., 1985). As far as the different pharmacokinetic parameters are concerned (i.e. rate and extent of absorption, volume of distribution and clearance) it appears that for some of these there is a much wider interspecies variability than for others. For example there do not appear to be profound

differences between species with respect to the absorption
parameters and the volume of distribution of several drugs
(Nau et al., 1985). On the other hand there are large
differences between species with respect to clearance, with
the understanding that in experimental animals drugs are
cleared much more rapidly than in man (Table 1).

**Table 1. Comparison of clearance values of drugs
(ml/min/kg) in several animal species and in man[1]**

Species	Caffeine	Trimethadione	Valproic acid
Mouse	12	12	7-15
Rat	13	5	14
Hamster		7	4
Guinea Pig			
Rabbit	5.9	6	
Dog			
Monkey	3.1		2-3
Man	2.0		0.2

1 Data from: Bonati et al., 1985; Tanaka et al., 1983; Nau
et al., 1985

This generalisation holds true not only for lipophilic
drugs which are eliminated predominantly by metabolism but
also for hydrophilic drugs which are efficiently excreted
by renal pathways. As a result of the generally higher
clearances the elimination half-lives of most compounds are
also much shorter in experimental animals compared to man
(Table 2).

Due to these differences in pharmacokinetics, the
concentration versus time profiles that are obtained upon
certain dosing regimens may differ significantly between
species. Upon single dose administration of a compound in
a fixed dose (adjusted for body weight), quite comparable
peak concentrations may be expected in various species
since the volumes of distribution are similar. However
due to the differences in elimination half-life, there will
be quite signigicant differences in the duration of the
exposure. Upon chronic dosing by means of a zero order
infusion, there will be significant differences in the
steady-state concentrations, due to the difference in
clearance, which means that in principle the maintenance

dose of a compound in toxicity testing should be adjusted to the clearance, such as to obtain comparable concentrations in different species. The situation that

Table 2. Comparison of elimination half-lives of drugs in animal species and man [1]

Drug	Half-life, hours					
	Mouse	Rat	Rabbit	Dog	Monkey	Man
Valproic acid	0.8	1-4		1-4		8-16
Primidone	1-3					3-17
Phenobarbital	3-4					50-150
Diazepam	1.1	1	3	8		20-50
Hexobarbital	0.3	2	1	4		3-7
Phenylbutazone		6	3	2-6	8	72
Oxyphenyl- butazone		6	3	0.5-6	8	72
Antipyrine				1-2	1-2	12

1 Data from Ritschel, 1970; Klotz et al., 1976; Nau et al., 1981 and references therein.

is encountered upon repetitive dosing is even more complicated, since here not only the difference in clearance resulting in different average steady-state concentrations is of importance, but also the difference in elimination half-life. As was discussed above, many drugs exhibit much shorter half-lives in animals than in man. This means that in experimental animals upon repetitive dosing, whereby usually drugs are administered on a once or twice daily basis, a concentration versus time profile is obtained that is characterized by a series of narrow and high drug concentration-time peaks, while in man the fluctuations are usually much less pronounced (Figure 5). It appears that such widely different concentration versus time profiles in comparison to the human situation, can have significant implications in the safety evaluation of xenobiotics.

In addition to the existence of wide species differences in pharmacokinetics pronounced interindividual variability within one given species has been shown to exist. It appears that there is particularly a wide

variability in the rate of drug metabolism in humans due to
genetic variables, and pathophysiological circumstances.
This may well have implications for the toxicity of
compounds, and should therefore be taken into account in

**Figure 5. Schematic representation of the influences of
difference in elimination half-life on the exposure profile
upon once daily administration of a compound.**

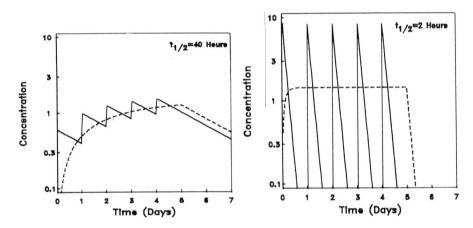

Left Panel:half-life of 40 hours; gradually increasing
concentration with relatively small differences between
maximal and minimal concentrations. Right panel: half-life
of 2 hours; profile characterized by a series of narrow and
high drug concentration peaks. The dotted line represents
the situation upon continuous infusion (Collins 1985;
reproduced with permission).

the safety evaluation (Breimer, 1983).

POTENTIAL PHARMACOKINETIC COMPLICATIONS IN CHRONIC DOSING

From the foregoing it appears that ideallyin the
safety evaluation of xenobiotics, the (chronic) dosing
regimen should be adjusted to the species diffferences in
pharmacokinetics (i.e. clearance). Generally the
concentration versus time profile obtained upon a certain
chronic dosing regimen can be predicted on the basis of the
values of the pharmacokinetic parameters determined
following single dose administration. However there are
quite a few situations in which this is not the case, due
to the fact that upon chronic dosing the values of the
pharmacokinetic parameters can change or can be different

from the ones obtained upon single dose administration. In these situations, the dosing of a compound in safety evaluation tests requires special attention. Briefly, these situations are the following:

a. Enzyme saturation

Assuming Michaelis-Menten enzyme kinetics, the clearance of a compound can be related to the enzyme kinetic parameters according to equation 2. From this equation it can be seen that at low concentrations, relative to the K_m value (approximately $<0.1K_m$), the clearance is independent of the plasma concentration. In this concentration range there is a linear relationship between the maintenance dose administered and the steady-state plasma concentration. However at higher concentrations the clearance becomes concentration dependent owing to saturation of the enzymes involved in the elimination, with the understanding that clearance decreases at increasing plasma concentrations. This implies that under these conditions a certain increment of the dose may result in a disproportionate increase of plasma concentration making the dosing under these conditions very delicate. Generally, for most compounds no enzyme saturation occurs when administered in "therapeutic" doses to humans. However, exceptions occur, as has been demonstrated to be the case for phenytoin and salicylate (Richens and Dunlop, 1975; Levy, 1965). In animal studies on the other hand, non-linear pharmacokinetics may be expected to occur more readily, especially upon repetitive dosing according to a once or twice daily regimen, since under these conditions relatively high peak concentrations may occur as was discussed in the foregoing (Figure 5).

b. Enzyme induction

The development of enzyme induction during chronic administration can have different effects on the values of the various pharmacokinetic parameters of a drug, depending upon the pharmacokinetic properties of the compound under investigation and the route of administration. As can be seen from equation 1, the value of the clearance of a compound is among other factors dependent on both the intrinsic clearance (Cl_{int}) and the blood flow to the organ of elimination (Q). Each of these processes can be rate-limiting in the elimination and on the basis thereof drugs can be divided into compounds of which the rate of elimination is mainly determined by Cl_{int} (generally designated as compounds with a **low** extraction

ratio, E) on one hand and compounds of which the rate of
elimination is determined mainly by Q (generally designated
as compounds with a **high** extraction ratio). Development of
enzyme induction means an increase in the intrinsic
clearance of the compound. This may therefore, depending
on the value of the extraction ratio, result in an increase
in the overall clearance of the compound. In order to
determine the effect of enzyme induction on the
pharmacokinetic parameters however, the route of
administration also needs to be taken into account.
Generally these effects can be summarized as follows.

Upon oral adminstration the clearance of both compounds
with a high, as with a low extraction ratio, is determined
by the intrinsic clearance. Thus upon the development of
enzyme induction there will always be an increase in the
overall clearance. This means that upon chronic dosing,
when enzyme induction occurs the ultimate steady-state
plasma concentrations will be lower than the ones
predicted on basis of single dose experiments. Upon iv
administration a somewhat different situation is
encountered. For a drug with a low extraction ratio, in
this situation the overall clearance is again mainly
dependent on the intrinsic clearance and thus sensitive to
enzyme induction. For a drug with a high extraction ratio
however, the clearance following iv administration is
determined largely by the blood flow and thus insensitive
to enzyme induction. This means that under these
circumstances enzyme induction will have no effect on the
steady-state concentrations that are reached upon a certain
dosing regimen.

With regard to elimination half-life the effects of
enzyme induction are as follows. For a compound with a low
extraction ratio the half-life is determined mainly by the
intrinsic clearance. In this situation an increase in the
intrinsic clearance due to enzyme induction results in a
lower value for the elimination half-life. For a compound
with a high extraction ratio, the elimination half-life is
determined mainly by the value of the blood-flow to the
organ of elimination and is thus insensitive to enzyme
induction.

For several drugs it has been demonstrated that they
are able to cause induction of drug metabolizing enzymes,
upon chronic administration. This means that such
compounds may also enhance their rate of metabolism, as
has, for example, been demonstrated for carbamazepine
(Eichelbaum, 1975). Therefore, the chronic dosing of such
compounds requires special attention, particularly in
situations in which it is desirable to maintain the steady-

state concentrations within relatively narrow limits.

c. Enzyme inhibition

Although rare, enzyme inhibition can also occur upon chronic administration of certain compounds. This has for example been demonstrated to occur with orphenadrine (Labout et al., 1982). Upon chronic administration of this compound, significantly higher steady-state plasma concentrations are observed, than predicted on basis of data obtained following single dose administration, as the result of a decrease in intrinsic clearance. It appeared that this decreased intrinsic clearance can be explained by the accumulation of the N-demethylated metabolite of orphenadrine, which causes inhibition of the enzymes involved in the metabolism of the parent compound. So far, such a mechanism has not been described for many other drugs. Nevertheless it cannot be excluded that similar situations exist for other compounds. It has for example been demonstrated that a variety of hydroxylated metabolites can upon injection inhibit the metabolism in vivo of their precursors as well as other drugs (Soda and Levy, 1975).

RATE CONTROLLED DRUG DELIVERY

In the foregoing it was discussed that in laboratory animals drugs generally are cleared at a much higher rate and also exhibit much shorter elimination half-lives than humans. This means that in conventional toxicity testing, whereby drugs are administered by gavage once or twice daily, grossly different concentration versus time profiles are seen compared to the ones observed in the human situation (see also Figure 5), and this may well have toxicological consequences. Ideally, the drug concentration versus time profile should resemble the human situation as much as possible. However, there are numerous practical problems involved with achieving this. One way in which this can be achieved is to administer the drug more frequently. However, if for example the drug level fluctuations are not to exceed 50%, the dosing interval must not exceed the time of one half-life of the drug. For drugs with short half-lives this would result in much too frequent and therefore impractical dosing. Another possibility is to incorporate the drug in the food or to dissolve it in the drinking water. Measurement of the food or water consumption would then yield the dose of the drug. However, since the times of food and water consumption of animals are quite unpredictable and in the case of rodents mainly confined to the night hours, great variations of drug levels must also be expected with this mode of administration.

A more practical approach, to obtain stable concentrations of a drug over prolonged periods of time, is by the use of implantable osmotic mini-pumps, which deliver drugs at a zero order rate. In Figure 6 a schematic diagram of the components of an osmotic minipump is shown. Briefly, the system consists of a reservoir surrounded by an osmotic driving agent which is encapsulated in a semi-permeable membrane. This membrane serves as a rigid housing and contains an orifice for delivery of drug solution or suspension. The system can be filled through the orifice with the drug solution or suspension to be investigated using a blunted needle. After filling, insertion of a flow moderator is desirable to prevent uncontrolled loss of drug through the orifice. In operation, the osmotic agent imbibes water across the semi-permeable membrane to displace an equal volume of drug solution from the reservoir. This results then in a zero order delivery of the compound from the system (Theeuwes and Bayne, 1981).

It has now been clearly demonstrated that with the osmotic minipumps, stable concentrations of drugs can be maintained in vivo over prolonged periods of time (Breimer et al., 1985), which indicates that these devices can prove to be a valuable tool in the toxicity testing of xenobiotics.

The idea of using osmotic minipumps in the toxicity testing of drugs was for the first time applied by Nau and his colleagues in their studies into the possible embryotoxic effects of valproic acid (Nau et al., 1981).

Valproic acid is an example of a drug which exhibits a much shorter elimination half-life in small animals (0.8 hours in mice) than in man (8 to 16 hours). Therefore in mice there are markedly exagerated peak and trough concentration patterns upon once or twice daily injections, whereas the therapeutic concentration range in humans is relatively narrow. Also it appears that upon administration of once daily injections, peak concentrations can be reached that are an order of magnitude higher than the therapeutic concentrations in humans (Nau et al., 1981). This raises the question of whether these relatively high peak concentrations reached in mice may have implications for the outcome of the toxicity testing. In studies that were designed to answer this question, valproic acid was administered by two different regimens in the same total dose range to pregnant mice from day 7-15 of gestation, by

Figure 6. Schematic diagram of the components of an osmotic drug delivery system.

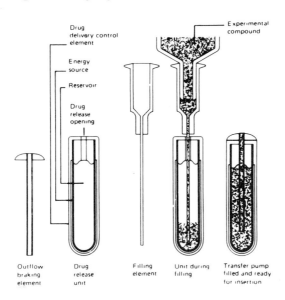

once daily injections on one hand or by constant rate infusions from implanted osmotic pumps on the other. It appeared from these studies that with the infusion a significantly higher total dose was required to produce both fetal resorptions and exencephaly than with the once daily injections. In other words the dose-response curves for both fetal death and exencephaly were shifted dramatically to the right when valproic acid was given by infusion instead of once daily injection. However the concentration-response relationships were quite similar for both regimens, at least when steady-state levels after infusion were compared with the peak level after injections. Thus, for valproic acid it appears that a particular threshold concentration must be reached, either by a series of short lived concentration peaks or by steady-state concentrations of the same magnitude, in order to induce fetal malformations (Nau et al., 1985). This example shows very convincingly that the artificially high peak concentrations, that are obtained upon once daily administration of a compound to experimental animals, markedly influences the outcome of the toxicity testing, and these in principle should be avoided.

Thus, in the safety evaluation not only the dose of the compound that is administered is important, but that also the rate at which it is administered may have consequences

for the outcome of the test. This emphasizes the need for
rate controlled drug delivery in safety evaluation, for
which purpose osmotic mini pumps (and other devices) may
prove to be very valuable tools.

CONCLUSION

The concentration versus time profiles of xenobiotics
can differ markedly upon different dosing regimens. Also
upon distinct dosing regimens, there are pronounced
differences between various animal species and man, due to
the species differences in pharmacokinetics. This has
important implications for safety evaluation studies, since
the outcome of the toxicity can be expected to be related
to the "exposure" of the compound under investigation. In
principle therefore, a dosing regimen has to be designed
that results in a concentration versus time profile that is
relevant with regard to the toxicity testing. In addition,
in animal experiments, the dosing regimen should be such
that the concentration time profile resembles the profile
obtained in the human situation. The design of such dosing
regimens requires detailed knowledge of the pharmacokinetic
properties of the compound under investigation (in
particular the clearance and the elimination half-life),
the species differences in the values of the
pharmacokinetic parameter, and the changes in these
parameters that may occur upon chronic dosing.

In principle, the maintenance dose of the compound has
to be adjusted to the species difference in clearance, such
as to obtain average steady-state plasma concentrations in
the same concentration range as are obtained in humans. In
addition the occurence of high peak concentrations upon
repetitive dosing, should also ideally be avoided. For
this purpose the osmotic minipump may prove a valuable
tool in the dosing of the compound.

To date, only very few studies have been published in
which the influence of the concentration versus time
profile of a compound on the outcome of the toxicological
evaluation has been examined. The studies with valproic
acid, described in the foregoing, demonstrate clearly, that
there may be a marked influence. It is to be expected
therefore, that control of the concentration versus time
profile in the safety evaluation of a compound, and thus
implementation of the above mentioned principles, may
contribute significantly to the understanding to its toxic
potential.

REFERENCES

Bonati, M., Latini, R., Tognoni, G., Young, J.F. and
    Garratini, S. (1985) Drug Metab. Rev. 15, 1355.
Breimer, D.D. (1983) Clin. Pharmacokin 8, 371.
Breimer, D.D., de Leede, L.G.J. and de Boer, A.G. (1985)
    In:"Rate control in Drug Therapy," (Eds. Prescott,
    L.F. and Nimmo, W.S.,) Churchill Livingstone,
    Edingburgh,p.54
Collins, J.M. (1985) in "Topics in Pharmaceutical Sciences
    1985" (Eds. D.D. Breimer and P. Speiser).
    ElsevierScience Publishers, Amsterdam, p. 133.
Eichelbaum, M., Ekbom, K., Bertilsson, L., Ringbergen, V.A.
    and Rane, A. (1975) Europ. J. Clin. Pharmocol. 8, 337
Klotz, U., Antonin, K-H., and Bieck, P,R. (1976) J.
    Pharmacol. exp. Ther. 199, 67.
Labout, J.J.M., Thyssen, C.T., Keijser, G.G.J. and Hespe,
    W. (1982), Europ. J. Clin. Pharmacol, 21, 343.
Levy, G. (1965) J. Pharm. Sci. 54, 959
Nau, H., Zierer, R., Spielmann, H., Neubert, D. and Gansau,
    C. (1981) Life Sci, 29, 2803.
Nau, H., Trotz, M. and Wegner, C. (1985) In: "Topics in
    Pharmaceutical Sciences 1985" (Eds. D.D. Breimer
    and P. Speiser). Elsevier Science Publishers,
    Amsterdam,   p.143.
Richens, A. and Dunlop, A. (1975) Lancet 2, 247.
Ritschel, W.A. (1970) Drug Intell. Clin. Pharmacy 4, 332.
    Rowland, M. and Tozer, T.N. (1980). "Clinical
    Pharmacokinetics," Lea and Febiger, Philadelphia.
Soda, D.M.and Levy, G. (1975) J. Pharm. Sci. 64, 1928.
    Tanaka, E., Kinoshita, H., Yoshida, T. and Kuroiwa, Y.
    (1983) J. Pharm. Dyn. 6, 481.
Theeuwes, F. and Bayne, W. (1981) In "Controlled-release
    Pharmaceuticals. (Urquhart, J., ed) American
    Pharmaceutical Association, Washington, D.C., p.61.

EFFECT OF EXPOSURE ROUTE ON METABOLISM AND KINETICS

J. Brian Houston

Department of Pharmacy, University of Manchester,
Manchester, M13 9PL, UK

INTRODUCTION

Any considerations on the effect of exposure route on drug disposition can only evolve from a detailed consideration of the absorption process. Absorption of drug from most sites of adminstration is a complex process involving both permeability and metabolism. Both factors govern the rate and extent of input into the body and hence may influence the metabolic and pharmacokinetics behaviour observed. The main emphasis of this chapter is concerned with metabolic barriers to drug input.

First it is necessary to clearly define the absorption process. There are at least four possible definitions which may be adopted according to the investigator's area of interest. Absorption may be considered to have occured when either 1) drug is lost from the site of input e.g., the gastrointestinal tract following oral administration; 2) drug appears in blood system efferent to the site of input e.g., the hepatic portal vein following oral administration; 3) drug appears in the systemic circulation; or 4) drug reaches the site of action. For the majority of disposition studies definition 2 would be ideal, but as blood sampling is normally limited to peripheral vessels, definition 3 is the most appropriate. Therefore, the absorption process encompasses all events occuring between site of input and site of sampling. In the case of oral administration, absorption would include the first pass of drug through the liver. The importance of first pass or pre-systemic hepatic metabolism has been realised for many years (Riegelman and Rowland, 1973; Gibaldi and Perrier, 1974), however the extent of first pass metabolism by other tissues is poorly defined.

PULMONARY FIRST PASS METABOLISM

Figure 1 illustrates various sites of input which are

used in drug therapy. Also shown are cetain sites of input
which are experimentally useful in characterising the
absorption process; of particular relevance to the present
discussions are the intra-arterial (IA), intravenous (IV),
hepatic portal venous (HPV) and oral (PO) routes.

**Figure 1. Sites of drug input used therapeutically and
experimentally to elucidate the absorption process.**

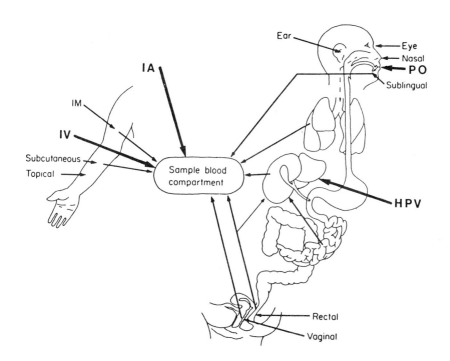

For all the routes shown in Figure 1 with the exception
of IA, there is the potential for first pass metabolism in
at least one tissue, the lung (Cassidy and Houston, 1980).
Until a drug enters the arterial system and is distributed
to the various tissues of the body, its concentration in
blood leaving the site of absorption is high. Thus for
many routes of administration the lungs receive a
concentrated pulse of drug and the potential exists for
extensive first pass metabolism.
    A quantitative description of the absorption process
requires estimates of both the rate and the extent of input
into the body. Both parameters need to be evaluated with

respect to a standard route of administration using a
standard site of sampling. The importance of these latter
two points can be appreciated by considering a series of
studies on naphthol and phenol (Mistry and Houston, 1985;
Cassidy and Houston, 1984 and 1980). Both compounds are
metabolised almost exclusively by glucuronidation and
sulphation and both glucuronyltransferease and
sulphotransferase are found in extrahepatic tissues
including the lung and intestinal mucosa (Gram, 1980).
Concentration-time profiles for naphthol and phenol
obtained employing different routes of administration and
different sampling sites are shown in Figures 2 - 4.

**Figure 2. Naphthol plasma concentration-time profiles
following either IA or IV administration of naphthol to
male rats.**

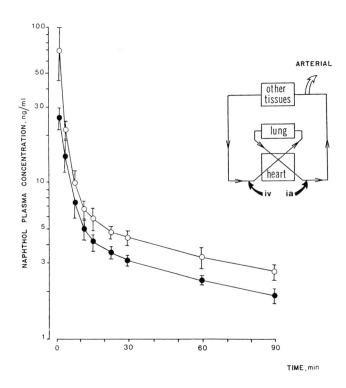

Arterial samples were taken and AUCs were 727 and 420
ng.ml^{-1}.min for IA (O) and IV (●) routes, respectively.
The insert illustrates schematically the sites of input
and sampling with respect to the cardiopulmonary circuit.

Figure 3. Naphthol plasma concentration-time profiles obtained from either venous or arterial samples following IV administration of naphthol to male rats.

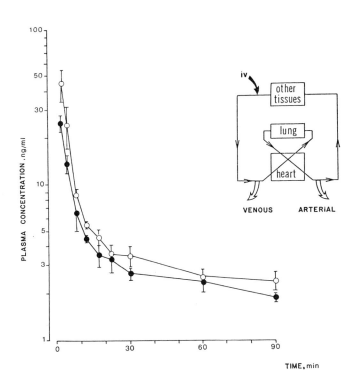

AUCs were 684 and 423 $ng.ml^{-1}.min$ for venous (O) and arterial (●) sampling, respectively. The insert illustrates schematically the sites of sampling and input with respect to the cardiopulmonary circuit.

The unique anatomical position of the lungs dictates that complete systemic availability of a compound may only result when that compound is administered into or very near to the left ventricle. From this site the drug may then be distributed to the various tissues of the body in accordance with the respective cardiac output. In contrast the use of any intravenous site involves transit to the right atrium and circulation through the lungs prior to reaching the general arterial system. Figure 2 shows the difference between the arterial plasma concentration-time curves when naphthol is administered either side of the

Figure 4.   Phenol blood concentration-time profiles
following either IA, IV, HPV or PO administration of phenol
to male rats.

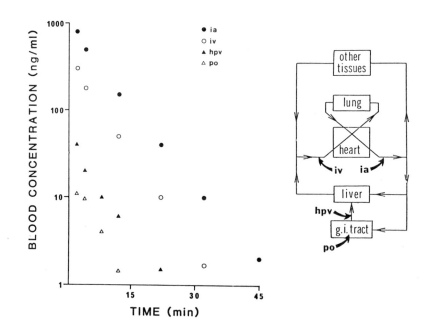

Arterial samples were taken and AUCs were 6.03, 2, 0.29 and
0.11 $\mu g.ml^{-1}.min$ for the IA(●), IV(○), HPV (▲)and PO (△)
routes, respectively. The insert illustrates schematically
these routes of input.

cardio-pulmonary circuit (IA and IV). The non-equivalence
of these curves may be explained by pulmonary first pass
metabolism which decreases the systemic availability to 42%
based on the ratio of the two areas under the curve.
     The   use   of the IA route of administration and
arterial sampling may present practical or ethical
problems.   The IV route of administration with venous
sampling is a more standard protocol for disposition
studies.   The area under the plasma concentration-time
curve (AUC) for naphthol under these conditions (Figure 3)
does not differ from that calculated from the IA/arterial
sampling in Figure 2. However as one might predict IV
administration/arterial sampling results in lower plasma
concentrations as the result of the first pass pulmonary
effect.   There is good agreement between the two methods of
assessing pulmonary first pass conjugation of naphthol

shown in Figures 2 and 3 (Mistry and Houston, 1985).

ORAL ADMINISTRATION

The above approaches for assessing first pass metabolism in an individual tissue may be extended to situations where more than one site of metabolism exists and these sites are arranged anatomically in one series. For example, in order to assess the extent of oral absorption, the role of the intestinal mucosa, liver and lung as potential sites of first pass metabolism should be considered. The oral availability (F_{PO}) is dependent on the individual fractions of drug escaping metabolism in each tissue (f_G, f_H, f_L for gut mucosa, hepatic and lung fractions, respectively).

Hence $$F_{PO} = f_G \cdot f_H \cdot f_L \qquad (1)$$

In Figure 4, arterial blood concentration-time profiles for phenol after IA and PO administration are shown. F_{PO} is very low and using the ratio of AUCs for PO and IA a systemic availability of 7% is obtained. The contribution of the individual 3 potential sites of first pass metabolism may be assessed by additional experiments involving intravenous administration into either the hepatic portal vein (HPV) or the jugular vein (IV)

$$f_G = AUC_{PO}/AUC_{HPV} = 0.14 \qquad (2)$$

$$f_H = AUC_{HPV}/AUC_{IV} = 0.12 \qquad (3)$$

$$f_L = AUC_{IV}/AUC_{IA} = 0.42 \qquad (4)$$

From these data it may be concluded that conjugation of phenol by the enzymes in the gut mucosa and liver is extensive and comparable. The role of the pulmonary enzymes is less yet its contribution to phenol conjugation is still substantial. There is a lack of route dependence on the qualitative nature of phenol disposition as the metabolite AUCs for all routes do not differ. Thus incomplete uptake from the site of absorption would appear not to contribute to the low availability of phenol by the routes discussed. The differences in the slopes of the profiles shown in Figure 4 result from systemic rather than first pass events (Cassidy and Houston, 1984).

The basis of the equations 2-4 have been discussed (Cassidy and Houston, 1980; Gibaldi and Perrier, 1974) and the relationship between AUC and availability fraction is shown below:

$$AUC = \frac{F \cdot Dose}{CL_S} \qquad (5)$$

Thus when dose and systematic clearance (CL_S) remain constant any difference in AUC reflects a difference in F between the two routes of administration.

An analogous situation exists for steady-state drug concentrations following a constant rate of input (R):

$$CSS = \frac{F \cdot R}{CL_S} \qquad (6)$$

Therefore an alternative approach to the assessment of first pass metabolism involves use of the ratio of C_{SS} for different sites of input or for different sites of sampling. Examples of the use of these methods include the investigations of Mulder et al (1984a; 1984b) and Wedlund et al (1983) using harmol, methylumbelliferone and carbamazepine, respectively. However the application of equation (6) has not been as extensive as equation (5) (Pond and Tozer, 1984).

RELATIONSHIP BETWEEN ENZYME ACTIVITY, TISSUE BLOOD FLOW AND DRUG BINDING

It should be realised that although F is a useful parameter to assess the extent of input of drug into the systemic evaluation, it is not a pure measure of enzymic activity even when uptake from the absorption site is complete. Other factors contribute to the availability fraction for a given tissue including blood flow through the tissue (Q) and binding of drug within the blood (fu). The interrelationship between these factors can be summarised by the following equation:

$$F = \frac{Q}{Q + CL_{int} \cdot fu} \qquad (7)$$

where CL_{int} is a measure of the intrinsic metabolising ability of the tissue. Equation (7) is based on a perfusion rate limited model for tissue disposition of drug where the enzyme distribution within the tissue is assumed to be homogenous and only unbound drug is available to be metabolised (Rowland et al. 1973; Wilkinson and Shand 1975). Despite the physiological shortcomings of this type of model it has proved useful in rationalising many data.

From equation (7) it can be seen that unless the value of CL_{int} is similar to or larger than Q the availability across the tissue will be reasonable. Hence the methods discussed above are only useful for high clearance compounds (see Table 1). For example when blood binding is negligible then a CL_{int} of 0.5 will result in a F of 0.67. When blood binding is important then a higher CL_{int} is needed before significant losses in availability are evident. The resulting availability for several combinations of CL_{int} and blood binding are listed in Table 1 (note that CL_{int} is expressed in units of blood flow which allows application to any tissue).

Intrinsic clearance has units of flow and relates the rate of metabolism to the unbound drug concentration leaving the tissue. It may be conceptualised in terms of Michaelis Menten parameters:

$$CL_{int} = \sum_k \frac{V_{max\,i}}{K_{m\,i}} \qquad (8)$$

where V_{max} is the maximal rate of metabolism and K_m the Michaelis constant for each of the pathways is operating for the drug under study.

Table 1. Effect of intrinsic clearance and unbound fraction in blood on systemic availability.

	Availability fraction[*]		
CL_{int}[+]	fm = 1	fm = 0.5	fm = 0.1
0.05	0.95	0.98	0.99
0.1	0.91	0.95	0.99
0.5	0.67	0.80	0.95
1	0.50	0.67	0.91
5	0.20	0.28	0.67
10	0.09	0.17	0.50
50	0.02	0.04	0.16

[*] Calculated using equation (7).
[+] Expressed as multiples of blood flow.

Clearly the Michaelis Menten parameters operating <u>in vivo</u> are not completely synonymous with those determined <u>in vitro</u>. However one might expect that at least a good rank order exists between intrinsic clearance in vivo and intrinsic activity in vivo. Figure 5 substantiates this for the liver and intestine using morphine, naloxone and buprenorphine, three compounds which are essentially only subject to glucuronidation. The in vitro activity was obtained using native microsomal preparations and the V_{max} to K_m ratio has been corrected for microsomal yield. In vivo intrinsic clearance was obtained using AUCs and correcting the availability fraction for the role of blood flow and drug blood binding using equation (7) (Mistry and Houston, 1986). Other similar successful comparisons of in vitro and in vivo data have been made with phenacetin (Klippert et al, 1983) and benzo(a)pyrene (Wiersma and Roth, 1983).

NON LINEAR FIRST PASS METABOLISM

In the studies involving morphine and structural analogues low doses were employed and linearity in pharmacokinetics was validated. However it may not always be possible due to analytical constraints to investigate first pass metabolism under first order conditions. Thus a more appropriate equation for intrinsic clearance would be:

$$CL_{int} = \frac{V\ max}{K_m + C} \qquad (9)$$

where C is the unbound drug concentration leaving the tissue. Under such non-linear conditions, CL_{int} will be sensitive to changes in concentration entering the tissue particularly during absorption when concentrations are high and may exceed the K_m (Riegelman and Rowland, 1973). Thus unequivocal determination of the availability fraction may be difficult or even impossible when more than one metabolising tissue exist in series and the actual concentration within each tissue cannot be assessed with confidence. Figure 6 illustrates the AUC/dose relationships for phenol over a range of doses administered by the IA, IV, HPV and PO routes (Cassidy and Houston, 1984). For the IA route this relationship (which is equivalent to CL_S) is dose independent. The other three routes show varying degrees of dose dependency. At the lowest dose each tissue availability fraction may be estimated with reasonable confidence, however as the doses increase the ability to factor out the individual contributions of each tissue becomes difficult and the validity of these values must be carefully considered.

The IV route provides a direct measure of the extent of

Figure 5. Relationship between in vivo intrinsic clearance and in vitro intrinsic activity to glucuronidate morphine, naloxone and buprenorphine in the intestine (o) and liver (●) of female rats. For each tissue and each method the rank order of glucuronidation is buprenorphine > naloxone > morphine.

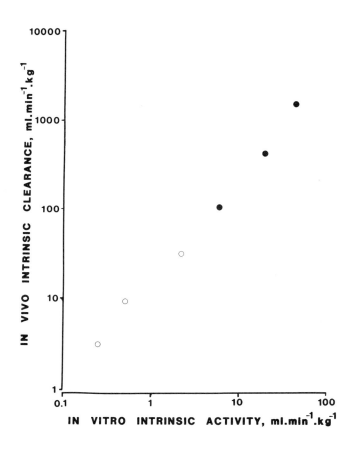

pulmonary metabolism which is constant at the two lower doses. The HPV route when compared to the IA route assesses the contribution of both pulmonary and hepatic metabolism. The hepatic contribution is extensive at 0.4 mg/kg but only minimal at 1.5 mg/kg. As these tissues are inseries, the amount of phenol entering the lung after HPV will be less than after IV at a given dose level. Since pulmonary metabolism is constant below 1.5 mg/kg, both f_L and f_H may be considered accurately estimated. The gut mucosa appears to have a greater capacity to conjugate phenol than the other two tissues. Even at the highest dose where both pulmonary and hepatic first pass metabolism is negigible, the availability by the oral route is only 0.33. As a consequence of the large capacity of the gut mucosal enzymes, the amount of phenol presented to the liver after PO will be at most one-third of that from direct HPV administration of the same dose. It is therefore difficult to accurately estimate f_G at the intermediate doses; F_{PO} will represent the lower limit (approximately 0.1) and 0.33, the upper limit. Despite these problems in quantifying f_G accurately there is no doubt that the gut mucosa possess the largest capacity to conjugate phenol during the first pass following PO administration.

Figure 6 . **Metabolite concentration-time profiles following oral administration of drug computer simulated according to scheme in text.**

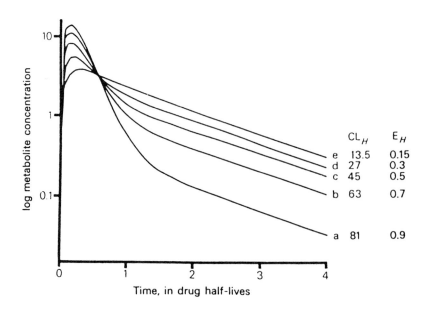

		CL_H	E_H
e	13.5	0.15
d	27	0.3
c	45	0.5
b	63	0.7
a	81	0.9

For each curve all pharmacokinetic parameters are held constant except hepatic clearance (and hence F) which is altered as indicated.

FIRST PASS METABOLITE PRODUCTION

Another aspect of first pass metabolism can often be seen when metabolite concentration-time profiles following two routes of drug administration are compared. Consequent with the clearance of drug during first pass is the generation of substantial amounts of metabolite. There are many examples of metabolites which retain the pharmacological activity of the parent drug, possess different pharmacological activity (in certain cases these metabolites are associated with the side effects of the drug) or display reactivity with tissue macromolecules (Drayer, 1982). Thus the surge of metabolite which may result during a first pass transit may be of great consequence either within the tissue where it is generated or within the circulating blood which perfuses other tissues.

A scheme which describes the impact of route of administration on metabolite concentration-time profiles is shown below (Houston and Taylor, 1984).:

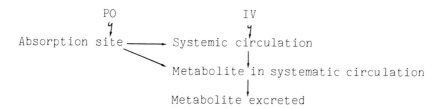

PO and IV routes will be compared and for simplicity the liver will be the only site of metabolism. The drug is completely converted to a single metabolite which is excreted per se by an efficient renal clearance mechanism. Both chemical entities show rapid distribution dynamics, minimal protein binding and linear kinetics with respect to concentration and time.

After IV administration of drug, the metabolite is generated acccording to the systemic clearance of the drug and is eliminated rapidly such that its kinetics are formation rate limited (Houston, 1982). After PO administration, uptake of drug from the absorption site is complete but varying degrees of first pass metabolism result in the dose appearing in the systemic circulation in the form of both drug and metabolite. As the liver is the only site of metabolism, the F can be varied by altering the hepatic clearance relative to hepatic blood flow and hence the hepatic extraction (E_H):

$$F = 1 - E_H = 1 - \frac{CL_H}{Q_H} \qquad (10)$$

The consequences of varying F on the metabolite concentration-time profile can be seen in Figure 6. In order to aid comparison of the different metabolite curves, which were computer simulated (Houston and Taylor, 1983) the time scale is expressed in terms of the parent drug half-life.

For the low clearance case (curve e) the metabolite concentration-time profile is biexponential and no route dependence would be evident. As the clearance is increased and the F is decreased a distinct triexponential curve becomes apparent. The maximum metabolite concentration increases progressively by up to four-fold and the time to achieve this maximum decreases. The marked effect seen in curves a-e is only apparent for the oral route as it results from first pass metabolism; for the IV route all metabolite curves would be similar in nature to curve e. The curves in Figure 6 have the same AUC; for a metabolite this is determined by the fraction of dose converted to the metabolite (fm) and the metabolite's own clearance (CLm):

$$AUC \ (m) = \frac{fm \ . \ Dose}{CLm} \qquad (11)$$

Neither parameter in equation (11) is altered by the first pass effect. The extent of metabolism is the same for all cases, only the residence time as the parent compound and as the metabolite in the body alters.

The metabolite kinetic behaviour in Figure 6 may be rationalised in the following manner. After oral administration only a certain fraction of the dose escapes first pass metabolism (F) and is metabolised subsequently in an analogous manner to an intravenous drug dose. The remaining fraction of the oral dose (1-F) appears in the systemic circulation as the metabolite. Viewed from the systemic circulation the metabolite formed during the first pass will behave kinetically as if the metabolite per se had been administered. Thus when there is substantial first pass metabolism, the initial decay in metabolite concentrations is influenced largely by the metabolite's own half-life. As formation rate limited metabolite kinetics most frequently occurs, the systematically formed metabolite displays the drug half-life and the metabolite concentration-time profile declines in a biphasic manner.

The discussions above provide an explanation for certain anomalies in the literature concerning the effect of route of administration (Houston and Taylor, 1982). For example, certain drugs have been reported to form particular metabolites only after oral administration since plasma metabolite concentrations were evident following parenteral administration. An alternative explanation for this finding is that the analytical procedure used is only sensitive enough to detect the surge in metabolite plasma concentrations following first pass formation. A similar rationale may explain why certain high clearance drugs show a greater pharmacological response after PO administration than following parenteral administration.

REFERENCES

Cassidy, M.K., Houston, J.B. (1980) J. Pharm. Pharmac. 32, 57.

Cassidy, M.K., Houston, J.B. (1984) Drug Metab. Dispos. 12, 619

Drayer, D.E. (1982) Drugs 24, 519

Gibaldi, M.and Perrier, D. (1974) Drug Metab. Rev. 3, 185.

Gram, T., ed. (1980) Extrahepatic Metabolism of Drugs and other Foreign Compounds, MTP Press, Lancaster.

Houston, J.B. (1982) Pharmac. Therap. 15 521.

Houston, J.B., Taylor, G. (1984) Br. J. Clin. Pharmac. 17, 385.

Klippert, P., Brom, P., Noorhoek, J. (1982) Biochem. Pharmac. 31, 2545.

Mistry, M., Houston, J.B. (1985) Drug Metab. Dispos. 13, 781.

Mistry, M., Houston, J.B. (1986) submitted for publication.

Mulder, G.J., Weitering, J.G., Scholtens, E., Dawson, J.R., Pang, K.S. (1984a) Biochem. Pharmac. 33, 3081.

Mulder, G.J., Brouwer, S., Scholtens, E. (1984b) Biochem. Pharmac. 33, 2341.

Pond, S.M., Tozer, T.N. (1984) Clin. Pharmacokin. 9, 1.

Riegelman, S., Rowland, M. (1973) J. Pharmacokin. Biopharm. 1 419.

Rowland, M., Benet, L.Z., Graham, G. (1973) J. Pharmacokin. Biopharm. 1, 123.

Wedlund, P.J., Chang, S.L., Levy, R.H. (1983) J. Pharm. Sci. 72, 860.

Wiersma, D.A., Roth, R.A. (1983) Mol. Pharmac. 24, 300.

Wilkinson, G.R., Shand, D.G. (1975) Clin. Pharmac. Therap. 18, 377.

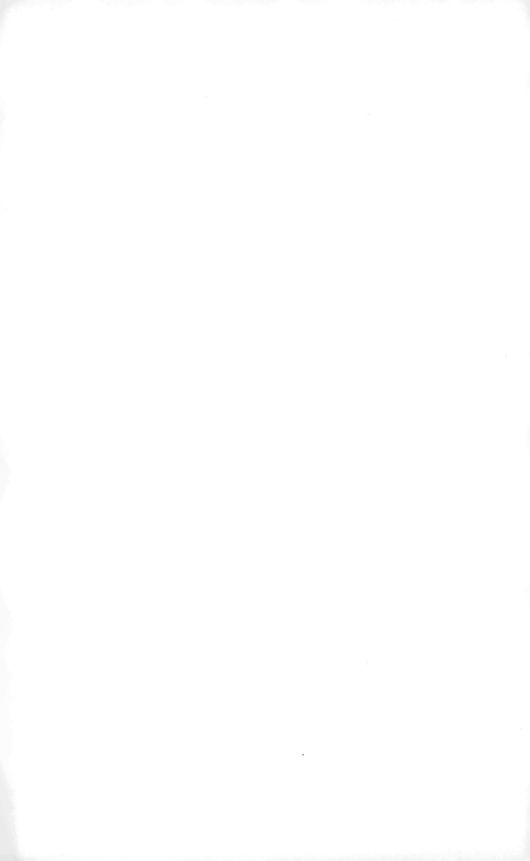

10. Metabolic fate of particular classes of compound.

RECENTLY DISCOVERED ROUTES OF METABOLISM

Bernard Testa

School of Pharmacy, University of Lausanne, Place du Chateau 3. CH-1005 Lausanne, Switzerland

INTRODUCTION

The number of xenobiotics being investigated for their biotransformation has been growing rapidly for many years, and this trend is likely to continue. Furthermore, our fundamental knowledge expands while instrumentation and experimental skills reach high levels of sophistication. An obvious consequence of these progresses can be found in the number of compounds being discovered either as metabolites or newly investigated xenobiotics, or as novel metabolites of previously studied substrates.

While most of these products arise from known pathways of metabolism, a number of studies report the discovery of novel metabolic routes. However, a semantic problem is evident here since the concept of metabolic routes may not have the same meaning for all workers in the field. In the present review, a broad meaning is chosen; although there is some overlap, the following cases will be documented and discussed:
a) Classical metabolic reactions mediated by alternative enzymes.
b) Metabolism of novel substrates and especially unexpected functional groups by classical pathways;
c) Novel non-enzymatic and post-enzymatic reactions;
d) Novel metabolic routes stricto sensu.
Clearly, notions such as "classical", "alternative", "novel" and "unexpected" are somewhat arbitrary. Their application may lead to disagreement between readers and the reviewer, a stimulating and thought-provoking situation.

Two reviews published a number of years ago (Jenner and Testa, 1978; Testa and Jenner, 1978) have presented an extensive coverage of novel pathways and novel metabolites. The present chapter is intended as an update of these two reviews, duplication being avoided unless necessary.

PHASE I (FUNCTIONALISATION) REACTIONS

Cases a) and b) above are considered in the following section, while cases c) and d) are discussed later.

Metabolite reactions mediated by alternative enzymes, and metabolism of novel substrates by classical routes

In recent years, a number of classical phase I metabolites have been found to be produced not only by traditional enzymes, but also by other systems designated here as alternative enzymes. For example, the oxidation of numerous xenobiotic substrates can also be mediated by prostaglandin hydroperoxidase by a process know as cooxidation and aptly reviewed by Eling et al (1983). Cytochrome P-450 functioning in the hydroperoxidative mode is able to mediate a number of reactions previously known only for the monooxygenase mode, as illustrated in Table 1.

The generation of iminium ions as metabolites of N-alkyl compounds is a well-known pathway of monooxygenases (for a review, see Overton et al, 1985). Rather unexpected, therefore was the recent discovery that MPTP (1-methyl-4-phenyl-1,2,3,6-tetrahydropyridine) is aromatized by monoamine oxidase (mainly MAO-B) in a two-step reaction first yielding the iminium ion MPDP+ (1-methyl-4-phenyl-2,3-dihydropyridinium) which then disproportionates to MPTP and MPP+ (1-methyl-4-phenylpyridinium) (Figure 1). This reaction has attracted enormous interest after Langston et al (1983) reported that MPTP is a neurotoxin inducing Parkinson-like symptoms. There is now conclusive evidence that MPP+, is in fact, the toxic metabolite causing nigrostriatal neuronal damage (e.g. Markey et al, 1984).

Another relevant reaction is the hydrolysis of various esters mediated by serum albumin, in particular human serum albumin, as recently discussed in the context of enzymatic versus non-enzymatic biotransformation (Testa, 1983).

A some-what different situation occurs when novel substrates or unexpected functional groups are metabolized by well-known pathways. A few such cases are reported in Figure 2 although the selection is rather arbitrary. Thus, the two-step oxidation of methylene to carbonyl groups is a very classical pathway, but its occurence at methylene groups alpha to a nitrogen atom is prevented by the instability (C-N cleavage) of the carbinolamine intermediate resulting in N-dealkylation or deamination. However there may be a few instances where the carbinolamine is sufficiently stabilized for

Table 1 Classical Phase I metabolites generated by alternative enzymes

Enzymes	Reactions	Substrates	Ilustrative references
Prostaglandin hydroperoxidase	Cooxidation	Polycyclic aromatic hydrocarbons Aromatic amines Various drugs	Eling et al, 1983
Various peroxidases Cytochromes P-450 (peroxidative function)	N-Demethylation N-Debenzylation N-Depropargylation N-Oxidation	Tertiary amines Pargyline	Hollenberg et al, 1985; Weli and Lindeke, 1986
Monoamine oxidase (B > A)	Aromatization	1-Methyl-4-phenyl-1,2,3,6-tetrahydropyridine (MPTP)	Chiba et al, 1985; Gessner et al, 1984; Peterson et al, 1985; Salach et al, 1984
Serum albumin	Hydrolysis	Various esters	Kuruno et al, 1979,1983

Testa

Figure 1. Monoamine oxidase-mediated oxidation of MPTP to the iminium ion MPDP+ which then disproportionates to MPTP and MPP+ (Chiba et al, 1985; Gessener et al, 1984; Peterson et al, 1985; Salach et al, 1984).

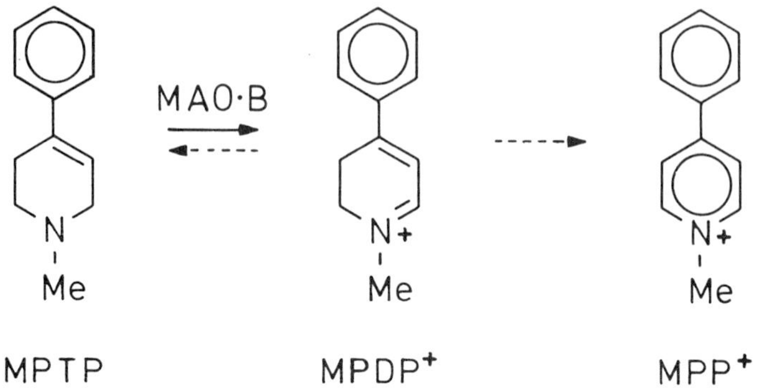

Figure 2. Some novel substrates of classical oxidation and reduction pathways.

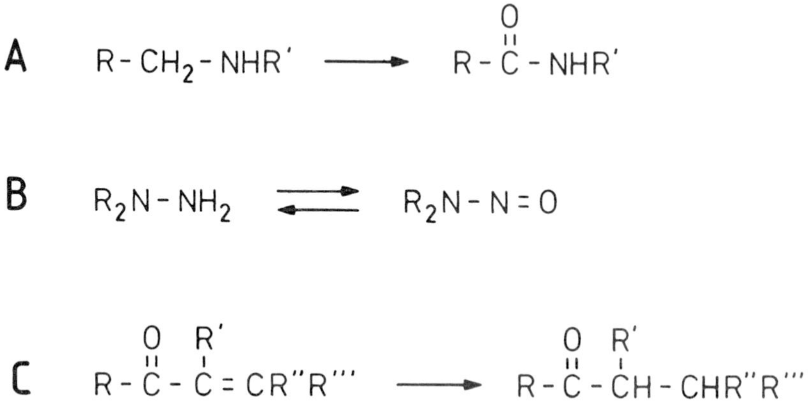

A: Formation of amides from CH_2-N groups. B: Formation of nitrosamines from 1,1-disubstituted hydrazines. C: α,β - Ketoalkene reduction. See text for substrates and references.

dehydrogenation to take place. The oxidation of an N-methyl to an N-formyl group in lieu of N-demethylation could be such an instance (for a review see Jenner and Testa, 1978). An N-formyl metabolite of methadone has recently been characterized in the rat in vivo (Abbot et al, 1985); this paper also contains a lucid discussion on various reaction mechanisms believed to lead to formamide metabolites. Gorrod and Gooderham (1985) report what may well be another interesting case of amide formation. Indeed, N-benzylanilines were found to be oxidized to N-phenylbenzamides (see Figure 2A) in·hepatic microsomes of various species. Although the actual reaction mechanism was not established (carbinolamine and nitrone were the two intermediates considered most likely), a competition between deamination/dealkylation and amide formation is indicated in this study.

The biological oxidation of nitrogen atoms in organic molecules is a topic of considerable interest and relevance (Gorrod and Damani, 1985). The chemical complexity of N-oxidation and N-reduction metabolites is great indeed, and as a consequence the discovery of novel intermediates, rearrangement products and metabolites should continue. An interesting recent finding is the in vitro metabolic conversion of a 1,1-disubstituted hydrazine to the corresponding nitrosamine (see Figure 2B) (Tatsumi et al, 1984). The reverse reaction has also been characterized in vivo and in vitro (Tatsumi et al, 1983)

There are a few examples in the literature of metabolic carbon-carbon double bond reduction, but much fundamental knowledge is missing on this reaction. The characterization of an α,β-ketoalkene reductase activity (see Figure 2C) in the cytosol of mammalian tissues is therefore of interest (Lindstrom and Whitaker, 1984a, 1984b). The same reaction was found to occcur with digoxin, which in humans is reduced to (20R)-dihydrodigoxin (Reuning et al, 1985).

Novel metabolic routes

A number of functionalization reactions have been uncovered in recent years which must be viewed as genuinely novel and were quite unexpected. In most cases, little is known regarding their chemical and enzymatic mechanism, suggesting that we can look forward to interesting findings. A selection of such novel routes is presented below.

Aromatic heterocycles have been found to be subject to novel oxidation routes, as illustrated with imidazole and

furan derivatives.   Thus, the antiprotozoal agent
tinidazole exhibited the first reported case of nitro group
migration (Figure 3), presumably by a mechanism analogous
to the NIH shift (Chasseaud et al, 1984; Wood et al, 1985).
The new metabolite, the structure of which was proven by X-
ray crystallography, accounts for approximately 20% of
dose in humans.   Two toxic furan derivatives, 2-methyl-and
3-methylfuran, were found to undergo oxidative ring
opening (Figure 4) resulting in highly reactive
electrophiles (Ravindranath et al, 1984).   A number of
medicinal furan derivatives are potential substrates for
this novel route of toxication.

Figure 3.   Metabolic ring hydroxylation of tinidazole
involving a novel nitro group migration (Wood et al, 1985).

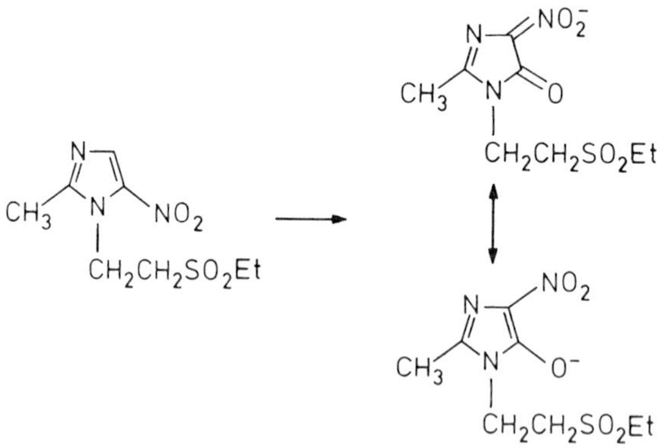

Figure 4   Toxication of methylfurans by oxidative ring
opening (Ravindranath et al, 1984).

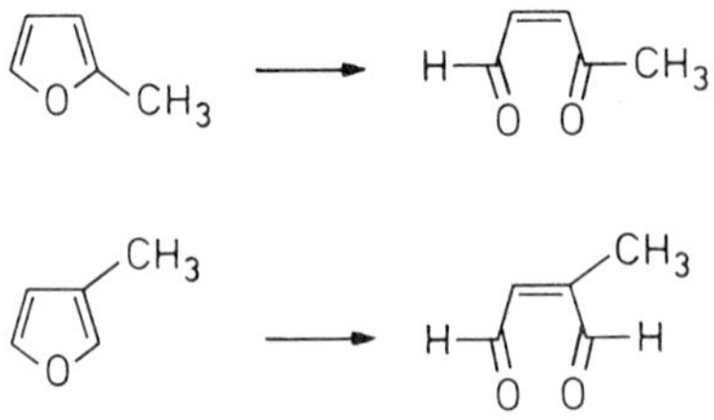

   Reactions of N- and O-dearylation (Figure 5) have been
known for a number of years, but until now have received
only limited interest.   In 1971, Heykants et al reported

that the butyrophenone derivative azaperone undergoes loss of the α-pyridyl moiety (Figure 5B), this route accounting for approximately 50% of the dose in rats. This early finding is gainfully compared with N-dephenylation reaction such as the cytochrome P-450-mediated conversion

Figure 5. Examples of N- and O-dearylation reactions. See text for references.

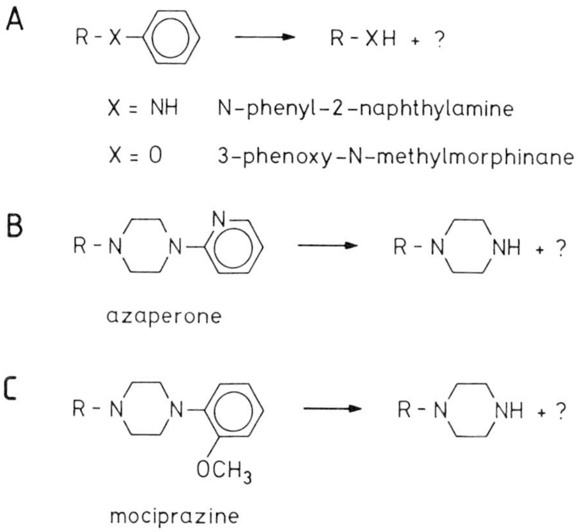

A

R - X —◯ ⟶ R - XH + ?

X = NH   N-phenyl-2-naphthylamine

X = O   3-phenoxy-N-methylmorphinane

B

R - N⟩N—◯(N) ⟶ R - N⟩NH + ?

azaperone

C

R - N⟩N—◯ ⟶ R - N⟩NH + ?
          OCH₃

mociprazine

of N-phenyl-2-naphthylamine to the carcinogenic 2-naphthylamine (Batten and Hathway, 1977; Anderson et al, 1982; Laham and Potvin, 1983) (see Figure 5A). A reaction similar to that occurring in azaperone, namely N-dephenylation of a piperazinyl moiety, has just been reported for the antiemetic agent mociprazine (Pognat et al, 1986) (see Figure 5C). We note that both compounds have one unsubstituted carbon atom in the ortho position of the aromatic ring.

O-Dephenylation is documented for 3-phenoxy-N-methylmorphinane, the reaction being a diaryl ether cleavage (Leinweber et al, 1981) (see Figure 5A). The mechanism is postulated to involve epoxidation of the phenyl ring, which is reasonable in view of the arguments noted above, followed by glutathione addition and cleavage of the ether bridge (Kamm et al, 1979). Clearly such

dearylation reactions are challenging from a mechanistic
point of view and in some cases have pharmacodynamic
consequences.   They should not be confused with the
presumably hydrolytic deamination reaction exhibited by 1-
hydrazinophthalazines such as hydralazine.

Other significant oxidation or reduction reactions have
received rather recent recognition.   Let us simply mention
the activation of the prodrug nabumetome to its
antiinflammatory metabolite by an oxidation shortening of
the 3-oxobutyl side chain to an acetyl moiety (Haddock et
al, 1984).   Also, much has been recently uncovered
regarding cycling of, and free radical formation from,
quinone xenobiotics and metabolites (e.g. Chesiset al,
1984; Hochstein, 1983; Oldcorneet al, 1984).
Unfortunatley, these reactions cannot be considered here
due to space limitations.

Among metabolic reactions occurring without change in
the degree of oxidation, we mention a non-enzymatic lactam-
lactone tautomeric equilibrium which has intrigued several
groups including our own.   This reaction is illustrated in
Figure 6A with proxibarbal, a non-hypnotic barbiturate
containing a β -hydroxylated side-chain.

Figure 6. Reversible lactam ring opening and lactone ring
formation as occurring in, e.g., the metabolism of
proxibarbal (A) and phenylbutazone (B). See text for
references.

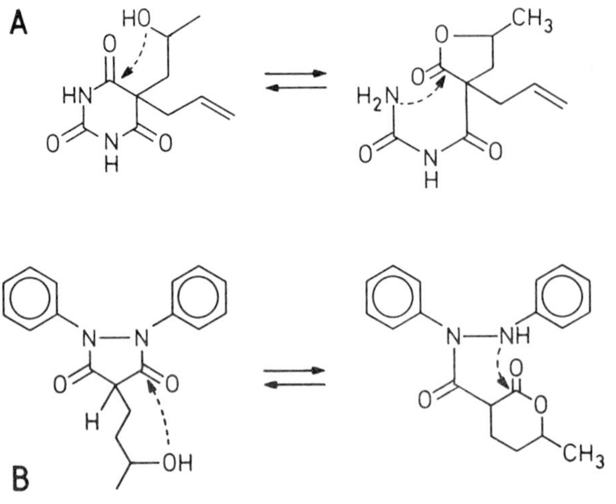

This drug is in a pH-dependent equilibrium with its lactonic tautomer, known as valofan (Wittekind and Testa, 1979; Wittekind et al, 1984; and ref. therein). Lactam ring opening and lactone ring formation occur by a nucleophilic attack of the OH group on a carbonyl group; at physiological pH, the proxibarbal/valofan equilibruim is 84/16. Valofan then undergoes irreversible hydrolytic removal of its allophanyl side-chain.

A number of hyponotic barbiturates undergoing metabolic side-chain β-hydroxylation can conceivably display this reaction, but results are scarce. One noteworthy case is α-phenyl- γ-valerolactone, a metabolite excreted following phenobarbital intoxication and presumably arising after β-hydroxylation of the ethyl group and lactone formation (Andersen et al, 1976). Interestingly, the same reaction has just been characterized for phenylbutazone (Alexander et al, 1985); following administration to the rat, the drug yields among others a γ-hydroxylated metabolite which was shown to slowly isomerize to a δ-lactone (Figure 6B).

A totally different and as yet unclassified reaction has been discovered in the metabolism of n-butylglycidyl ether, which inrats is transformed via epoxide ring opening into an N-acetylamino acid derivative (Figure 7) (Eadsforth et al, 1985).

Figure 7. Hypothetical mechanism for the biotransformation of n-butylglycidyl ether into 3-butoxy-2-acetylamino propionic acid (Eadsforth et al, 1985).

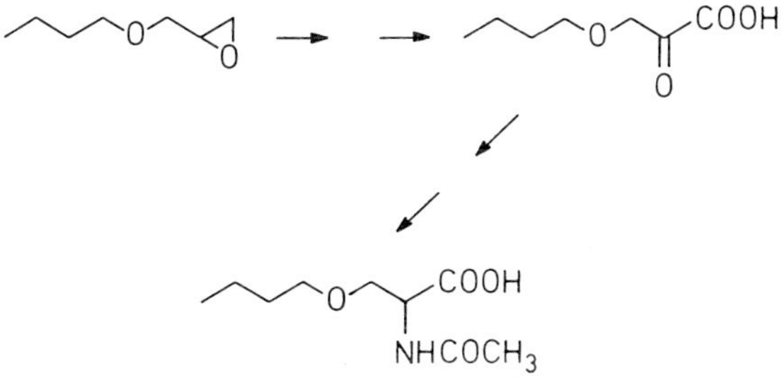

This novel metabolic route of an aliphatic epoxide could be due to a primary reaction of aminolysis, but is more likely to involve hydrolysis, formation of 3-butoxypyruvic acid, and finally transamination and N-acetylation (Figure 7). But whatever its mechanism, this route is intriguing and its occurrence in the metabolism of other oxiranes should be investigated.

The metabolic chiral inversion of antiinflammatory 2-arylpropionates is a novel route with important pharmacokinetic and pharmacodynamic consequences (Hutt and Caldwell, 1983). It is discussed by Vermeulen elsewhere in this volume and will not be considered here.

PHASE II (CONJUGATION) REACTIONS

In this section cases, b), c) and d) (see Introduction) are discussed, case a) having no relevance to conjugation reactions

Novel substrates of classical transferases

Cyanamide ($NC-NH_2$), an alcohol deterrent, undergoes in vitro and in vivo N-acetylation as a major metabolic reaction in several species including man (Shirota etal, 1984). The reaction is catalyzed by an N-acetyltransferase, and this novel substrate thus shows a metabolic reactivity similar to that of aromatic amines.

Reactions of sulphoconjugation have recently been shown to involve the N-oxide and secondary amine functional groups, two rather unexpected findings. The vasodilator agent minoxidil is thus conjugated to its N-oxide group, yielding small amounts of the zwitterionic N-O-sulphate ester (Figure 8A) (Johnson et al, 1983). As regards the antiinflammatory drug tiaramide (Figure 8B), it undergoes two distinct sulphoconjugation reactions. First, it is a direct substrate for sulphotransferase, yielding the alkylsulphate ester which was characterized following incubations with rat and mouse hepatic cytosol (Iwasaki et al, 1983a), and which is a potential alkylating agent. Additionally, tiaramide is N-dealkylated to the secondary amine, and the latter is then N-sulphoconjugated in rat and mouse hepatic cytosol. The sulphamate metabolite has also been detected in the urine of mice dosed with the drug (Iwasaki et al., 1983a, 1983b). Formation of sulphamates from primary amines is a known, albeit rare metabolic pathway (Jenner and Testa, 1978), but we are not aware of any previously reported N-sulphoconjugation of a secondary amine.

Novel non-enzymatic and post-enzymatic reactions

A number of acidic drugs are conjugated by UDP-glucuronyltransferase to yield 1-O-acyl glucuronides which in recent years have received marked attention. Indeed,

Figure 8. Novel sulphoconjugates.

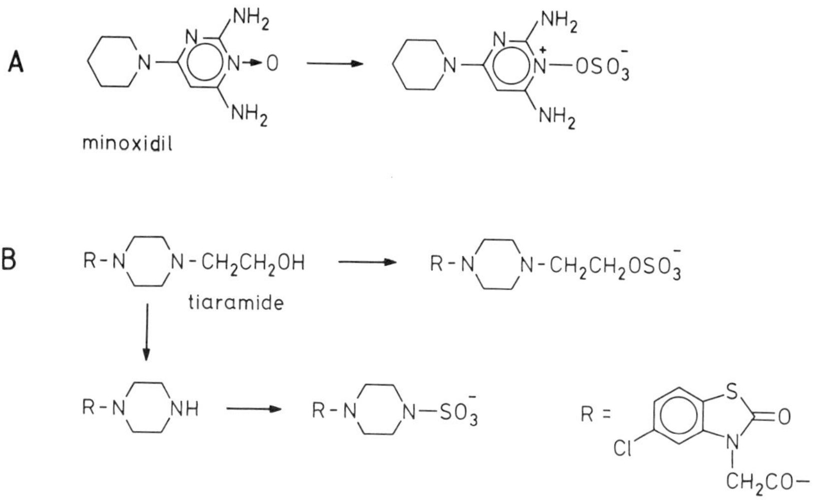

A: N-O-sulphate ester formed from the N-oxide minodixil; B: Formation of a sulphamate from the secondary amine metabolite of tiaramide. See text for references.

these metabolites display a remarkable reactivity, the pharmacokinetic and pharmacodynamic consequences of which are progressively being assessed (for a good review see Faed, 1984). Thus, they isomerize in a pH-dependent manner to β-glucuronidase-resistant forms (see for example studies with furosemide (Rachemel et al, 1985) and valproic acid (Dickinson et al, 1985)). The reaction is an intramolecular migration of the acyl moiety leading to the 2-0, 3-0 and 4-0 positional isomers, and possibly also to various furanose isomers. Additionally, the 1-0 acyl glucuronides are electrophilic, acylating agents able to react with some endogenous nucleophiles such as thiol groups in albumin (van Breemen and Fenselau, 1985).

Non-enzymatic reactions of glutathione (GSH) have been characterized in a number of instances (for a review see Testa, 1983). Recent findings increase the range of these reactions and show that other endogenous thiols may also be involved. The thiol-containing drug captopril (CapSH) is particularly illustrative. This compound is oxidized by glutathione disulphide (GS-SG) via thiol/disulphide exchange to form the mixed disulphide CapS-SG and then dimer CapS-SCap; formation of other mixed disulphides with thiol-containing amino acids, peptides and proteins also occurs (Rabenstein and Theriault, 1985; Drummer and Jarrott, 1986). Similar reactions are documented for alacepril, an analogue of captopril (Matsumoto et al, 1986), while N-(2-mercapto-2-methylpropanoyl)-L-cysteine, a dithiol compound, undergoes cyclization by intramolecular SS formation (Horiuchi et al, 1985).

An interesting non-enzymatic reaction involving GSH or cysteine has been characterised in the metabolism of aromatic sulphonamides (Conroy et al, 1984). Nucleophile attack on the ipso-carbon results in replacement of the sulphamoyl group by the glutathionyl or cysteinyl moiety with loss of SO_2 and NH_3. A series of aromatic heterocyclic derivatives were examined, and the reaction rate was found to be correlated with the pK_a of the sulphamide.

Novel conjugates

In animals, formation of glycosides other than glucuronides is a rare but genuine metabolic route (Jenner and Testa, 1978) which recent findings have helped to better document and understand. For example, one quarter of a dose of phenobarbital administered to human subjects is recovered in urine as the N-glucoside (Tang et al, 1984), showing that this route can hardly be considered as negligible in some cases.

Similarly, conjugation with a single amino acid such as glycine, glutamine, taurine, ornithine or arginine is well established, but conjugation with polypeptides (excepting GSH) is infrequent (for a brief review see Waring and Mitchell, 1985). it is therefore interesting that a number of polypeptide conjugates were detected in the urine of calves dosed with phenothiazine, an anthelmintic agent (Waring and Mitchell, 1985). Four major N-conjugates were characterized as having the glu-glu, gly-pro-gly, ala-pro-pro-ala-glu, and thr-lys-gly-ser-ser-gly chains, respectively.

When trichloroethylene was administered to rats and mice, a metabolite accounting for 5-7% of urinary radioactivity was isolated and found to be N-(hydroxyacetyl)-aminoethanol (Dekant et al, 1986) (see Figure 9A). The metabolic sequence was postulated to involve activation by cytochrome P-450, covalent binding of a reactive intermediate with membrane phospholipids, liberation of the phosphatidylethanolamide of glyoxylic acid, and further biotransformation to the novel conjugate. Formation of the latter, if the postulated sequence is

Figure 9. Two novel and borderline cases of conjugation reactions.

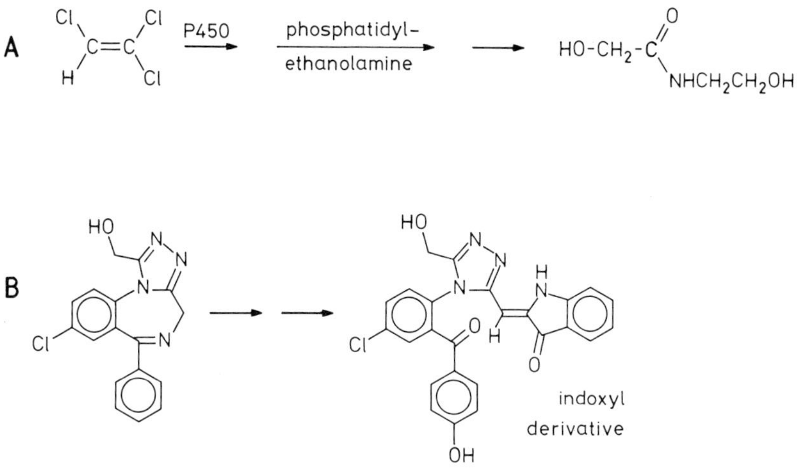

A: Formation of N-(hydroxyacetyl)-aminoethanol from trichloroethylene following a sequence postulated to involve covalent binding to membrane phospholipids. B : Formation in urine of indoxylidene derivatives of aldehydic drug metabolites. See text for details and references.

genuine, must be considered more as an index of chemical insult to membranes than as an actual metabolic route, although the difference between these two reaction pathways is more superficial than fundamental.

Another borderline case, although conceptually different, is found in the formation of indoxyl derivatives of drug metabolites. Faigle et al (1985), while investigating the metabolism of two triazolobenzodiazepine analogues in rats and dogs, found urinary compounds characterized as indoxylidene derivatives (see Figure 9B). Evidence indicates that the reaction sequence involves opening of the diazepine ring with oxidation of C-3 to an aldehyde function, and non-enzymatic condensation of the latter with indoxyl. Interestingly, the indoxyl conjugate is not found in freshly voided urine collected at 0°C, but only in urine samples stored for a few hours at room temperature. This indicates that the condensation reaction occurs only in the bladder (if the urine is stored long enough) and/or extracorpeally after micturition. Whether such a borderline case can be still considered as a metabolic reaction remains to be decided.

A conceptual breakthrough of recent years is certainly the awareness that a considerable number of xenobiotics can enter pathways of lipid biosynthesis, exhibiting significant pharmacokinetic and pharmacodynamic impact, e.g. formation of tissue residues and disturbance of membrane structure and function. The xenobiotics involved are mainly carboxylic acids, but also some alcohols and aldehydes. Their metabolic interrelationships with lipids have been pioneered and reviewed by Caldwell (Caldwell and Varwell Marsh, 1983; Caldwell, 1984) and are summarized in Table 2. Recent examples include conjugation of fatty acids to ethanol (Mogelson and Lange, 1984) and codeine (Leighty and Fentimen, 1983), synthesis of 3-phenoxybenzoic acid-containing lipids via the monoacylglycerol pathway (Imhof et al 1985), cholesterol ester formation by transesterification of chlorambucil (Gunnarsson et al, 1984), and carnitine conjugation of pivalic acid (Vickers et al, 1985).

MACROMOLECULAR ADDUCTS AS NOVEL CONJUGATES

Covalent binding of xenobiotics to endogenous compounds, particularly macromolecules such as proteins and nucleic acids, is a molecular phenomenon attracting considerable attention and resources due to its toxicological significance (Hemminki, 1983; Martin and de la Iglesia, 1983). Considered in a metabolic context, macromolecular adduct formation is distinct by a number of criteria from both functionalisation and conjugation reactions, and shows characteristic aspects some of which are briefly mentioned here:
- The reaction may be non-enzymatic (e.g. covalent binding of cisplatin to DNA), post-enzymatic (e.g. binding of a reactive intermediate formed by either phase I or phase II enzymes), or enzymatic as for suicide substrates.
- The covalent bond formed may be strong (e.g., C-N bonds) or of medium energy (e.g., S-S bonds), and as such adduct formation is at least conceptually distinct from reversible, non-covalent binding to circulating and tissular macromolecules.
- The adducted macromolecules may be soluble (e.g., serum albumin), membranal, or located within organelles (nucleic acids).
- The fate of macromolecular adducts can hardly be expected to resemble that of phase I and phase II metabolites, but our ignorance of the topic is almost complete.

Table 2. Xenobiotic metabolism pathways involving lipid biosynthesis reactions (Caldwell and Varnell Marsh, 1983; Caldwell, 1984)

Functional group in xenobiotic	Reaction
Alcoholic hydroxyl group group	Esterification with fatty acids
Aldehyde group	Addition of one 2-carbon unit (Synthesis of acrylic acids)
Carboxylic group	Addition of single or multiple 2-carbon units (Formation of hybrid fatty acids) Incorporation of xenobiotic or hybrid fatty acids into hybrid di- and triglycerides Esterification with cholesterol or bile salts (Formation of 3-0-sterol esters) Conjugation with carnitine.

The above suggests that macromolecular adducts of xenobiotics should be viewed as a third group of metabolites, the biochemical and metabolic study of which has just begun. Sufficient data must accumulate before the relevant reactions can be classified according to substrates, functional groups, chemical mechanisms, acceptors, etc, in analogy with functionalisation and conjugation reactions.

CONCLUSION

As stated in the introduction, there is an element of arbitrariness in deciding whether a given metabolite is "novel", i.e. "recently discovered", or has a flavour of deja vu. However, this formal and superficial discrimination is not at issue here. Rather, this review attempts to illustrate the richness and steady maturation of the science of xenobiotic metabolism. Particularly striking is the growing awareness of the interrelationships between xenobiotic and endobiotic metabolism, a field where fascinating developments and breakthroughs can be expected. Indeed, xenobiotics may thus become a new means of exploring metabolic pathways not so much at the reduced level of biochemical reactions than at a higher level of physiological regulations and homeostasis.

REFERENCES

Abbott, F.S., Slatter, J.G., Burton, R. and Kang, G.I. (1985) Xenobiotica 15, 129.

Alexander, D.M., Mathew, G.E.A. and Wilson, B.J. (1985) Xenobiotica 15, 123

Anderson, M.M., Mitchum, R.K. and Beland, F.A. (1982) Xenobiotica 12, 31.

Andresen, B.D. Davis, F.T., Templeton, J.L., Hammer, R.H. and Panzik, H.L. (1976) Res. Comm. Chem. Path. Pharmacol.15, 21.

Batten, P.L. and Hathway, D.E. (1977) Br. J. Cancer 35, 342.

Caldwell, J. (1984) Biochem. Soc. Trans. 12, 9.

Caldwell, J. and Varwell Marsh, M,. (1983) Biochem. Pharmacol. 32, 1667.

Chasseaud, L.F., Henrick, K., Matthews, R.W., Scott, P.W. and Wood, S.G. (1984) J. Chem. Soc. Chem. Comm. 491.

Chesis, P.L., Levin, D.E., Smith, M.T., Ernster, L. and Ames, B. (1984)Proc. Nat. Acad. Sci.(USA) 81, 1696.

Chiba, K., Peterson, L.A., Castagnoli, K.P., Trevor, A.J. and Castagnoli, N. Jr. (1985) Drug Metab. Disp. 13, 342

Conroy, C.W., Schwam, H. and Maren, T.H. (1984) Drug Metab. Disp. 12, 614.

Dekant, W., Schulz, A., Metzler, M. and Henschler, D. (1986) Xenobiotica 16, 143.

Dickinson, R.G., Kluck, R.M., Eadie, M.J. and Hooper, W.D. (1985) J. Pharmacol. Exp. Ther. 233,214.

Drummer, O.H. and Jarrott, B. (1986) Med. Res. Rev. 6, 75.

Eadsforth, C.V., Logan, C.J., Page, J.A. and Regan, P.D. (1985) Drug Metab. Disp. 13, 263.

Eling, T., Boyd, J., Reed, G., Mason, R. and Sivarajah, K. (1983) Drug Metab. Rev. 14, 1023.

Faed, E.M. (1984) Drug Metab. Rev. 15, 1213.

Faigle, J.W., Stierlin, H., Mory, H., Winkler, T. and Kriemler, H.P. (1985) Experientia 41, 476.

Gessner, W., Brossi, A., Shen, R.-s., Fritz, R.R and Abell, C.W (1984) Helv. Chim.Acta 67, 2037

Gorrod, J.W. and Damani, L.A., (1985) eds. "Biological Oxidation of Nitrogen in Organic Molecules. Chemistry, Toxicology and Pharmacology", Ellis Horwood,

Chichester.

Gorrod, J.W. and Gooderham, N.J (1985) Xenobiotica 15, 1021.

Gunnarsson, P.O., Johansson, S.A. and Svensson, L. (1984) Xenobiotica 14, 569.

Haddock, R.E., Jeffery, D.J., Lloyd, J.A and Thawley, A.R. (1984) Xenobiotica 14, 327.

Hemminki, K. (1983) Aech. Toxicol. 52, 249.

Heykants, J., Pardoel, L. and Janssen, P.A.J. (1971) Arzneim. Forsch. (Drug Res.) 21, 982.

Hochstein, P. (1983) Fund. Appl. Toxicol. 3, 215.

Hollenberg, P.E., Miwa, G.T., Walsh, J.s., Dwyer, L.A., Rickert, D.E.and Kedderis, G.L. (1985) Drug Metab. Disp.13, 272

Horiuchi, M., Takashina, H., Iwatani, T. and Iso, T. (1985) J. Pharm. Soc. Jap. 105, 665.

Hutt. A.J. and Caldwell, J. (1983) J. Pharm. Pharmacol. 35 693.

Imhof, D.A., Logan, C.J. and Dodds, P.F. (1985) Biochem. Pharmacol. 34, 3009.

Iwasaki, K., Shiraga, T., Noda, K., Tada, K. and Noguchi, H. (1983a) Xenobiotica 13, 273.

Iwasaki, K., Shiraga, T., Noda, K., Tada, K. and Nogichi, H. (1983b) Xenobiotica 13, 565.

Jenner, P. and Testa, B. (1978) Xenobiotica, 8 1.

Johnson, G.A., Barsuhn, K.J. and McCall, J.M (1983) Drug Metab. Disp. 11, 507.

Kamm. J.J., Szuna, A. and Mohacsi, E. (1979) Pharmacologist 21, 173.

Kuruno, Y., Maki, T., Yotsuyanagi, T. and Ikeda, K. (1979) Chem. Pharm. Bull. 27, 2781.

Kuruno, Y., Kondo, T. and Ikeda, K. (1983) Arch. Biochem. Biophys. 227, 339.

Laham, S. and Potvin, M. (1983) Drug Chem. Toxicol. 6, 295.

Langston, J.W., Ballard. P., Tetrud, J.W. and Irwin, I. (1983) Science 219, 979.

Leighty, E.G. and Fentiman, A.F.Jr (1983) J. Pharm. Pharmacol. 35, 260.

Leinweber, F.J., Szuna, A.J., Williams, T.H., Sasso, G.J. and DeBarbieri, B.A. (1981) Drug Metab. Disp. 9, 284.

Lindstrom, T.D. and Whitaker, G.W. (1984a) Xenobiotica 14, 503.

Lindstrom, T.D. and Whitaker, G.W. (1984b) Drug Metab. Disp. 12, 72.

Markey, S.P., Johannessen, J.N., Chiueh, C.C., Burns, R.S. and Herkenham, M.A. (1984) Nature 311, 464.

Martin, R.A. and de la Iglesia, F.A. (1983) Drug Metab. Rev. 14, 513.

Matsumoto, K., Miyazaki, H., Fujii, T., Yoshida, K., Amejima, H. and Hashimoto, M. (1986) Arzneim.-Forsch. (Drug Res.) 36, 40.

Mogelson, S. and Lange, L.G. (1984) Biochemistry 23, 4075.

Oldcorne, M.A., Brown, J.R. and Patterson, L.H. (1984) Biochem. Soc. Trans. 12, 681.

Overton, M., Hickman, J.A., Threasgill, M.D., Vaughan, K. and Gescher, A. (1985) Biochem. Pharmacol. 34, 2055.

Peterson, L.A., Caldera, P.S., Trevor, A., Chiba, K. and Castagnoli, N. Jr. (1985) J. Med. Chem. 28, 1432.

Pognat, J.F., Enreille, A., Chabard, J.L., Bush, N and Berger, J.A. (1986) Drug Metab. Disp. 14, 147.

Rabenstein, D.L. and Theriault, Y. (1985) Can. J. Chem. 63, 33.

Rachmel, A., Hazelton, G.A., Yergey, A.L. and Liberato, D.J. (1985) Drug Metab. Disp. 13, 705.

Ravindranath, V., Burka, L.T. and Boyd, M.R. (1984) Science 224, 884.

Reuning, R.H., Shepard, T.A., Morrison, B.E and Bockbrader, H.N. (1985) Drug Metab. Disp. 13, 51.

Salach, J.I., Singer, T.P., Castagnoli, N. Jr. and Trevor, A. (1984) Biochem. Biophys.Res. Comm. 125, 831.

Shirota, F.N., Nagasawa, H.T., Kwon, C.H. and Demaster, E.G. (1984) Drug Metab. Disp. 12, 337.

Tang, B.K., Yilmaz, B. and Kalow, W. (1984) Biomed. Mass Spectrom. 11, 462.

Tatsumi, K., Yamada, H. and Kitamura, S. (1983) Arch. Biochem. Biophys. 226, 174.

Tatsumi, K., Kitamura, S. and Sumida, M. (1984) Biochem. Biophys. Res. Comm. 118, 958.

Testa, B. (1983) in "Biological Basis of Detoxication" (Ed. by Caldwell, J. and Jakoby, W.B.), Academic Press, New York, p.137.

Testa, B. and Jenner, P. (1978) Drug Metab. Rev., 7, 325.

Van Breemen, R.B. and Fenselau, C. (1985) Drug Metab. Disp. 13, 318.

Vickers, S., Ducan, C.A.H., White, S.D., Ramjit, H.G., Smith, J.L., Walker, R.W., Flynn, H. and Arison, B.H. (1985) Xenobiotica 15, 453.

Waring, R.H. and Mitchell, S.C. (1985) Xenobiotica 15, 459.

Weli, A.M. and Lindeke, B. (1986) Xenobiotica 16, 281.

Wittekind, H.H and Testa, B. (1979) J. Chromatog. 179, 370.

Wittekind, H.H., Testa, B. and Balant, L.P (1984) Eur. J. Drug Metab. Pharmacokin. 9, 117.

Wood, S.G., Scott, P.W., Chasseaud, L.F., Faulkner, J.K., Matthews, R.W. and Henrick, K. (1985) Xenobiotica 15, 107.

METABOLISM OF SULPHUR-CONTAINING DRUGS

L.A. Damani

Chelsea Department of Pharmacy, King's College London (KQC), Chelsea Campus, Manresa Road, London. SW3 6LX.

INTRODUCTION

This review outlines how organosulphur compounds are metabolically handled by mammalian systems, with particular emphasis on sulphur-containing medicinal agents. There were two options open to the reviewer in writing this article. The first option was to classify the organosulphur compounds used as medicinal agents into various pharmacological or therapeutic classes, and to arbitrarily outline the biological fate of a selected number of compounds from each class. The only advantage of this approach would be the portrayal of the importance of organosulphur compounds in medicinal chemistry (Table 1). This is often not recognised and there are literally hundreds of such compounds, either in use or under development. The second option was to classify organosulphur drugs according to the type of sulphur functionality present in the molecule (Table 2) to examine how such groups (e.g. thiols, sulphides etc) are handled metabolically, and attempt to relate this to the known chemistry of the functionalities. This latter approach seemed more desirable, since it may enable general principles to be explored, as well as give the opportunity of presenting compound-specific data. Consequently, this review will describe the biochemistry of various sulphur functionalities, exemplifying specific reactions with reference to well known drugs, and will indicate the significance of appropriate reactions to the disposition and biological activity of various drugs.

IMPORTANCE AND USES OF ORGANOSULPHUR COMPOUNDS

There are several sources of interest in organosulphur compounds. Sulphur is essential to the life and growth of all organisms - from microbes to man. It is a constituent of vitamins (e.g. biotin, thiamine), co-enzymes (e.g. -

Table 1. Clinically used sulphur-containing drugs[1]

PHARMACOLOGICAL/ THERAPEUTIC CLASS	EXAMPLES OF DRUG(S) IN EACH CLASS THAT CONTAIN A SULPHUR FUNCTIONAL GROUP
Antipsychotics, CNS drugs	Phenothiazines (eg chlorpromazine), dothiepin
Histamine H_2-receptor antagonists (antiulcer)	Cimetidine, ranitidine
Mucolytics	S-Carboxylmethyl-L-cysteine (carbocisteine)
Anthelmintics	Thiabendazole, phenothiazine
Hypnotics	Chlormethiazole
Antirheumatics	Sulindac
Anti-platelet aggregation (also an uricosuric agent)	Sulphinpyrazone
Antimicrobials	Dapsone, sulphadimidine (and other related sulphones & sulphonamides)
Antihypertensive	Captopril
Cytotoxic agents	Thioguanine, mercaptopurine
Chelating agent (also an antirheumatic agent)	Penicillamine
Treatment of alcoholism	Disulfiram
Intravenous anaesthetics	Thiopentone
Antithyroid agents	Carbimazole, Propylthiouracil
Antitubercular drugs	Ethionamide
Anti-infective skin/scalp preparations	Malathion, Pyrithione

---

[1]There are a large number of other clinically used sulphur-containing drugs where the sulphur plays no appreciable role in disposition and/or bioactivation/inactivation. These drugs are not listed in this table.

Table 2. Types of sulphur functionalities common in sulphur-containing drugs[1]

SULPHUR FUNCTIONALITY[2]	POTENTIAL METABOLITE(S)[2]	EXAMPLE OF DRUG(S) THAT AFFORD THESE METABOLITES IN VITRO AND /OR IN VIVO.
Thioether (sulphide) $R - S - R$ (0)	Sulphoxide $R - \overset{O}{\underset{}{S}} - R$ (0) Sulphone $R - \overset{O}{\underset{O}{S}} - R$ (+2)	Chlorpromazine (Aromatic sulphur heterocycle) Chlormethiazole (thiazole ring system) (see text) Thioridazine (Aromatic sulphur heterocycle and an alkylaryl sulphide side chain) Dothiepin (thiepin ring system)
Sulphoxide $R - \overset{O}{\underset{}{S}} - R$ (0)	Sulphide $R - S - R$ (-2) Sulphone $R - \overset{O}{\underset{O}{S}} - R$ (+2)	Sulphinpyrazone, Sulindac (alkylaryl sulphoxides)
Sulphone $R - \overset{O}{\underset{O}{S}} - R$ (+2)	Metabolically stable (sulphonamides attacked at the amido group	Dapsone (diaryl sulphone) Sulphadimidine (a sulphonamide)
Thiol (mercaptan) (oxidations) $R-SH$ (-2)	Sulphenic acid $[R-SOH]^{[3]}$ (0) Sulphinic acid $R-SO_2H$ (+2) Sulphonic acid $R-SO_3H$ (+4) Disulphide $R-S-S-R$ (-1) (also mixed di-sulphides see text)	Methimazole (mercaptoimidazole-thiocarbamide type structure) Methimazole, carbimazole Pyrithione (Pyridine-2-thiol-N-oxide) (arylmercaptan) Captopril, penicillamine (alkyl-mercaptans)
Thiol (mercaptan) (conjugations) $R-SH$ (-2)	Sulphide (methylation) $R-S-CH_3$ (-2) S-Glycoside $R-S-C_6H_9O_6$ (-2) (a glucuronide)	Captopril, Thioguanine, mercaptopurine Disulfiram, pyrithione

Cont'd

Table 2 (Cont'd)

SULPHUR FUNCTIONALITY[2]	POTENTIAL METABOLITE(S)[2]	EXAMPLE OF DRUG(S) THAT AFFORD THESE METABOLITES IN VITRO AND/OR <u>IN VIVO</u>.
Thione	desulphurated oxo-derivative	See (a) - (c) below
(a) thioamide $R - \overset{\overset{\text{S}}{\parallel}}{C} - NH_2$ (-2)	S-Oxide (sulphine) $R - \overset{\overset{\text{S}}{\parallel}\rightarrow O}{C} - NH_2$ (0)	Ethionamide (2-ethylthioisonicotinamide)
	di-S-Oxide (sulphene) $O=\overset{\overset{O}{\parallel}}{S}$ $R-C-NH_2$ or $R-\overset{\overset{SO_2H}{\vert}}{C}=NH$ (+2)	Ethionamide (?) (no direct evidence for sulphene- postulate toxic intermediate)
	Amide $R - \overset{\overset{O}{\parallel}}{C} - NH_2$	Ethionamide (desulphuration to amide similar to that in other thioamides)
(b) phosphorothionate $R - \overset{\overset{S}{\parallel}}{\underset{\underset{OR^1}{\vert}}{P}} - OR^2$ (-2)	Phosphate $R - \overset{\overset{O}{\parallel}}{\underset{\underset{OR^1}{\vert}}{P}} - OR^2$	Malathion (O,O-dimethyl-1,2-bis-ethoxycarbonylethyl phosphoro-dithionate)
(c) thiocarbamide (2-mercaptoimidazoles, 2-thiopyrimidines)	desulphurated oxo metabolite	Thiopentone (metabolised to pentobarbitone)
	imidazole sulphenic & sulphic acids (see above for thiols), and imidazole i.e. desulphation.	Methimazole, Carbimazole
(thiol) (thione)		

1-Thiocarbamates are not used as drugs and are not therefore represented in this table. 2-The numbers in parenthesis refer to the oxidation number of the sulphur, computed according to rules described by Pauling and Pauling (1975). 3-Unstable or postulated intermediates are in square brackets.

lipoic acid) and proteins containing sulphur amino acids e.g. cysteine). Sulphur is also present in a large number and variety of naturally occurring compounds of nutritional value. For example, propyl mercaptan ($CH_3CH_2CH_2SH$) is one of the volatile compounds evolved from freshly chopped onions. In the genus Allium, to which both onion and garlic belong, the precursors of the odoriferous and flavour constituents are a series of alkyl or alkenyl cysteine sulphoxides. Similarly, the olfactory characteristics of food crops in the Brassica genus (cabbage, mustard) is due to isothiocyanates, generated enzymatically from glucosinolate precursors (Fenwick et al, 1983).

A large number of organosulphur compounds are also used as industrial and agricultural chemicals, e.g. carbon disulphide (solvent), phosphorothionate triesters (insecticides), thio- and dithiocarbamates (herbicides) (Rosen et al, 1981). More pertinent to the present review is the fact that in the last two decades, an ever increasing number of sulphur compounds have been introduced into medicine. It is this use more than anything else, that has resulted in an increased interest in the biotransformation pathways of organosulphur xenobiotics. In the sulphur-containing medicinal agents, almost all pharmacological or therapeutic classes are represented (Table 1). These medicinal agents in turn represent a spectrum of chemical classes or functionalities, with the sulphide (-S-), sulphoxide (-SO-), sulphone ($-SO_2-$), thiol (-SH) and thione ($>C=S$ or $>P=S$) groups particularly common (Table 2).

METABOLISM OF ORGANOSULPHUR COMPOUNDS

As in the case of most other foreign compounds, organosulphur xenobiotics undergo oxidations, reductions, carbon-sulphur bond formation and fission, depending on the reaction conditions and the type of sulphur-containing functional group(s) in the molecule. Table 2 lists the type of functionalities that are commonly found in sulphur medicinal agents and their potential metabolites; functional groups such as disulphides, thiocarbamates etc, that are not normally present in many medicinal agents are excluded from the table. However, for completeness, their biotransformation is briefly discussed in appropriate sections (see later). The most common metabolic pathway for sulphur xenobiotics appears to be S-oxidation; this is not surprising in view of the readily accessible lone pair of electrons on the divalent sulphur of most sulphur compounds. S-Oxidation either affords S-oxygenated metabolites (e.g. sulphoxides, sulphones, sulphonic acids, etc) or disulphides (probably via reactive S-oxygenated intermediates). Reductions appear to be less predominant, but as will be seen later, sulphoxide and disulphide reduction may be an important event in the bioactivation of certain drugs.

Carbon-sulphur bond formation occurs during conjugation of foreign thiols (mercaptans). S-Methylation of thiol groups, particularly in aryl thiols, is common and is followed by S-oxygenation to water-soluble sulphoxides, and in some cases sulphones. This probably represents the most important detoxication pathway for foreign thiols, and for thiols generated in vivo from cysteine conjugates of non-sulphur drugs via the C-S lyase pathway (Tateishi et al, 1978). S-Glycosylation of mercaptans is another important detoxication pathway, with S-glucuronidation particularly important in mammals. The role of S-acylation reactions in the metabolism of mercaptans is uncertain. Acetylation of various aliphatic thiols, by an acetyl-CoA-dependent enzyme, has been described in vitro with pigeon liver homogenates (Brady and Stadtman, 1954). The donor molecule, acetyl CoA, certainly has a high acetyl group-transfer potential, but competition with endogenous substrates probably limits the importance of this metabolic route in vivo for thiols. It is likely that labile, short-lived derivatives of thiols are formed via S-sulphation, S-phosphorylation etc, but these are not seen as the ultimate excretion products (see review by Mannervik, 1982).

Carbon-sulphur bond fission occurs during metabolic S-dealkylation and desulphuration reactions. Alkyl and alkylaryl sulphides may undergo S-dealkylations in addition to the S-oxygenations outlined in Table 2. S-Dealkylation involves an initial oxidative attack by cytochrome P-450 at the carbon atom alpha to the divalent sulphur; the unstable hydroxyalkyl derivative is then converted to the thiol and the corresponding aldehyde. The mechanism therefore appears to be similar to that described for O- and N-dealkylations, but few detailed studies have been carried out since the work of Mazel et al (1964). Desulphuration of thiones to the corresponding oxo-derivatives involves direct oxidative attack at the thione sulphur ($>C=S$ or $>P=S$). The reactive "S-oxides" ($=S^{\nearrow O}$ or $=S{\nwarrow_O^O}$) are thought to be the intermediates that subsequently afford the oxo-metabolites ($>C=O$ or $>P=O$) and reactive sulphur [S] (see section on thione-desulphuration).

The subsequent sections of this review will in turn describe each of the above metabolic pathways in more detail, illustrating reactions with reference to drug molecules.   The enzyme systems involved in each reaction, and the toxicological implications of certain reactions (e.g. oxidative desulphuration) will also be discussed.

METABOLISM OF SULPHIDES

Most alkyl, alkylaryl, aryl and heterocyclic sulphides are nucleophilic, and they are readily oxidised to sulphoxide and sulphone metabolites in vitro or in vivo (Table 2, Ziegler, 1982; Damani and Case, 1984, Mitchell and Waring, 1985).   For example, S-carboxymethyl-L-cysteine (carbocisteine) and cimetidine (both alkyl sulphides) give sulphoxide metabolites as urinary excretion products in man (Figure 1).   Carbocisteine (Mucodyne[R]), a thiol substituted derivative of the amino acid L-cysteine, is used as a mucolytic in the supportive treatment of chronic asthma and bronchitis.   Metabolic studies have revealed that this compound yields a variety of chemically modified forms as urinary excretion products in various mammalian systems. Oxidation at the divalent sulphur is the major metabolic pathway in man, four of the eight identified metabolites being sulphoxides (Waring, 1978; Waring, 1980; Waring and Mitchell et al, 1982).   With cimetidine, a histamine H_2-receptor antagonist, the sulphoxide only accounts for about 7.4% of the dose excreted in urine in 24 hours in man (Mitchell et al, 1982).   In this case however the drug appears to be metabolically largely stable, around 63% of the dose is eliminated unchanged in urine.   Therefore, sulphoxidation still represents the major route of metabolism for this drug.

Figure 1. Sulphoxidation of carbocisteine and cimetidine

carbocisteine

sulphoxide metabolite

cimetidine

sulphoxide metabolite

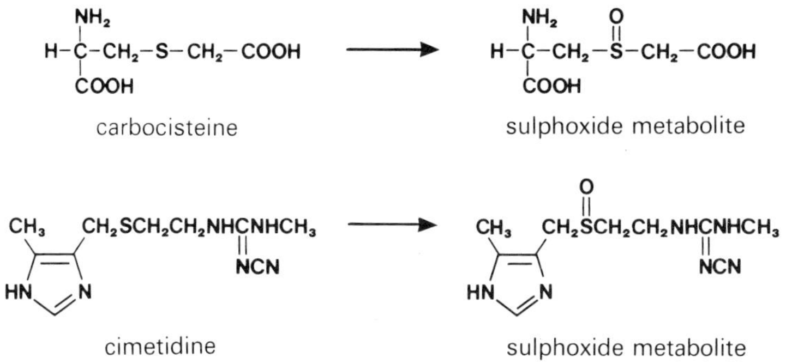

The phenothiazine derivative, thioridazine (Figure 2), is an interesting molecule since it contains two sulphur centres, an aromatic heterocyclic sulphur and an alkylaryl side-chain sulphur, both of which can potentially be oxidised to sulphoxides and sulphones. Ring-S-oxidation, which is quantitatively an important route of metabolism, leads to pharmacological inactivation; this is in common with most other phenothiazines (Papadopoulos and Crammer, 1986). Side-chain S-oxidation is also important in man, and leads to products that are pharmacologically active; the side-chain sulphoxide (mesoridazine) and sulphone (sulphoridazine) have been demonstrated to possess significant antipsychotic effects in man (Axelsson, 1977). Whereas the antipsychotic activity of the sulphoxide might have been explained by a possible *in vivo* reduction to the sulphide (c.f sulindac and sulphinpyrazone), the activity of the sulphone (sulphoridazine) is unlikely to be due to this mechanism, sulphones being metabolically resistant to reduction. The side-chain sulphoxidation products may therefore possess intrinsic pharmacological activity, the initial S-oxidation therefore being a "bioactivation" pathway.

Ring sulphoxidations have been reported in a few other sulphur heterocyclic drugs (Figure 3). Dothiepin (Prothiaden[R]), a drug used in the treatment of depression, is an interesting example of an oxidation in a dibenzthiepin ring (Maguire et al, 1981), since this ring system is only rarely encountered in sulphur chemistry. A recent study (Offen et al, 1985) has described a novel S-oxidation in a thiazole ring system. Chloromethiazole [5-(2-chloroethyl)-4-methylthiazole] is widely used as a sedative, hypnotic and anticonvulsant. Although this compound has been extensively studied and various metabolites previously reported (Pal and Spiteller, 1982), Wilson and co-workers have recently reported 4,5-dimethylthiazole-N-oxide-S-oxide as a urinary metabolite in man (Figure 3, Offen et al, 1985). These workers tentatively suggest that this metabolite may be in the same order of quantitative importance as the major C-oxidation metabolites previously reported. The N-oxide-S-oxide metabolite is unique in two respects; firstly it is the first instance of a sulphoxidation of a thiazole sulphur, and secondly it is the first reported example of two heterocyclic atoms in the same aromatic ring undergoing oxidation. The compound is evidently produced metabolically in a multistep reaction, but the enzyme systems involved are not yet known. The chemistry and biochemistry of such thiazole metabolites would seem to be

Figure 2. Metabolism of thioridazine to sulphoxides and sulphones in man.

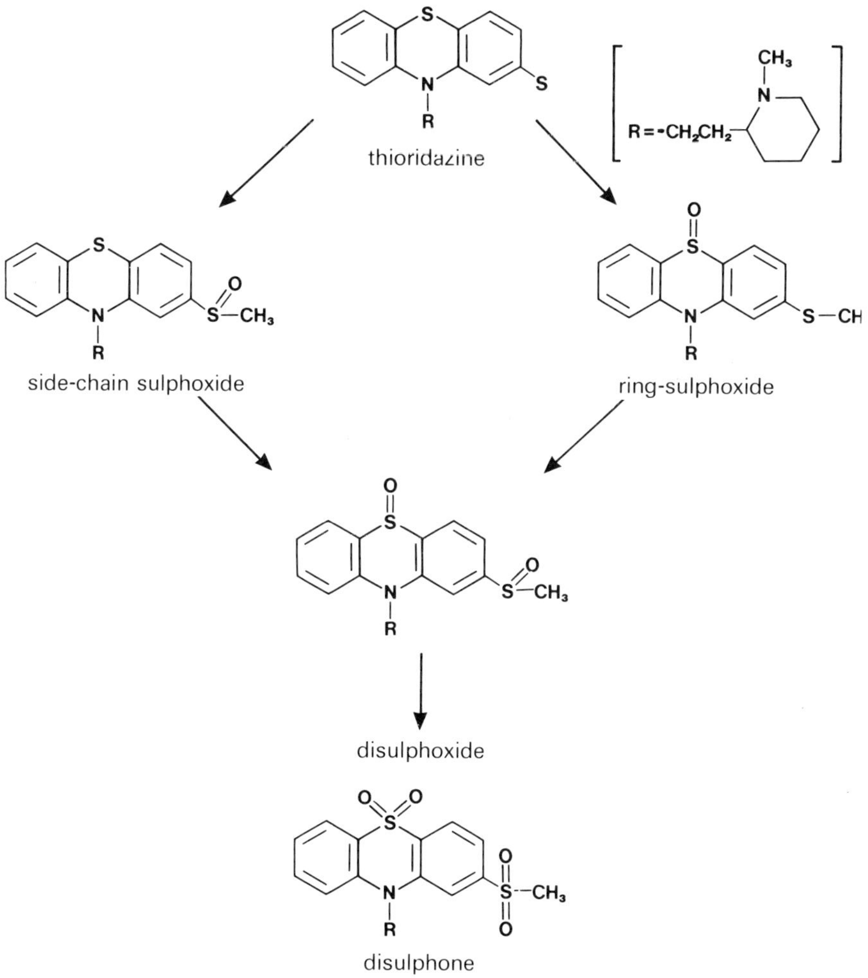

thioridazine

R = -CH₂CH₂-

side-chain sulphoxide

ring-sulphoxide

disulphoxide

disulphone

a very attractive area for future research.

Sulphoxide and sulphone metabolites are hydrophilic and usually chemically stable, and are therefore readily detected in the urine of animals treated with sulphide drugs. The amount of sulphone formed in vivo or in vitro is usually less than that of the sulphoxide. This is probably due to the water-solubility of the sulphoxides, which presumably limits their partitioning into the catalytic sites on the microsomal monooxygenases. The

Figure 3.   Novel sulphoxidations in thiazole (chlormethiazole) and dibenzthiepin (dothiepin) ring systems.

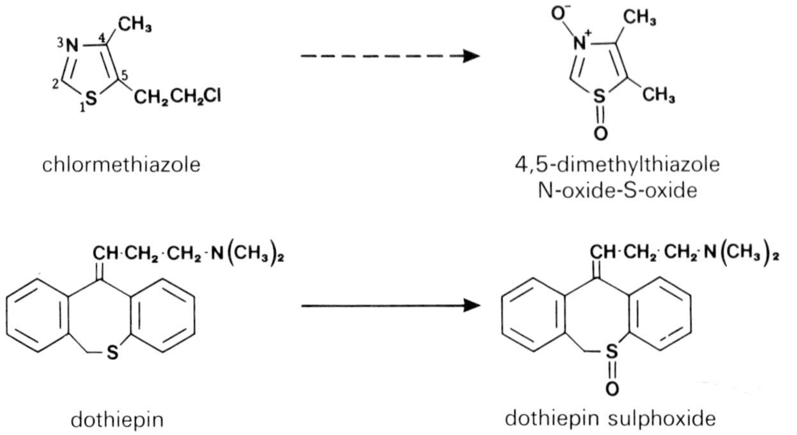

chlormethiazole   4,5-dimethylthiazole
                                   N-oxide-S-oxide

dothiepin   dothiepin sulphoxide

first oxidation at sulphur in sulphides, i.e. sulphoxide
formation, is reversible, but the subsequent reaction to
sulphones is irreversible.   At least three different enzyme
systems have been reported to catalyse sulphoxide
formation, cytochrome P-450, the flavin-containing
monooxygenase and the microsomal prostaglandin synthetase.
Any particular compound may be a substrate for more than
one enzyme, a major determinant being the electromolecular
environment in which the sulphur occurs (Hunt et al, 1982).
For example, the more nucleophilic divalent sulphur atoms
in aliphatic and alicyclic sulphides (e.g. diethylsulphide
and tetrahydrothiophene, respectively) (Figure 4) are
oxidised exclusively by the flavin monooxygenase.   The
sulphur in aromatic heterocyclic rings (e.g.
dibenzothiophene), where there is partial delocalisation
due to the aromatic rings, is oxidised exclusively by
cytochrome P-450 (Hoodi and Damani, 1984; Houdi, 1986).   It
is of interest that p-tolylethylsulphide, an alkylaryl
sulphide, is oxidised to a chiral sulphoxide by both the
monooxygenases (Waxman et al, 1982).   The more nucleophilic
sulphides can also function as cosubstrate reductants for
the endoperoxide precursors of prostaglandins and
thromboxanes, during the prostaglandin synthetase mediated
reactions (Egan et al, 1979).   However, the in vivo
significance of this type of S-oxygenation for the sulphide
drugs (Table 2) is unclear.   Indeed, most of the
mechanistic/enzymology studies have been carried out in

Figure 4. Structures of some non-drug model thioethers.

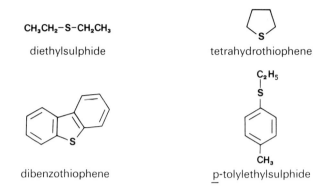

$CH_3CH_2-S-CH_2CH_3$

diethylsulphide

tetrahydrothiophene

dibenzothiophene

p-tolylethylsulphide

vitro with model sulphides (Figure 4). The contribution of the various S-oxygenases to sulphoxidation of drugs and foreign sulphides in vivo is unknown. The thiocarbamate group (R-S-C$\overset{O}{-}$N<) is not present in any medicinal agents, but is common in many herbicides. These compounds can form sulphoxides and sulphones, but the products are very much more reactive than sulphide S-oxygenated metabolites (Rosen et al, 1981).

METABOLISM OF SULPHOXIDES

In addition to the metabolic formation of sulphoxides from sulphides (see above), a sulphoxide functional group may itself be incorporated in a drug molecule. The uricosuric and platelet anti-aggregation agent sulphinpyrazone is a sulphoxide, as is sulindac, an antirheumatic agent (Figure 5). There are two metabolic options open to the sulphoxide funtionality - a further two electron oxidation to a sulphone, or a reduction to the more lipophilic sulphide. As a rule, sulphone formation from sulphides and sulphoxides is a minor route of metabolism, but there are some exceptions. For example, whereas the sulphoxide is the major S-oxygenated urinary product of tetrahydrothiophene in the rat, the sulphone is the predominant urinary metabolite of its acyclic analogue, diethylsulphide (Hoodi and Damani, 1983). The mechanism of sulphone formation and the nature of the enzyme systems involved have not yet been reported.

Reduction of the sulphoxide functionality appears to be a more common route of metabolism for sulphoxides. This reduction may be mediated by microbes in the gastrointestinal tract, or by hepatic and extrahepatic

Figure 5. Sulphinpyrazone and sulindac - examples of sulphoxide drugs undergoing sulphoxide reduction.

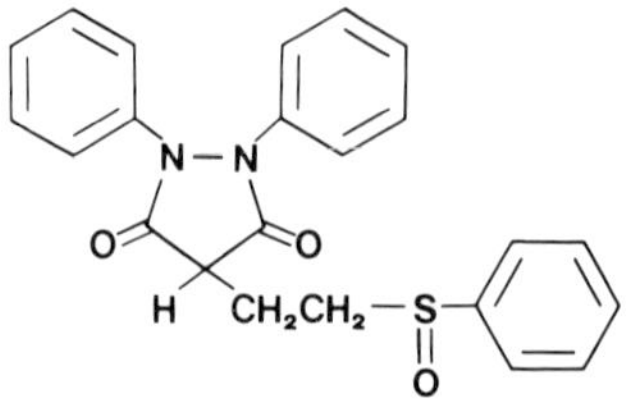

sulphinpyrazone 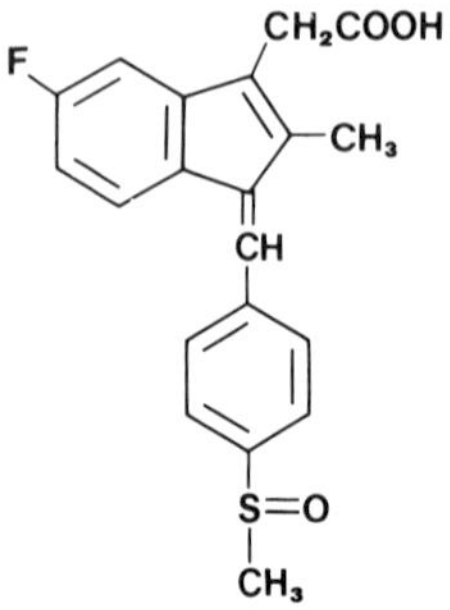   sulindac

mammalian sulphoxide reductases. For the two sulphoxide drugs (Figure 5), this enzymatic reduction is an important bioactivation pathway, the pharmacological activities of both drugs being due to the sulphide reduction products. After oral or parenteral administration of sulphinpyrazone to man and other mammalian species, the sulphide is the major circulating metabolite (Dieterle et al, 1980). Since this metabolite has a longer half-life (Schlicht et al, 1985) and is considerably more potent than sulphinpyrazone, a clear understanding of the site and mechanism of sulphoxide reduction may have important clinical implications. The gut microorganisms appear to be the major, if not the sole, site of conversion of sulphinpyrazone to its active sulphide in man and experimental animal models (Renwick et al, 1982; Renwick et al, 1986; Strong et al, 1984). Biliary excretion is apparently the route by which the orally or parenterally administered drug enters the hind gut, where it is reduced by microflora to the active sulphide. Entero-hepatic circulation and gut microflora-mediated sulphoxide reduction are therefore responsible for the prolonged action of sulphinpyrazone. The reduction of sulindac appears to take place in the liver; studies in rats show that sulindac is rapidly reduced to the sulphide, peak plasma levels of the pharmacologically active metabolite occurring around 2 hours after dosing sulindac (Duggan et al, 1978). The mammalian enzymes which catalyse sulindac reduction are located both in the microsomes and in the cytosol (Kitamura and Tatsumi, 1982). Sulindac reduction by gut microflora in vitro has also been described (Strong et al, 1983) and it may be that this mechanism of reduction is also important in man.

METABOLISM OF SULPHONES AND SULPHONAMIDES

The sulphone functional group in the antileprotic drug dapsone (Figure 6) is metabolically stable; metabolism in this drug, and in the related sulphonamides, is directed at the $-NH_2$ groups, affording N-acetyl, N-hydroxy and N-glucuronide metabolites. The sulphone group is stable to further oxidation, and does not appear to be reduced back to the sulphoxide. Sulphonal, trional and tetronal (Figure 6) were at one time used as hypnotics, but are no longer used because of their toxicities. These aliphatic disulphones were purported to require metabolic conversion to some pharmacologically active species (Baumann and Kast, 1890), but no definitive reports have appeared on the nature of these metabolites.

Figure 6. Structures of some medicinal sulphones.

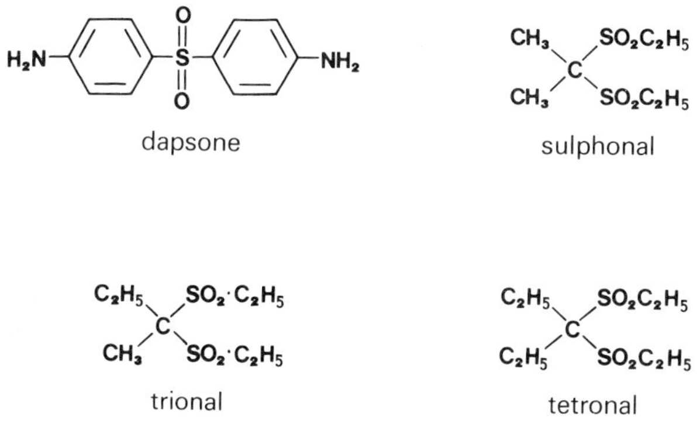

dapsone

sulphonal

trional

tetronal

Whereas most sulphonamides mainly afford N-acetylated metabolites, the thiazole- and imidazole-2-sulphonamides are interesting examples where there is cleavage of the ring carbon-sulphur bond. For example, the sulphonamide group in 2-benzothiazolesulphonamide (Figure 7) is readily displaced by glutathione; this GSH-conjugate is then converted to a mercapturic acid, a thiol and a S-glucuronide (Clapp, 1956; Colucci and Buyske, 1965). The latter two metabolites presumably involve further cleavage of the cysteine conjugate by C-S lyases to the thiol, followed by S-glucuronidation. The initial nucleophilic displacement of the sulphonamido-group by glutathione is not unexpected, in view of the reported chemical reactivity of such 2-substituted aromatic heterocyclic sulphonamides (Stirling, 1974).

Figure 7. Biotransformation of benzothiazole-2-sulphon-
amide involving nucleophilic displacement of the
sulphonamide-group to afford mercapturic acid, mercaptan
and S-glucuronide metabolites.

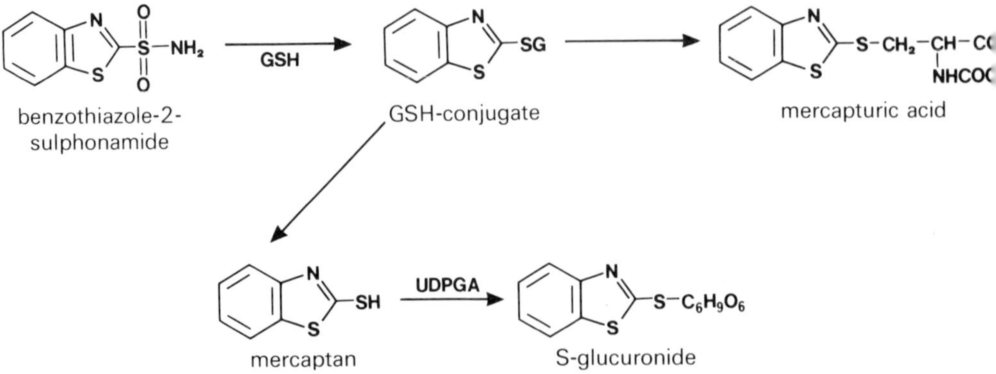

benzothiazole-2-   GSH-conjugate   mercapturic acid
sulphonamide

mercaptan   S-glucuronide

METABOLISM OF THIOLS AND DISULPHIDES

The alkyl and aryl mercaptan drugs (e.g. captopril and
6-mercaptopurine, respectively) can undergo many reactions
at the thiol functional group. The reactivity of the
thiols is due to the fact that most thiols are readily
ionised at physiological pH to the nucleophilic thiolate
anion. Enzymic oxygenation of thiols affords reactive
sulphenic acids (R-SOH) and then sulphinic acids (R-SO$_2$H).
The antithyroid drug methimazole (Figure 8) is metabolised
by these pathways in vitro, although the intermediate
sulphenic acids are not directly demonstrable (Poulsen et
al, 1979).
The sulphenic acids can react with excess thiols to
afford disulphides as below :

$$RSH \xrightarrow{[O]} [RSOH] \xrightarrow{RSH} RSSR + H_2O$$

$$RSSR \xrightarrow{[O]} R\overset{O}{\overset{\|}{S}}SR \xrightarrow[H_2O]{[O]} RSO_2H \xrightarrow{[O]} RSO_3H$$

The disulphides can either be reduced back to thiols,
or be converted to sulphonic acids via the intermediate
thiosulphenic and sulphinic acids. It is not clear how
many thiol drugs and other foreign thiols actually undergo
these elegant sequences of reactions proposed by Ziegler
(1984). Oxidation to the highest oxidation state (+4) is

Figure 8. Structures of some drugs containing a thiol functional group.

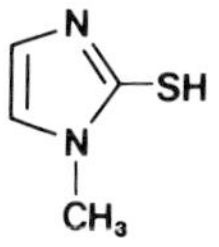

methimazole

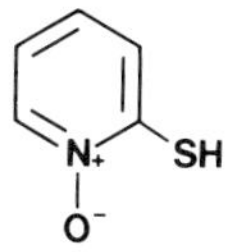

pyridine-2-thiol-1-oxide

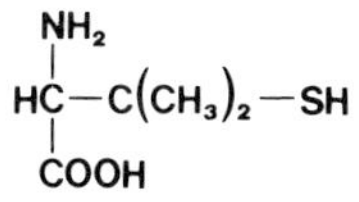

penicillamine

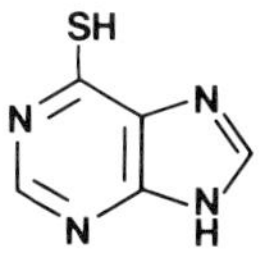

6-mercaptopurine

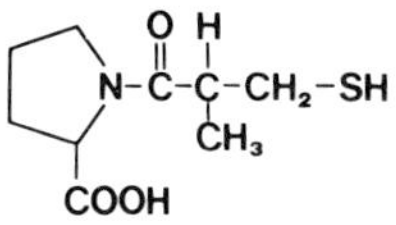

captopril

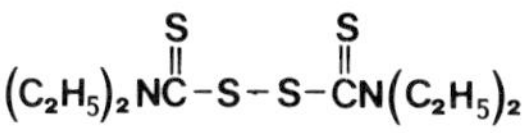

disulfiram

not often seen with thiols and pyridine-2-thiol-N-oxide (Figure 8) is an interesting example. This aryl thiol, used as a scalp antiseptic in man, gave rise to the corresponding sulphonic acid as the major metabolite in rats after dermal administration (Min et al, 1970); the disulphide was also present in smaller amounts. The metabolism after intravenous administration is completely different, the major metabolite being a S-glucuronide (Wedig et al, 1978a and 1978b). The thiol drugs captopril and penicillamine afford disulphides as the main metabolites. In both these drugs, the free thiol group is the only functional group that undergoes biotransformation to disulphides, mixed disulphides with glutathione or other endogenous mercaptans, and drug-protein disulphides. The thiol drugs and their disulphides probably undergo ready interconversions, but even the formation of these relatively short-lived drug-plasma protein conjugates may be of relevance to the toxicity of these thiols (Crawhall et al, 1979; Park and Yeung, 1983).

Conjugation reactions of thiol drugs are probably more relevant to their detoxication and removal from the body. The excretion products normally seen with thiol drugs are S-methyl and S-glucuronide metabolites. Thiol methyltransferases are present in human erythrocytes that methylate captopril (Drummer et al, 1983) and 6-mercaptopurine (Weinshilboum and Sladek, 1980). Thiol methyltransferase activity has also been demonstrated in many other mammalian tissues (see review by Weisiger and Jakoby, 1980). Genetic deficiency of thiol methyltransferase activity, particularly of the erythrocyte enzyme(s), may be relevant to the toxicity of 6-mercaptopurine and related mercaptan drugs in certain individuals in a population. The cytotoxic thiopurines rely on S-methylation for detoxication. On a genetic basis approximately one in 300 subjects lack thiopurine methyltransferase activity, and 11% of the subjects have intermediate activities (Lennard et al, 1987). In these deficient individuals, larger amounts of the putative toxic thiopurine nucleotides are generated, and there appears to be a good correlation with risk for the development of toxicities to the thiopurine drugs.

Thiol drugs also undergo conjugation with glucuronic acid to afford S-glucuronides. Pyridine-2-thiol-1-oxide is mainly metabolised to the S-glucuronide in swine and rats after intravenous injection. However, the main metabolite after dermal application is the corresponding sulphonic acid (Wedig et al, 1978a and 1978b). Disulfiram, a compound used in the treatment of chronic alcoholism, is a dithioic acid. The -S-S- bond is reductively cleaved to diethyldithiocarbamate, which is then susceptible to S-conjugation. S-Methylthiocarbamate (Gessner and Jakubowski, 1972) and the S-glucuronide metabolite (Kaslander, 1963) have both been identified as major metabolites in man.

METABOLISM OF THIONES

Metabolic Desulphuration

The metabolic conversion of a carbon-sulphur double bond (i.e. thione, $>C=S$), or a phosphorus-sulphur double bond (i.e. phosphorothione, $\rightarrow P=S$), to the corresponding oxo-derivative (ketone and phosphate, respectively) is referred to as desulphuration. In view of the toxicity and reactivity of various °thiones' such as thioamides (e.g. thioacetamide), phosphorothionate triesters (e.g. parathion), thiocarbamides (e.g. methimazole) and thio-carbamate (e.g. molinate), interest in 'desulphuration' has been extensive (see reviews by Neal, 1980; Halpert and Neal, 1982; Ziegler, 1982 and 1984). The initial event in desulphuration appears to be an enzymic oxygenation at the sulphur to a 'S-oxide' (sulphine). Cytochrome P-450 and the flavin- containing monooxygenases have both been implicated in this oxidation, depending on the substrate and the reaction conditions (e.g. substrate concentration). The S-oxides of some thiones are stable, and in many instances authentic crystalline materials have been synthesised. Enzymic desulphuration probably involves conversion of the S-oxide to a three membered thioxirane ring; this is then cleaved rapidly to afford the oxo-derivative and atomic sulphur as a highly electrophilic singlet. This reactive form of sulphur can form hydrodisulphides (protein - S-S-H) with protein thiol group (protein-SH), and this may be the initial biochemical lesion responsible for the subsequent tissue necrosis. An alternate mechanism for toxicity of other 'thiones' (e.g. thioacetamide - a thioamide) is the further oxidation of S-oxides to S,S-dioxides (sulphenes). The biotransformation of 'thiones' is however far more complex than indicated above, and there are important mechanistic differences between the various groups of compounds involved.

Medicinal Thioamides

The only thioamides that have been used clinically are ethionamide (Figure 9) and related pyridino-compounds that are used in the treatment of tuberculosis. In fact the availability of better tuberculostatic medicinal agents have resulted in the decline in use of these toxic isonicotinothioamides.

Figure 9. Structures of drug 'thiones' that undergo desulphuration.

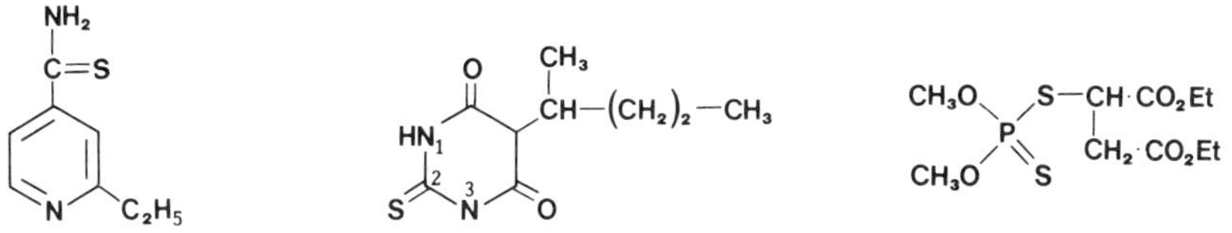

ethionamide   thiopentone   malathion

The mechanism of hepatic injury with these medicinal agents appears to be similar to that elucidated for the two well known toxicants, thioacetamide and thiobenzamide. The initial oxidative conversion to the S-oxide (sulphine) is mediated by the flavin-containing monooxygenase, but the biochemical mechanism for the second oxidative step to the dioxygenated product (sulphene) has not been resolved; the following sequence of reactions has been proposed (Ziegler, 1982 and 1984).

$$\underset{R-\overset{\displaystyle S}{\overset{\|}{C}}-NH_2}{} \xrightarrow{[O]} \underset{R-\overset{\displaystyle \overset{\nearrow O}{S}}{\overset{\|}{C}}-NH_2}{} \xrightarrow{[O]} R-\overset{\displaystyle SO_2H}{C} \equiv NH + 1/2\ H_2O \rightarrow R-\overset{\displaystyle O}{\overset{\|}{C}}-NH_2 + 1/2\ H_2S_2O_3$$

The sulphene is best represented as the iminosulphinic acid (see above), and it is probably this reactive intermediate that is responsible for the covalent binding. The sulphenes can also undergo conversion in water to the amide i.e. desulphuration with the concomitant release of sulphur as thiosulphate (Porter and Neal, 1978; Hanzlik et al, 1980). Ethionamide presumably undergoes the above reactions, since it is extensively metabolised in man, and 2-ethylisonicotinic acid is an important urinary metabolite (Putter, 1972).

Medicinal Phosphorothionates

The phosphorothionate triesters (e.g. parathion) are widely used as pesticides, but are extremely toxic. Malathion is one of the few such compounds that shows sufficient selectivity to be used in man in anti-infective skin preparations. Malathion, which is 0,0-dimethyl-S-1,2-bisethoxycarbonylethyl) phosphorodithionate (Figure 9), has two safety features. Firstly, it is rapidly de-esterified in mammals by carboxyesterases to a non-toxic malathionic acid. Secondly, in insects there is little de-esterification, but the compound is oxidatively attacked at the P=S sulphur via insect microsomal monooxygenases and converted to an S-oxide. This is then converted to the oxo-metabolite malaoxon. The actual toxicant, i.e. the acetylcholinesterase inhibitor, is malaoxon, and therefore, in addition to distributional factors (i.e. external application), selective metabolic activation is responsible for the safety of this phosphorothionate (Kruegar and O'Brien, 1959). The oxidative desulphuration of phosphoroethionates such as parathion is catalysed by cytochrome P-450 (Neal et al, 1977) and the covalent binding of released sulphur is responsible for the inactivation of the P-450 enzymes. However, the hepatotoxicity in vivo is more likely to be due to covalent binding of intermediate S-oxides (Halpert and Neal, 1980 and 1982).

Medicinal Thiocarbamides

Several thiocarbamides, which includes 2-mercaptoimidazoles (e.g. methimazole, carbimazole) and 2-mercaptopyrimidines (e.g. methyl and propylthiouracils), reduce the synthesis of thyroxine, and are therefore used in the treatment of hyperthyroidism. As in the case of acyclic thiocarbamide moieties (e.g. in α-naphthylthiourea, phenylthiourea), the aromatic heterocyclic thiocarbamide groups can exist in both the thiol and thione forms (Table 2). Carbimazole, the 2-ethoxycarbonyl-derivative of methimazole (Figure 8), appears to be a pro-drug, and is rapidly metabolised to methimazole in man (Skellern et al, 1973). Oxygenation at the 2-mercapto group undoubtedly occurs in the disposition of methimazole, but the full metabolic profile in man and other mammals is far from clear (Skellern and Steer, 1981). In vitro studies with the purified flavin-containing monooxygenase show that methimazole can be S-oxygenated to the sulphenic (R-SOH) and sulphinic (R-SO$_2$H) acids (Poulsen et al, 1979). The reactivity of the sulphenic acids of these heterocyclic derivatives is similar to those of the acyclic thiocarbamides (thioureas), i.e. they can react with thiol groups of mixed-disulphides, or protein mixed-disulphides. However, this is unlikely to be a significant reaction for disposition in vivo since the sulphenic acid would be preferentially reduced by glutathione (Ziegler, 1982). The dioxygenated metabolites, i.e. the heterocylic sulphinic acids, are readily hydrolysed, liberating sulphite and the desulphurated heterocycle. This reaction may well occur in vivo, since 1-methylimidazole is a reported urinary metabolite of methimazole in the rat (Skellern and Steer, 1981). This is an interesting "desulphuration" since the end product is not an oxo-derivative. However, 1-methylhydantoin is also a urinary metabolite, and therefore a classical $>$C=S → $>$C=O reaction may still be operative. In contrast to the reactions described above for heterocyclic sulphine acids, the formamidinesulphinic acids of the acyclic thioureas can form covalent links with cell constituents, via nucleophilic displacement of the -SO$_2$H group by amines, to form stable guanidine adducts. The toxicity of the thioureas may be due to this type of covalent binding (Ziegler, 1984). Thiopentone (Figure 9) has been widely used as an intravenous anaesthetic.

Although it has long been known to be metabolised by desulphuration to the corresponding oxo-derivative, pentobarbitone, in vivo (Winters et al, 1955), mechanistic in vitro data are not available. The enzymology of the reaction has never been fully studied, nor the nature of the released sulphur elucidated (Gorrod, 1979).

CONCLUDING REMARKS

This review on the metabolism of sulphur-containing drugs demonstrates that the sulphur functionality can contribute to disposition in one of four ways. Firstly it may be present as a relatively inconsequential structural feature insofar as metabolism and excretion are concerned, as in the case of sulphones and most sulphonamides. Secondly, the sulphur functionality may limit drug disposition, by being converted to a metabolite that is more lipophilic, as in the case of sulphoxides that are reduced to sulphides. In this instance it is noteworthy that the sulphur group is the centre for "bioactivation", since the sulphides (e.g. sulindac sulphide) are very often more pharmacologically active than the sulphoxide drugs. Thirdly, the sulphur functionality may be a centre for detoxication, as in the case of thiol-conjugations, the S-methyl and S-glucuronide conjugates being more water-soluble and less toxic than the parent thiols. Lastly, the sulphur group may be a centre of metabolic activation to reactive/toxic metabolites, as in the case of thioamide metabolism to sulphenic and sulphinic acids. Reactions at sulphur groups in drugs and other xenobiotics are many and varied, and considerably more studies are required to fully characterise the mechanisms and enzymology of all the reactions. For example, S-oxygenation is a quantitatively important route of metabolism for many drugs. In these instances, it is important that efforts be directed towards determining the enzymic basis for these reactions. Clearly any information on the influence of environmental, physiological or genetic factors on such S-oxygenation reactions would be extremely useful in understanding and explaining interindividual differences in drug effects and/or drug disposition. A further discussion of approaches to elucidating the relative roles of cytochrome P-450 and the flavin-monooxygenase in the metabolism of thioethers is given elsewhere (Damani, 1987).

REFERENCES

Axelsson, R. (1977). Current Therapeutic Trends, 21, 587.

Baumann, E. and Kast, A. (1890). Hoppe-Seyl. Z, 14, 52.
Brady, R.O. and Stadtman, E.R. (1954). J. Biol. Chem, 211, 621.
Clapp, J.W. (1956). J. Biol. Chem, 223, 207.
Colucci, D.F. and Buyske, D.A. (1965). Biochem. Pharmacol, 14, 457.
Crawhall, J.C., Lecavalier, D. and Ryan, P. (1979). Biopharmaceutics and Drug Dispos, 1, 73.
Damani, L.A. (1987). Pharmaz. ztg, in press.
Damani, L.A. and Case, D.E. (1984). in "Comprehensive Heterocyclic Chemistry" (Ed. O-Meth-Cohn, Series ed. A.R. Katritzky and C.W. Rees), Pergamon Press, Oxford, p.223.
Dieterle, W., Faigie, J.W. and Moppert, J. (1980). Arzneimitel Forsch/Drug Res, 30, 989.
Drummer, O.H., Miach, P. and Jarrott, B. (1983). Biochem. Pharmacol, 32, 1557.
Duggan, D.E., Hooke, K.F., Noll, R.M., Hucker, H.B. and van Arman, C.G. (1978). Biochem. Pharmacol, 27, 2311.
Egan, R.W., Gale, P.H. and Kuehl, Jr. F.A. (1979). J. Biol. Chem, 254, 3295.
Fenwick, G.R., Heaney, R.K. and Mullin, W.J. (1983). CRC Crit. Rev. Food Sci. Nutrition, 18, 123.
Gorrod, J.W. (1979). in "Drug Toxicity" (Ed. J.W. Gorrod), Taylor & Francis Ltd, London, p.1.
Gessner, T. and Jakubowski, M. (1972). Biochem. Pharmacol, 21, 219.
Halpert, J. and Neal, R.A. (1980). J. Biol. Chem, 255, 1080.
Halpert, J. and Neal, R.A. (1982). in "Biological Reactive Intermediates II. Chemical Mechanisms and Biological Effects" (Eds. R. Snyder, D.V. Parke, J.J. Kocsis, D.J. Jollow, G.G. Gibson, and C.M. Whitner, Plenum Press, New York, p.1037.
Hanzlik, R.P., Cashman, J.P. and Traiger, G.J. (1980). Toxicol. Appl. Pharmacol, 55, 260.
Hoodi, A.A. and Damani, L.A. (1983). in "Sulphur in Xenobiotics" (Eds. S.C. Mitchell and R.H. Waring), Birmingham University Press, Birmingham, England, p.131.
Hoodi, A.A. and Damani, L.A. (1984). J. Pharm. Pharmacol, 36 (Suppl), 63P.
Houdi, A.A. (1986). PhD Thesis, University of Manchester, England.
Hunt, P.A., Mitchell, S.C. and Waring, R.H. (1982). in "Biological Reactive Intermediates II - Chemical Mechanisms and Biological Effects", (Eds. R. Snyder, D.V. Parke, J.J. Kocsis, D.J. Jollow., G.G. Gibson and

C.M. Whitmer), Plenum Press, New York, p.1255.

Kaslander, J. (1963). Biochim. Biophys. Acta, 71, 730.

Kitamura, S. and Tatsumi, K. (1982). Jap. J. Pharmacol, 32, 833.

Krueger, H. and O'Brien, R. (1959). J. Econ. Entamol, 53, 25.

Lennard, L., Van Loon, J.A., Lilleyman, J.S. and Weinshilboum, R.M. (1987). Clin. Pharmacol. Therap, 41, 180.

Maguire, K.P., Burrows, G.D., Norman, T.R. and Scoggins, B.A. (1981). Br. J. Clin. Pharmacol, 12, 405.

Mannervik, B. (1982). in "Metabolic Basis of Detoxication" (Eds. W.B. Jakoby, J.R. Bend and J. Caldwell). Academic Press, New York, p.185.

Mazel, P., Henderson, J.F. and Axelrod, J. (1964). J. Pharmac. Exp. Ther, 143, 1.

Min, B.H., Parekh, C., Golberg, L. and McChesney, E.W. (1970). Food Cosmetics Toxicol, 8, 161.

Mitchell, S.C., Idle, J.R. and Smith, R.L. (1982). Xenobiotica, 12, 283.

Mitchell, S.C. and Waring, R.H. (1985). Drug Metab. Rev, 16, 255.

Neal, R.A. (1980). in "Reviews in Biochemical Toxicology Vol 2" (Eds. E. Hodgson, J.R. Bend and R. Philpot), Elsevier, New York, p.131.

Neal, R.A., Kamataki, T., Hunter, A.L. and Catignani, G. (1977). in "Microsomes and Drug Oxidations" (Eds. V. Ullrich, A. Hildebrandt, J. Roots, R.W. Estabrook, and A.H. Conney). Pergamon Press, New York, p.467.

Offen, C.P., Frearson, M.J., Wilson, K. and Burnett, D. (1985). Xenobiotica, 15, 503.

Pal, R. and Spiteller, G. (1982). Xenobiotica, 12, 813.

Papdopoulus, A.S. and Crammer, J.L. (1986). Xenobiotica, 16, 1097.

Park, B.K. and Yeung, J.H.K. (1983). in "Sulphur in Xenobiotics" (Ed. by S.C. Mitchell and R.H. Waring), Birmingham University Press, Birmingham, England, p.97.

Pauling, L. and Pauling, P. (1975). in "Chemistry", Freeman, San Francisco, California, p.186.

Porter, W.R. and Neal, R.A. (1978). Drug Metab. Dispos, 6, 379.

Poulsen, L.L., Hyslop, R.M. and Ziegler, D.M. (1979). Arch. Biochem. Biophys, 198, 78.

Putter, J. (1972). Arzneim-Forsch. Drug Research, 22, 1027.

Renwick, A.G., Evans, S.P., Sweatman, T.W., Cumberland, J. and George, C.F. (1982). Biochem. Pharmacol, 31, 2649.

Renwick, A.G., Strong, H.A. and George, C.F. (1986).

Biochem. Pharmacol, 35, 64.

Rosen, J.D., Magee, P.S. and Casida, J.E. (eds.) (1981). "Sulphur in Pesticide Action and Metabolism", ACS Symposium Series, American Chemical Society, Washington, D.C.

Schlicht, F., Staiger, C., De Vries, Jan X., Geudert-Remy, U., Hildebrandt, R., Harenberg, Job., Wang, N.S. and Weber, E. (1985). Eur. J. Clin. Pharmacol, 28, 97.

Skellern, G.G. and Steer, S.T. (1982). Xenobiotica, 11, 627.

Skellern, G.G., Stenlake, J.B. and Williams, W.D. (1974). Xenobiotica, 3, 121.

Stirling, C.J.M. (1974). Int. J. Sulphur, Chem, 6, 277.

Strong, H.A., Oates, J., Sembi, J., Renwick, A.G. and George, C.F. (1984). J. Pharmacol. Exp. Ther, 230, 726.

Strong, H.A., Renwick, A.G. and George, C.F. (1983). in "Sulphur in Xenobiotics" (Eds. S.C. Mitchell and R.H. Waring), Birmingham University Press, Birmingham, England, p.83.

Tateishi, M., Suzuki, S. and Shimizu, H. (1978). J. Biol. Chem, 253, 8854.

Waring, R.H. (1978). Xenobiotica, 8, 265.

Waring, R.H. (1980). Eur. J. Drug Metab. Pharmacokinet, 5, 49.

Waring, R.H. and Mitchell, S.C. (1982). Drug Metab. Dispos, 10, 61.

Waxman, D.J., Light, D.R. and Walsh, C. (1982). Biochemistry, 21, 2499.

Wedig, J.H., Mitoma, C., Howd, R.A. and Thomas, D.W. (1978a). Toxicol. Appl. Pharmacol, 43, 373.

Wedig, J.H., Wentwort, R.A., Gallo, M.A., Babish, J.G. and Henion, J.D. (1978b). Food. Cosmet, 16, 553.

Weinshilboum, R.M. and Sladek, S.L. (1980). Am. J. Human Genet, 32, 651.

Weisiger, R.A. and Jakoby, W.B. (1980). in "Enzymatic Basis of Detoxication" (Ed. W.B. Jakoby), Academic Press, New York, p.131.

Winters, W.D., Spector, E., Wallach, D.P. and Shideman, F.E. (1955). J. Pharmac. Exp. Ther, 114, 343.

Ziegler, D.M. (1982). in "Metabolic Basis of Detoxication" (Eds. W.B. Jakoby, J.R. Bend and J. Caldwell). Academic Press, New York, p.171.

Ziegler, D.M. (1984). in "Drug Metabolism and Drug Toxicity" (Eds. J.R. Mitchell and M.G. Horning). Raven Press, New York, P.33.

DELIVERY, DISTRIBUTION, CLEARANCE AND DEGRADATION: KEY FACTORS IN THE DESIGN AND DEVELOPMENT OF PEPTIDE AND PROTEIN DRUGS.

Colin McMartin

Research Centre, Ciba-Geigy Pharmaceuticals,
Horsham, Sussex.

INTRODUCTION

The short plasma half-lives and poor oral bioavailability of many peptide and protein hormones create major problems for their development and application in therapy. It is frequently difficult to obtain reliable and effective time profiles of drug concentration in the circulation let alone at the site of action where slow penetration and local degradation may reduce bioavailability still further. In addition these same factors of high clearance and poor bioavailability necessitate the use of large doses of products which are extremely costly to produce in a pure and adequately characterised form. Understanding the processes which determine the distribution and fate of these products is therefore of crucial importance for the design and testing of new drugs and novel delivery systems.

Peptides and proteins do not cross cell membranes unless specific mechanisms make this possible. As a result, the distribution of these molecules is restricted to those compartments in the body which can be accessed by the available transport processes· for each type of molecule. This is fortunate because a large number of peptidases with a broad range of specificities are present but they are highly compartmentalised. If a peptide or protein had access to all of these enzymes degradation would be rapid, the pattern of breakdown would be complex and the prospect of making stable analogues would be correspondingly daunting.

It will be evident however that to understand the fate of these molecules in biological systems it is essential to know about transport as well as degradative mechanisms and this overview therefore places emphasis on both aspects.

For a detailed recent review of peptide metabolism see Humphrey and Ringrose. 1986).

GENERAL PROPERTIES OF PEPTIDES AND HORMONES

Molecular Structure

Peptides are molecules formed by linkage of two or more amino acids of amide bonds. The amide bond, which is formed between a carboxylic acid and an amino group attached to the respective alpha-carbons of the amino acids, is known as a peptide bond. These bonds are metastable in an aqueous environment but hydrolyse extremely slowly unless assisted by enzymes. The alpha-carbons of all amino acids except glycine are chiral and mammalian peptides have all the amino acids in the L form. Changing from the L to the D form often has dramatic effects on biological properties and on stability to enzymic hydrolysis.

Peptides can be of a wide range of molecular weights - from dipeptides (MWt ca. 250) to molecules like insulin (MWt 6000). They are often flexible linear molecules (a peptide backbone carrying amino acid side chains with a range of functional groups of differing polarity) but they can contain loops and more complex cross-linkages formed by bonds between sulphur atoms on the side-chains of cysteine amino acids residues. Proteins are large molecules similar in basic composition to peptides. The molecular weights are usually greater than 10,000 and the folding of the greater part of the peptide chain is well determined.

Physico-Chemical Properties

The peptide back-bone is hydrophilic and peptide hormones are usually water soluble. Although proteins will often have a large total hydrophobic amino acid content, the hydrophobic side-chains tend to be buried leaving a preponderence of hydrophilic surface groups.

Peptides and proteins are usually not lipid soluble and for this reason once these molecules are in the extracellular compartments of the body they will not enter cells unless specific cellular uptake mechanisms enable this to take place.

Susceptibility to Enzymatic Degradation

Peptide and protein metabolism usually involves the cleavage of peptide bonds. The hydrolysis is catalysed by a wide range of enzymes (peptidases) each with its own specificity for the side-chains present on adjacent amino acids and sometimes the neighbours of these amino acids. These enzymes have well formed binding pockets and require the peptide and side-chains to be in the correct conformation. Examples of peptidases or classes of peptidases and their specifications are given in Table 1.

Table 1. Examples of peptidases of different specificity

ENZYME	SUBSTRATE
Aminopeptidases	NH_2X^a ↟ X---
Carboxypeptidases	---X ↑ XCOOH
Angiotensin converting enzyme	---X ↑ X.XCOOH
Elastase	---Gly^b ↑ X---
Chymotrypsin	---Phe^c ↑ X---
Trypsin	---Arg^d ↑ X---
Thrombin	---Arg ↑ Gly---

a) X is usually an L-amino acid other than proline; b) can be Ala; c) can be Tryp or Try; d) can be Lys.
↑ Site of cleavage.

Many of these enzymes do not cleave bonds where one of the adjacent amino acids is in the D configuation or is a proline. Common strategies in the design of analogues are therefore, replacement of L by D amino acids, replacement by proline, N-methylation of the peptide nitrogen, or replacement of the peptide bond by a pseudo-peptide bond with similar stereochemical properties.

Linear peptides can usually readily adopt the required conformation for cleavage but with cyclic peptides restriction may result in the stabilisation of bonds which would otherwise be quite unstable (Allen et al, 1984).

Proteins with a well defined three-dimensional structure are less accessible to peptidase attack although certain links may be presented in a manner which makes them extremely liable to specific enzymes. The possibilities arising from this phenomenon are widely exploited in natural biological mechanisms involving activation of proenzymes and prohormones (e.g. prothrombin, plasminogen, trypsinogen, angiotensinogen) and it seems likely that

locally acting protein factors (interferons, interleukins)
are also structured for ready local inactivation.

Behaviour of Endogenous Peptides and Proteins

The compartmentalisation of peptides and proteins and
their ready activation or deactivation by peptidases makes
them ideal candidates for the role of extracellular
messengers. The properties can be used either for systemic
distribution of a transient message or for localised
signalling between cells.

In the first case the hormone message is distributed
throughout the body and is delivered when the hormone has
passed into the interstitial space and activated receptors
on the outside face of the membrane of the appropriate cell
(sometimes the receptors are on the luminal surface of
blood vessels and extravasation is not necessary). In the
case of a distributed message it is important that the
hormone should be rapidly cleared from the circulation and
this is accomplished by peptidases and the other processes
described below.

Locally acting molecules may be expected to be
characterised by the presence of local inactivation
mechanisms, slow exit from the site of action, efficient
removal from the circulation of any material which does
leave the site of action. Products of this sort present
the greatest difficulties for therapeutic use unless local
delivery or targeting can be achieved.

DISTRIBUTION AND METABOLISM

This section considers the main processes which apply
to a peptide or protein once it is in the circulation,
administration being considered in a later section.

The processing of molecules can be ordered from the
vascular space outward as shown in Figure 1. Within the
vasculature degradation can be caused by plasma enzymes or
by enzymes lining the luminal surface of vascular
endothelium. Further clearance involves passage across the
endothelium or uptake by endothelial cells. Degradation
may occur in the interstitial space or the molecule may be
taken up by cells. Once inside the cell, transfer to the
lysosome may occur with subsequent digestion by lysosomal
peptides or the molecule may be excreted for instance into
the bile. In addition to these processes, peptides and
small proteins are filtered at the glomerulus of the kidney
and pass into tubules where degradation can occur at the
luminal surface, uptake into the cell may take place
followed by lysosomal digestion or the product may simply

Figure 1. Transport and degradation of peptides and proteins in different compartments of the body.

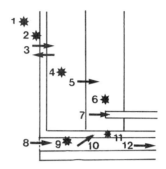

1. Degradation in plasma.
2. Degradation at the luminal surface of the vascular endothelium.
3. Passive diffusion across the vascular endothelium.
4. Degradation in the interstitial space.
5. Uptake by cells.
6. Degradation inside the cell.
7. Excretion into bile.
8. Glomerular filtration.
9. Degradation of the luminal border of the kidney tubule.
10. Uptake into cells of the tubule.
11. Degradation within the cells of the tubule.
12. Excretion into urine.

pass unchanged into the urine.

The relative importance of these processes varies from one product to another. In view of the variety of processes and the sequential nature of some of them it is normally helpful to concentrate only on the rate controlling steps likely to be of major quantitative significance for the specific application in hand. The application of certain general principles may help to simplify the situation for a given product and to identify key questions or possibilities to be probed in experimental work. Carefully planned experimentation is usually essential since many aspects of the handling of these products are highly specific.

Extravasation

A number of studies have shown that the vascular endothelium of most tissues except brain is highly permeable to polar molecules of low to moderate molecular weight (Crone and Levitt, 1984). Molecules larger than 50,000 molecular weight leave the vasculature more slowly except in the liver, spleen and bone marrow. As an indication of the times involved, the distribution half-life for hirudin (MWt 10,800) in man is 9 min. (Markwardt et al, 1984) whereas that for albumin is around 1 day (Schultze and Heremans, 1966a). The exchange is reversible and so small peptides and fragments will be able to leave the interstitial space quite fast. Larger molecules will leave much more slowly and in fact mainly return to the circulation through the lymphatic route which involves passage through lymph nodes.

Glomerular Filtration

This process is also of low specificity apart from a marked molecular weight dependence. Molecules up to 10,000 molecular weight are rapidly cleared. Dextrans of greater than 20,000 molecular weight show progressively reduced filtration efficiencies starting at about 20% (Wallenius, 1954). Albumin (MWt 65,000) is filtered so slowly and is so resistant to other clearance processes that it has an elimination half-life in excess of 20 days (Schultze and Heremans, 1966a).

Clearance By Active Uptake Into Cells

This form of transport tends to be specific for individual compounds or classes of compounds. Several examples are given in Table 2. It is important to note that uptake by the renal tubule occurs after glomerular filtration. Filtration is irreversible and cellular uptake is usually followed by lysosomal degradation. Therefore, stabilising a product which is filtered against this type of uptake is unlikely to effect the circulating half-life of the product although it will reduce the potential accumulation in the kidney.

In contrast to this, clearance of TPA by the liver is the rate determining step which determines the plasma half-life of this molecule and functional hepatectomy results in stable blood levels for at least 45 minutes in rabbits (Korninger et al, 1981).

Local Enzymatic Degradation

Table 3 lists some of the main types of peptidases involved in inactivating and activating peptides and proteins and indicates their site of action. The blood-borne, endothelial and interstitial enzymes are obviously the only ones likely to play a part in influencing availability at extracellular sites of action. Lysosomal

Table 2. Uptake of peptides and proteins by cells

SITE	COMPOUNDS	FATE
Liver	Asialoglycoproteins Tissue plasminogen activator Minisomatostatin	Degradation[a] Degradation[b] Biliary[c]
Kidney Tubule	Peptide and Proteins	Degradation[d]

a) Morell et al, 1971; b) Korininger et al, 1981; c) Baker et al, 1984; d) Baker et al, 1977.

enzymes can be expected to play a terminal role in digesting products which have been selectively taken up by the appropriate cell. The rate of degradation by extracellular enzymes varies greatly from one compound to another whereas lysosomal enzymes in the slightly acidic environment of the lysosome are capable of totally degrading many natural peptide and protein sequences.

IMMUNOGENICITY

Modified peptides and proteins are potentially immunogenic. Although the immunogenicity arises from the fact that foreign features have been introduced into the molecule the metabolic processing of the molecule plays an essential role in the initial triggering of an immune response. The immunogen must be taken up to antigen presenting cells and then partially degraded into fragments which are then displayed on the surface of the antigen presenting cell (Gray and Chestnut, 1985). If the initial uptake or the partial enzymic hydrolysis could be avoided the molecules would not trigger a primary immune response.

ROUTES OF ADMINISTRATION

Provided solubility is adequate and local irritation is not a problem the intravenous route can provide controlled input to match pharmacological requirements and pharmacokinetic behaviour. Alternatives to this route are

Table 3. Peptidases involved in the metabolism of endogenous peptides and proteins

SITE	EXAMPLES
Plasma	Aminopeptidase, ACE[a]
Vascular endothelium	ACE
Interstitial space	Aminopeptidase
Small intestine: human	Endopeptidases
brush border	Aminopeptidases
cytosol	Di- and tri-peptidases
Kidney/liver lysosomes	Endopeptidases
Kidney tubule brush-border	Aminopeptidase

a) Antiotensin converting enzyme.

essential for wide-spread application and some of these are now considered.

Sub-Cutaneous Injection
    For molecules up to the size of insulin, sub-cutaneous injection will normally provide input into the systemic circulation over a period of 30-60 min. Certain somatastatin analogues have proved to be exceptions to this rule and prolonged input has been observed at the appropriate dose (Baker et al, 1984). Proteins may leave the site of injection very slowly over periods of longer than one day and travel through the lymphatics (Schultze and Heremans, 1966b).

Oral Administration
    Peptides and proteins are generally very poorly absorbed from the gastrointestinal tract even when stable analogues have been prepared and in this respect they are similar to many polar drugs. Specific pathways do however exist. Di- and tri- peptides are very efficiently transported across the mucosal membrane of the small intestine and this has been exploited in the design of antibacterial phosphonic peptide analogues which have a high oral bioavailability in man (Allen et al, 1979).

The Nasal Route
    This route has recently been the subject of considerable investigation (Chien and Chang, 1985).

Successful treatment of diabetic patients for 3 months with
an intranasal insulin spray using deoxycholate as a
permeation enhancer has been reported (Salzman et al,
1985). In addition a survey of results obtained in several
species with 25 different compounds has shown that there is
a sharp change in availability at molecular weights greater
than 1000 (McMartin and Peters, 1986). Below this
reproducible uptake of an average 70% can be obtained and
uptake does not appear to be independent of such factors as
charge and hydrophobicity (Hutchinson et al, 1986).

Rectal Delivery

The uptake of peptides and proteins by this route
appears to require the use of adjuvants and this topic is
being actively investigated. (Nishihata et al, 1983).

EXAMPLES OF INDIVIDUAL COMPOUNDS OR CLASSES

Bradykinin

Bradykinin is a nonapeptide with very potent vasoactive
properties. It is produced locally at sites of injury by
the action of kallikreins on kininogen. It is rapidly
degraded in many tissue beds and 80% is degraded to
fragments in a single passage through the lungs by the
enzymes of the luminal surface of the capillaries of this
tissue (Ferriera and Vane, 1967). This is a good example
of a locally acting peptide.

Corticotrophins

Adrenocorticotrophin is 39 amino acids long and it is
released from the pituitary into the circulation. Its
major target is the adrenal. Corticotrophins are stable in
blood in vitro but have short half-lives in vivo and
rapidly leave the circulation. 40% of the dose enters
muscle and skin and is almost immediately degraded by a
variety of enzymes. Aminopeptidase is evidently important
because molecules with a D-residue at the N-terminus are
found intact in the muscle and skin and give much higher
blood levels. For these reasons it appears that
degradation by aminopeptidase probably occurs in the
interstitial space (Bennett and McMartin, 1979).

Desamino-D-Arginine Vasopressin

Vasopressin is an octapeptide with a short half-life in
vivo. The removal of the amino group and replacement of
arginine with the D isomer give a product with a longer
half-life, greater potency and greater specificity
(Anderson and Arner, 1972). This product , given by the

nasal route has been used successfully in the treatment of diabetes insipidus since 1968.

Tissue Plasminogen Activator
This is a protein of molecular weight 70,000. It is produced locally and facilitates lysis of fibrin clots. Its clearance from the circulation in the rabbit (plasma half-life 2 minutes) is due almost entirely to uptake by the liver by a selective mechanism which is not blocked by asialoglycoproteins. Functional heptatectomy results in steady plasma concentrations for at least 45 minutes (Korninger et al, 1981).

Proteins Modified With Polyethylene Glycol
The clearance of proteins from the circulation and their immunogenicity can be profoundly modified by coupling polyethylene glycol chains of 5000 to 10,000 molecular weight. This apparently confers inertness thus rendering the molecule non-immunogenic and in addition greatly reducing the rate of clearance (Abuchowski et al, 1977).

CONCLUSIONS

Peptides equilibrate rapidly throughout the extracellular space (except for the brain) and their removal from this space depends not only on degradation by peptidases but on other processes such as renal filtration and biliary clearance.

Although considerable increases in potency may result from the design of stable analogues, the non-enzymatic processes of clearance continue to operate and the half-lives are usually not extended beyond one or two hours. The results might be improved by designing molecules with a high volume of distribution or a high degree of plasma protein binding.

Proteins of molecular weight greater than 50,000 will not be filtered rapidly at the glomerulus and so there is a prospect of obtaining products with prolonged plasma half-lives provided degradation and specific clearance processes can be avoided. Because of the much slower equilibration time of these products with the interstitial space in the body, if an extravascular site of action is envisaged it will be necessary either to target, to administer locally or to obtain a prolonged period in the circulation and to minimise local degradation.

REFERENCES

Abuchowshi, A., McCoy, J.R., Palczuk, N.C., Van Es, T. and Davis, F.F. (1977). J. Biol. Chem., 252, 3582

Allen, J.G., Havas, L., Leicht, E., Lenox-Smith, J. and Nisbet, L.J. (1979). Antimicrob. Agents Chemo., 16, 306.

Allen, M., McMartin, C., Peters, G.E. and Wade, R. (1984). Reg. Peptides, 10, 29.

Anderson, R.E. and Arner, B. (1972). Acta. Med. Scand., 192, 21.

Baker, J.R.J.., Bennett, H.P.J., Christian, R.A. and McMartin, C. (1977). J. Endoc., 74, 23

Baker, J.R.J., Kemmenoe, B.H., McMartin, C. and Peters, G.E. (1984). Reg. Peptides, 9, 213

Bennett, H.P.J and McMartin, C. (1979). Pharmacol. Rev., 30, 248.

Chien, Y.W.and Chang, S.F. (1985). In "Transnasal Medical Systems" (ed. Y. W. Chien) Elsevier, Amsterdam.

Crone, C. and Levitt, D.G. (1984). Handbook on Physio., 6, 411.

Ferreira, S.H. and Vane, J.R. (1967). Br. J. Pharmacol., 30, 417.

Grey, H.M.and Chestnut, R (1985).Immunology Today, 6, 101.

Humphrey, M.J. and Ringrose, P.S (1986). Drug. Met, Rev., in the press.

Hutchinson, L.E.F., Hyde, R., Metcalfe, J.B., McMartin, C. and Peters, G.E. (1986). In preparation.

Korninger, C., Stassen, J.M and Collen, D. (1981). Thromb. Haemostas., 46, 658.

McMartin, C. and Peters, G.E (1986). In "Advanced Drug Delivery Systems for Peptides and Proteins". (Eds. Davis. S.S., Illum, L. and Tomlinson, E.) Plenum Press, New York.

Markwardt, F., Nowak, G., Sturzebecher, T. Griessbach, V., Walsman, P. and Vogel, G. Thromb. Haemostas., 52, 160.

Morell, A.G., Gregoriadis, G., Scheinberg, I.H., Hickman, J. and Ashwell, G. (1971). J. Biol. Chem., 246, 1461.

Nishihata, T., Kim, S., Morishita, S., Kamada, A., Yata, N. and Higuichi, T. (1983). J. Pharm. Sci., 72 280.

Salzman, R., Manson, J.E., Griffing, G.T., Kimmerle, R., Rudderman, N., McCall, A., Stolz, E.I., Mullin, C., Small, D., Armstrong, J. and Melky, J.C. (1985). New Eng. Med. J., 312, 1078.

Schultze and Heremans (1966a). In "Molecular Biology of Human Proteins. Elsevier, Amsterdam, 452.

Schultze and Heremans (1966b). In "Molecular Biology of Human Proteins". Elsevier, Amsterdam, 590.

Wallenius, G. (1954). Acta Soc. Med. Upsalen. Suppl., 4, 1.

STEREOSELECTIVITY IN THE ENZYMATIC BIOTRANSFORMATION OF DRUGS AND OTHER XENOBIOTICS

Nico P.E. Vermeulen

Department of Pharmacochemistry (Molecular Toxicology), Free University, De Boelelaan 1083, 1081 HV Amsterdam (The Netherlands).

INTRODUCTION

Nowadays it is increasingly recognised that stereochemical factors play a significant role in the disposition and action of drugs and other xenobiotics in living organisms (Ariens, 1983; Albert, 1985). Desired and undesired effects of xenobiotics may be influenced by stereoselectivity at the level of their absorption and distribution (Van Ginneken et al, 1983; Simonye et al, 1986), metabolism (Vermeulen and Breimer, 1983; Vermeulen, 1986; Testa, 1986a) and excretion. Stereoisomerism is a rather broad phenomenon and manifests itself in various forms, such as the occurrence of enantiomers, epimers, diastereoisomers, meso compounds, geometrical isomers etc. Such isomers may bind differently to optically active macromolecules and as a result of this (for example in the case of binding of enantiomers to an enzyme or a receptor protein) two different diastereomeric complexes with different physical and chemical properties may arise. Consequently, in the case of a metabolic reaction, the nature of the rate of the reaction may become quite different for enantiomers, whereas in the case of binding of enantiomers to a receptor the intensity or even the nature of the action may become different.

Generally speaking, the consequences of stereoisomerism for disposition and action of xenobiotics in living organisms are still difficult to predict, because they are complex and of a multifactorial origin. Nevertheless, there is growing interest among researchers to set up experiments in such a way that beneficial or detrimental consequences of stereoselectivity become clear as early as possible. Recent developments in analytical techniques, enabling the simultaneous separation of enantiomers with HPLC (Special issue, J.Liq.Chrom, 1986), GLC (Testa,

1986b), chiral antisera (Cook, 1985) and GLC-MS with the use of stable isotopes (Baillie, 1981), as well as in stereocontrolled synthesis (Beld and Zwanenburg (1986) certainly have contributed to the increased interest in this aspect of drug disposition.

In this chapter a number of examples of stereoselective biotransformation of drugs and other xenobiotics is discussed. Special attention is paid to those examples which illustrate the stereoselective action of important enzymes, to the resulting consequences for drug disposition and to examples in which stereoselectivity is used as a tool to study mechanisms of biotransformation.

IMPORTANCE OF STEREOSELECTIVE METABOLISM

From a quantitative point of view, stereoselective metabolism of drugs and other xenobiotics is an extremely important phenomenon, as may be derived from the many examples described in the literature (Testa and Jenner, 1980; Vermeulen, 1986). Both pharmacological and toxicological consequences of stereoselective metabolism have been reported. As to pharmacological consequences, the examples of hexobarbital (HB), at present mainly used as model-substrate, can be looked upon as illustrative (Van der Graaff, 1985). Apart from a large difference between the intrinsic hypnotic activities of the enantiomers of this highly lipophilic chiral drug, the S-(+)-enantiomer being far the most active enantiomer in most species, substrate- and product-stereoselective metabolism is involved (Figure 1).

In vitro studies with hepatic microsomes of several species have demonstrated pronounced differences in the rate of oxidative degradation of the enantiomers; in rat liver microsomes this was mainly ascribed to a lower K_m value (Miyano et al, 1980). With microsomes of untreated rats, S-(+)-HB was predominantly found to be metabolised to 3'-β-hydroxy-S-(+)-HB, whereas the other enantiomer was preferentially metabolised to 3'-α-hydroxy-R-(-)-HB. Loss of this form of product-stereoselectivity upon treatment of rats with the enzyme inducer phenobarbital (PB) and the enzyme inhibitor SKF-525A (Miyano et al, 1980), as well as significant gender and species differences observed in other studies, might lead to the suggestion that different forms of cytochrome P-450 could be involved in the hydroxylation of the HB-enantiomers. Apart from their stereoselective formation, 3'-α-hydroxyl-(-)- and 3'-β-hydroxy-(+)-HB were also shown to be preferentially glucuronidated and dehydrogenated (Miyano et al, 1981).

Figure 1. Chemical structure of S-(+)- and R-(-)- Hexo-barbital and major primary metabolic pathways in the rat.

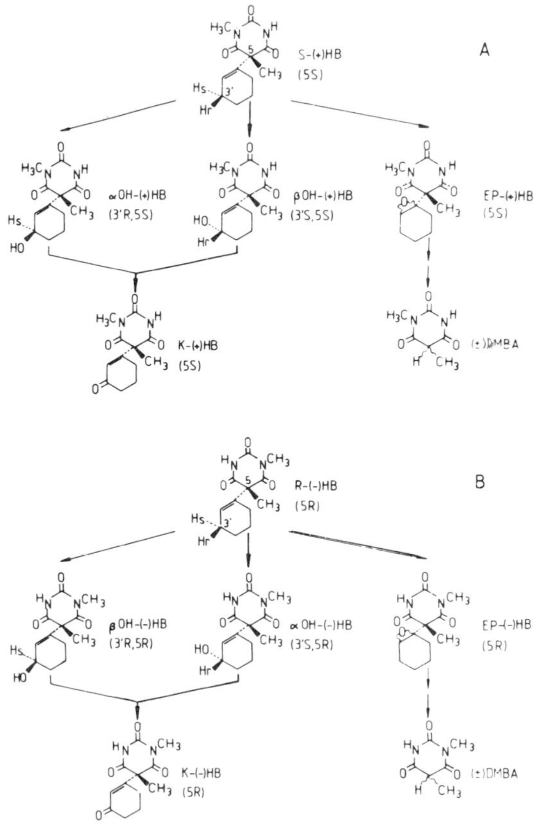

Secondary conjugation reactions are not included (adapted from Van der Graaff, 1985.

The formation of 1,5-dimethyl-barbituric acid, the end product of the epoxide-diol pathway in HB (Van der Graaff et al, 1983), did not appear to be dependent on the configuration of the parent compound. Recently, a comparable product stereoselectivity in the epoxidation, hydroxylation and dehydrogenation steps was observed in vivo in rats treated orally with the pure enantiomers of HB (Table 1).

Using a pseudoracemic mixture of HB, consisting of a mixture of S-(+)- and N_1-trideutero-R-(-)-HB, and an analytical procedure based on mass fragmentography (Van der

Table 1. Pharmacokinetic parameters and recoveries of unconjuated metabolites in urine of S(+)HB and R(-)HB after p.o. and i.a. administration of 25mg/k^{-1}.

	S(+)HB p.o.	S(+)HB i.a.	R(-)HB p.o.	R(-)HB i.a.
$t_{1/2}$ (min)	13.4±0.8	15.7±1.5	16.7±0.6	13.3±0.4
AUC ($\mu g.min^{-1}.ml^{-1}$)	16.4±2.2	366±37	129±22	444±30
CL ($ml.min^{-1}.kg^{-1}$)	1621±197	73.9±7.5	226±36	54.4±2.4
V ($ml.kg^{-1}$)		1670±233		1042±56
E	0.94±0.01		0.68±0.03	
OH-HB (% dose)	15.6±0.9	20.6±2.2	10.9±1.3	16.9±2.3
K-HB "	19.3±0.8	17.3±1.7	56.2±1.8	54.9±9.0
DMBA "	9.1±1.4	7.8±1.2	11.8±1.9	11.6±4.8
Total "	44.0±1.8	45.7±3.3	78.9±2.9	83.4±6.6

Values (n=6) represent the mean ± S.E.M.

Graaff et al, 1986), the stereoselective disposition of HB-enantiomers was studied upon simultaneous administration to the rat. It was found that the disposition of the pseudoracemic mixture of enantiomers was not essentially different from that of separately administered enantiomers (Van der Graaff et al, 1986). With respect to pharmacokinetics, the difference in intrinsic clearances between S-(+)- and R-(-)-HB, as reflected by the difference in the areas under their respective blood concentration time curves after oral administration to the rat, (AUC_{oral}) was about sevenfold (Van der Graaf et al, 1983 and 1986). It was, however, far larger than the difference between the corresponding elimination half lives ($t_{1/2}$) or systemic clearances (CL_S) as estimated upon intra-arterial administration (Figure 2). The observed discrepancies in the pharmacokinetic parameters (Table 1) are to be attributed to hepatic bloodflow limited metabolism of HB (Van der Graaff, 1985; Vermeulen et al, 1983), a phenomenon which was further substantiated by the relatively high hepatic extraction ratios of the enantiomers, viz extraction ratio E = 0.68 for R-(-)- and 0.95 for S-(+)-HB. As a result of the relatively high presystemic elimination of the S-(+)-enantiomer, its contribution to the total AUC upon administration of racemic HB is only limited when compared to that of the R-(-)-enantiomer.

Figure 2. Blood concentration-time profiles of Hexo-barbital-enantiomers in the rat upon oral administration of 25mg/kg S-(+)- or R-(-)-HB.

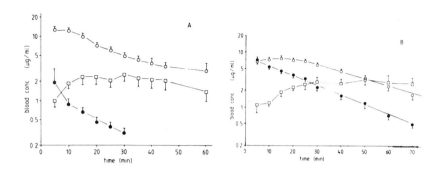

A) S-(+)-HB and B) R-(-)-HB.   ● = HB, O = 3'OH-HB and □ = 3'-K-HB, respectively (adapted from Van der Graaff, 1985.

Considering the relatively high presystemic elimination of S-(+)-HB as well as the facts that in untreated, PB- and 3-methylcholanthrene (3MC) -treated rats, $CL_{intrinsic}$ of S-(+)- and D_3-R-(-)-HB have been found to correlate strongly upon oral administration of pseudoracemic HB (r = 0.89, n=22) and that the above mentioned inducers did not significantly influence the metabolic pattern of the respective enantiomers of HB, it has been concluded that $CL_{intrinsic}$ of racemic HB can be seen as a relatively accurate reflection of (PB-inducible) hepatic cytochrome P-450 activity (Van der Graaff, 1985). The measurement of sleeping times for this purpose, theoretically speaking, preferentially done by making use of the far more active S-(+)-enantiomer, however is complicated by hepatic bloodflow limitations.

Product-stereoselective metabolism may also be important from a toxicological point of view. This was for example illustrated by the mutagenic behaviour of cis- and trans-1,2-dichlorocyclohexane with and without metabolic activation (Van Bladeren et al, 1979). Using the Ames-test with Salmonella typhimurium it was shown that, in contrast to the trans-isomer, the cis-isomer demonstrated mutagenic activity that was significantly increased upon addition of 9,000g and 100,000g supernatant of a rat liver homogenate. The explanation of this stereoselective effect was given in terms of a stereospecific action of glutathione transferase present in liver homogenate fractions and catalysing the substitution of the vicinal chlorine atoms according to a SN2-substitution mechanism. Only in the cis-1,2-dichlorocyclohexane isomer can this conjugation reaction lead to the formation of a reactive thiiranium-ion, which is suspected to be responsible for the mutagenic activity (Figure 3).

Figure 3.   Conjugation of cis- and trans- 1,2-dichloro-cyclohexane to glutathione.

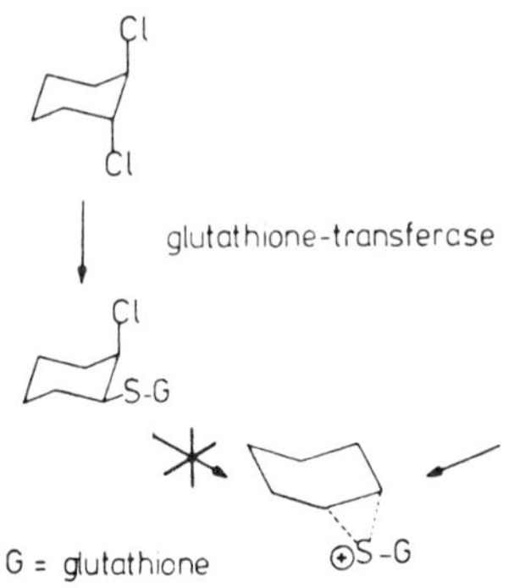

Formation of the reactive thiiranium-ion is only possible with the cis-isomer (taken from Van Bladeren et al, 1979).

There exist many other examples illustrating various consequences of stereoselectivity in the biotransformation of drugs and other xenobiotics. Some of them, e.g. propranolol, warfarin, nicotine and tocainide have been reviewed elaborately recently (Vermeulen, 1986).

STEREOSELECTIVITY IN OXIDATIVE BIOTRANSFORMATION : MIXED-FUNCTION OXIDASES (MFO).

One of the most important drug and xenobiotic metabolising enzyme systems in mammalian and non-mammalian systems is the MFO-system, consisting of a family of cytochrome P-450 isoenzymes which, in general, exhibit a broad range of substrate- and product selectivity. The multiplicity and the widely varying substrate selectivity complicate considerably the study of the stereoselectivity as such, as well as the correlation of stereoselectivities in different species.

Among the best documented examples illustrating the

stereoselective action of cytochrome P-450 isoenzymes, as well as approaches to using stereoselectivity in bio-transformation as a tool for different purposes, are provided by studies on the stereoselective bioactivation of polycyclic aromatic hydrocarbons (PAHs) to carcinogens by cytochrome P-450c (Jerina et al, 1985). This isoenzyme was found to highly stereoselectively catalyze the epoxidation of benzo(a)pyrene (BP) to (+)-7R,8S-arene oxide, which upon stereoselective hydrolysis by epoxide hydrolase to (-)-7R,8R-dihydrodiol-BP is converted by the same former isoenzyme to BP-7R,8S-dihydrodiol-9S,10R-epoxide, in which the benzylic hydroxyl group and epoxide are trans, in over 85% diastereomeric excess (Figure 4). The latter diol-epoxide was demonstrated to be a considerably more potent initiator of lung tumours than its stereoisomers.

Figure 4. Formation and absolute stereochemistry of benzo(a)pyrene metabolism by cytochrome P-450c and epoxide hydrolase.

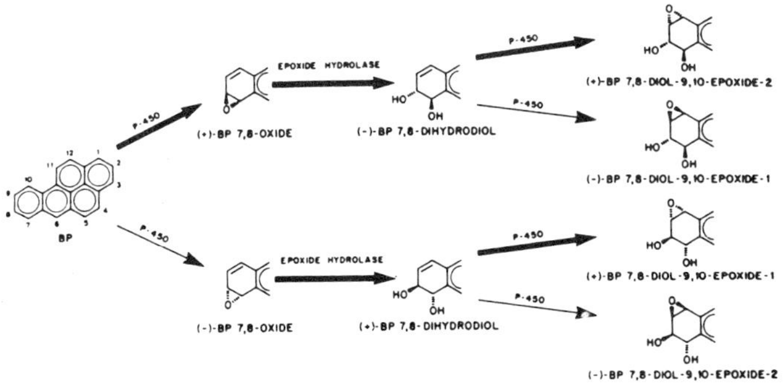

Heavy arrows indicate the major metabolic pathways (adapted from Van Bladeren et al, 1984).

By studying the stereospecificity of various PAHs in detail, Jerina and coworkers were able to propose a model for the steric requirements of the catalytic site of the cytochrome P-450c involved (Figure 5), predicting a)- the regio-isomeric epoxidation, b)- the fact that the arene-oxides formed should have the R-absolute configuration at the benzylic centers and the S-absolute configuration at the allylic centers. In addition the model could predict, realising that epoxide hydrolase converts the configuration of the allylic center in forming trans-dihydrodiols, that c)- R,R-dihydrodiols should be preferentially formed from R,S-arene oxides as well as d)- the preferential formation of trans-dihydrodiols from R,R-dihydrodiols with "bay-region" double bonds. The model was demonstrated to be also valid in predicting the stereoselective metabolism of PAHs like phenanthrene, chrysene and benzanthracene (e.g. Van Bladeren et al, 1984).

Figure 5. Nine membered ring model for the substrate binding site of cytochrome P-450c.

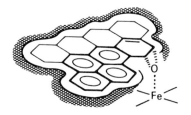

B(a)P is represented in the binding site in such a way that B(a)P-9S,10R-oxide is obtained. By turning B(a)P in the model it is possible to rationalise also the stereoselective formation of B(a)P-(4S,5R)-oxide and B(a)P-(7R,8S)-oxide (taken from Jerina et al, 1982).

Numerous drugs are known to be metabolised, at least partly, by this cytochrome P-450c, e.g. phenacetin, propranolol and warfarin. The model developed for PAHs is as yet not applicable, however, to the biotransformation of other compounds.

CHIRAL SULPHOXIDATIONS

Some studies on the chirality of sulphoxidation by FAD-containing microsomal monooxygenase and cytochrome P-450 oxygenase isoenzymes have been published (Waxman et al, 1982; Light et al, 1982). The latter enzyme system can oxygenate carbon, nitrogen and sulphur atoms, the former only nitrogen and sulphur but not carbon. Using 4-tolyl ethyl sulphide as a prochiral model compound (Figure 6), rat liver microsomal FAD-containing monooxygenases yielded predominantly the R-(+)-enantiomer of 4-tolylethyl sulphoxide, whereas rat liver microsomes (containing FAD- as well as the cytochrome P-450 monooxygenase) yielded both the R-(+)- and S-(-)-enantiomers (46 vs 54%). The formation of the S-(-)-enantiomer was mainly carried out by PB-inducible cytochrome P-450 isoenzymes as was demonstrated by using two purified cytochrome P-450 isoenzymes isolated from PB induced rat livers.

Figure 6. Oxidation pathway of the pro-chiral p-tolyl ethyl sulphide to enantiomeric sulphoxides by NADPH-dependent cytochrome P-450 oxygenase or FAD-containing monooxygenase (adapted from Waxmann et al, 1982).

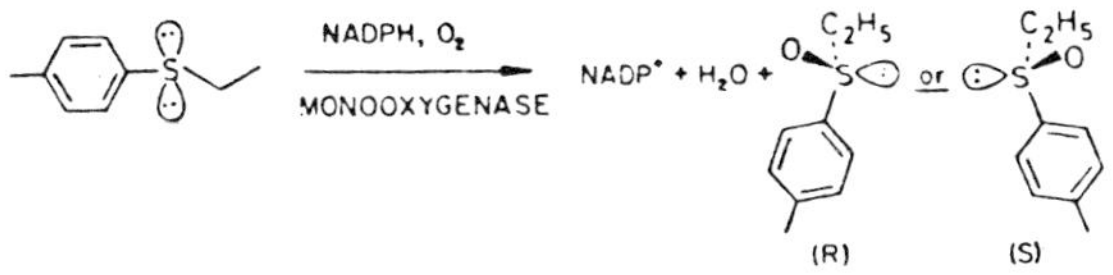

Benzylic carbon oxidation was only carried out by microsomal cytochrome P-450 and as to be expected not by the FAD-monooxygenase. Lack of absolute stereo- and/or regioselectivity is apparently typical of P-450-isoenzymes as it was also noted previously in PAH and warfarin metabolism. The extent of product stereoselective sulphoxidation was strongly dependent on substituents at the sulphur atom (Waxman et al, 1982; Light et al, 1982) and on the relative participation of cytochrome P-450, FAD-monooxygenases or even other sulphur oxygenating enzymes such as the copper dependent dopamine-β-hydroxylase. A drug in which sulphur oxygenation (and reduction of a sulphoxide) is of importance, is sulindac sulphide, a non-steroidal anti-inflammatory agent which is delivered therapeutically as the sulphoxide prodrug (Rosenkranz et al, 1983). The low stereoselectivity in sulindac sulphide oxygenation in ram seminal vesical microsomes has been suggested to be the net result of prostaglandin cyclooxygenase (generating preferentially the S-(-)-sulphoxide) and of FAD-containing monooxygenases (probably generating the R-(+)-sulphoxide in this tissue).

CHIRALITY AND OXIDATION POLYMORPHISMS

Biotransformation by hepatic cytochrome P-450 containing monooxygenases is a major determinant of interindividual differences in the rate of elimination of numerous drugs and other xenobiotics and, consequently, in their pharmacological or toxicological responses.

Amongst compounds whose oxidation has been reported to be impaired in poor metaboliser phenotypes (representing approximately 10% of the European population) is the β-adrenoceptor antagonist bufuralol (Buf). It is a chiral drug for which 1'-hydroxylation (Figure 7) is under genetic

control and selective for the (+)-isomer. Aromatic Buf 4-
and 6-hydroxylations are under the same genetic control but
selective for the (-)-isomer. The selectivity for the
aliphatic and aromatic oxidations is virtually abolished in
poor metaboliser phenotypes. Apart from these oxidation
reactions, glucuronidation of the hydroxyl group in the
side chain and elimination appeared to be stereoselective
for (+)-Buf and particularly important in poor
metabolisers. Due to a concerted action of the various
pathways of metabolism/elimination, plasma concentration
ratio's of (-)-Buf and (+)-Buf in vivo are only slightly
different, viz. 1.6 in extensive and 2.6 in poor
metabolisers.

**Figure 7.   Chemical structure of bufuralol and the 1'-
hydroxylated metabolite (adapted from Boobis et al, 1985).**

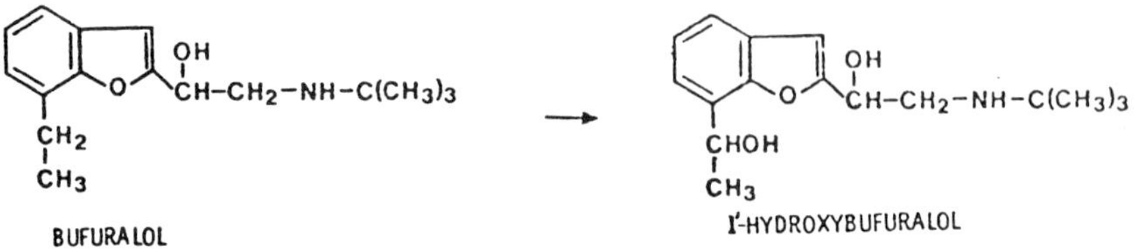

BUFURALOL   1'-HYDROXYBUFURALOL

Meyer et al (Dayer et al, 1984 and 1985) assessed the
stereoselectivity of Buf-1'-hydroxylation in liver
microsomes of extensive and poor metabolising humans, as
well as in a reconstituted system of a purified cytochrome
P-450 isoenzyme isolated from a liver of an extensive
metaboliser. Poor metaboliser microsomes were demonstrated
to possess a slightly lower V_{max}, a much high K_m and a
largly abolished substrate stereoselectivity. Since there
was no overlap between V_{max} and K_m values for the
1'hydroxylation of (+)-Buf as to the poor and extensive
metabolisers tested, it was suggested that these two
parameters in combination with the enantiomeric ratio,
$V_{max}(-)/V_{max}(+)$, could be used as a tool to phenotype
individuals in vitro.

Various recent investigations (including those with a
purified human isoenzyme) have provided evidence for the
hypothesis that 1'hydroxylation of Buf is mediated by a
polymorphic cytochrome P-450 isoenzyme, which also
catalyses the 4-hydroxylation of debrisoquine, oxidation of
sparteine, E-10-hydroxylation of nortriptyline, O-
demethylation of dextrometorphan, trans-4'-hydroxylation of
perhexiline, α-hydroxylation of (+)-metoprolol and several
others (Boobis et al, 1985; Distlerath et al, 1985). Meyer
et al proposed a model for the active site of the isoenzyme
involved in this type of polymorphic oxidation (Kronbach et

al, 1985) on the basis of structural and reaction characteristics of several substrates. Specific aspects of this model are: 1) a distance of about 7Å from a basic nitrogen to the reaction site; 2) nearly planar aromatic or aliphatic rings; 3) a non-enantioselective protein binding site; 4) a chiral center, which in the case of Buf confers the oxidation regioselectivity and 5) the substrate binding site, the lipophilic plane and the reaction site are not in one plane.

5-Substituted 5-phenylhydantoins represent another class of drugs, showing an oxidation polymorphism involving stereoselectivity. Examples are mephenytoin (N-methyl-5-ethyl-5-phenyl-hydantoin, nirvanol (5-ethyl-5- phenyl-hydantoin) and phenytoin (5,5-diphenylhydantoin). In the case of mephenytoin (Kupfer et al, 1981), aromatic 4-hydroxylation is the preferred metabolic reaction in man for S-mephenytoin ($t_{1/2} \sim 1hr$), whereas N-demethylation is the preferred reaction for the R-isomer. Furthermore, only the S-mephenytoin 4-hydroxylation reaction is genetically deficient. The R-enantiomer was found to be excreted much slower ($t_{1/2} \sim 70$ hr) and is therefore likely to contribute most to the well-known accumulation of 5-phenyl-5-ethyl-hydantoin during chronic anticonvulsant therapy. In so-called poor metabolisers, S-mephenytoin is not significantly para-hydroxylated, has a $t_{1/2} \sim 70$ hr, and, like the R-enantiomer is then available for N-demethylation. As in the case of mephenytoin, aromatic 4-hydroxylation of prochiral phenytoin and nirvanol were found to yield stereoselective para-hydroxy-derivatives with an S-configuration. Whether the aromatic hydroxylation reactions in the phenyl-substituted hydantoins are mediated by the same cytochrome P-450 isoenzyme(s) therefore seems likely.

It is interesting to observe that stereoselectivity in the oxidation of Buf, other β-blocking agents and other drugs were used in an attempt to characterise the polymorphic enzymes involved or even to elucidate the possible shape of the active site of a particular isoenzyme, which, due to its polymorphic nature, can have such important consequences for drug therapy. Successful modelling of the active site of such enzymes, i.e. with a predictive value for other substrates might have substantial advantages in the development of new drugs, not suffering from such polymorphisms in biotransformations.

STEREOSELECTIVITY IN EPOXIDE HYDROLASES

Epoxide hydrolases are enzymes which catalyse the

hydrolysis of alkene oxides into diols and of arene oxides into dihydrodiols (Figure 8; Oesch, 1979). Although specific examples are known in which bioactivation was evident, epoxide hydrolases generally inactivate electrophilic epoxides formed during metabolism. Epoxides have been identified as metabolites of a wide variety of substrates possessing olefinic or aromatic groups, such as endogenous steroids, environmental xenobiotics as well as clinically used drugs such as tricyclic antidepressants (Frigerio et al, 1976). Two different epoxide hydrolases have been isolated and identified, namely a microsomal membrane bound (Oesch, 1979) as well as a cytosolic soluble form (Hammock et al, 1980). Substrate selectivities of both hydrolases are large and overlap, although the cytosolic hydrolase seems to possess a higher activity towards aliphatic epoxides. Mechanistically, the enzymatic hydration of epoxides most probably proceeds according to a base-catalysed nucleophilic addition of "activated water" (Hanzlik et al, 1976). A simple electrophilic (acid-catalysed) mechanism was ruled out by experiments with $^{18}OH_2$, which demonstrated regiospecific hydration at the 2-position of unlabelled styrene- and naphthalene oxides (Hanzlik et al, 1976; Jerina et al, 1970).

Figure 8. Stereo- and enantioselective formation of trans-diols by epoxide hydrolase (EH) from cyclohexeneoxide and naphthalene-oxide.

(-)-trans-1R,2R-
(70%)

(-)-trans-1R,2R-
(40%)

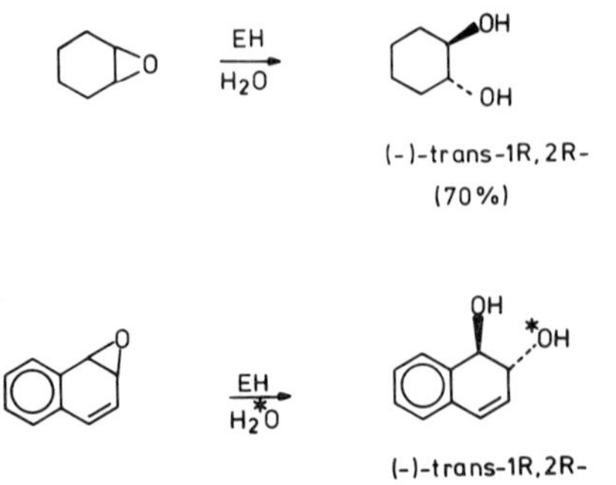

Enzymatic hydrolysis of naphthalene-oxide in a $^{18}OH_2$-medium ($H_2{}^*O$) resulted in the regiospecific introduction of ^{18}O at the 2-position (taken from Jerina et al, 1970).

Stereochemical studies have shown that epoxide hydrolases hydrate epoxides of cyclic olefins including

arene oxides, in such a way that trans-diols with varying
degrees of enantiomeric homogeneity are formed (Figure 8;
Armstrong et al, 1981). Geometric isomers of aliphatic
epoxides have also been shown to undergo trans-hydration,
which means that trans-epoxides yield erytho-glycols and
cis-epoxides threo-glycols.

Low and high substrate enantioselectivity have been
described for microsomal epoxide hydrolases. For example,
for 4,5-benzo(a)pyrene oxide, a biphasic first-order
kinetic behaviour reflecting a 40-fold difference in the
rates of hydration of the (+)- and (-)enantiomers was
observed under certain in vitro conditions (Armstrong et
al, 1980). The enantioselectivity and positional
selectivity of the microsomal epoxide hydrolase have been
studied in greater depth with stereoisomeric 3-tert-butyl-
1,2-epoxy cyclohexanes (Belluci et al, 1982) as well as
tetrahydro- and diol-epoxides derived from benz(a)-
anthracene (Sayer et al, 1985). From these and other
studies, authors have deduced a geometry of the active site
where a hydrophobic pocket directs the binding of
the stereoisomers in a proper orientation for the
nucleophilic attack of water (Figure 9, Armstrong et al,
1981).

Figure 9. Proposed transition state for the reaction of
the epoxide hydrolase-substrate-water complex.

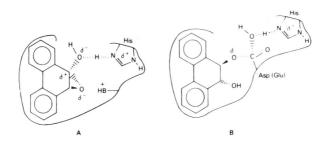

Apart from a certain hydrophobic pocket directing the
stereoselective orientation of the binding of substrates, a
base-catalysed nucleophilic attack or "activated" water is
generally believed to be important in this enzymatic
reaction (adapted from Armstrong et al, 1980).

STEREOSELECTIVITY IN GLUTATHIONE-TRANSFERASES (GSH-t)

Drugs and other xenobiotics possessing an electrophilic

center (i.e. pre-existing or as a result of
biotransformation) often undergo conjugation with the
optically active tripeptide glutathione (GSH, γ-glu-cys-
gly). Apart from aliphatic and aromatic epoxides, GSH-
transferases catalyse the conjugation of GSH to many other
hydrophobic substrates possessing leaving groups, such as
phosphates, sulphates and halides (Arias and Jakoby, 1976).
The mechanism of the conjugation reaction, which is
generally catalysed by a cytosolic system of GSH-
transferases is consistent with a SN2 type substitution
mechanism involving a direct attack of the sulphydryl group
of GSH at the electrophilic atom of the substrate.

    With regard to the stereoselectivity of GSH conjugation
to rigid epoxides it was, for example, found by identifying
and quantifying mercapturic acids excreted in urine of rats
treated with the model compound cyclohexane, that only two
trans-2-hydroxycyclohexyl-mercapturic acids and no cis-
isomers were found in vivo (Van Bladeren et al, 1981;
Vermeulen et al, 1980). Regarding the enzymatic reaction
for alkylhalides rat liver cytosolic GSH transferases were
found to conjugate chiral α-phenylethyl-chloride and
-bromide with a high degree of substrate-stereoselectivity
(Mangold and Abdel-Monem, 1980). S-enantiomers were far
better substrates than R-enantiomers. A trans-addition
mechanism involving SN2 substitution was also found for the
enzymatic conjugation of (+)-B(a)-4,5-oxide using rat liver
cytosol as a source of transferase activity. Apparently,
both positional isomers (at C_4 and C_5; Figure 10) were
produced, however, with a preference for two
diastereoisomers. Subsequent investigations with optically
active (+)-4S,5R and (-)-4R,5S-B(a)P-4,5-oxides (Armstrong
et al, 1981) have shown that the rat liver cytosol GSH-
transferases preferentially catalyse the formation of the
5-glutathionyl-isomer (4S,5S) from the (+) and the 4-
gluthionyl-isomer (4S,5S) from the (-)-B(a)P-4,5-oxide
isomer. Apparently, these GSH-transferases prefer to
attack the oxirane carbon of the B(a)P-4,5-oxide, which has
the absolute R-configuration.

    Unless different isoenzymes possess the same kind of
stereoselectivity towards a substrate, it may be
anticipated that a mixture of isoenzymes will exhibit a
diminished stereoselective metabolism. In the case of GSH-
transferases the stereoselection is even more complicated
since one isoenzyme may exist as a homo- or heterodimeric
protein of two subunits, each of the subunits potentially
having structurally different active sites apart from their
GSH-binding site. By studying the stereoselectivity of a
heterodimeric isoenzyme C towards various K-region arene

Figure 10.   Chemical structures of four possible
glutathione (GSH) conjugates from (+)- and (-)-
benzo(a)pyrene-4,5-oxide.

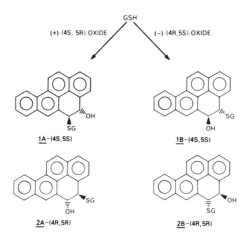

Cytosolic rat liver GSH-transferase preferentially forms
the conjugates IA and IB from racemic benzo(a)pyrene-4,5-
oxide (taken from Armstrong et al, 1981b).

oxides and azarene analogues, Cobb et al (1983) confirmed a
high stereoselectivity with predominant (> 95%) attack at
the oxirane carbon of R-absolute configuration to give S,S-
products. Their results further suggested that hydrophobic
interactions between the substrate and the enzyme surface
distal to the oxirane ring, rather than electronic
differences between the two oxirane carbons, are important
in determining the stereoselectivity of the isoenzyme C
(Figure 11).
    More recently, the existence of microsomal GSH-
transferases has been firmly established (Morgenstern et
al, 1983). Apart from the usual substrates for the
cytosolic GSH-transferases, compounds like the nephrotoxins
hexachloro-1,3-butadiene and tetrafluorethene seem to be
the better substrates for the microsomal enzymes (Wolf et
al, 1984). Dohn et al, (1985) were the first to show with
^{19}F-NMR a stereochemical control of an enzymatic addition
(and no addition-elimination) reaction of chlorotrifluoro-
ethene with GSH. Using rat liver microsomal fraction,
predominantly one diastereomeric GSH-conjugate was formed,
whereas a cytosolic fraction produced an equimolar fraction
of two diastereomeric S-(2-chloro-1,1,2-trifluorethyl)
glutathione conjugates. Further studies on the (regio-

Figure 11. Possible asymmetries in the active site of the
C subunit of GSH-transferase isoenzyme C.

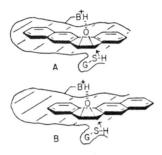

Differences in hydrophobic overlap between enzyme and
substrate and/or in efficiency of protonation of the
leaving group dictate the stereo- and regioselectivity of
the GSH-attack (taken from Cobb et al, 1983).

and) stereospecifities of GSH-transferases might revea_
information on the respective mechanisms of the reactions.

STEREOSELECTIVITY IN CYSTEINE-CONJUGATE β-LYASE

Several cysteine-conjugates are metabolised by β-lyase
to produce thiols, ammonia and pyruvate (Tateishi, 1983).
Cytosolic β-lyases have been isolated from the kidney,
liver and from intestinal microflora. Since it has become
clear that β-lyases can play a decisive role in the
bioactivation of cysteine conjugates to nephrotoxic agents,
such as those from hexachloro-1,3-butadiene or other
halogenated alkenes, the scientific interest in this enzyme
has increased considerably (Elfarra and Anders, 1984).
As to its stereoselectivity, relatively little is known
as yet except that the natural S-configuration in the
cysteine residue is a prerequisite for cysteine-conjugates
to be a substrate of β-lyases. This fact has been used as
a tool to ascertain the role of β-lyase in the development
of nephrotoxicity by cysteine conjugates. No data are
available as yet with regard to substrate-stereoselective
effects of the non-cysteine part of thioether substrates of
β-lyase.

STEREOSELECTIVITY IN GLUCURONIDATION

β-D-glucuronic acid is an important optically active
cofactor for the microsomal UPD-glucuronyltransferases,
which catalyse the conjugation of this glucuronic acid to

substrates containing O-,N- or C-atoms.

Apart from substrate-stereoselective glucuronidation of hydroxylated hexobarbital, considerable enantioselective differences have been shown in vitro for propranolol (Vermeulen, 1986), fenoterol (Koster et al, 1986) and oxazepam (Table 2) (Sisenwine et al, 1982). Some detergents (e.g. Triton X-100) were found to inhibit glucuronidation in dog liver microsomes and caused a substantial decrease in stereoselectivity, whereas others (e.g. Brij 35) stimulated the glucuronidation without affecting stereoselectivity. Apparently, changes in lipid or membrane environment may influence the stereoselectivity of this type of biotransformation reaction. In vivo, enantioselectivity is often less pronounced. It is conceivable that such differences may be a result of other competing stereoselective reactions or of biliary excretion of glucuronides, subsequent enterohepatic circulation and de-/reconjugation in the intestine and/or intestinal mucosa. The lack of an in vivo - in vitro correlation as well as the observed species dependent variations in stereoselectivity considerably complicates the selection of a proper model system for glucuronidation in humans. It is intriguing to speculate that the species dependent variations in stereoselectivity are related to varying populations of glucuronyltransferase isoenzymes, each possibly exhibiting a high stereoselectivity. Recently, support for this hypothesis was obtained by studies in which the influence of more or less selective inducers on the formation of two diastereomeric glucuronides from racemic oxazepam in hepatic microsomes of rabbits was

Table 2. In vitro glucuronidation of oxazepam-enantiomers (nmol/hr/g liver).

SPECIES	S (+)	R(-)	RATIO S/R
Rhesus monkey	238	596	0.4
Dog	826	43	19.1
Miniature swine	41	29	1.4
Rabbit	178	92	1.9
Rat	424	22	19.3

investigated (Yost and Finley, 1985). 3MC, β-naphthoflavone (usually seen as inducers of a so-called GT_1-isoenzyme) and ethanol produced a large increase in enantioselectivity, whereas inducers of the GT_2-isoenzyme, such as PB only increased oxazepam glucuronidation activity without affecting enantioselectivity. Inducers of forms other than GT_1 and GT_2, such as trans-stilbene oxide and clofibric acid generally caused increases coupled with increases in R/S ratios. Measurement of enantiomeric selectivity in the glucuronidation of racemic oxazepam was suggested to be a useful tool to characterise the nature and selectivity of inducers of the glucuronyltransferase system (Yost and Finley, 1985). Possible racemization of oxazepam in aqueous solution, however, is a complicating factor in using the compound for this purpose.

STEREOSELECTIVITY IN SULPHATE CONJUGATION

Until recently, no evidence was available for stereoselective sulphate conjugation. Generally speaking, conclusions regarding stereoselective sulphation in vivo are difficult to draw, because of the fact that competition exists between (stereoselective) glucuronidation and sulphation of the same substrates. Recently, however, stereoselective sulphation of 4'-hydroxypropranol enantiomers was demonstrated in vitro in hepatic tissue of various species (Christ and Walle, 1985). Enantiomeric (-/+)-4'-hydroxypropranolol sulphate ratios varied from 1.07 in the rat to 0.73 in the dog to 0.62 in the hamster. Both the species-dependent preference as well as the degree of apparent stereoselectivity may be due to the activity of multiple sulphotransferase isoenzymes present in the supernatant preparations. At least three isoenzymes have been isolated from rat liver.

Stereoselective sulphate conjugation may be of great therapeutic importance, if it also applies to phenolic drugs such as adrenergic antagonists, e.g. labetolol, and adrenergic agonists, e.g. salbutamol and fenoterol.

METABOLIC INVERSION OF CONFIGURATION

An interesting type of biotransformation with in some cases important consequences for pharmacological action is metabolic inversion of configuration. Epimerization of enantiomeric cyclo alkanols via a reversible enzymatic alcohol-alkanone equilibrium represents one example. Another type of substrate-and/or product stereoselective metabolic inversion reaction was observed in oral nonsteroidal anti-inflammatory drugs with a chiral 2-arylpropionic acid moiety, such as ibuprofen (2-(4-isobutylphenyl) propionic acid; Figure 12, Cox et al, 1985), cycloprofen (α-methylfluorene-2-acetic acid), benoxaprofen (4-chlorophenyl-5-benzoxazol-2-propionic acid), fenoprofen (α-methyl-3-phenoxy-benzene-acetic acid, Rubin et al, 1985). In vitro, the enantiomers with a S-(+)-configuration were found to be more potent inhibitors of the fatty acid cyclo-oxygenase system for blood platelets, a system which is often used to detect anti-inflamatory activity. On the basis of 50% inhibition, S-(+)-fenoprofen, for example, was two times more active than the racemate and about 35 times the R-(-)-enantiomer. In vivo, however, no differences were observed in the pharmacological and toxicological activities in several species. These findings were associated with a rapid and essentially complete inversion of the R-(-)-fenoprofen to the active S-(+)-enantiomer.

Figure 12. Metabolic configurational inversion of anti-inflammatory 2-arylpropionates (taken from Testa, 1986).

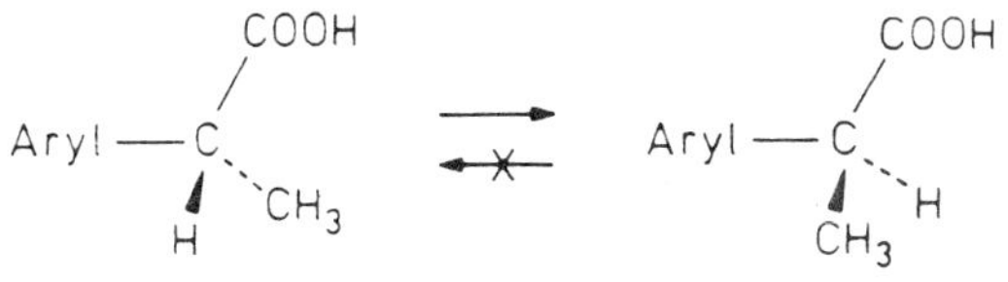

nonsteroidal anti-inflammatory 2-arylpropionates (taken from Testa, 1986).

The mechanism of the metabolic inversion is still uncertain. The involvement of lipid metabolising enzymes essentially causing the loss of the chiral center by dehydrogenation and subsequent reduction of the intermediate by an enoyl reductase that stereospecifically converts the S-enantiomer has been proposed (Hutt and Caldwell, 1983).

Recently, perfused rat liver has been used to define more clearly the role of the liver in the clearance of ibuprofen stereoisomers (Cox et al, 1985). Hepatic clearance of R-(-)-ibuprofen by chiral inversion was observed and it was about 2 times greater than the clearance due to non-inversion (oxidation and conjugation) processes. The overall clearance of the R-(-)-isomer was about 2.5 times larger than the clearance of S-(+)-ibuprofen. Interpretation of these results, however, is limited by the lack of (potentially stereoselective) plasma protein binding data.

STEREOSELECTIVITY AND MONO AMINO OXIDASE INTERACTIONS

Mono amino oxidase (MAO) is a flavine containing enzyme, localised mainly in the outer mitochondrial membrane. There is now solid evidence available for the existence of MAO in two distinct forms, commonly called MAO-A and MAO-B. Some substrates are more or less specifically oxidatively degraded by the form MAO-A, e.g. 5-hydroxytryptamine and noradrenaline, whereas others are better substrates for MAO-B, e.g. benzylamine and phenylethylamine. Selective reversible or irreversible inhibition of MAO may have important pharmacological or toxicological consequences.

Stereochemical aspects of MAO-inhibition have recently been reviewed (Strolin-Benedetti and Dostert, 1985). The phenylethyl amines, S-(+)-amilflamine and S-(+)-amphetamine have been found to be more potent and selective MAO-A inhibitors than their R-(-)-enantiomers. The reason for this has been due to a stereoselective removal of the α-hydrogen in the S-enantiomers by MAO. From representatives of the oxazolidinone series, such as cimoxatone and toloxatone, the R-isomers (with the same absolute configuration as R-(-)-noradrenaline) show the highest affinity for MAO-A. Analogues of cimoxatone, methylated at the α-position to the oxazolidinone and thus giving rise to the existence of erythro- and threo-diastereoisomers, have also been tested. Erythro-isomers had an inhibitory potency, which was comparable to that of cimoxatone. The threo-enantiomers were practically devoid of inhibitory activity. Apparently a spatial arrangement similar to that present in S-(+)-amphetamine is a prerequisite for the inhibitory potency. From these and other studies it seems clear that the active centre present in MAO-A is sensitive to stereoisomerism of the β -centre of alcohol or ether inhibitors in the oxazolidinone series, whereas the MAO-B active centre is not.

STEREOSELECTIVITY AND PREVENTION OF TOXICITY BY CYSTEINE

L-cysteine is utilised for the bio-synthesis of cosubstrates for several conjugation reactions, such as glutathione, sulphate and taurine. The unphysiological isomer D-cysteine has been used frequently to investigate mechanistic aspects of physiological processes involving cysteine.

In rats, sulphoxidation rates of L-and D-cysteine as

well as sulphation rates of the test substrate harmol to inorganic sulphate were found to be very similar, so that stereoselectivity for the amino acid seems not to play a role in these reactions (Glazenburg et al, 1984). Since D-cysteine, in contrast to the L-isomer, did not increase taurine concentration in serum, this type of stereoselectivity can be used to selectively enhance sulphate availability in vivo.

Glutathione, as the main intracellular non-protein sulphydryl, plays an important role as a co-substrate or a reductant in the detoxication of electrophilic compounds in organisms as well as in the repair of various kinds of cellular injury. Consequently, increased levels of glutathione may exert beneficial effects in some cases. Administration of L-cysteine, an obvious precursor in glutathione biosynthesis, is not ideal to increase glutathione levels, because this amino acid is rapidly metabolised and exerts extracellular toxic effects. N-acetyl-L-cysteine, which is rapidly hydrolysed to L-cysteine, more successfully promotes synthesis in vivo and is known to protect against paracetamol induced hepatoxicity. Alternatively, however, 2-alkyl- or 2-aryl-substituted thiazolidine-4-R-carboxylic acids (especially those derived from the condensation of L-cysteine with even alkyl carbon aldehydes, i.e. aldehydes that are readily metabolised to endogenous or nontoxic products) can more successfully serve as prodrugs of L-cysteine and can protect against paracetamol toxicity (Nagasawa et al, 1984). The proposed mechanism is as follows: the sulphydryl-masked prodrug form of L-cysteine in vivo, releases the amino acid intracellularly by non-enzymatic ring opening followed by solvolysis. Incorporation into glutathione and not the liberation of sulphydryl groups per se appears to be important, since analogues with 4-S-configuration, which dissociate to the unphysiological D-cysteine, were found to be totally ineffective as protective agents (Nagasawa et al, 1984).

CONCLUSIONS

This review has demonstrated that it is now becoming increasingly recognised that stereochemical factors play a significant role in the disposition and the pharmacological or toxicological action of drugs and other xenobiotics. Stereoselectivity may occur at the level of absorption, distribution, biotransformation, excretion and at the level of receptor interaction. Consequences of this for biological action in general are difficult to predict because of the complex regulation of the biological activities.

In recent years, however, considerable progress has been made in the elucidation of stereochemical mechanisms of several important biotransformation enzymes, despite the fact that their multiplicity and widely varying substrate-selectivities as well as secondary metabolism (which in itself can be stereoselective) complicate considerably the study of such mechanisms. In principle, the same factors complicate the correlation of data on stereoselective effects obtained in vitro with those obtained in vivo, even though it concerns the same species. Prediction of stereoselective effects from one species to another or from one drug to another is even more difficult.

Nevertheless, as this review has demonstrated in some cases, further insight into stereochemical mechanisms at a molecular level (i.e. at the level of binding of substrate molecules to active (or binding) sites of isolated and purified (iso-)enzymes (or other proteins) provided a simplified model or a working hypothesis that might help predict stereoselective processes. Progress in research along these lines will be most promising, not only from an academic but also from a more practical view.

From a drug development point of view it is important to stress that knowledge of stereoselective effects at different levels of drug disposition should be obtained as early as possible. Without this knowledge it is almost impossible to interpret the pharmacodynamics and pharmacokinetics of a chiral drug. Whether this should lead to the development of pure stereoisomers as drugs or other biologically active compounds is a question, which is difficult to answer in general terms. Neglecting the existence of stereoselectivity in this regard, however, can lead to studies which have been qualified as "expensive highly sophisticated pseudoscientific nonsense" (Ariens, 1984).

REFERENCES

Albert, A., "Steric Factors" (1985). In : "Selective Toxicity". The physicochemical basis of therapy". 7th Ed., (Ed. A. Albert) p.490.

Arias, I.M. and Jakoby, W.R. eds. (1976). "Glutathione, Metabolism and Function". Raven Press, New York.

Ariens, E.J. (1983). In : "Stereochemistry and biological activity of drugs". (Eds. E.J. Ariens, W. Soudijn and P.B.W.M.M. Timmermans). Blackwell, Oxford, p.11.

Ariens, E.J. (1984). Eur. J. Clin. Pharmacol, 26, 663.

Armstrong, R.N., Kedzierski, B., Levin, W. and Jerina, D.M.
    (1981). J. Biol. Chem, 256, 4726.
Armstrong, R.N., Levin, W. and Jerina, D.M. (1980). In
    "Microsomes, Drug Oxidations and Chemical
    Carcinogenesis" (Eds. M.J. Coon, A.H. Conney, R.W.
    Estabrook, H.V. Gelboin, J.R. Gillette and P.J.
    O'Brien.). Academic Press, New York.
Armstrong, R.N., Levin, W., Ryan, D.E., Thomas, P.E., Duck
    Mah, H. and Jerina, D.M. (1981). Biochem. Biophys. Res.
    Commun, 100, 1077.
Baillie, T.A. (1981). Pharmacol Rev, 33, 81.
Beld, A.J. and Zwanenburg, B. (1986). In : "Innovative
    Approaches in Drug Research". (Ed. A.F.Harms). Elsevier
    Science Publishers B.V., Amsterdam, p.331.
Belluci, G., Berti, G., Bianchini, R., Cetera, P. and
    Mastrorilli, E. (1982). J. Org. Chem, 47, 3105.
Boobis, A.R., Murray, S., Hampden, C.E. and Davies, D.S.
    (1985). Biochem. Pharmacol, 34, 65.
Christ, D.D. and Walle, T. (1985). Drug Metab. Dispos, 13,
    380.
Cobb, D., Boehlert, C., Lewis, D. and Armstrong, R.N.
    (1983). Biochem, 22, 805.
Cook, C.E. (1985). TIPS, 6, 302.
Cox, J.W., Cox, S.R., Van Giessen, G. and Ruwart, M.J.
    (1985). J. Pharmacol. Exp. Ther, 232, 636.
Dayer, P., Gasser, R., Gut, J., Kronbach, T., Roberts, G.-
    M., Eichelbaum, M. and Meyer, U.A. (1984). Biochem.
    Biophys. Res. Comm, 125, 374.
Dayer, P., Leemann, T., Gut, J., Fronbach, T., Kupfer, A.,
    Francis, R. and Meyer, U. (1985). Biochem. Pharmacol,
    34, 399.
Dohn, D.R., Quebbeman, A.J., Borch, R.F. and Anders, M.W.
    (1985). Biochemistry, 24, 5137.
Distlerath, L.M., Reilly, P.E.B., Martin, M.V., Wilkinson,
    G.R. and Guengerich, F.P. (1985). In : "Microscomes and
    Drug Oxidations" (Eds. A.R. Boobis, J. Caldwell, F. De
    Matteis and C.R. Elcombe). Taylor and Francis, London,
    p.380.
Elfarra, A.A. and Anders, M.W. (1984). Biochem. Pharmacol,
    33, 3729.
Frigerio, A., Cavo-Briones, M. and Belverdere, G. (1976).
    Drug Metab. Rev, 5, 197.
Glazenburg, E., Jekel-Halsema, I.M.C., Baranczyk-Kuzma.,
    Krijgsheld, K.R. and Mulder, G.J. (1984). Biochem.
    Pharmacol, 33, 525.
Hammock, B., Ratcliff, M. and Schooley, D.A. (1980). Life
    Sci, 27, 1635.
Hanzlik, R.P., Edelman, M., Michaely, W.J. and Scott, G.

(1976). J. Am. Chem. Soc, 98, 1952.
Hutt, A. and Caldwell, J. (1983). J. Pharm. Pharmacol, 35, 693.
Jerina, D.M., Ziffer, H. and Daly, J.W. (1970). J. Am. Chem, Soc, 92, 1056.
Jerina, D.M., Michand, D.P., Feldman, R.J., Armstrong, R.N., Vatsis, K.P., Thakker, D.R., Yagi, Y., Thomas, P.E., Ryan, D.E. and Levin, W. (1982). In : "Fifth International Symposium on Microsomes and Drug Oxidations". (Eds.R. Sato and K. Kato,), Japan Scientific Societies Press, p.195.
Jerina, D.M., Sayer, J.M., Yagi, H., Van Bladeren, P.J., Thakker, D.R., Levin, W., Chang, R.L., Wood, A.W. and Conney, A.H. (1985). In : Microsomes and Drug Oxidations". Taylor and Francis, London, p.310.
J. Liq. Chromatogr. 9 (1986). Special Issue.
Koster, A.S., Frankhuyzen-Sierevogel, A.C. and Mentrop, A. (1986). Biochem. Pharmacol, 35, 1981.
Kronbach, T., Dayer, P. and Meyer, U.A. (1985). Abstract 17th Ann. Meeting of USGEB/USSBE, Geneva, Experienta in press.
Kupfer, A., Roberts, R.K., Schenker, S. and Branch, R.A. (1981). J. Pharmacol. Exp. Ther, 218, 193.
Light, D.R., Waxman, D.J. and Walsh, C. (1982). Bichemistry, 21, 2490.
Mangold, J.B. and Abdel-Monem, M.M. (1980). Biochem. Biophys. Res. Commun, 96, 333.
Miyano, K., Fujii, Y. and Toki, S. (1980). Drug Metab. Dispos, 8, 104.
Miyano, K., Ota, T. and Toki, S. (1981). Drug Metab. Dispos, 9, 60.
Morgenstern, R., Guthenberg, C., Mannervik, B. and Depierre, J.W. (1983). FEBS, 160, 264.
Nagasawa, H.T., Coon, D.J.W., Muldoon, W.P. and Zera, R.T. (1984). J. Med. Chem, 27, 591.
Oesch, F. (1979). In : "Progress in Drug Metabolism", Vol 3 (Eds. J.W. Bridges and L.F. Chasseaud). Wiley, Chichester, p.253.
Rosenkranz, B., Fisher, C., Jacobsen, P., Pedersen, K., Frohlich, J.C. (1983). Eur. J. Clin. Pharmacol, 24, 231.
Rubin, A., Knadler, M.P., Ho, P.P.K., Bechtol, L.D. and Wolen, R.L. (1985). J. Pharm. Sci, 74, 82.
Sayer, J.M., Yagi, H., van Bladeren, P.J., Levin, W. and Jerina, D.M. (1985). J. Biol. Chem, 260, 1630.
Sisenwine, S.F., Tio, C.O., Hadley, F.V., Lin, A.L., Kimmel, H.B. and Ruelius, H.W. (1982). Drug Metab. Dispos, 10, 605.

Simonye, M., Fitos, I. and Visy, J. (1986). TIPS, 7, 112.
Strolin-Benedetti, M. and Dostert, P. (1985). TIPS, 6, 246.
Tateishi, M. (1983). Drug Metab. Rev, 14, 1207.
Testa, B. and Jenner, P. (1980). In : "Concepts in Drug Metabolism", Part A, (Eds. P. Jenner and B. Testa) Marcel Dekker Inc. New York, p.75.
Testa, B. (1986a). TIPS, 7, 60.
Testa, B. (1986b). Xenobiotica, 16, 265.
Van Bladeren, P.J., van der Gen, A., Breimer, D.D. and Mohn, G.R. (1979). Biochem. Pharmacol, 28, 2521.
Van Bladeren, P.J., Breimer, D.D., van Huijgenvoort, I.A.T.C.M., Vermeulen,, N.P.E. and van der Gen, A. (1981). Biochem. Pharmacol, 30, 2499.
Van Bladeren, P.J., Vyas, K.P., Sayer, J.M., Ryan, D.E., Thomas, P.E., Levin, W. and Jerina, P.M. (1984). J. Biol. Chem, 259, 8966.
Van der Graaff, M., Vermeulen, N.P.E., Joeres, R.P. and Breimer, D.D. (1983). Drug Metab. Dispos, 11, 489.
Van der Graaf, M. (1985). "Characterisation and Prediction of in vivo Oxidative Drug Metabolising Enzyme Activity", PhD Thesis, University of Leiden.
Van der Graaf, M., Vermeulen, N.P.E., Hofman, P.H., Breimer, D.D., Knabe, J. and Schamber, L. (1986). Biomed. Mass Spectrom, 12, 464.
Van Ginneken, C.A.M., Rodriques de Miranda, J.F. and Beld, A.J. (1983). "Stereochemistry and Biological Activity of Drugs". (Eds. E.J. Ariens, W. Soudijn and P.B.W.M.M. Timmermans). Blackwell Oxford, p.55.
Vermeulen, N.P.E. and Breimer, D.D. (1983). In : "Stereochemistry and Biological Activity of Drugs". (Eds. E.J. Ariens, W. Soudijn and P.B.W.M.M. Timmermans). Blackwell Oxford, p.33.
Vermeulen, N.P.E., Cauvet, J., Luijten, W.C.M.M. and van Bladeren, P.J. (1980). Biomed. Mass Spectrom, 7 413.
Vermeulen, N.P.E., Danhof, M., Setiawan, I. and Breimer, D.D. (1983). J. Pharmacol. Exp. Ther, 226, 201.
Vermeulen, N.P.E. (1986). in : "Innovative Approaches in Drug Research". (Eds. A.F. Harms). Elsevier Science Publishers B.V. Amsterdam, p.393.
Waxman, D.J., Light, D.R. and Walsh, C. (1982). Biochemistry, 21, 2499.
Wolf, C.R., Berry, P.N., Nash, J.A., Green, T. and Lock, E.A. (1984). J. Pharmacol. Exp. Ther, 228, 202.
Yost, G.S., Finley, B.L. (1985). Drug Metab. Dispos, 13, 5.

ORAL BIOAVAILABILITY OF THE LLL AND LDL DIASTEREOMERS OF PYROGLUTAMYL-(2-PYRIDYLALANYL)-PROLINEAMIDE IN RAT AND DOG.

Gary D. Bowers[1], Barry Kaye and David J.Rance[2]

Pfizer Central Research, Department of Drug Metabolism, Sandwich, Kent, U.K. [1] Present address : Glaxo Group Research (Greenford), Greenford, Middlesex, U.K.[2] To whom correspondence should be addressed.

INTRODUCTION

Pyroglutamyl-(2-pyridylalanyl)-prolineamide (P;I), a synthetic analogue of the tripeptide thyrotropin releasing hormone (TRH ; II), is a 1:1 mixture of diastereomers, one of which (P-LLL) is believed to have the "natural" stereochemistry (as in TRH) while the other (P-LDL) has the "unnatural" configuration. The in vitro and in vivo metabolism of (^{14}C)-P was investigated, the compound being labelled in the D and L pyridylalanine residues. In addition, the oral bioavailability of the intact peptides P-LLL and P-LDL was determined from their urinary excretion following oral and intravenous administration to rat and dog.

I; R = - CH₂—pyridyl ; P (1:1 mixture of P-LLL and P-LDL)
* position of ^{14}C atom

II; R = - CH₂—imidazole ; TRH

RESULTS AND DISCUSSION

Assessment of the in vitro stability of (^{14}C)-P (initial concn. 10μg/ml) showed that the P-LLL component was completely degraded within 0.5h at 37° in rat plasma but was stable (for 16h) in dog plasma; a similar species difference has previously been noted for the metabolism of TRH (Brewster and Waltham, 1981) which has LLL configuration. The degradation of P-LLL in rat plasma contrasts with the reported stability of other TRH analogues in which L-histidine is replaced by alternative L-amino acids (e.g. ornithine, arginine; Oliver et al, 1978). P-LDL was not degraded in plasma from either species so that contrary to the situation with the LDL isomer of TRH, which is unstable in rat serum (Oliver et al, 1978), substitution of D- for L-pyridylalanine apparently conferred stability towards plasma enzymes. Urine was the principal route of excretion (> 75% dosed radioactivity) following intravenous dosing of (^{14}C)-P to rats and dogs (Table 1).

Table 1. Excretion of radioactivity for rats and dogs over five days following administration of pyroglutamyl-(2-pyridylalanyl)-prolineamide as a 1:1 mixture of diastereomers (LLL and LDL)

Sample	RAT		DOG	
	Oral (40mg/kg)	Intravenous (1mg/kg)	Oral (40mg/kg)	Intravenous (0.1mg/kg)
Urine	28.4	76.3	36.9	85.1
Faeces	52.8	9.1	47.7	8.0
Carcass	2.6	7.6	N.D.	N.D.
Total	83.8	93.0	84.6	93.1

N.D. indicates not determined
Results expressed as percentages of dosed radioactivity; values for rat are mean (n=3)

The differences in stability of the two isomers to metabolism in vitro correlated with their apparent stability in vivo, with urinary recovery of intact P-LLL and P-LDL comprising 16% and 72% of the isomer doses

respectively in rat, and 58% and 72% respectively in dog
(Figure 1). After oral administration, urine contained a
similar proportion of the dose in rat (28%) and dog (37%),
but whereas urinary radioactivity for rat comprised mainly
pyridylalanine, in dog urine there were much larger
proportions of the intact peptides.

Comparison of the oral and intravenous data (Figure 1)
indicated that both P-LLL and P-LDL had appreciable oral
bioavailability in dog (21-24%) but this was much lower in
rat (4%). TRH itself has higher oral bioavailability in dog
(up to 12.6%) than rat (up to 1.5%) (Yokohama et al,
1984a), and the same is true for γ-butyrolactone-γ-
carbonyl-L-His-L-ProNH$_2$ (DN1417), a TRH analogue which is
more resistant to metabolism, for which the corresponding
values for bioavailability were 10% and 1% respectively
(Yokohama et al, 1984b). For both species, the oral
bioavailability of P-LLL is similar to that of P-LDL which
suggests that the absorption characteristics of these
molecules are not affected by their stereochemical
differences; this may imply that both isomers are absorbed
by a passive diffusion, as is the case for DN1417, rather
than the active transport process described for TRH
(Yokohama et al, 1984a, b).

Figure 1. Calculation of oral bioavailability of P-LLL and
P-LDL in rat and dog from urinary excretion of intact
peptides following oral (open bars) and intravenous
(hatched bars) administration

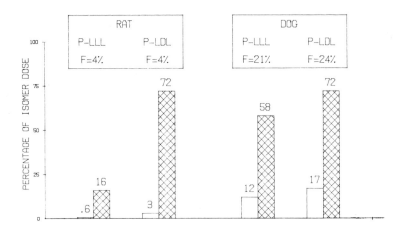

ORAL BIOAVAILABILITY OF P-LLL AND P-LDL
IN RAT AND DOG

In both rat and dog, urinary excretion of pyridylalanine as a proportion of dosed radioactivity was somewhat higher following oral compared to intravenous dosing suggesting that some of it was produced presystemically. Although first pass metabolism may contribute to the limited oral bioavailability, particularly for the P-LLL component in the rat, the major determinant is likely to be the inherently poor absorbability of these polar molecules. Thus, the species difference between rat and dog in the oral bioavailability of TRH and its analogues probably reflects a difference in absorption.

ACKNOWLEDGEMENT

The authors acknowledge Mr. A.R. Mollatt and Mr. V. F. Voss for the synthesis of (^{14})-P.

REFERENCES

Brewster, D. amd Waltham, K. (1981). Biochem. Pharmacol. 30, 619.

Oliver, C., Gillioz, P., Giraud, P. and Conte-Devolx, B. (1978). Biochem. Biophys. Res. Comm. 84, 1097.

Yokohama, S., Yasmashita, K., Toguchi, H., Takeuchi J., and Kitamori, N. (1984a). J. Pharm. Dyn. 7, 101.

Yokohama, S., Yoshioka, T. and Kitamori, N. (1984b). J. Pharm. Dyn. 7, 527.

CYTOCHROME P-450 DEPENDENT DENITROSATION OF DIPHENYLNITROSAMINE: A POSSIBLE BIOACTIVATION PATHWAY

K.E.Appel[1], S. Gorsdorf[1], T.Scheper[1], H.H. Ruf[2], M.Schoepke[1] C.S.Ruhl[1] and A.G. Hildebrandt[1]

[1]Max von Pettenkofer Institute, German Federal Health Office, D-1000 Berlin 33, F.R.G and 2 Institute for Physiological Chemistry, University of the Saarland, D-6650 Homburg, F.R.G.

INTRODUCTION

Nitrosodiphenylamine (NDphA) possesses no oxidizable hydrogens on the carbon atoms in α-position to the N-nitroso function. Therefore the molecule is not susceptible to the generallly accepted oxidation bioactivation pathway of N-nitrosamines. Based on earlier studies in rats and mice, NDphA had been classified as a non-carcinogen (Argus et al. 1961; Druckrey et al. 1967; Boyland et al. 1968). However, more recent studies have shown that it induced transitional cell carcinomas in the bladders of rats and lung adenomas when painted on the skin of hairless mice (Cardy et al. 1979; Iversen 1980). NDphA failed to induce DNA repair in rat hepatocytes, was non-mutagenic in both mammalian and microbial cells and did not induce transformation in mammalian cells (Jones et al. 1980). However, NDphA was recently shown to be active in the induction of morphological transformation of hamster embryo cells (Schuman et al. 1981). In addition, it could be demonstrated that NDphA was mutagenic to TA98 when norharman was present (Wakabayashi et al. 1981).

In order to evaluate the mechanism by which NDphA might exert its toxic effects, its metabolism was investigated and the compound was tested for induction of DNA damage with the alkaline elution assay in rat heptaocytes and Chinese hamster V79 cells.

RESULTS AND DISCUSSION

Figure 1 represents the elution profiles of rat hepatocyte DNA after treatment with NDphA at different doses. 1mM NDphA led to a significantly increased elution rate of the DNA indicating that NDphA by itself or a metabolite produced DNA single-strand breaks. This is in accordance with the results of Bradley et al. (1982)

Figure 1. Elution of rat hepatocyte DNA after treatment with NDphA at different doses:

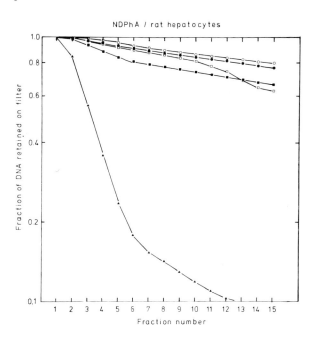

o control, □ 500 μM N-nitroso-di-n-butylamine (positive control), ● 300 μM NDphA, ■ 600 μM NDphA, ▲ 1 mMNDphA. Each profile represents the mean value of two equally treated samples (treated cells). The alkaline elution assay was performed according to Kohn et al. (1981) with modifications. Isolated hepatocytes were cultured in 5 cm dia. Nunclon plastic Petri dishes in the same medium as V79 cells and did not attach to these dishes during the 2 hour incubation period with the test compound.

In order to clarify if the unaltered molecule or a metabolite produced DNA damage, NDphA was tested in Chinese hamster V79 cells which do not possess measurable microsomal monooxygenase activities. In this system, all doses of NDphA employed (0.3 - 3.0 mM) did not lead to any detectable DNA damage. With respect to the chemical structure, reductive denitrosation (Appel et al. 1980, Appel and Graf 1982; Appel et al. 1986) and ring-hydroxylation might be the main metabolic pathways of

NDphA. Thus NDphA (1 mM) was incubated with liver microsomes from NMR1 mice pretreated with phenobarbital (PB) in order to determine the metabolites resulting from these pathways. Besides the parent compound, three metabolites were found one of which is diphenylamine (DphA). The two other metabolites are suspected to be 4-hydroxydiphenylamine and its oxidised product, the corresponding quinoneimine. When DphA was incubated with liver microsomes the ring-hydroxylated metabolite and the corresponding quinoneimine were also found to have identical retention times and UV spectra. This indicates that both metabolites derive from the DphA structure.

When testing DphA in V79 cells, the single-strand breaks observed could not be related directly to the substance. Obviously they strictly correlated with the DphA-induced cytotoxity as was evaluated by trypan blue exclusion. Also nitrite or nitrate up to 1 mM were unable to produce DNA damge in V79 cells under experimental conditions. However, DphA was unable to produce single-strand breaks in rat hepatocytes (Gorsdorf et al., in preparation).

N-hydroxylation, not ring-hydroxylation, is recognised as the initial step in the bioactivation of carcinogenic arylamines, although the nature of the ultimate carcinogen, possibly a free radical or a nitrenium ion, which will lead to DNA-adducts and DNA damage, is still under debate (Frederick et al. 1985; Lai et al. 1985; Moller et al. 1984; Stier et al. 1982).

Therefore, the N-hydroxy-derivative of DphA may be a potential metabolite which may explain the toxic effects of NDphA as e.g. carcinogenesis, morphological transformation of hamster embryo cells and DNA single strand breaks in rat hepatocytes. This possible metabolite, however, has not yet been detected by us in microsomal incubations. However, from studies of Alexander et al. (1965) it seems likely that N-hydroxylation of DphA might occur. Although these authors were also unable to detect this metabolite in the urine of rats or rabbits under the conditions used, oral administration of DphA to a single cat caused considerable methaemoglobin formation which might be indicative of the formation of the N-hydroxyderivative. Administration of diphenylhydroxylamine (DphAOH) produced severe cyanosis in the rat, indicating methaemoglobin production. This indirect evidence suggests that DphA may be partially metabolised via DphAOH. We have therefore synthesised this putative metabolite for testing in the same system. As can be seen from Figure 2. DphAOH is an active agent in producing DNA single-strand breaks in V79

Figure 2. Elution profiles of Chinese hamster V79 DNA after treatment with DphAOH at different doses:

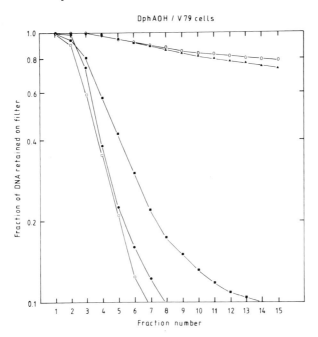

DphAOH / V 79 cells

o control, □ 100 μM MNNG, ▲ 300 μM DphAOH.
■ 600 μM DphAOH, ● 1 mM DphAOH.

o control, □ 100μM MNNG (positive control), ▲ 300 μM NDphA,
■ 600 μMDphAOH, ● 1 mM DphAOH. Results are the means of
two equally treated samples . V79 cells were grown as a
monolayer culture in 25 cm² Nunclon flasks in Earle's MEM
supplemented with 10% heat-inactivated fetal calf serum,
penicillin (100 units/ml) and streptomycin (100 μg/ml) at
37° C, 5% CO_2 and a 100% humidified atmosphere. Cells were
treated with the test compound for 2 h at 37° C.

cells.
    The mechanism by which the substance is able to produce
this genotoxic effect is not known. Covalent binding
through the intermediary formation of a nitrenium ion in
analogy to primary aromatic amines seems to be unlikely
from a chemical standpoint but cannot be fully excluded.
The nitrenium ion (if formed at all) would be very stable
with respect to the chemical nature of the secondary aryl
amine. A possible explanation comes from the observation
that after incubation of DphAOH with microsomes and NADPH,
an ESR spectrum was obtained (Figure 3) with ESR lines
being identical to those obtained with the native

diphenylnitroxide. Further investigations showed, however, that the formation of the nitroxide radical is not due to enzymatic catalysis but rather to an autoxidation process. It was shown by Nakayama et al. (1983) that autoxidation of N-hydroxymetabolites of naphthylamine and aminoazo dyes generated reactive oxygen species like hydrogen peroxide and the superoxide anion radical and a good parallelism was found between the active oxygen formation and convertibility to free radicals suggesting a possible role of free radicals in aromatic amine carcinogenesis. Furthermore it was shown that DNA lesions could be detected in cultured human fibroblasts induced by active oxygen species generated from N-hydroxy-2-naphthylamine (Kaneko et al. 1984; Kaneko et al. 1985).

Figure 3. ESR spectrum (A) obtained after incubation of DphAOH (1 mM) with rat liver microsomes (PB-pretreated, 24 mg prot./ml; 2.3 nmol P-450/mg) and NADPH (1 mM).

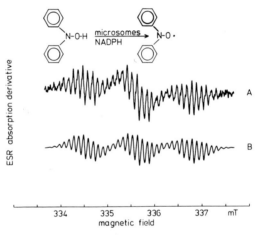

After 5 min incubation, the ESR spectrum was recorded (gain 4×10^4). After 30 min, 3 µl of an unknown concentration of the diphenylnitroxide radical was added and the spectrum (B) was recorded (gain 1×10^3). ESR was measured with a Varian E-spectrometer at $22°C$ (microwave frequency 9.5 GHz, power 2mW, modulation amplitude 40µT). ESR spectra were stored on-line in a digital computer (Data General Nova) for baseline corrections and double integrations.

Therefore the autoxidation process of DphAOH may lead to H_2O_2, O_2-, and the nitroxide radical. If it occurs in the nucleus of the cell, thus in the absence of protective enzymes like superoxide dismutase and catalase, the reactive oxygen species formed might lead to the observed genotoxic effects. Mello Filho et al. (1984) concluded from their results that the formation of DNA single strand breaks produced by H_2O_2 is mediated by hydroxyl radicals formed when H_2O_2 reacts with chromatin-bound Fe^{2+} according to a Fenton-like reaction. In this sense, denitrosation of NDphA would represent a bioactivation rather than an inactivation pathway. (Figure 4). The relatively weak carcinogenic potential of NDphA might therefore depend on the amount of metabolic DphAOH formed reaching the nucleus. The involvement of further metabolites in the generation of these genotoxic effects cannot be excluded and is under investigation

Figure 4. Proposed scheme of metabolism of N-nitroso-diphenylamine.

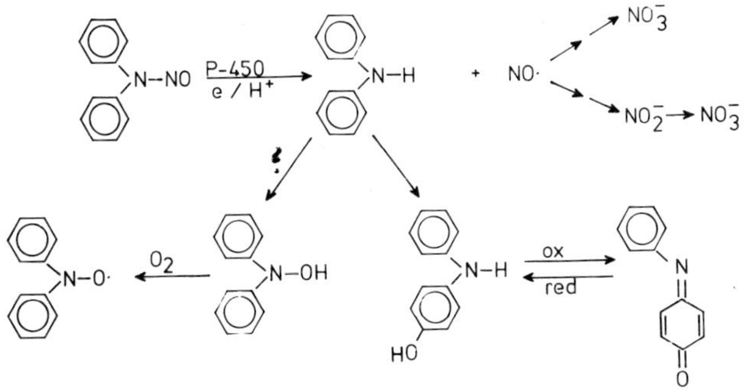

ACKNOWLEDGEMENTS

This work was supported by the Deutsche Forschungsgemeinschat. We wish to thank Mrs. Weispfenning for preparing the manuscipt.

REFERENCES

Alexander, W.E., Ryan, A.J., Wright, S.E (1965) Fd. Cosmet. Toxicol. 3, 571
Appel, K.E., Schrenk, D., Schwarz, M., Mahr, B., Kunz, W. (1980). Cancer Lett. 9, 13
Appel, K.E., Graf, H. (1982) Carcinogenesis 3, 293
Appel, K.E., Wiessler, M., Schoepke, M., Ruhl, C.S., Hildebrandt, A.G. (1986) Carcinogenesis 7,659
Argus, M.F., Hoch-Ligeti, C. (1961) J. Natl. Cancer Inst. 27, 695

Boyland, E., Carter, R.L., Gorrrod, J.W., Roe, F.J.C. (1986) Eur. J. Cancer 4, 233

Bradley, M.O., Dysart, G., Fitzsimmons, K., Harback, P., Lewin, J., Wolf, G.(1982) Cancer Res. 42, 2592

Cardy, R.H., Lijinsky, W., Hildebrandt, P.K. (1979) Ecotoxicol. Environm. Safety 3, 29

Druckrey, H., Preussmann, R., Ivankovic, S., Schmahl, D. (1967)Z. Krebsforsch. 69, 103

Frederick, C.B. Weis, C.D., Flammang, T.J., Martin, C.N., Kadlubar, F.F (1985) Carcinogenesis 6, 959

Iversen, O.H. (1980) Europ. J. Cancer 16, 695

Jones, C.A., Hubermann, E. (1980) Cancer Res. 40, 406

Kaneko, M., Nakayama, T., Kodama, M., Nagata, Ch. (1984) Gann. 75, 349

Kaneko, M., Nagata, Ch., Kodama, M. (1985) Mutat. Res. 143, 103

Kohn, K.W., Ewig, R.A.G., Erickson, L.C., Zwelling, L.A. (1981) .In: "DNA repair" (Eds. Friedberg, E.D., Hanawalt, P.C.), Marcel Dekker, New York: p379

Lai, C.C., Miller, J.A., Miller, E.C., Liem, A. (1985) Carcinogenesis 6, 1037

Mello Filho, A.C., Hoffmann, M.E., Meneghini, R. (1984) Biochem. J. 218, 273

Moller, M.E., Glowinski, I.B., Thorgeirsson, S.S (1984) Carcinogenesis 5, 797

Nakayama, T., Kimura, T., Kodama, M., Nagata, Ch. (1983) Carcinogenesis 4, 765

Schuman, R.F., Lebher+, W.B., Pienta, R.J., (1981) Carcinogenesis 2, 679

Stier, A., Clauss, R., Lucke, A., Reitz, I. (1982) "Free Radicals, Lipid Peroxidation and Cancer", (ed. McBrien D.C.H.M., Slater, T.F.) Academic Press, p 329

Wakabayashi, K., Nagao, M., Kawachi, T., Sugimura, T.(1981) Mutation Res. 80, 1

METABOLIC ACETAL SPLITTING OF BUDESONIDE - A NOVEL INACTIVATION PATHWAY FOR TOPICAL GLUCOCORTICOIDS.

Staffan Edsbacker[1], Paul Andersson[1], Claes Lindberg[1], Jan Paulson[1], Ake Ryrfeldt[1] and Arne Thalen[2]

[1]Pharmacokinetics and [2]Organic Chemistry Laboratories, Research and Development Department, AB Draco (subsidiary of AB Astra), Lund, Sweden.

INTRODUCTION

Budesonide (Pulmicort[R], Rhincort[R]) is a potent glucocorticoid, used clinically in the local treatment of skin and respiratory diseases. The drug deviates structurally from the common topical $16\alpha,17\alpha$-acetonide glucocorticoids by a new type of nonsymmetric acetal substituent (Figure 1). This chemical modification improves the topical antiinflammatory potency at least five-fold as commpared with the symmetric acetonide analogue (Brattsand et al, 1982). The symmetric $16\alpha,17\alpha$-isopropylidene-dioxy substituent, present in e.g. desonide, flunisolide and triamcinolone acetonide seems to be metabolically stable (Kripalani et al, 1975, Chu et al, 1979, Edsbaker et al, 1983). The $16\alpha,17\alpha$-butylidenedioxy substituent of budesonide, giving two epimers 22R and 22S at a 1:1 ratio, provides however sites for metabolic inactivation in the liver.

Budesonide may be pharmacokinetically characterised as a high hepatic clearance drug with no or negligible extrahepatic elimination (Ryrfeldt et al, 1982; Edsbacker, 1986). The present study was undertaken to elucidate the metabolic pathways of budesonide, focusing on the metabolic consequences of the modified acetal side chain. The drug epimers were separately studied using liver 9000g supernatant fraction from rat, mouse and man. Metabolite identification was performed with LC-MS using stable isotopes and with ^{1}H-NMR (Edsbacker, 1986).

RESULTS AND DISCUSSION

The major metabolite in human liver preparations and in plasma and urine after administration to man was 16α-hydroxyprednisolone (Figure 1) Only epimer 22R of

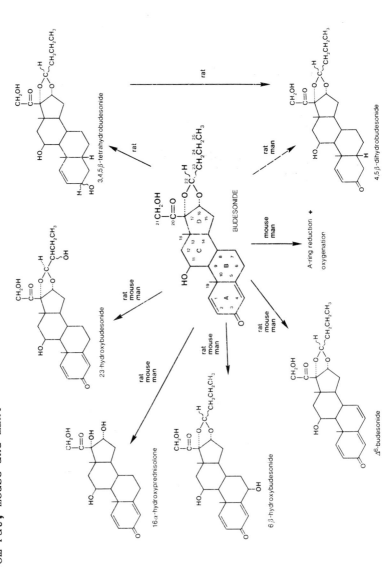

Figure 1. Suggested metabolic pathways for budesonide in liver 9000g supernatant fraction from rat, mouse and man.

budesonide is involved in this metabolic pathway, which requires NADPH, is catalyzed by microsomal enzymes and is inhibited by SKF 525-A. Liver monooxygenases generally have these features, but an oxidation reaction cannot in a simple way explain the molecular events of the biotransformation.

Budesonide, being chemically stable against hydrolysis, may theoretically be enzymatically hydrolyzed to 16α-hydroxyprednisolone and butyraldehyde. However, incubation experiments with budesonide labelled with deuterium in the acetal side chain ($(^2H_8)$-budesonide), showed that the formation of butyric acid was an intergral part of the biotransformation.

If esterase inhibitors were added to the liver preparation prior to incubation, the formation of 16α-hydroxyprednisolone was completely inhibited, and a previously unknown compound was formed in equivalent amounts. The compound was identified as the butyric acid ester of 16α-hydroxyprednisolone. Similar experiments, performed under ^{18}O-atmosphere with $(^2H_8)$-budesonide, showed that oxygen had been incorporated at the 22-carbon of budesonide. The data are in accordance with the mechanism shown in Figure 2. Atmospheric oxygen is incorporated at the 22-carbon by the liver cytochrome P-450 system. The resulting hypothetical hemiorthoester intermediate is chemically labile and will rearrange to the energetically more favourable ester isomer. Similar labile hemiorthoester intermediates are suggested to be formed in the acyl migration of glucocorticoid 17- and 21-esters (Bundgard and Hansen, 1981, Misaki et al, 1982). In the presence of liver esterase activity, the ester is instantaneously hydrolysed to 16α-hydroxyprednisolone and butyric acid. The acetal cleavage of (22R)-budesonide was especially prominent in the mouse and human livers.

The 22S-epimer of budesonide was not biotransformed by acetal side chain cleavage. Instead 23-hydroxylation of (22S)-budesonide occured, particularly in rat liver.

The metabolic pathways of budesonide in liver homogenates from rat, mouse and man is summarised in Figure 1. Apart from the pathways involving the acetal side chain, the metabolism was similar to that of other synthetic glucocorticoids (Fotherby and James, 1972). Thus oxidative metabolism predominated, 6β-hydroxybudesonide and Δ^6-budesonide being identified in all investigated species. A-ring reduction was most pronounced in the rat. $4,5\beta$-Dihydro- and $3,4,5\beta$-tetrahydrobudesonide were formed and further metabolised by oxidative pathways. In the rat, there was a marked sex difference in the budesonide

Figure 2. Suggested mechanism for the $16\alpha, 17\alpha$-acetal splitting of (22R)-budesonide. Structure in brackets denotes a postulated hemiorthoester intermediate.

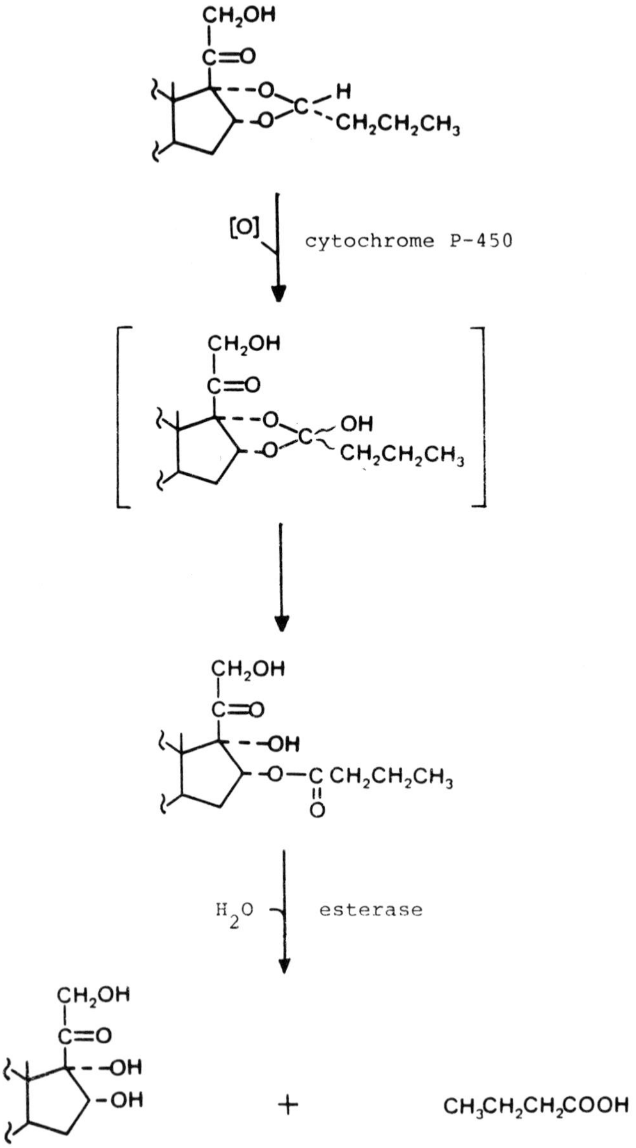

metabolism, mainly due to the much lower 6β-hydroxylase activity of the female rat. No sex difference was apparent in the mouse and human livers. When the rates and routes of budesonide metabolism were compared in the three species, mouse and man were most similar. The identified metabolites had reduced glucocorticoid activity as compared with budesonide (Dahlberg et al, 1984, Edsbacker, 1986)

The extensive liver biotransformation of budesonide to metabolites of low glucocorticoid activity may partly explain the favourable ratio between local therapeutic effect and systematic side effects noted for the drug in clinical studies.

REFERENCES

Brattsand, R, et al, (1982),J. Steroid Biochem., 16, 779.
Bundgard, H. and Hansen, J., (1981), Int. J. Pharm., 7, 197.
Chu, N.I., et al, (1979), Drug Metab. Disp., 7, 81.
Dahlberg, E., et al, (1984), Mol. Pharmacol., 25, 70.
Edsbacker, S., et al, (1983), Drug Metab. Disp., 11, 590
Edsbacker, S., (1986), "Studies on the Metabolic Fate and
    Human Pharmacokinetics of Budesonide"
    (Thesis), Studentlitteratur, Lund.
Fotherby, L. and James, F., (1972) in "Advances in Steroid
    Biochemistry and Pharmacology" (Eds. Briggs, M.H.,
    and Christie, G.A.), Academic Press, New York, p67
Kripalani, K.J., et al, (1975), J. Pharm. Sci., 64, 1351.
Misaki, T., et al, (1982), Yakuzaigaku, 42, 92.
Ryrfeldt, A., et al, (1982), J. Steroid Biochem 10, 317.

11. Metabolism and toxicity.

METABOLISM AND MECHANISMS OF TOXICITY - AN OVERVIEW

Laurence J. King

Department of Biochemistry, University of Surrey,
Guildford, Surrey, GU2 5XH, U.K.

INTRODUCTION

In 1949, R. Tecwyn Williams in the first edition of his book "Detoxication Mechanisms" noted that his chosen title, convenient for its brevity, was not entirely true because it implied a process whereby the toxicity of a chemical compound was reduced or abolished. He acknowledged that these processes could also increase the toxicity of a compound. He went on to say that, at that time, the primary objectives of most research workers in the field was to elucidate the catabolic processes of the foreign compounds and that for many of these, the relative or absolute toxicities of their metabolites were not of immediate importance, but that this was an aspect which merited more attention in the future. This session, and several others at this meeting and many others elsewhere witness that this advice has been taken.

I mention R T Williams because he was not only one of the most important early pioneers in this field but he was also the teacher and mentor of Professor Dennis V. Parke, whose continued work in this field we are honouring at this meeting. By the time D.V. Parke came to write his first book, "The Biochemistry of Foreign Compounds" in 1968, the distinction between detoxication and intoxication was becoming much clearer such that in the opening chapter he gave the now classic examples presented in Figure 1. There are also numerous other examples cited throughout the book where metabolism results in increased reactivity of the molecule and is the possible cause of toxicity.

The nature of cytochrome P-450 was also becoming apparent about this time and although all the complexities of the different isoenzymes were not entirely apparent, it was being realised that the same enzyme may inactivate one compound but activate another. In this overview some of the better understood activation processes are reviewed, hopefully to provide a basis for the later more detailed contributions.

Figure 1. Detoxication and intoxication by metabolic transformations.

Detoxication: Phenobarbitone —hydroxylation→ p-Hydroxyphenobarbitone
                     (active drug)   (inactive metabolite)

Activation: Prontosil —reductive scission→ Sulphanilamide
                     (inactive "pro-drug")   (active drug)

Intoxication: Parathion —desulphuration→ Paraoxon
                     (inactive insecticide)   (active insecticide)

     In many people's minds, metabolic activation of xenobiotics is synonymous with the formation of reactive intermediates which react non-specifically with cellular nucleophiles such as nucleic acids, proteins and lipids. Such interactions have been detected as covalent binding of the reactive metabolite with these nucleophiles and this is certainly good evidence for the formation of a reactive intermediate. However, the automatic association of such covalent binding with the toxicity ultimately expressed is not valid and careful investigation is required to identify a particualr interaction as being a means of combatting the effects of reactive electrophiles and in many cells the most abundant nucleophile is glutathione which provides a means of detoxifying many of these reactive intermediates. In several instances it has now been established that the cellular glutathione has to be depleted by reaction with reactive, electrophilic intermediates before the electrophile is able to interact with the crucial target for toxicity.

THE SITE OF ACTION OF REACTIVE INTERMEDIATES.

     An important consideration with regard to where, within the cell, the tissue and the body, the reactive metabolite may act is determined by the half-life of the reactive entity. The broad possibilities are outlined in Table 1. Very reactive entitities of ultra-short half-life will not escape their site of formation and most likely will interact with the enzyme molecule that has produced it. Such entities are therefore likely to be suicide inhibitors of the activating enzyme. Progressively less reactive intermediates will travel further before interaction with a tissue component such that some may reach other organs of the body to express their toxicity. In the extreme case of the most stable intermediates, those of so-called ultra-long half-life, they may be excreted in the urine or bile and therefore may express their toxic potential in the kidney or bladder, or the small intestine.

The actual site of toxic action will also be dependent upon other pharmacokinetic and metabolic considerations. For toxicity to occur a tissue must receive a sufficient dose of the parent compound or the reactive metabolite. If the tissue is exposed to the parent compound, the activating enzyme system must be present and the expression of toxicity will be determined by the balance between enzymic activation and detoxication, either by competing metabolic transformations or protection by glutathione and glutathione-dependent enzymes such as glutathione S-transferases, glutathione peroxidase and glutathione reductase.

Table 1. Potential distribution of reactive metabolites

METABOLITE HALF-LIFE	SITE OF ACTION
Ultra-short	Site of formation - 'suicide inhibitors'
Short-lived	Within the cell of formation
Intermediate	Within neighbouring tissue and blood cells - confined to the activating organ
Long-lived	Potentially all organs of the body
Ultra-long	Potentially all organs of the body. Their accumulation in urine or bile may predispose the kidney and bladder or small intestine to toxicity.

ACTIVATION DURING PHASE I METABOLISM

Since the microsomal mono-oxygenase system incorporating cytochrome P-450 plays such an important role in the first phase of metabolism of so many lipophilic xenobiotics, it is not surprising to find that this system has been implicated in so many metabolic activation reactions. One of the features of this system is that the electrons, derived principally from NADPH, are donated to the enzyme-substrate complex one at a time. Such a mechanism provides the opportunity for the formation of radical species, which for some substrates may result in very reactive entities. However the existence of a transient radical intermediate does not automatically mean that a toxic event will result. Figure 2 shows two possible mechanisms, the concerted mechanism and the radical mechanism, by which the ultimate reactive form of cytochrome P-450, the perferryl oxygen complex ($Fe^{V}O$), may effect a normal aliphatic hydroxylation. The existence of an isotope effect for some substrates has been cited as evidence for the radical mechanism (Groves et al., 1978) but this should not be viewed as a potentially toxic reaction as the radical is constrained within the reaction site and does not have an independent existence.

In the cytochrome P-450-mediated oxidative metabolism of some substrates, for example cyclopropylamines, phenethylhydrazine and dihydropyridines, free radicals of ultra-short half-life are released. The possible reaction sequence for a dihydropyridine is outlined in Figure 3. In the reaction sequence that may be expected to lead to N-hydroxylation of the substrate, a transient nitrogen-centred radical reaction may be formed. Instead of oxygenation occuring at this centre, the radical aromatizes with the release of a proton and an ethyl radical, which reacts immediately with a pyrrole nitrogen of the cytochrome-P450 haem (De Matteis et al., 1981; Ortiz de Montellano et al., 1981). These dihydropyridines are therefore suicidal substrates of cytochromeP-450 resulting in its destruction. This interaction accounts for this destructive aspect of the toxicity of dihydropyridines but not for the associated porphyria which develops. This is attributable to the subsequent effects of the N-ethylporphyrin which is released from the cytochrome P-450 active site and is a potent inhibitor of ferrochelatase in the haem biosynthesis pathway (De Matteis et al., 1980).

The dihydropyridines provide an example of where the radical is generated in the final stages of the cytochrome P-450 oxygenation cycle, but perhaps the best known examples are those where the radical is formed at the beginning of the cycle, at the initial reductive stage. The halogenated hydrocarbons, particularly carbon tetrachloride and halothane, provide perhaps the best known examples yielding the trichloromethyl (Poyer et al., 1980)

Figure 2. Possible mechanisms of cytochrome P-450-mediated aliphatic hydroxylation.

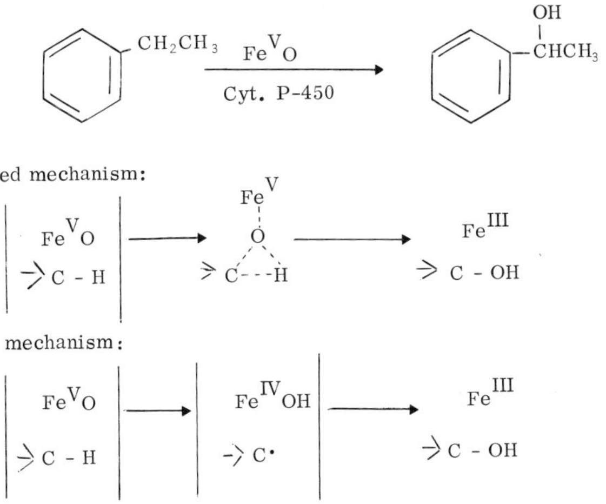

$Fe^{V}O$ represents the perferryl oxygen complex of cytochrome P-450 which effects the oxygenation reaction and Fe^{III} the normal oxidised state of the cytochrome.
$\geqslant$C-H represents the aliphatic carbon atom which is ultimately hydroxylated.

and 1,1,1-trifluoro-2-chloroethyl (Poyer et al., 1981) radicals respectively. These radicals and the subsequently produced peroxy radicals, from reaction with dioxygen, not only result in inactivation of cytochrome P-450 but also escape to initiate damage at other sites within the cell (Slater, 1972). This is consistent with them being termed short-lived radicals.

The escape of the trichloromethyl radical results in a plethora of radical initiated reactions including covalent binding to membrane lipids and proteins, cofactor depletion and initiation of lipid peroxidation (Recknagel and Glende, 1977). The process of lipid peroxidation itself also leads to other reactive entities such as hydroxyaldehydes and malondialdehyde. Such a spectrum of effects has provided a classic example of the problem of identifying which event is directly responsible for the ultimate hepatotoxicity; a problem which is not yet finally resolved. One theory that is popular at present is the failure of the endoplasmic reticulum to sequester calcium ions and the sequence of events that follows from the loss of homeostatic control of cytosolic calcium. (Moore, 1980).

Figure 3. Possible mechanism for suicidal radical formation from dihydropyridines by the perferryl oxygen complex of cytochrome P-450.

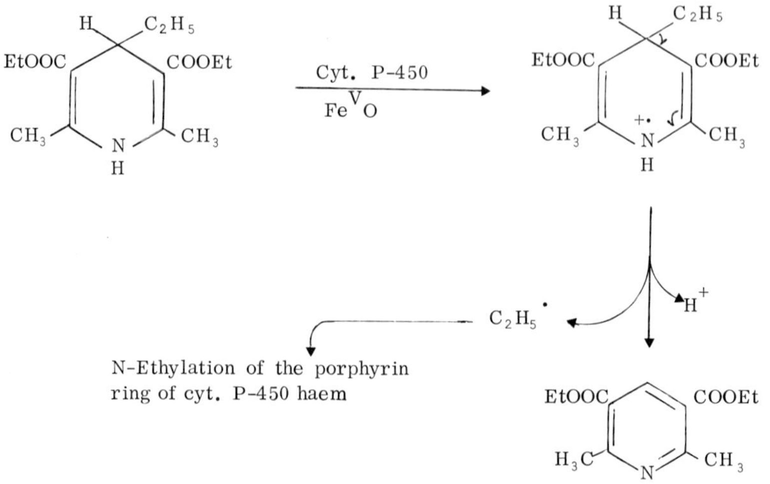

H   C₂H₅
EtOOC   COOEt

Cyt. P-450
Fe^V O

CH₃   N   CH₃
      H

H   C₂H₅
EtOOC   COOEt

CH₃   +·N·   CH₃
      H

N-Ethylation of the porphyrin
ring of cyt. P-450 haem

C₂H₅·   H⁺

EtOOC   COOEt

H₃C   N   CH₃

The metabolism of halothane and its relevance to the occasionally observed hepatoxicity is intriguing because there are two alternative cytochrome P-450-mediated pathways (Figure 4), both of which operate in vivo. The reductive pathway produces the radical intermediate, a relatively stable cytochrome P-450-carbanion complex and ultimately the volatile, exhaled metabolites of halothane (Ahr et al., 1982). By analogy with carbon tetrachloride, the radical may initiate the damage ultimately responsible for the toxicity (De Groot and Noll, 1983). Alternatively, the predominating oxidative pathway, leading to trifluoroacetic acid, proceeds via the acyl chloride intermediate which may acylate proteins resulting in the proposed immunological aspects of halothane hepatotoxicity (Vergani et al., 1980).

In addition to the formation of radicals derived from the xenobiotic, the cytochrome P-450 system may, under some circumstances, release the bound dioxygen as the superoxide anion radical, O_2^- (Khutan et al., 1978). This is claimed to be the case with the particular isoenzyme of cytochrome P-450 synthesised in response to repeated dosing with ethanol (Ingelman-Sundberg and Johansson, 1984). Again, the crucial sequence of events leading to the ultimate hepatotoxicity is not yet clearly established but a primary role for the superoxide radical is very likely.

Figure 4. Cytochrome P-450-mediated and reductive metabolism of halothane

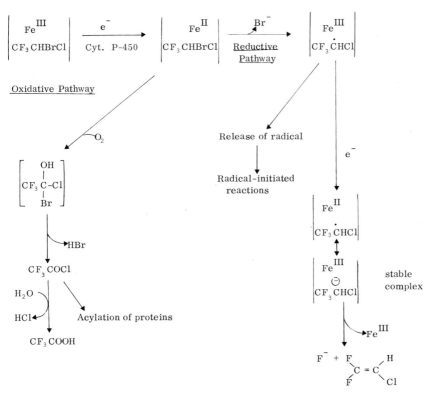

It is proposed that the superoxide radical gives rise to increased cytosolic hydrogen peroxide through the action of superoxide dismutase, and may also reduce some postulated cytosolic chelate of ferric ion to the ferrous form. The ferrous chelate supports a Fenton reaction with the hydrogen peroxide to produce the highly reactive hydroxyl radical which is likely to be the direct cause of cellular damage and lipid peroxidation, as well as initiating a radical oxidation of the ethanol.

Apart from these cytochrome P-450-mediated radical reactions, the microsomal monooxygenase system can generate other reactive products and the most common of these is the formation of epoxides in the metabolism of alkenes and aromatic compounds. The half-life and reactivity of these depend upon the structure of the substrate and range from ultra-short for ethylene oxide formed from ethylene, which is therefore a suicide substrate (Ortiz de Montellano et al., 1981), to long-lived for bromobenzene-3,4-epoxide (Lau et al., 1984). The half-life of bromobenzene-3,4-epoxide in blood, following its formation in the liver of rats, was estimated to be approx. 14 sec, sufficient time to allow it to reach most organs of the body, as the mean circulation time of the blood in rats is less than 10 secs.

ACTIVATION DURING PHASE II METABOLISM

For many years, the second phase of xenobiotic metabolism, the conjugation reactions, were viewed as true detoxication mechanisms. This still holds true for the large majority of compounds but there are notable exceptions. The metabolism of 2-acetamidofluorene (AAF) to its ultimate carcinogenic form is one well studied example. AAF may be metabolised by two major pathways. The first is the non-toxic pathway of hydroxylation of the unsubstituted aromatic ring and subsequent formation of the corresponding O-glucuronides. The second pathway leading to the toxic metabolites commences with the formation of N-hydroxy-AAF. Investigation of this substrate showed that it was not sufficiently reactive to account for the interaction with DNA. However either enzyme-mediated transfer of the acetyl group to the N-hydroxyl group or conjugation of the N-hydroxy group with sulphate provides conjugates with better leaving groups, acetate and sulphate respectively (Figure 5) (Meerman et al ., 1981). The electrophilic carbon centres are indicated by the structures of the glutathione conjugates produced in vivo (Meerman et al., 1982). The role of such conjugates in toxicity can generally only be inferred from indirect experiments because they must be generated within the cell to reach their site of action. In addition they usually react too rapidly with aqueous solvents for any in vivo experimentation.

N-Hydroxylation may also be the crucial activation reaction in the hepatotoxicity arising from paracetaamol overdose (Miner and Kissinger, 1979), The quinone-imine reactive intermediate produced formally by loss of water from the N-hydroxy metabolite, does not cause toxicity until the majority of the cellular glutathione has been depleted through conjugation to the quinone-imine (Figure 6) (Mitchell et al., 1973). This provides a good example of the protective, detoxicating role of this cellular nucleophile. The majority of this glutathione metabolite is ultimately excreted from the body as the N-acetylcysteine-S- and cysteine-S-conjugates of paracetamol (Figure 7). However not all of the metabolic products are

Figure 5.   Activation of N-hydroxy-2-acetamidoflurorene by conjugation of the N-hydroxyl group. Glutathione provides some protection by conjugating to the reactive intermediates.

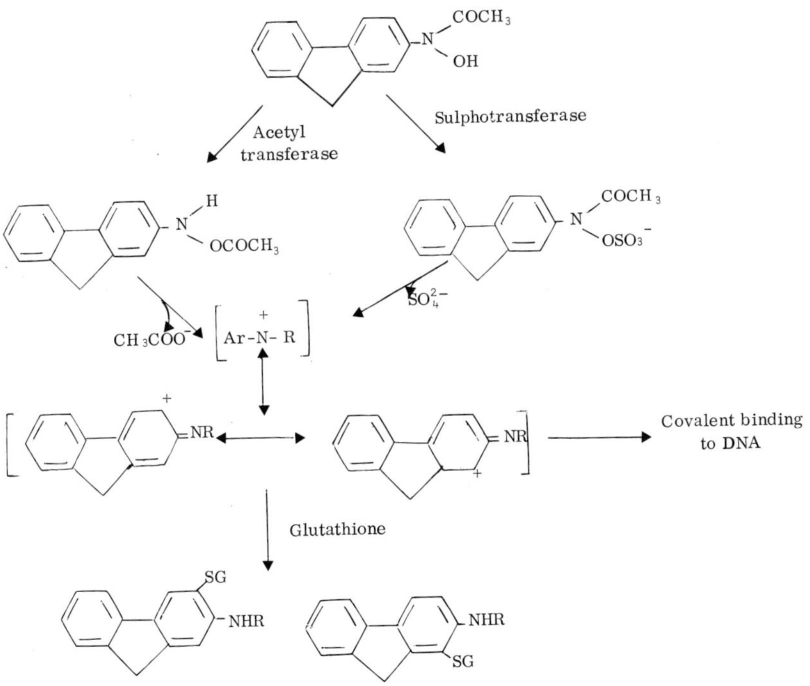

eliminated this way and a small amount of the cysteine conjugate undergoes further metabolism by, as yet, not clearly defined enzymes with β-C-S lyase activity (Warrender et al., 1985).   In the case of the paracetamol metabolite this results in the probable formation of paracetamol-3-thiol, the existence of which is inferred from the detection of the subsequent 3-thiomethyl and corresponding sulphoxide metabolites. Whether the putative thiol contributes to the toxicity of paracetamol is not known but it is now clearly established that renal C-S lyase activity is responsible for the toxicity of glutathione conjugates of a number of halogenated aliphatic hydrocarbons (Elfarra and Anders, 1984.)

This brief overview has sought to exemplify how the enzymes concerned with the metabolism of xenobiotics may in

some instances result in the formation of reactive
intermediates and metabolites which are responsible for the
toxicity caused by some xenobiotics in vivo. There are
many other equally good examples which have not been
mentioned. A feature of many of these enzymes of
xenobiotic metabolism is their relatively low substrate
specificity, necessary to enable them to cope with the
range of naturally occurring xenobiotics, let alone the
additional burden provided by man's activities in synthetic
chemistry. The benefit accruing from this broad substrate
specificity is one of cellular economy while maintaining a
wide range of protection for the cell and tissue. The
price to pay is that eventually a substrate will be found
that is unfortunatley converted to a more reactive entity
and this may ultimately result in toxicity.

Figure 6. Detoxication and activation of paracetamol.

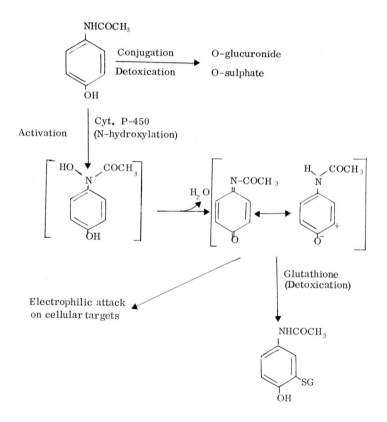

Figure 7. Further metabolism of 3-glutathionyl paracetamol.

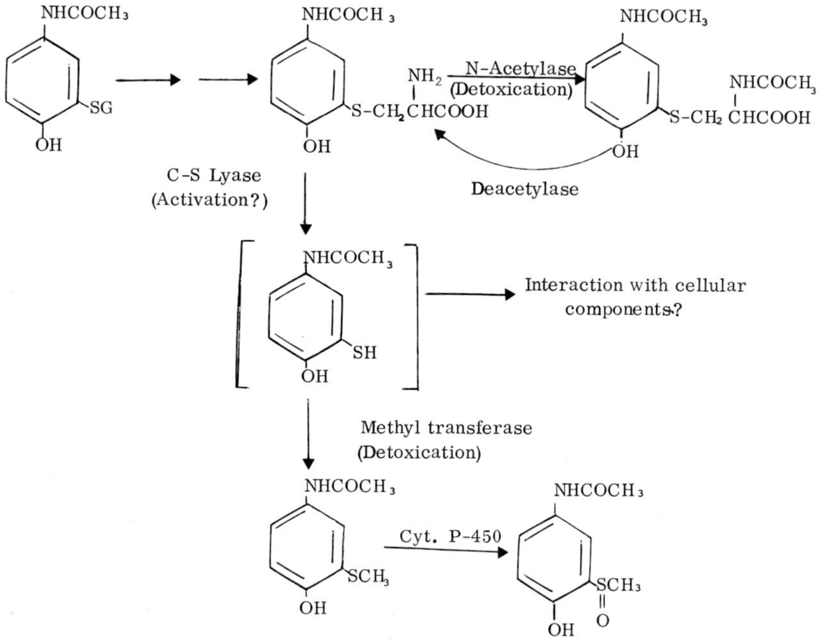

REFERENCES

Ahr, H.J., King, L.J., Nastaincyk, W. and Ullrich, V. (1982) Biochem. Pharmacol, 31, 383.

De Groot, H. and Noll, T. (1983) Hepatology, 3 601.,

De Matteis, F., Gibbs, A.H., Farmer, P.B. and Lamb, J.H. (1981) FEBS Letts,129,328

De Matteis, F., Gibbs, A.H. and Smith, A.G. (1980) Biochem. J., 189,645

Elfarra, A.A. and Anders, M.W. (1984) Biochem Pharmacol, 33, 3729

Groves, J.T., McClusky, G.A., White, R.E. and Coon, M.J. (1978) Biochem. Biophys. Res. Commun 81, 154

Ingelman-Sundberg, M. and Johansson, I (1984) J. Biol. Chem, 259, 6447

Khutan, H., Tsuji, H., Graf, H., Ullrich, V., Werringloer, J. and Estabrook, R.W. (1978) FEBS Lett, 91 343

Lau, S.S., Marks, T.J., Greene, K.E and Gillette, J.R (1984) Xenobiotica, 14, 539

Meerman, J.H.N., Boland, F.A., Ketterer, B., Srai, S.S.,

Bruins, A.P. and Mulder, G.J. (1982) Chem-Biol. Interact,39, 149.

Meerman, J.H.N., Boland, F.A. and Mulder, G.J. (1981) Carcinogenesis, 2, 413.

Miner, D.J. and Kissinger, P.T. (1979) Biochem. Pharmacol, 28 3285.

Mitchell, J.R., Jollow, D. J., Potter, W.Z., Gillette, J.R. and Brodie, B.B. (1973) J. Pharmacol. Exp. Ther. 187 211.

Moore, L., (1980) Biochem Pharmacol, 29, 2505.

Ortiz de Montellano, P.R., Beilan, M.S. and Kunze, K.L., (1981) J. Biol. Chem., 256, 6708.

Ortiz de Montellano, P.R., Beilan, H.S., Kunze , K.L., and Mico, B.A. (1981) J. Biol. Chem, 256, 4395

Parke, D.V. (1968) in "The Biochemistry of Foreign Compounds", Pergamon, Oxford, p.7

Poyer, J.L., McCay, P.B., Lai, E.K., Janzen, E.G and Davis, E.R. (1980) Biochem. Biophys. Res. Commun, 94, 1154.

Poyer, J.L. McCay, P.B., Weddle, C.C. and Downs, P.E. (1981) Biochem Pharmacol, 30 1517.

Recknagel, R.O. and Glende, E.A. (1977) in "Handbook of Physiology, Reactions to Environmental Agents" (Eds. Lee, D.H.K., Falk, H.L., Murphy, S.D and Geiger, S.R.), Williams and Wilkins, Baltimore, p.591

Slater, T.F. (1972) in "Free Radical Mechanisms in Tissue Injury", Pion Ltd., London.

Vergani, D., Mieli-Vergani, G., Alberti, A., Neuberger, J., Eddleston, A.L.W.F., Davis, M. and Williams, R., (1980), New England J. Med, 303, 66.

Warrender, A., Allen, J.M. and Andrews, R.S. (1985), Xenobiotica, 15 891.

Williams, R.T. (1949) in "Detoxication Mechanisms," John Wiley, New York, p.1.

A CHEMICAL APPROACH TO REACTIVE METABOLITES

Daniel Mansuy

Laboratoire de Chimie et Biochimie Pharmacologiques et
Toxicologiques, Unite Associee au C N R S en Developpement
Concerte avec l' INSERM, UA 400, 45 rue des Saints Peres,
75270 PARIS Cedex 06, France.

INTRODUCTION

It is now generally accepted that the hepatotoxic
effects induced by the administration of exogenous
compounds are very often not due to the parent compound
itself but to reactive metabolites formed in situ inside
the cell. In the case of hepatotoxic compounds, two kinds
of toxicity may result from the formation of reactive
metabolites: a direct toxicity which is related to the
dose of the starting exogenous compound and, especially in
man, an immunoallergic toxicity which is very rare
(typically 1 case in 10,000), very dependent on the
individual and not clearly related to the dose. Most
reactive metabolites are formed inside the cells by
cytochrome P-450-dependent monooxygenases. They are very
often strongly electrophilic and lead to irreversible
alkylations of cell macromolecules which are the first
events in the reaction chain responsible for the toxic
effects (scheme 1). In some patients suffering from
immunoallergic hepatitis after administration of certain
exogenous compounds including drugs, circulating antibodies
directed against cell organelles appear (Homberg et al.,
1985; Mackay, 1985).

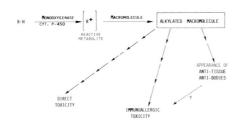

Scheme 1

Two main questions that are important in order to understand the detailed mechanisms of appearance of such toxic effects will be discussed in the following: Is it possible to interpret or to predict the nature of the reactive metabolites formed upon activation of a given exogenous compound, by considering the present knowledge of the detailed mechanisms of cytochrome P-450-dependent reactions?

How are these reactive metabolites related to toxic effects and, in particular, what are the steps involved in the appearance of immunoallergic hepatitis? Even more particularly, what are the nature of the antigens for the anti-organelle antibodies appearing in certain drug induced hepatitis?

MECHANISM OF SUBSTRATE OXIDATIONS BY CYTOCHROME P-450 AND FORMATION OF REACTIVE METABOLITES.

The catalytic cycle of dioxygen activation and substrate oxidation by microsomal cytochromes P-450 is indicated on Figure 1. The nature of all, except one, of the iron intermediates of this catalytic cycle is now clear. The only intermediate iron complex of this cycle whose structure is not completely known presently is the so called active oxygen complex, the hydroxylating species. From much indirect evidence, it seems to be a high-valent iron-oxo complex having a free radical-like reactivity. Two intermediates of this catalytic cycle are able to activate substrates. Cytochrome P-450-Fe(II) which is an electron transferring agent is involved in the reductive metabolism of halogenated compounds and nitroaromatics for instance. The active oxygen complex is the key intermediate for metabolic oxidation of almost any organic compound. This highly oxidizing species is able to insert its oxygen atom into the C - H bond of alkanes, to epoxidize alkenes and aromatic rings and to transfer its oxygen atom on heteroatoms. Most reductive or oxidative activations of substrates by cytochrome P-450 involve intermediate free radicals derived from these substrates which are more or less efficiently controlled by the iron inside the hydrophobic pocket of the hemoprotein (Mansuy and Battioni, 1985).

For instance, the reduction of reactive halogenated compounds such as CCl_4 starts with a one electron reduction of a C - Cl bond by P-450Fe(II). The CCl_3 radical formed in close proximity to the iron can either escape from the active site leading to lipid peroxidation and covalent binding to macromolecules which are mainly responsible for

Figure 1. Catalytic cycle of cytochrome P-450. The particular case of reductive and oxidative activation of halothane.

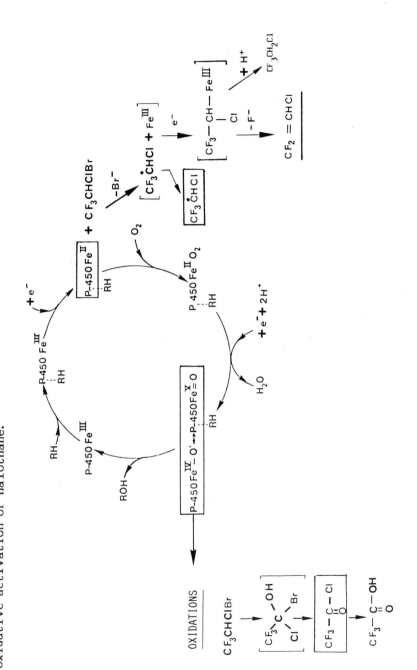

the hepatotoxic effects of CCl_4, or be reduced by the iron(II) state of cytochrome P-450 leading to $CHCl_3$ after protonation.

Aliphatic C - H bonds are activated by the $Fe(IV)-O^•$ species of the active oxygen cytochrome P-450 complex by hydrogen atom abstraction. This leads to the free radical derived from the substrate and P-450 Fe(IV)-OH. This free radical is very efficiently controlled by the iron in this high oxidation state. It has no chance to escape from the active site because of this very efficient control which is possibly due to the formation of a transient σ-alkyl iron complex. The hydroxylated metabolite is eventually formed by reductive elimination of the OH and σ-alkyl ligands which are in the cis position on the iron (eq.1).

$$\underset{}{\geq}C-H \;+\; Fe \overset{IV}{-} O^• \longrightarrow \left[Fe\overset{IV}{-}OH \;+\; {}^•C\overset{}{\leq}\right] \rightarrow \left[Fe\overset{V}{\underset{OH}{\overset{C}{\leq}}}\right] \longrightarrow Fe \overset{III}{} + \underset{}{\geq}C-OH \tag{eq.1}$$

Such hydroxylations of C - H bonds do not produce intermediate free-radicals able to give toxic effects. However, the final alcohol metabolite can be, in particular cases, a reactive metabolite. This occurs when the starting product is of the $RCHX_2$ type (X=Cl, Br or I) since the RCX_2OH metabolite rapidly loses HX leading to a reactive acylating agent R-CO-X (eq.2) This was reported to occur upon $CHCl_3$ metabolism, phosgene being the reactive metabolite in this case (Mansuy et al., 1977; Pohl et al., 1977).

$$RCX_2H + Fe\overset{IV}{-}O^• \xrightarrow{\;-Fe^{III}\;} \left[RCX_2OH\right] \xrightarrow{\;-HX\;} R - \underset{O}{\overset{\|}{C}} - X \tag{eq.2}$$

Addition of the $Fe(IV)-O^•$ species to double bonds of alkenes or aromatic rings leads to an intermediate free radical also very efficiently controlled by Fe(IV). Its intramolecular oxidation, presumably via a four membered metallocycle (Mansuy and Battioni, 1985) leads to the epoxide metabolite. This epoxide may be reactive and alkylating for cell macromolecules when it bears electron-donor substituents as in the case of chloro-olefin epoxide and aflatoxin epoxide, or when it is an arene oxide.

MECHANISM OF HALOTHANE HEPATOTOXICITY

Two patterns of hepatic damage have been encountered in patients exposed to the anaesthetic halothane. A relatively frequent benign direct toxicity with minor elevations in serum transaminases and focal hepatocellular necrosis and a severe hepatitis with a very low incidence (about 1 case in 30,000). Several features of the severe hepatitis suggest an immunological origin. Moreover, about 25% of the patients suffering from this severe hepatitis have anti-organelle antibodies called anti-LKM$_1$ since they seem directed in in vitro experiments against components of liver and kidney microsomes (Mackay, 1985).

Halothane is metabolized by a reductive and an oxidative pathway, both processes producing reactive metabolites (Figure 1) (Sipes, 1981). Cytochrome P-450 Fe(II) reduces the C -Br bond of halothane leading to the $CF_3^{\bullet}CHCl$ radical which may escape from the active site and bind covalently to cell macromolecules. This radical may also lead to metabolites derived from the possible evolution of an intermediate P-450 Fe(III)-CHClCF$_3$ complex (Ruf et al., 1984) : CF_3CH_2Cl and $CF_2=CHCl$. This reductive metabolism is favoured under hypoxic conditions and direct hepatotoxicity has been obtained in animals treated by halothane under low oxygen pressure. Nevertheless, halothane undergoes reductive metabolism in man albeit to a small degree under normal oxygen pressure.

Halothane is also oxidized by the active oxygen complex of cytochrome P-450 with insertion of an oxygen atom into its C - H bond. This gives the electrophilic acylating metabolite CF_3COCl which may bind covalently to cell macromolecules or be hydrolyzed to trifluoroacetic acid, a major metabolite of halothane in vivo (Sipes, 1981). Several indirect evidences suggest that this oxidative metabolism is involved in the severe immunoallergic hepatotoxicity observed in very rare cases after halothane administration (Davis, 1983). As far as the possible role of the anti-LKM$_1$ antibodies appearing in patients suffering from halothane-induced hepatitis is concerned, it has been shown that these antibodies bind specifically to hepatocytes from rabbits pretreated by halothane. This specific binding results in the activation of these hepatocytes towards destruction by lymphocytes (induced cytotoxicity assay) (Vergani et al, 1980).

The human liver antigen for anti-LKM$_1$ antibodies is not known so far. However, recent results in rats using antibodies raised against tri-fluoroacetylated albumin show that these antibodies bind specifically to hepatocytes from rats pretreated by halothane. Moreover, these antibodies specifically recognise two liver microsomal proteins from rats pretreated by halothane, one of them being a cytochrome P-450 (Satoh et al, 1985a and b). These data suggest that the C_3COCl reactive metabolite formed upon oxidation of halothane by rat liver binds to two microsomal proteins of rat liver and that the antigenic determinant $COCF_3$ is also present in the outer hepatocyte membrane. In man, binding of circulating anti-LKM$_1$ antibodies to hepatocytes bearing this antigen could lead to their destruction by lymphocytes. However, the direct involvement of these antibodies as a cause more than a consequence of severe halothane-induced hepatitis remains to be established.

THE CASE OF TIENILIC ACID

Tienilic acid is an uricosuric diuretic drug (See Figure 2) which has not led to any direct hepatotoxic effects but which has led as halothane, to rare cases (1 in 10,000) of immunoallergic heptotoxic effects. In some patients suffering from tienilic acid-induced hepatitis, circulating anti-organelle autoantibodies have been found. They seem directed against components of liver and kidney microsomes and have been called anti-LKM$_2$ antibodies (Homberg et al, 1985).

Metabolic Oxidation of Tienilic Acid

Tienilic acid is extensively metabolised in man and rat and its major metabolite in urine is a compound derived from the hydroxylation of its thiophene ring in position 5 (Figure 2) (Mansuy et al, 1984). This oxidative metabolism also occurs in vitro upon incubation of tienilic acid with rat or human liver microsomes in the presence of NADPH (HPLC technique with detection of radioactive metabolites from tienilic acid ^{14}C-labelled on its keto group).

Figure 2. Main metabolites of tienilic acid in man.

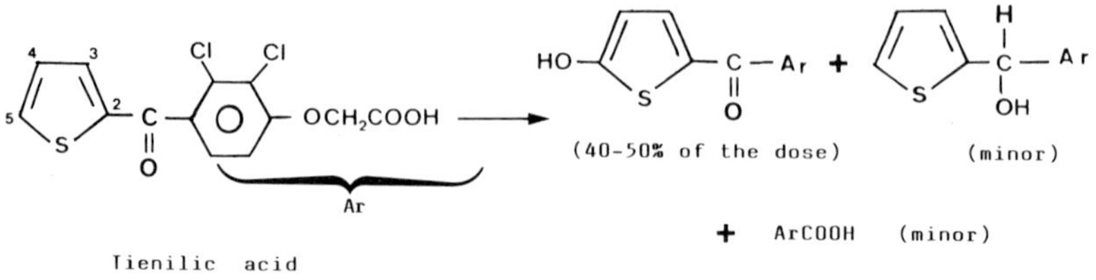

Besides the formation of 5-OH-tienilic acid which is also the major metabolic transformation of tienilic acid in vitro, covalent binding of reactive metabolites of tienilic to microsomal proteins was also observed (Dansette et al, in preparation).

Determination Of The Human Liver Antigen For Anti-LKM$_2$ Antibodies

A recent immunoblot analysis of human liver microsomes and some purified human liver cytochromes P-450, called P-450-5, P-450-8 and P-450-9 (Wang et al, 1983), using human sera containing anti-LKM$_2$ antibodies showed us that these antibodies recognised only one protein of human liver microsomes. This protein was found electrophoretically and immunologically identical to a previously purified human liver cytochrome P-450 called cytochrome P-450-8 (Beaune et al, submitted for publication). Accordingly, sera containing anti-LKM$_2$ antibodies led to immunoblot recognition patterns identical to those obtained with anti-cytochrome P-450-8 antibodies but very different to those obtained with antibodies raised against another purified human liver cytochrome P-450, called cytochrome P-450-5. Moreover, sera containing anti-LKM$_2$ antibodies as well as anti-cytochrome P-450-8 antibodies failed to recognise any component of fetal human liver microsomes which were previously shown to be devoid of cytochrome P-450-8 (Cresteil et al, 1985).

Analagous immunoblot analyses were performed with 40 sera from patients or volunteers. From the 20 tested sera from patients suffering from hepatitis and containing anti-LKM$_2$ antibodies, 12 sera recognised almost exclusively cytochrome P-450-8 in human liver microsomes. The 20 control tested sera which did not contain anti-LKM$_2$ antibodies failed to recognise cytochrome P-450-8.

These results strongly suggest that anti-LKM$_2$ antibodies are specifically directed against one protein of human liver: the cytochrome P-450-8 isoenzyme.

Nature Of The Human Liver Cytochrome P-450 Responsible For Tienilic Acid Hydroxylation.

5-Hydroxylation of tienilic acid by human liver microsomes is greatly inhibited by anti-cytochrome P-450-8 antibodies as well as by sera containing anti-LKM$_2$ antibodies (80 to 100%). The observed inhibition of tienilic acid hydroxylation by human sera containing antibodies is not due to a general non specific inhibitory effect of these sera on microsomal cytochrome P-450-dependent activities since they gave no inhibition of ethoxycoumarin deethylation, a classical microsomal reaction which does not seem to depend on cytochrome P-450-8. All the sera containing anti-LKM$_2$ antibodies which could be tested (11) were found to inhibit 5-hydroxylation of tienilic acid with ID$_{50}$ values between 2 and 50 µl of serum per nmole of cytochrome P-450. All the 20 tested control sera which did not contain anti-LKM$_2$ antibodies gave no or very low inhibitory effects toward 5-hydroxylation of tienilic acid by human liver microsomes (Beaune, et al, submitted for publication).

   These results provide the <u>first</u> <u>evidence</u> <u>for</u> <u>the</u> <u>existence</u> <u>in</u> <u>humans</u> <u>of</u> <u>circulating</u> <u>antibodies</u> <u>raised</u> <u>against</u> <u>a</u> <u>cytochrome</u> <u>P-450</u>. This is also the first indication that antibodies appearing in the serum of patients suffering from a drug-induced hepatitis is directed against a human liver cytochrome P-450 which is responsible for the oxidative metabolism of this drug. From these results, it is tempting to propose a tentative mechanism for anti-LKM$_2$ antibody production after tienilic acid administration (scheme 2) : 1) hydroxylation of the drug mainly by cytochrome P-450-8, 2) formation of reactive metabolites during this process and subsequent covalent binding to liver proteins and particularly to cytochrome P-450-8, 3) immunological response and production of antibodies against cytochrome P-450-8 alkylated by a tienilic acid metabolite.

Tienilic acid ⟶ [Reactive metabolite] ⟶ [Alkylated P-450-8]
                                +   ↓
                      5-OH-tienilic acid   immune system
                                                             ↓
                                                  Appearance of anti-
                                                  LKM$_2$ antibodies

Scheme 2

   The fact that the anti-LKM$_2$ antibodies, as well as the anti-LKM[1] antibodies in the case of halothane, could be responsible for hepatitis observed in one case 10000 to 30000 patients having received either tienilic acid or halothane remains to be established. However the above results obtained on these two compounds provide a first approach to a detailed understanding of the molecular mechanism of some drug-induced immunoallergic hepatitis. In particular the following chain of events could be suggested from the presently available data :
1 - Oxidative activation of the drug by a cytochrome P-
         450

2 - Alkylation by a reactive metabolite of microsomal macromolecules and in particular of the cytochrome P-450 catalysing the oxidation
3 - Recognition of the alkylated cytochrome P-450, possibly after its passage in the outer membrane of hepatocytes, by the immune system
4 - Production of circulating antibodies able not only to recognise the hapten derived from the reactive metabolite but also the cytochrome P-450 carrier
5 - Activation of hepatocytes bearing the alkylated P-450 as an antigen after binding of the anti-LKM antibody
6 - Destruction of these hepatocytes by lymphocytes.

Naturally, much work is still necessary in order to confirm and to definitely establish this mechanism.

ACKNOWLEDGEMENTS

Laboratoire ANPHAR-ROLLAND (France) is acknowledged for providing tienilic acid and for a continous financial and scientific support during our work on tienilic acid.

REFERENCES

Cresteil, T., Beaune, P., Kremers, G., Guengerich, F.P., Leroux, J.P. (1985). Eur. J. Biochem, 151, 345.
Davis, M. (1983). in "Immunotoxicology" (Ed. G.G. Gibson., R. Hubbard and D.V. Parke), Academic Press, London. p.171.
Homberg, J.C., Abuaf, N., Helmy-Khalil, S. et al (1985). Hepatology, 722.
Mackay, I.R. (1985). Hepatology, 5, 904.
Mansuy, D. and Battioni, P. (1985). in "Drug Metabolism : Molecular Approaches and Pharmacological Implications" (Ed. G. Siest). Pergamon Press, Oxford, 195.
Mansuy, D., Beaune, P., Cresteil, T., Lange, M., Leroux, J.P. (1977). Biochem. Biophys. Res. Comm, 79, 513.
Mansuy, D., Dansette, P.M, Foures, C., Jaouen, M., Moinet, G. and Bayer, N. (1984). Biochem. Pharmacol, 33, 1429.
Pohl, L.R., Booshan B., Whittaker, N.F., Krishna, G. (1977). Biochem. Biophys. Res. Comm, 79, 684.
Ruf, H.H., Ahr, H., Nastainczyk, W., Ullrich, V., Mansuy, D., Battioni, J.P., Montiel-Montoya, R., Trautwein, A. (1984). Biochemistry, 23, 5300.
Satoh, H., Gillette, J.R., Davies, H.W., Schulick, R.D. and Pohl, L.R. (1985b). Molec. Pharmacol, 28, 468.
Satoh, H., Fukuda, Y., Anderson, D.K., Ferrans, V.J., Gillette, J.R. and Pohl, L.R. (1985a). J. Pharmacol.

Exp. Ther, 233, 857.

Sipes, I.G. (1981). in "Drug Reactions and the Liver". (Ed. M. Davis., J.M. Tredger and M.R. Williams), Pitman Medical, Tunbridge Wells, p.157.

Vergani, D., Miele-Vergani, G., Alberti, A., Neuberger, J.M., Eddleston A.L.W.F., Davies, M. and Williams, R. (1980). New Engl. J. Med, 303, 66.

Wang, P.P., Beaune, P., Kaminsky, L.S., Dannan, G.A., Kadlubar, F.F., Larrey, D. and Guengerich, F.P. (1983). Biochemistry, 22, 5375.

FREE RADICAL MECHANISMS IN RELATION TO CELL INJURY AND CELL DIVISION

Trevor F. Slater, Kevin H. Checseman, Michael J. Davies and John S. Hurst

Department of Biochemistry, Brunel University, Uxbridge Middx. UB8 3PH., U.K.

The importance of free radical reactions in chemistry and biochemistry was emphasised more than 50 years ago in the pioneering work particularly of Waters and Michaelis (see Waters, 1946; Michaelis, 1946). The extension of these early studies on reaction mechanisms, synthetic chemistry, enzymology and radiation chemistry followed relatively naturally and continously, and was helped particularly by the introduction of electron spin resonance (esr) spectroscopy in the 1940's (Zaviosky, 1945). The application of free radical concepts and techniques to studies on cell injury came later, and basically stemed from studies in the 1960's on the metabolic activation of CCl_4 and on the production and properties of $O_2^{\overline{\cdot}}$.

Carbon tetrachloride is a strong hepatotoxic agent, producing centrilobular necrosis and fatty degeneration of the liver in a wide variety of species (Cameron and Karunaratne, 1936). A variety of mechanisms have been proposed to explain its hepatotoxic action, ranging from a direct lipophilic solvent action (Wells, 1908; see Slater, 1971 and also Berger et al., 1986), through an effect on liver blood flow to cause hypoxia in cells of zone 3 (Himsworth, 1950), to effects on mitochondrial oxidation phosphorylation (Christie and Judah, 1954) or liver lysosomes (Beaufay et al., 1959). Some early studies even suggested that CCl_4 and $CHCl_3$ were changed in vivo to a more toxic substance such as hydrochloric acid (Graham, 1915) or phosgene (Muller, 1911); for a review of these early studies see Slater (1971). In 1961 Butler examined the metabolism of CCl_4 and $CHCl_3$ in dogs in vivo and also with mouse liver homogenates. He detected the conversion of CCl_4 to $CHCl_3$ in vivo, and obtained evidence in vivo for a possible mechanism for this reaction involving tissue thiols. No appreciable tissue specificity was observed for this reaction, which appeared largely non-enzymic in character. The most important aspect of this seminal study by Butler was his suggestion that CCl_4 and $CHCl_3$ are de-

degraded by reaction with tissue thiols and that an intermediate product is the trichloromethyl radical (see also Wirtschafer and Cronyn, 1964). Subsequent independent studies by Goshal and Recknagel (1965) and Slater (1966) provided a conceptual basis for the metabolic activation of CCl_4 to $CCl_3{}^\bullet$, and the importance of this free radical in the ensuing liver injury (for reviews see Recknagel, 1967; Slater, 1971; Recknagel et al., 1977; Slater, 1982). The work on CCl_4 opened up a new area of study in biochemical pathology, and many toxic substances are known now to be metabolically activated to free radical intermediates that have significant roles in the development of the cell and tissue injury associated with such substances.

The studies with CCl_4, outlined above, have led to the introduction of a number of important concepts of rather general application in relation to free radical-mediated cell injury. For example: the importance of the NADPH-P450 electron transport chain in the production of free radical intermediates by metabolic activation (Slater, 1966); the relationship between chemical reactivity and diffusion radius in relation to free radical intermediates (Slater, 1976); the importance of breakdown products arising from lipid peroxidation to the spreading consequences of an initial lesion (Slater, 1976) and the relative importance of aldehydes in this process (Benedetti et al. 1980; Esterbauer, 1982); the effects of local concentrations of O_2 on free radical reactivity, especially in relation to halogenated carbon-centered radicals (Packer et al. 1978); and the major criteria for protecting against such types of damage by free radical scavenging processes (Slater, 1981). In addition, the detailed study of the hepatotoxity of CCl_4 has led to an understanding of the multicausal nature of such free radical-mediated events (see Slater, 1982; Dianzani and Poli, 1985).

Another major discovery with considerable importance to biochemical pathology in general was made also in the 1960's: this stemmed from the work of Fridovich and colleagues and concerned the superoxide anion radical $O_2{}^-$ (see McCord and Fridovich, 1977). These early studies have led to a remarkable and important proliferation of research on the production and properties of $O_2{}^-$ in a wide variety of cell injuries and diseases, and on the essentially protective nature of superoxide dismutase. Their perceptive work has led to to the widespread interest currently taken in 'activated oxygen species', a class of reactive intermediates that includes not only free radicals such $O_2{}^-$, $HO^\bullet$ alkoxy-and peroxy-species but also the non-radical species singlet oxygen (for recent studies see

Sies, 1985; Fridovich, 1986).

The studies initiated on CCl_4 and on O_2^- have led over the last 10 years or so to the realisation that a number of important human diseases may have significant features that arise from free radical-mediated disturbances. Table 1 gives some examples.

TABLE 1. Some diseases and toxic injuries where free radical intermediates have a significant role in the early disturbances.

Toxic liver injuries	Inflammation
Recycling of redox-active agents	Arthritis
Radiation injury	Atherosclerosis
Photosensitisation	Reperfusion injury
Alcoholism	Some aspects of tumour promotion and carcinogenesis
Some nutritional disorders	Ageing

Studies on free radical-mediated reactions in biological materials are complicated by a number of difficult problems: (i) how to establish that a free radical intermediate is indeed produced, and which one?; usually, the concentration of the free radical intermediate is very low and its life-time transient. (ii) What is the chemical reactivity of the free radical intermediate with neighbouring biomolecules. (iii) How can the primary mechanisms of damage be clearly separated from secondary consequences; this is particularly difficult since many of the primary free radical species have half-lives in the μs-ms range. Some brief comments on these particular problems are given below using CCl_4 as a model example.

DETECTION AND IDENTIFICATION

Direct esr spectroscopy is not often useful as most reactive free radical intermediates are present at steady state concentrations that are too low for adequate resolution with the esr technique (see Borg, 1976). The introduction of spin trapping in biological situations has provided a valuable technique for demonstrating the production of free radicals and, on occasion, identifying the particular radical species involved. Early applications of the technique were by Harbour et al (1974); Lai and Piette, 1974; Saprin and Piette (1977); Lown

(1978); Poyer et al (1978) and Ingall et al (1978). The technique requires care in interpretation of the results (see Janzen, 1980; Schaich and Borg, 1980); recent reviews that may be consulted are by Cheeseman et al (1985) and Mason (1984). The production of the $CCl_3 \cdot$ radical from CCl_4 in vitro and in vivo has been demonstrated using the spin trap -phenyl-N-t-butylnitrone, PBN (Poyer et al., 1978; Lai et al., 1979 and Albano et al., 1982). An interesting observation has been made by Connor et al. (1986) that CCl_4 is also oxidised to the CO_2^- species, which can be spin trapped.

Free radicals like $CCl_3 \cdot$ can be generated photolytically and the charateristics of the spin trap adducts readily studied (Davies and Slater, 1986a); the same procedures can be used to study the spin trap adducts of alkoxy- and peroxy-radicals (Davies and Slater, 1986b).

CHEMICAL REACTIVITY

Since many free radicals have short life-times in solution, it is necessary to use rapid reaction techniques for studying the kinetics of free radical reactions; a convenient system that is flexible and has considerable powers of resolution is pulse radiolysis (see Willson, 1978).

When this technique was applied to $CCl_3 \cdot$ (Packer et al., 1978) it was found that relatively speaking the $CCl_3 \cdot$ radical is not very reactive (second order rate constants with many biomolecules less than $10^5 M^{-1} s^{-1}$). With O_2, however, there is a very rapid reaction (K approximately $10^{10} M^{-1} s^{-1}$; to form the $CCl_3 OO \cdot$ species that has a much higher reactivity. Table 2 summarises a few values found by the Brunel group to illustrate this point. It is now known that this O_2-effect is a rather general phenomenon with halogenocarbon-centered radicals; thus the 'concentration' of O_2 in the micro-environment around the site of formation of a radical such as $CCl_3 \cdot$ can be of considerable importance to what reactions then occur.

REACTIONS OF REACTIVE RADICALS

The formation of reactive free radicals such as $HO \cdot$, alkoxyl ($RO \cdot$) or peroxyl ($ROO \cdot$) inside a cell can produce a wide spectrum of metabolic and structural perturbations. For example, initiation of lipid peroxidation; covalent binding to unsaturated molecules (nucleic acids, proteins, lipids); changes in redox status of $NAD(P) \cdot / NAD(P)H$ and SH/disulphide (see Slater, 1984). Obviously, when a

Table 2. Selected second-order rate constants for reactions
of $CCl_3OO^{\bullet}$; data from the Brunel Free Radical Group (see
Slater, 1984; Willson, 1978; Packer et al., 1978).

Interacting substance	Rate constant $(M^{-1} sec^{-1})$
Promethazine	4.5×10^8
Propyl gallate	2×10^8
Glutathione	1.4×10^7
Tryptophan	1.2×10^8
Arachidonic acid	7×10^6
Indomethacin	1×10^8
α-tocopherol	5×10^8
β-carotene	1.5×10^9

reactive free radical intermediate is produced in a
membrane system such as the endoplasmic reticulum then
primary disturbances will be essentially local due to the
small diffusion radius of the primary reactive species
(Slater, 1976). With CCl_4 this analysis has led to much
attention concerning the relative contributions of lipid
peroxidation and covalent binding to the initial cellular
disturbances, some arguing the case for lipid peroxidation
being of major importance (see Recknagel et al., 1977) and
others for covalent binding (see Castro, 1984). Within
the time frames of the primary mechanisms of injury (µs-ms)
it appears to us likely that both (and additional)
mechanisms are important contributors to early metabolic
perturbations. In fact, the view that CCl_4 produces its
damaging effects on the liver cell by a multicausal
mechanism (see Slater, 1982) is now becoming widely
accepted.

It is important to note that covalent binding itself
involves the formation of a new radical species that, in
principle, can itself initiate new chain reactions (Figure
1). The situation in practice, however, is more
complicated for a number of reasons. Firstly, with a free
radical species such as $CCl_3^{\bullet}$ it is known that this can
covalently bind at a relatively slow rate, but does not
react very effectively with polyunsaturated fatty acids
(PUFA) to initiate lipid peroxidation (Forni et al., 1983).
$CCl_3^{\bullet}$ will form $CCl_3OO^{\bullet}$ very easily, however, and this can
readily initiate peroxidation of PUFA (Forni et al., 1983);

Figure 1. Major pathways for the covalent binding of a
reactive free radical R. to an unsaturated compound A-
CH=CH-B.   Also shown are some reactions with oxygen to
yield peroxyl-radicals, and the initiation of new radical
processes by the covalently-bound adducts.

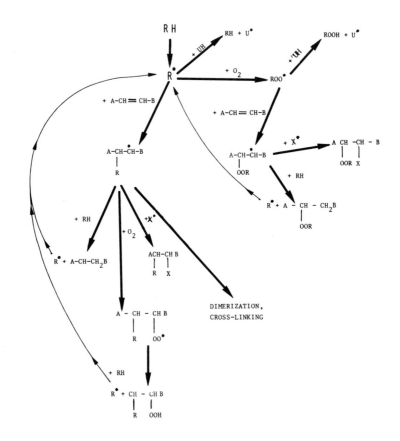

covalent binding of $CCl_3OO\cdot$, which may well occur in situ
may not survive experimental work-up procedures (Slater,
1982) due to the relatively weak C-O-O-C bond.   Free
radical scavengers such as promethazine react rapidly with
$CCl_3OO\cdot$ but not with $CCl_3\cdot$ (Packer et al., 1978), and
strongly inhibit lipid peroxidation stimulated by CCl_4, but
not covalent binding (Cheeseman, 1982).   These data
indicate the complexity of free radical events in the early
stages of liver cell injury and the participation of more
than one free radical intermediate in the first stages of
metabolic perturbation.
    A particular consequence of lipid peroxidation is the

formation of a large variety of biologically active products that ensue a diffusion of the initial lesion (Slater, 1976); these products include lipid hydroperoxides, epoxy fatty acids and aldehydes (see Slater, 1984; Esterbauer, 1985). The production of such products can have rapidly diversifying consequences for metabolic control by affecting secondary messenger cascades such as the cyclic nucleotide system (Paradisi et al., 1985) and prostaglandin synthesis. In the latter context, for example, it has been shown that CCl_4 affects arachidonate metabolism in peritoneal leucocytes (Lynch et al., 1985) and leukotrienes are aggravating to the liver injury (Keppler et al., 1985). We have studied the effects of CCl_4 on ^{14}C-arachidonate metabolism in rat liver homogenates, microsomal suspension, isolated hepatocytes and in vivo (S. Hewertson, R.G. McDonald-Gibson, J.S. Hurst and T.F.Slater, to be published). There is no doubt that CCl_4 has important early effects on this aspect of liver cell metabolism; some illustrative data are in Figure 2.

Although the evidence supporting the view that the hepatotoxicity produced by CCl_4 is largely the result of metabolic activation to the trichloromethyl free radical is now overwhelming, in many other instances the linkage between tissue injury and free radical production is circumstantial. One such instance concerns reperfusion injury to various tissues, including heart. An attractive hypothesis (see McCord, 1985) is based on a modification to the enzyme xanthine dehydrogenase during a period of hypoxia such that it then exhibits oxidase activity. In consequence, when reperfusion commences, and oxygen is carried back to the previously hypoxic tissue, electron transfer to O_2 occurs producing $O_2^{\overline{\cdot}}$. If the local environmental is significantly acidic, which is a normal consequence of ischaemic anoxia mainly due to lactate production, then $O_2^{\overline{\cdot}}$ can be protonated to the more reactive $HO_2^{\cdot}$ species. Moreover, tissue disturbance associated with ischaemia can be expected to change intracellular and extracellular compartmentation of iron. This could facilitate production of the very toxic $HO^{\cdot}$ species from $O_2^{\overline{\cdot}}$. In consequence, reperfusion injury may result from free radical mediated disturbances, at least in part. There is strong circumstantial evidence for this : the iron-chelator desferal has been reported to be strongly protective against reperfusion injury to the heart in dogs (Aust and White, 1985); free radical scavengers protect against reperfusion-induced heart arhythmias in rats and addition of substances known to stimulate radical productive aggravate the arrhythmias (Bernier et al, 1986).

Figure 2   The effect of CCl$_4$ (13nmol/kg, i.p.) on the
metabolism of (1^{14}C) arachidonate by liver homogenates
prepared from rats sacrificed 1 h following treatment.

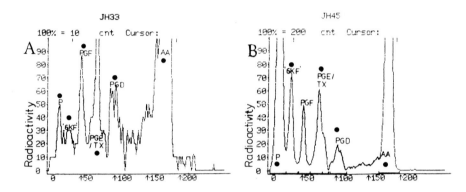

Data from radio-t.l.c.scans of extracted supernatants from
liver homogenate incubated with (^{14}C)-arachidonate (0.3
μCi, 30 μM) for 10 min at 37°C and HP 7.4. B is the
control. (Solvent system: the organic phase of ethyl
acetate/trimethyl pentane/acetic acid/water; 55:25:10:50,
v:v:v:v).

Direct evidence is so far not conclusive but spin trapping
studies have demonstrated the occurrence of a carbon-
centered radical in the effluent medium during the initial
minutes of reperfusion (M.J.Davies, P.B.Garlick, D.J.Hearse
and T.F.Slater, unpublished data.)
      The final examples to be discussed concern liver
tumours and regenerating liver. It is well known that many
liver tumours have a much reduced ability to undergo lipid
peroxidation stimulated by NADPH, NADPH-ADP-iron, NADPH-
ascorbate-iron and NADPH-CCl$_4$ (see Cheeseman et al., 1986),
or initiated by γ-radiation (Garner et al., 1986). The
reasons for this striking difference in free radical
reactivity have been analysed by Cheeseman et al (1986) for
the Novikoff tumour. The conclusion was that the main
contributory factor to the decreased rate of lipid
peroxidation is an increased content of the lipophilic
chain-breaking antioxidant α-tocopherol. The Novikoff
tumour cells have about 6-times the content of α-tocopherol
in relation to fatty acid allylic-methylenes compared to
that observed in normal rat hypatocytes. The question has
then to be asked : is this a specific feature of liver
tumour cells or is it a reflection of dividing liver cells?

To answer this question we turned to the study of liver regeneration after partial hepatectomy.

In rats entrained on a reversed light-dark cycle there is a marked periodicity in thymidine kinase activity and in DNA-synthesis (Hopkins et al., 1973). We have confirmed this and find, moreover, that there is a similar marked periodicity in the ability of microsomal fractions to undergo stimulated lipid peroxidation (Cheeseman et al., 1986). Associated with these cyclical changes in lipid peroxidation are changes in the content of α-tocopherol. It appears, therefore, that normal liver cells stimulated to divide have a marked ability to modulate their content of antioxidant material, and that this modulation produces a cyclical change in lipid peroxidation that is almost in phase with DNA-synthesis. Free radical-mediated reactions may thus have a role in the complex biochemical events leading to cell division (Slater et al., 1984).

ACKNOWLEDGMENTS: We are grateful to the National Foundation for Cancer Research, the Cancer Research Campaign and the Association for International Cancer Research for financial support.

REFERENCES

Albano, E., Lott, K.A.K., Slater, T.F., Stier, A., Symons, M.C.R. and Tomasi, A. (1982) Biochem. J., 204, 593.

Aust, S.D. and White, B.C (1985) Adv. Free Radical Biol. and Med 1, 1.

Beaufay, H., Van Campenhout, E. and de Duve, C. (1959) Biochem. J. 73, 617.

Benedetti, A., Comporti, M and Esterbauer, H. (1980) Biochim. biophys. Acta 620, 281.

Berger, M.L., Bhatt, H., Combeo, B. and Estabrook, R.W. (1986) Hepatology, 6, 36.

Bernier, M., Hearse, D.J. and Manning, A.S. (1986) Circulation Res. 58, 330.

Borg, D.C.(1976) in "Free Radicals in Biology" (ed. Pryor, W.A.) Academic Press, New York, 69.

Butler, T.C. (1961) J. Pharmacol. exp. Ther. 134, 311.

Cameron, G.R and Karunaratne, W.A.E (1936) J. Path.Bact. 42, 1.

Castro, J.A (1984)IUPHAR 9th Int. Cong. Pharmacology 2, 243

Cheeseman, K.H. (1982) in "Free Radicals, Lipid Peroxidation and Cancer" (Eds. McBrien, D.C.H. and Slater,   T.F.), Academic Press London, 197.

Cheeseman, K. H., Collins, M., Proudfoot, K., Slater, T.F.,

Burton, G.W. Webb, A.C. and Ingold, K.U. (1986) Biochem. J.235, 507.

Christie, G.S. and Judiah, J.D. (1954) Proc. Roy. Soc. B. 142, 421.

Connor, H.D., Thurman, R.G., Galizi, M.D. and Mason, R.P (1986) J. Biol. Chem. 261, 4542.

Davies, M.J. and Slater, T.F. (1986a) Chem. Biol. Interactions 58, 137.

Davies, M.J. and Slater, T.F. (1986b)Biochem. J. Submitted

Dianzani, M.U. and Poli, G. (1985) in "Free Radicals in Liver Injury" (Eds. Poli, G., Cheeseman, K.H., Dianzani, M.U. and Slater, T.F) IRL Press, Oxford, 149.

Esterbauer, H. (1982) in "Free Radicals, Lipid Peroxidation and Cancer" (Eds. McBrien, D.C.H. and Slater, T. F.) Academic Press, London, 101.

Esterbauer, H. (1985) in "Free Radicals in Liver Injury" (Eds. Poli, G., Cheeseman, K.H., Diaznani, M.U. and Slater, T.F.) IRL Press, Oxford, 29.

Fridovich, I. (1986) Archs. Biochem. Biophys. 247, 1.

Forni, L.G., Packer, J.E., Slater, T. F. and Willson, R.L. (1983) Chem. Biol. Interactions 45,171.

Garner, A., Jamal, Z. and Slater, T.F. (1986) Int. J. Rad. Biol. 50, 323.

Ghosal, A.K. and Recknagel, R.O. (1965) Life Sci. 4, 1521.

Graham, E.A. (1915) J. exp. Med. 22, 48.

Harbour, J.R., Chow, V. and Bolton, J. R. (1974) Canad. J. Chem. 52, 3549.

Himsworth, H.P. (1950) in The Liver and its Diseases" Blackwell, Oxford, 32.

Hopkins, H.A., Campbell, H.A., Barbiroli, B. and Potter, V.R. (1973) Biochem. J. 136, 955.

Ingall, A., Lott, K.A.K., Slater, T.F., Finch, S. and Stier, A. (1978) Biochem. Trans. 6, 962.

Janzen, E.G. (1980) in "Free Radicals in Biology" Vol 4 (Ed. Pryor, W.A.) Academic Press, New York, 116.

Keppler, D., Hagmann, W., Rapp, S., Denzlinger, C. and Koch, H.K. (1985) Hepatology, 5, 883

Lai, C-S. and Piette, L.H. (1974) Biochem. Biophys. Res. Commun., 78, 51.

Lai, E.K., McCay, P.B., Noguchi, T. and Fong, K.L. (1979) Biochem. Pharmacol. 28, 2231.

Lown, J.W., Sim, S-K. and Chen, H-H. (1978) Canad. J. Biochem, 56. 1042.

Lynch, T.J. Blackwell, G.J. and Moncada, S. (1985) Biochem. Pharmacol. 34, 1515.

Mason, R.P. (1984) in "Spin Labelling in Pharmacology" (Ed. Holtzmann, J.L.) Academic Press, New York, 87.

McCord, J.M. (1985) New Engl. J. Med. 312, 159

McCord, J. and Fridovich, I. (1977) in "Superoxide and Superoxide Dismutases" (Eds. Michelson, A.M., McCord, J.M. and Friedovich, I.) Academic Press, New York, 11.

Michaelis, L. (1946) in "Currents in Biochemistry" (Ed. Green, D.E) Interscience, New York.

Muller, R. (1911) Z. exp. Path. Ther. 9, 103.

Packer, J.E., Slater, T.F. and Willson, R.L. (1978) Life Sciences 23, 2617.

Paradisi, L., Panagini, C., Parola, M., Barrera, G. and Dianzani, M.U. (1985) Chem. Biol. Interactions 53, 209.

Poyer, J.L., Floyd, R.A., McCay, P.B., Janzen, E.G. and Davis, E.R. (1978) Biochim. biophys. Acta 539, 402.

Recknagel, R.O. (1967) Pharmacol. Rev. 19, 145.

Recknagel, R.O., Glende, E.A. and Hruszkewycz, A.M. (1977) in "Free Radicals in Biology" (Ed. Pryor, W.A), Academic Press, New York, 97.

Saprin, A.N. and Piette, L.M. (1977) Arch. Biochem. Biophys. 180, 480.

Schaich, K.M. and Borg, D.C. (1980) in "Autoxidation in Food and Biological Systems" (Eds. Simic, M.G. and Karel.)Plenum Press, New York, 45.

Sies, H. (1985)"Oxidative Stress" Academic Press, New York

Slater, T.F. (1966) Nature, Lond. 209, 36.

Slater, T.F. (1971) "Free Radical Mechanisms in Tissue Injury". Pion, Lond.

Slater, T.F. (1976) in "Recent Advances in Biochemical Pathology: Toxic Liver Injury" (Eds. Dianzani, M.U., Ugazio, G. and Sena, L.M.) Minerva Medica, Turin, 381.

Slater, T.F. (1981) in "International Workshop on (+)-cyanidanol-3 in diseases of the liver" (Ed. Conn, H.O.), Royal Society of Medicine, London, 11.

Slater, T.F. (1982) in "Free Radicals, Lipid Peroxidation and Cancer" Eds. McBrien, D.C.H. and Slater, T.F.) Academic Press, London ,243.

Slater, T.F. (1984) Biochem. J. 222, 1.

Slater, T.F., Benedetto, C., Burton, G.W. Cheeseman, K.U., Ingold, K.U. and Nodes, J.T. (1984) in "Icosanoids and Cancer" (Eds. Thaler-Dao, H., Crastes de Paulet, A. and Paoletti, R.) Raven Press, New York, 21.

Waters, W.A. (1946) in "The Chemistry of Free Radicals". Oxford.

Wells, H.G. (1908) Archs. intern. Med. 1, 589.

Willson, R.L. (1978) in "Biochemical Mechanisms of Liver Injury" (Ed. Slater, T.F.) Academic Press, London, 123.

Wirtschafter, Z.T.and Cronyn, M.W. (1964) Environ. Health 9, 186.

Zavoisky, E. (1945) J. Phys. U.S.S.R., 9, 211.

TISSUE DISTRIBUTION OF DRUG METABOLIZING ENZYMES IN RELATION TO TOXICITY

Gerald M. Cohen and Elizabeth J. Moss

Toxicology Unit, Department of Pharmacology, The School of Pharmacy, University of London, 29/39 Brunswick Square, London, WC1N 1AX, UK.

INTRODUCTION

A large number of different toxicities may be induced in various organs of the body by thousands of chemicals to which we are exposed. All tissues may be susceptible to these toxic effects but to varying degrees. Many chemicals damage particular organs perferentially. This phenomenon is known as target organ toxicity. Many factors, such as tissue distribution and metabolism of the chemical and response of the tissue will influence the susceptibility of particular organs to toxicity (Cohen, 1983;1986). In this review, we shall concentrate primarily on the importance of the tissue distribution of drug metabolism enzymes in determining the organ specific toxicity of chemicals. Many types of toxicity such as carcinogenesis, mutagenesis, teratogenesis, cell necrosis and hypersensitivity reactions may be mediated by reactive metabolites (Gillette et al, 1974). Such toxicities often result following the metabolism of xenobiotics to reactive electrophiles which combine covalently with critical cellular macromolecules such as DNA, RNA or proteins. (Miller and Miller, 1981).

Undoubtedly the metabolism of xenobiotics, in both hepatic and extrahepatic tissues, is of major importance in determining the relative susceptibility of these tissues to toxicity. In order to assess the contribution of tissue specific metabolism to toxicity, it is necessary first to consider whether the toxicity is mediated by one of the following: (a) the parent compound, (b) a chemically reactive metabolite(s), or (c) a chemically stable metabolite(s). Second, in those cases in which toxicity is mediated by a metabolite, consideration must be given to whether (1) the formation of the toxic metabolites occurs in one organ e.g. the liver, followed by transport to the target organs, (2) metabolic activation occurs in the target organ(s) or (3) the process requires a combination of both. These possibilities have been considered in detail by Boyd (1980a,b) and reviewed elsewhere (Cohen, 1983; 1986).

TOXICITY MEDIATED BY PARENT COMPOUND

If toxicity is mediated by the parent compound, then any factor such as metabolism or distribution which alters the effective concentration of a compound in the target organ(s) will cause a corresponding effect on its toxicity. In general, the role of the liver in metabolism is considered to be the most important in increasing water solubility and promoting rapid excretion of metabolites of toxic parent compounds. This is reflected by the very high levels of drug metabolizing enzymes in the liver compared to most other organs (Table 1).

TOXICITY MEDIATED BY REACTIVE METABOLITES

(1) Metabolite generated in one tissue and exerting its toxicity elsewhere.
The situation is more complex when toxicity is due to a metabolite. If the metabolite formed is chemically relatively stable, then it may be formed in one organ and transported by the systemic circulation to the target organ, as illustrated in Figure 1. Some examples of chemicals believed to exert their toxicity in this way are given in Table 2. Experimental evidence supports the suggestion that the pulmonary toxicity of the pyrrolizidine alkaloids, such as monocrotaline, is due to metabolic activation in the liver and then transport in the circulation to the lung (Figure 1) (Boyd, 1980a,b). This idea is supported by the observation that reactive metabolites may be formed by hepatic but not pulmonary enzymes, and that pulmonary endothelial toxicity produced by monocrotaline and the reactive pyrrole metabolite, dehydromonocrotaline are very similar. Work with enzyme inducers and inhibitors lends further support to this hypothesis. For example, pretreatment of rats with phenobarbitone increased liver microsomal enzyme activity in vitro and increased liver and lung concentrations of reactive pyrrole derivatives, which corresponded to the observed increase in liver and lung toxicity (Chesney et al, 1974).

(2) Toxic metabolite generated in target tissue.
In contrast, some metabolites may be chemically reactive, that is, their half-lives are very short. Such reactive metabolites would most likely react either

Table 1. Concentrations or activities of drug metabolising enzymes in different organs of the rat

Organ	Cytochrome P-450[1]	Cytochrome P-450 reductase[2]	Epoxide hydrolase[3]	Glutathione S-transferase[4] Microsomal	Cytosolic
Liver	0.73	181	6.39	126	1400
Lung	0.046	42	0.36 (6)*	15.4 (12)*	78.8 (6)*
Kidney	0.135	41	0.71 (11)	8.54 (7)	336 (24)
Intestine	0.042	50	0.13 (2)	60.2 (48)	429 (31)
Adrenal	0.5	-	0.26 (4)	51.9 (41)	253 (18)
Testis	0.1	-	1.47 (23)	129 (102)	3850 (275)
Spleen	-	-	0.14 (2)	9.01 (7)	55.7 (4)
Brain	0.025	26	0.10 (1.6)	7.95 (6)	190 (14)
Heart	-	-	0.02 (0.3)	7.23 (6)	92.6 (7)
Thymus	-	-	0.11 (1.7)	4.37 (4)	46.3 (3)
Mammary gland	0.001	-	-	-	-,)

[1] nmol/mg microsomal protein. [2] nmol cytochrome c reduced/min/mg microsomal protein.
[3] nmol 4,5-dihydro-4,5-dihydroxybenzo(a)pyrene formed/min/mg microsomal protein. [4] nmoles conjugate formed/min/mg protein using 1-chloro-2,4-dinitrobenzene as the second substrate.
*Results in brackets are expressed as percentage of liver values.
Values from Wolf, 1984; Oesch et al, 1977; dePierre and Morgenstern, 1983; Sesame et al, 1977.

Table 2. Compounds believed to exert their toxicity by reactive metabolites generated in an organ other than the target organ.

Compound	Metabolising Organ	'Active Species'	Target Organ or Toxicity
Monocrotaline	Liver	Dehydromonocrotaline	Lung
Tetraethyl lead	Liver	Triethyl lead	Nervous system
n-Hexane	Possibly liver	2,5-Hexanedione	Nervous system
2-Methoxyethanol	Liver and others	Methoxyacetic acid	Testis
3,3'-Dimethyl-1-phenyltriazene	Possibly liver	Monomethyl-1-phenyltriazene	Brain tumours
Vinyl Chloride	Liver	Chloracetaldehyde	Haemiangio-endotheliomas

Figure 1. Toxicity mediated by a toxic metabolite generated
in the liver and transported to the target organ.

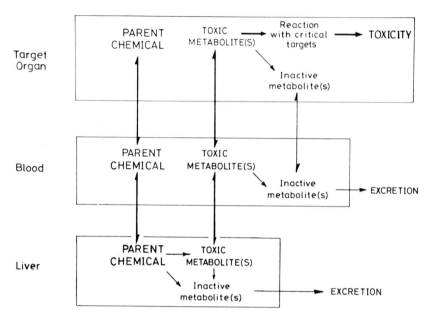

The toxic metabolite is formed in the liver and is
sufficiently stable that it may be transported via the
circulation to the target organ of toxicity. Examples of
chemicals believed to mediate their toxicity by this
mechanism are given in Table 2.

intracellularly, within the cell in which they were formed
or, if they escaped from the cells, with constituents of
blood. The liver is obviously a major target organ for
such compounds by virtue of its essential role in
metabolism. Hepatotoxins, such as aflatoxin B_1, can be
activated to very reactive short-lived intermediates by
cytochrome p-450 enzymes. The balance of activating and
detoxifying enzymes will be of critical importance. In
those species unable to deactivate such reactive
metabolites, e.g. by glutathione conjugation, high levels
of macromolecular binding and severe liver damage may
result (O'Brien et al, 1983). The extrahepatic toxicity of
these reactive metabolites will most likely be mediated by
short-lived intermediates generated in situ within their
target organs, as illustrated in Figure 2. This latter
case is particularly well exemplified by the work of Boyd

Figure 2. Toxicity mediated by reactive metabolites formed
in the target organ either from the parent chemical or from
a proximate toxic metabolite.

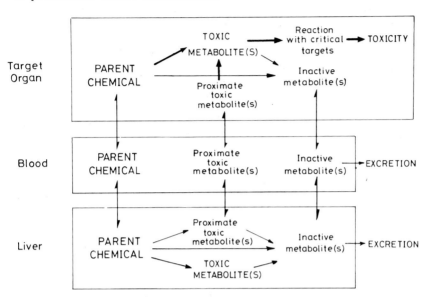

If the toxic metabolite is chemically very reactive, it may
have to be generated in situ in the target organ in order
to exert toxicity. Depending on the metabolite capability
of the tissue, the metabolic activation by parent chemical
may be completely carried out in the target organ.
Alternatively, part of the metabolic activation may be
carried out in other tissues, such as the liver, but the
ultimate toxic metabolites are formed in situ in the target
organ.

and colleagues with 4-ipomeanol which causes specific
damage to the Clara (nonciliated bronchiolar epithelial)
cells in a number of species (reviewed in Boyd, 1980b).
Following in vivo administration of (^{14}C)ipomeal to rats,
significantly more covalently bound radioactivity was
observed in lungs than any other tissues. Autoradiography
revealed that the covalently bound radioactivity was
predominantly associated with Clara cells (Boyd, 1977), and
in vivo studies suggested that a cytochrome P-450-dependent
monooxygenase was required to activate 4-ipomeanol to a
reactive metabolite(s) that bound covalently to
macromolecules. Both rat lung and liver were capable of
activating 4-ipoeanol to a binding species. However, when

the results were expressed on the basis of covalent binding per molecule of cytochrome P-450, the lung appeared approximately eightfold more active than the liver. Boyd (1977) and Serabjit-Singh et al (1979) have independently shown that at least one type of cytochrome P-450 is specifically localized in the Clara cells. These observations demonstrate the importance of the qualitative nature of the cytochrome P-450, and its tissue distribution, in determining cells in a specific organ that may be predisposed to toxicity.

(3) Proximate toxic metabolite formed in one tissue and ultimate toxic metabolite generated in the susceptible tissue.

Many toxic chemicals, require multistep metabolic activation before generating their ultimate toxic metabolites. Therefore it is conceivable that a stable proximate toxic metabolite may be initially formed in one tissue and then be transported to the target organ where it is metabolized to the ultimate toxic metabolite, as illustrated in Figure 2. The realization that many chemicals require such multistep activation suggests that this mechanism may be very important. Different enzymes could be involved at different stages of activation, and this may be of importance in target organ toxicity. For example, a target tissue may not be able to metabolize the parent compound to its proximate toxic metabolite but could convert the proximate toxic metabolite to the ultimate toxic metabolite. The metabolic activation of hexachlorobutadiene to a nephrotoxic metabolite appears to proceed by this mechanism, an initial conjugation with glutathione in the liver, followed by excretion, partial degradation, reabsorption, transport and activation in the kidney, where it is activated by C-S lyase to a toxic metabolite (Nash et al, 1984). Another example which might be considered to proceed by this mechanism is 2-naphthyl-amine, a bladder carcinogen. 2-Naphthylamine is metabolised in the liver to N-hydroxy-2-naphthylamine and its glucuronide conjugate. This may be reactivated in acidic urine to generate either reactive metabolites or compounds capable of being reactivated in bladder epithelial cells (Miller and Miller, 1981).

Several recent studies demonstrate that a number of extrahepatic tissues, whilst low in the activities of cytochrome P-450 dependent mixed function oxidases, may activate xenobiotics to reactive metabolites by a variety of different enzymes and mechanisms including prostaglandin endoperoxide synthetase, peroxidase, xanthine oxidase, tyrosinase and even byproducts derived during lipid peroxidation. In order to establish whether a compound is activated by either one or more of the previously discussed mechanisms, it is necessary to consider other factors, especially the tissue distribution of the xenobiotic enzymes, as illustrated in the following section.

TISSUE DISTRIBUTION OF XENOBIOTIC METABOLISING ENYMES

Whilst it is generally recognised that the liver is the major site of most xenobiotic metabolism, a significant amount of extrahepatic metabolism also takes place (Gram, 1980). The ability of extrahepatic tissues to metabolise xenobiotics has recently received more attention. Although quantitively the contribution of a particular extrahepatic tissue may represent only a small percentage of the overall metabolism, it may be of particular toxicological significance. The enzymes responsible for the activation of xenobiotics will often be the Phase I oxidative enymes but may in some cases be the Phase II conjugating enzymes, such as the activation of N-hydroxyacetylaminofluorene following sulphate conjugation (Miller and Miller, 1981). The tissue distribution of both Phase I and Phase II drug metabolising enzymes and the relative availabilities of their various cofactors are, therefore, vital factors in determining the relative susceptibilities of different tissues to toxic chemicals.

The wide tissue distribution of some of these xenobiotic metabolising enzymes and some of their cofactors are illustrated in Tables 1 and 3. It is the balance of the activities of the various activating and deactivating enzymes, which determines how much of a reactive metabolite will be formed in any particular cell or tissue and thus be available to exert its toxicity. The values shown in Tables 1 and 3 are representative ones taken from the literature and serve only as a very rough guide to differences in the various tissues. Careful perusal of the literature often shows substantial differences in many of the values shown in Tables 1 and 3, dependent on the method of preparation of the subcellular fraction, the strain of animal used etc. However, despite these disadvantages, certain generalisations may be made. An enormous variation of approximately 2-500 fold is observed between the concentration of cytochrome P-450 in the liver compared to other tissues (Table 1 and Wolf, 1984). A much smaller variation is noted in intertissue concentrations of other components of the mixed function oxidase system such as NADPH-cytochrome P-450 reductase (Table 1) and cytochrome

Table 3. Organ distribution of UDP glucuronyltransferase
and glutathione and related enzymes in rat tissues

Organ	UDP-Glucuronyl-transferase[1]	GSH mM	GSH Peroxidase[2]	GSSG Reductase[2] Se	non-Se
Liver	460	5.6	269	143	67
Lung	28 (6)	1.5	105	27	41
Kidney	150 (33)	2.8	146	66	146
Intestine	260 (57)	3.5	8	8	35
Adrenal	170 (37)	-	-		
Spleen	30 (7)	-	-		
Brain	0.8 (0.2)	1.8	33	12	-
Heart	1.4 (0.3)	1.1	225	0	9
Thymus	19 (4)	-			

[1] nmol 4-methylumbelliferyl glucuronide/g tissue wet weight.
[2] nmol of product/min/mg protein.
Values from Aitio and Marniemi, 1980; Ishikawa et al, 1986.

b_5 (Wolf, 1984). It has been noted that the concentration
of P-450 reductase relative to cytochrome P-450 is lower in
the liver than in any of the other tissues. Thus whereas
P-450 reductase may be rate limiting for certain
monooxygenase reactions in the liver, where each reductase
molecule reduces approximately 20 molecules of cytochrome
P-450, it may not be rate limiting in certain extrahepatic
tissues (Wolf, 1984). The concentrations of cytochromes b
$_5$ P-450 in the kidney are very similar suggesting a more
important role for cytochrome b_5 in monooxygenase reactions
in this tissue (Jones et al, 1980). Cytochrome b_5 in
kidney can be equally reduced by either NADH or NADPH and
NADH supports the monooxygenation of lauric acid in the
kidney (Ellin et al, 1972). Also particularly striking are
the high activities of epoxide hydrolase and glutathione S-
transferase in the testes (Table 1 and Oesch et al, 1977;
De Pierre and Morgenstern, 1983). Whilst our discussion
has centred mainly on the tissue distribution of drug
metabolising enzymes in the rat, there are important
species variations. For example in male NMR1-mice, the
tissue distribution of epoxide hydrolase was quantitatively

quite different from the rat and the highest activity was found in the testes, with a specific activity over 2-fold greater than liver (Oesch et al, 1977). The function(s) of the high epoxide hydrolase and glutathione S-transferase in the testes is not known but may be important in protection of germ cells against potential mutagens or in some endogenous function.

It should be stressed that although such extrahepatic metabolism may be demonstrated in vitro, it does not mean that these tissues will necessarily metabolise these compounds in vivo but it will depend on many factors such as blood flow, the nature of the substrate and its availability and supply of the necessary cofactors.

Important differences in the distribution of the drug metabolising enzymes in any particular tissue may also predipose particular cell types in a tissue to toxicity. Even in the liver, considered a relatively homogeneous tissue, large differences in the tissue distribution of cytochrome P-450 and glutathione have been observed using quantitative cytochemistry (Baron and Kawabata, 1983; Smith et al, 1979). Therefore, it is not suprising that in heterogeneous tissues, such as the lung, with more than forty cell types present, one observes an increased concentration of drug metabolising enzymes such as cytochrome P-450 in certain cell types. In addition to quantative differences in the distribution of these enzymes, important differences in isoenzymes, with different substrate specificities, may be observed which may also contribute to susceptibility to target organ toxicity.

The Clara (nonciliated bronchiolar epithelial) cells, which constitute only 1% of the cells of the lung, contain the majority of the pulmonary cytochrome P-450 (Boyd, 1977; Serabjit-Singh et al, 1979) and predisposes the Clara cells to chemical-induced damage (see later). Similarly a number of studies suggest that the highest activities of microsomal cytochrome P-450 mixed function oxidases in the kidney are found in the S_3 cells of the proximal tubules. The highest concentration of S_3 cells is found in the pars recta, that portion of the proximal tubule most susceptible to toxic damage.

From the above discussion, it is evident that tissue distribution and balance of the activating and detoxifying drug metabolising enzymes are key factors in determining organ specific toxicity of chemicals. Advances in the last few years on enzyme isolation and immunohistochemistry have given additional insight into substrate-, stereo- and regio-selectivity of different isozymes as well as the cellular distribution of the drug metabolising enzymes. Further advances, using immunochemical and electron microscopic techniques combined, will indicate the particular subcellular localisation of these key enzymes. The regulation of the drug metabolising enzymes in hepatic and extrahepatic tissues often appears to be under different control. For example, phenobarbitone is well documented as a classic inducer of mixed function oxidase activity in the liver but has no effect on this activity in the majority of extrahepatic tissues e.g. lung. Thus many factors affecting extrahepatic enzyme activity may also affect the toxicity of xenobiotics.

EXAMPLES OF TISSUE DISTRIBUTION OF DRUG METABOLIZING ENZYMES IN RELATION TO TOXICITY

A number of examples , of the importance of tissue distribution of drug metabolizing enzymes in the target organ toxicity of chemicals, is given in Table 4. This Table is not meant to be comprehensive but rather to illustrate that many different enzymes in a variety of tissues may contribute significantly to the organ specific toxicity of chemicals. In this last section we shall consider some examples in more detail.

(a) Lung
As with other extrahepatic tissues, the lung may metabolise many chemicals by a number of different pathways including oxidative, reductive, hydrolytic and conjugation reactions thereby modifying their pharmacological, therapeutic or toxicological activities (Bend et al, 1985; Cohen, 1981). The balance of activating and deactivating enzymes and their cofactors in a particular cell type in the lung may in part determine the cellular specificity of the toxic chemical (Minchin and Boyd, 1983). Using autoradiography, immunohistochemistry and isolated lung cells, most of the total lung content of cytochrome P-450 is concentrated in the Clara cells (Boyd, 1977; Serabjit-Singh et al, 1979) so providing a metabolic basis for the susceptibility of this cell type to many pulmonary toxins, including 4-ipomeanol, 3-methylfuran and naphthalene. Autoradiographic studies of animal lungs dosed in vivo with radiolabelled 4-ipomeanol showed specific localization of covalently bound radioactivity in the Clara cells (boyd, 1977). This was followed by Clara cell necrosis and then pulmonary oedema. A good correlation has been observed between the amount of pulmonary alkylation and the lung toxicity of 4-ipomeanol (Boyd, 1980b).

Table 4. Importance of tissue distribution of drug metabolising enzymes in the target organ toxicity of xenobiotics

Organ	Toxicity	Chemicals	Metabolic Basis of Susceptibility
Lung	Clara cell damage	4-ipomeanol, 3-methylfuran, naphthalene, CCl4.	Metabolic activation to toxic metabolites by specific form(s) of cytochrome P-450
Kidney	Pars recta of proximal Tubule	Hexachloro-1,3-butadiene, S-(1,2-dichlorovinyl) cysteine	C-S lyase in renal tubule metabolises cysteine conjugates to reactive thiols
Brain	Parkinson like syndrome	MPTP	Activation by MAO, selective uptake, redox cycling possibly catalysed by cytochrome P-450 reductase in substantia nigra.
Heart	Cardiomyopathy	Adriamycin	Heart deficient in enzymic defences (SOD and catalase) against oxidative stress. Adriamycin inactivates cardiac GSH peroxidase.
Cardiovascular system	Vascular and myocardial lesions	Allylamine	High activity of a particular amine oxidase in aorta, which converts allylamine to acrolein.
Eye	Cataracts	Naphthalene	High levels of catechol reductase in the rabbit lens.
Nose	Nasal tumours	Hexamethyl-phosphoramide	High level of cytochrome P-450 in olfactory epithelium.
Colon	Colonic tumours	Methylazoxymethanol	High activity of alcohol dehydrogenase in the colon.

A number of chemicals, including 4-ipomeanol, napthalene, 3-methylindole, 1,1-dichloroethylene and bromobenzene, has been shown to damage Clara cells. Many of these chemicals require metabolic activation to exert their toxicity and therefore the high concentration of cytochrome P-450 in these cells predisposes them to toxicity. However other factors must also be of importance in determining the marked susceptibility of the Clara cells to damage, as some chemicals e.g. methylcyclopentadienyl manganese tricarbonyl (Haschek et al,1982), do not appear to require metabolic activation by the Clara cells in order to exert their toxicity.

Mixed function oxidase activity is also found in other cell types in the lung including alveolar type II cells, tracheal and bronchial epithelial cells and the pulmonary alveolar macrophages of some species. Metabolic activation of some carcinogens, such as polycyclic aromatic hydrocarbons, by particular cell types may be important in certain respiratory tract cancers (Cohen and Ashurst, 1983).

(b) Nervous System

The levels of drug metabolizing enzymes in the nervous system are generally low. Few examples are known in which classical activation of compounds, by drug metabolizing enzymes within the nervous system results in selective toxicity to neuronal or glial cells. However the brain contains low levels of cytochrome P-450 (Table 1) which may activate some neurotoxins e.g. parathion (Norman and Neal, 1976). Cell selective toxicity within the nervous system is often the result of specific interaction of chemicals with receptors, enzymes and cellular uptake mechanisms. Even those cell selective toxins where metabolic activation is implicated may also involve a selective uptake mechanism. For example, 5,7-dihydroxytryptamine, a relatively selective toxin to serotoninergic neurones, is taken up by active transport into the target cell. The toxicity of 5,7-dihydroxytryptamine is reduced by pretreatment with monoamine oxidase (MAO) inhibitors, suggesting that in addition to selective uptake into the cell, the activation of 5,7-dihydroxytryptamine to a reactive intermediate by MAO may be involved (Creveling and Rotman, 1978; Cohen, 1985).

An intriguing example in which MAO activity is also implicated in nervous system toxicity is MPTP (Figure 3) (1-methyl-4-phenyl-1,2,3,6-tetrahydropyridine) a contaminant of a "designer drug synthesis". Following accidental ingestion by humans, this compound is selectively toxic to the dopamine neurones in the substantia nigra (Langston et al, 1983). The discovery of this selective toxicity in humans has caused great excitement due to the similarity of the MPTP effect to idiopathic Parkinson's disease. There is evidence that MPTP is activated to a metabolite, MPP^+ (Figure 3) and that this pyridinium species is the "ultimate" toxin (Markey et al, 1984). Both the formation of MPP^+ and the neurotoxicity can be blocked with monoamine oxidase inhibitors, such as pargyline and deprenyl (Markey et al, 1984; Heikkila, et al, 1984). MPP^+ accumulates in neuronal cells apparently by the transport system responsible for dopamine uptake. However, not all dopaminergic neurones are affected equally by MPTP (Burns et al, 1983) suggesting that the selective toxicity involves more than selective uptake. The metabolism of MPTP to MPP^+ is likely to occur within the brain. In this respect, MPTP is an example of target organ activation. However, in view of the involvement of dopamine uptake mechanisms (Javitch and Snyder, 1983), such activation is likely to be extracellular to the target cell. Recent histochemical observations have confirmed that oxidation of MPTP by MAO-B occurs in certain specific regions of the brain (e.g. the noradrenergic and serotoninergic neurones of the brainstem and the histamine neurones of the caudal hypothalamus) but not in the dopamine neurones (Nakamura and Vincent, 1986). These histochemical results show reasonable agreement with earlier immunohistochemical studies on the localization of MAO-B.

The fascinating problem that still remains is how does MPP^+ cause the observed neuronal degeneration and why are only certain of the cells with dopamine uptake mechanisms affected. Two main theories have been proposed, one involving an interaction with neuromelanin and the other involving redox cycling. The redox cycling of MPP^+ has been demonstrated in vitro in the presence of NADPH and NADPH cytochrome P-450 reductase (Sinha et al, 1986). It is interesting to note that this reductase is found at relatively high concentrations in brain (Table 1) and has been shown by immunohistochemical methods (Haglund et al, 1983) to be mainly localised in several discrete areas including the substantia nigra, the area of the brain most susceptible to MPTP toxicity.

(c) Organ Specific Carcinogenesis

One of the most widely studied aspects of the tissue distribution of drug metabolizing enzymes relates to target organ specificity in chemical carcinogenesis. Many carcinogens exhibit a very marked target organ specificity (Table 5), which has been extensively reviewed (Coombs, 1986, Langenbach et al, 1983). As with toxicity, the

Figure 3. Proposed mechanism of toxicity of MPTP (1-
methyl-4-phenyl-1,2,3,6-tetrahydropyridine).

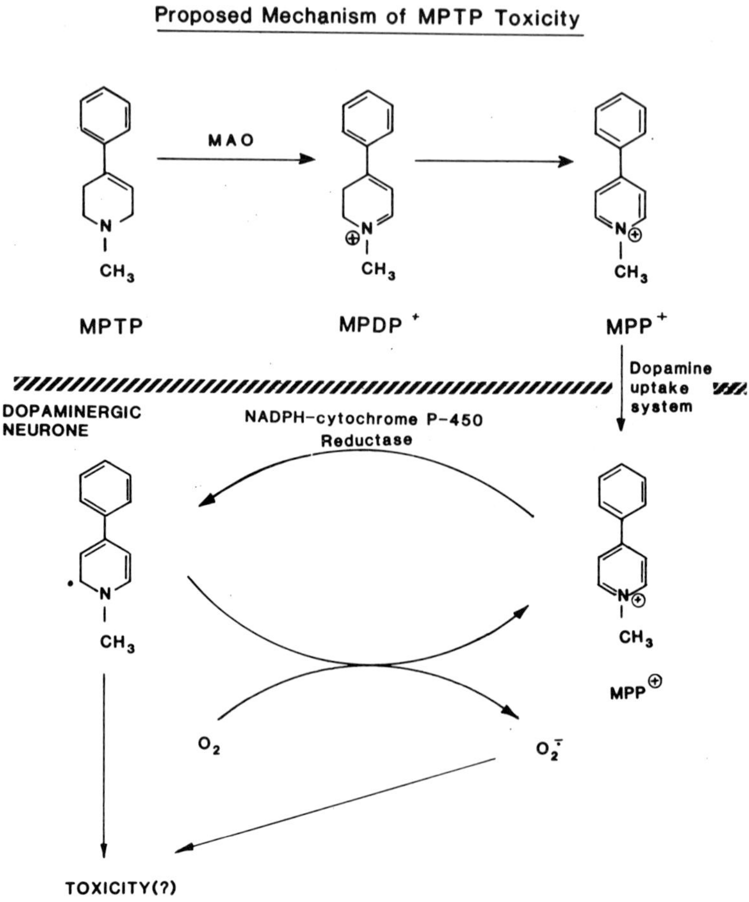

Proposed Mechanism of MPTP Toxicity

MPTP is metabolised to MPP$^+$ and is then taken up by a
specific uptake system into the substantia nigra, where it
may be further metabolized by cytochrome P-450 reductase,
setting up a redox cycle and generating superoxide anion
radical ($O_2^{\bar{\cdot}}$) and other active oxygen species.

mechanism for such specificity includes target cell
activation (e.g. aflatoxin B_1, dimethylhydrazine,
nitrosomorpholine) or transport of a proximate carcinogen
(2-naphthylamine). Both of these will be influenced by

Table 5. Organ specificity in carcinogenesis

Chemical	Target Tissue
Polycyclic aromatic hydrocarbons	Skin, respiratory tract
Aromatic amines	Bladder
Asbestos	Mesotheliomas
Vinyl chloride	Angiosacroma
1,2-Dimethylhydrazine	Colon
Dialkylnitrosamines (Symmetrical)	Predominantly liver
Dialkylnitrosamines (Asymmetrical)	Predominantly oesophagus

tissue distribution of 1) activating enzymes, 2) deactivating enzymes and 3) defence mechanisms and the balance of these within a target cell as already discussed. Factors, which influence this balance, such as species, age, sex, inducers, inhibitors and diet, will all contribute to the overall concentration of the ultimate carcinogen and its interaction with DNA. However, in addition to the role of drug metabolising enzymes in organ specific carcinogenesis, other host factors, such as DNA repair, may also play a key role. This is well illustrated by the organ specificity of certain nitrosamines and nitrosamides, where there is often a good correlation with the persistence of O^6-alkyl guanine and tumour susceptibility (Kleihues and Wiestler, 1986).

ACKNOWLEDGEMENTS
We thank Mrs M. Fagg for preparation and typing of the manuscript and Mr D. King for the preparation of the figures.

REFERENCES

Aitio, A. and Marniemi, J. (1980) In: "Extrahepatic Metabolism of Drugs and Other Foreign Compounds" (ed. Gram, T.E.) M.T.P. Press Ltd. England p.365
Baron, J. and Kawabata, T.T (1983) In: "Biological Basis of Detoxication" (eds Caldwell, J. and Jakoby, W.B.) Academic Press, New York. p105.
Bend, J.R., Serabijit-Singh, C.J. and Philpot, R.M. (1985) Ann. Rev. Pharmacol. Toxicol. 25, 97

Boyd, M.R. (1977) Nature 269, 713

Boyd, M.R. (1980a) Ciba Found. Symp. 76 (new ser.) 43.

Boyd, M.R. (1980b) Crit. Rev. Toxicol. 7, 103

Burns, R.S., Chiueh, C.C., Markey, S.P., Ebert, M.H., Jacobowitz, D.M. and Kopin, I.J. (1983) Proc. Natl. Acad. Sci. USA, 80, 4546.

Chesney, C.F., Jsu, I.C. and Allen, J.R. (1974) Res. Commun. Chem. Pathol. Pharmacol. 8, 567.

Cohen, G.M. (1981) In: "Scientific Foundations of Respiratory Medicine" (eds. Scadding, J.G., Cumming, G.and Thurlbeck, W.M.) W. Heinemann, London, p286.

Cohen, G.M. (1983) In: Biological Basis of Detoxication" (eds. Caldwell, J. and Jakoby, W.B.) Academic Press, New York, p325.

Cohen, G. (1985) (1985) In: "Oxidative Stress" (eds. Sies, H.) Acad. Press Inc (London) Ltd. p 383.

Cohen, G. M. (1986) In: " Target Organ Toxicity" Vol 1(ed. Cohen G.M.) CRC Press, Boca Raton, USA, p 1.

Cohen, G.M.and Ashurst, S.W. (1983) In: "Comparative Respiratory Tract Carcinogenesis" Vol. II (ed). Reznik-Schuller, H.M) CRC Press, Boca Raton, USA. p 135.

Coombs, M.M. (1986) In: "Target Organ Toxicity", Vol 2 (ed Cohen, G.M.) CRC Press, Boca Raton, USA, p 181.

Creveling, C.R and Rotman, A. (1978) In: "Serotonin neurotoxins" (eds. Jakoby, J.W. and Lytle, L.D.) New York Acad. Sci. 57.

DePierre, J.W. and Morgenstern, R. (1983) Biochem. Pharmac. 32, 721.

Ellin, A., Jakobsson, S.W., Schenkman, J.B. and Orrenius, S. (1972). Arch. Biochem. Biophys. 150, 64.

Gillette, J.R., Mitchell, J.R. and Brodie, B.B. (1974) Ann. Rev. Pharmacol. 14, 271.

Gram, T.E. (1980) In: "Extrahepatic Metabolism of Drugs and Other Foreign Compounds", (ed. Gram, T.E.) M.T.P. Press Ltd, England.

Haglund, L., Kohler, C., Haaparanta, T., Goldstein, M. and Gustafsson, J.A. (1983) In: "Extrahepatic Drug Metabolism and Chemical Carcinogenesis" (eds. Rydstorm, J., Montelius, J. and Bengtsson, M.) Elsevier Science Publishers B.V. p89.

Haschek, W.M., Hakkinen, P.J., Witschi, H.P., Hanzlik, R.P. and Traiger, G.J. (1982) Toxicol. Lett. 14, 85.

Heikkila, R.E., Manzino, L., Cabbat, F.S. and Duvoisin, R.C. (1984) Nature, 311, 467.

Ishikawa, T., Akerboom, T.P.M. and Sies, H. (1986) In: "Target Organ Toxicity Vol 1 (ed. Cohen, G.M.) CRC Press, Boca Raton, USA, p 129.

Javitch, J.J. and Synder, S.H. (1985) Europ. J. Pharamacol.

106, 455.

Jones, D.P. Orrenius, S., Jakobsson, S.W. (1980) In: "Extrahepatic Metabolism of Drugs and Other Foreign Compounds" (ed. Gram, T.E.) M.T.P. Press Ltd, England. p123.

Kleihues, P. and Wiestler, O. (1986) In: "Target Organ Toxicity" Vol 2 (ed. Cohen, G.M.) CRC Press, Boca Raton, USA, p 159.

Langenbach, R., Nesnow, S. and Rice, J.M. (1983) (eds) "Organ and Species Specificity in Chemical Carcinogenesis." Plenum Press, New York.

Langston, J.W., Ballard, P., Tetrud, J.W. and Irwin, I (1983) Science, 219, 979.

Markey, S.P., Johannessen, J.N., Chiueh, C.C., Burns, R.S. and Herkenham, M.A. (1984) Nature, 311, 464.

Miller, E.C., and Miller, J.A. (1981) Cancer 47, 2327.

Minchin, R.F. and Boyd, M.R. (1983) Ann. Rev. Pharmacol. Toxicol. 23, 217.

Nakamura, S. and Vincent, S.R. (1986) Neuroscience Lett. 65, 321.

Nash, J.A., King, L.J., Lock, E.A. and Green, T. (1984) Toxicol. Appl, Pharmacol. 73, 124.

Norman, B.J. and Neal, R.A. (1976) Biochem. Pharmac. 25, 37.

O'Brien, K., Moss, E., Judah, D. and Neal, G.E. (1983) Biochem. Biophys. Res. Comm. 114, 813.

Oesch, F., Glatt, H.R., Schmassmann, H.U. (1977) Biochem. Pharmac. 26, 603.

Sasame, H.A., Ames, M.M. and Nelson, S. (1977) Biochem. Biophys. Res. Comm. 78, 919.

Serabjit-Singh, C.J., Wolf, C.R., Philpot, R.M and Plopper, C.G. (1979) Science, 207, 1469.

Sinha, B.K., Singh, Y. and Krishna, G. (1986) Biochem. Biophys. Res. Comm. 135, 583.

Smith, M.T., Loveridge, N., Wills, E.D. and Chayen, J. (1979) Biochem. J. 182, 103.

Wolf, C.R. (1984) In: "Foreign Compound Metabolism" (eds. Caldwell, J. and Paulson, G.D.) Taylor and Francis, London.

12. Active metabolites and extrahepatic metabolism.

ACTIVE OXYGEN SPECIES AND TOXICITY

Helmut Sies

Institut fur Physiologische Chemie,
Universitat Dusseldorf, West Germany

INTRODUCTION

Reactive oxygen species have been shown to occur physiologically and can lead to toxicity in cells and organs. This is important in pathophysiological conditions such as inflammation, and also in drug and xenobiotic toxicity. Further, reactive oxygen species are generated in the process of redox cycling, as for use in chemotherapy.

The nature of these reactants and their effects on DNA, proteins, carbohydrates and lipids is briefly reviewed.

Toxicity can be influenced by a number of biological variables, as well as by the multiple lines of antioxidant defence.

REACTIVE OXYGEN SPECIES

The reactive species involved in biological systems are listed in Table 1. Most of them are free radicals, and it seems that the term oxygen free radicals is used more or less synonymously with reactive or aggressive oxygen species. However, it should be noted that ground state (triplet) molecular oxygen as a diradical is much less reactive than the excited state (singlet) molecular oxygen ($^1\Delta_g O_2$), which is diamagnetic, not of radical nature (see Wassermann and Murray, 1979). Thus, non-radical excited states of molecular oxygen and also of oxygen in organic compounds, such as excited carbonyls and dioxetanes (see Adam and Cilento, 1982;1983), and ozone fall into the category of reactive oxygen species of biological interest. The kinetic constants of the reactivity of $HO_2^{\bullet}/O_2^{\bullet-}$ with more than 300 organic and inorganic compounds in aqueous solution have been compiled (Bielski et al., 1985).

Formation of these species occurs by several pathways, enzymatic and nonenzymatic. One-electron reduction, initially leading to the formation of the superoxide anion radical, is a major source. Direct two-electron reduction

Table 1. Reactive Oxygen Species of Interest in Oxidative
          Stress (From Sies, 1985)

Compound	Remarks
$O_2^{\bar{\cdot}}$, superoxide anion	One-electron reduction state, formed in many autoxidation reactions (e.g. flavoproteins; redox cycling
$HO_2^{\cdot}$, perhydroxy radical	Protonated form of $O2^{\bar{\cdot}}$, more lipid-soluble
H_2O_2, hydrogen peroxide	Two-electron reduction state, formed from $O_2^{\bar{\cdot}}$ ($HO_2^{\cdot}$) by dismutation, or directly from O_2
HO· (OH·), hydroxyl radical	Three-electron reduction state, formed by Fenton reaction, metal(iron)-catalyzed Haber-Weiss reaction;highly reactive.
RO·,alkoxy radical	Oxygen-centered organic (e.g. lipid) radical
ROO·, peroxy radical	Formally formed from organic (e.g. lipid) hydroperoxide, ROOH, byhydrogen abstraction
ROOH	Organic hydroperoxide (e.g. lipid-,thymine-OOH)
$^1\Delta_g O_2$ (also O_2^*)	Singlet molecular oxygen, first excited state, 22kcal/mol above ground state (triplet)$^3O_2$;red (dimol) or infrared (monomol) photoemission.
^3RO(also RO^*)	Excited carbonyl, blue-green photoemission (e.g., formed via dioxetane as intermediate)

generates hydrogen peroxide: an example for this is given
by the fatty acyl-CoA oxidase in the peroxisome. The
formation of the hydroxyl radical may occur directly
through radiolysis of water, and also via the Fenton
reaction.

The cellular sources of superoxide produced via one-
electron reduction of molecular dioxygen include the
mitochondrial and microsomal respiratory chains and the
bacterial activity of leukocytes and macrophages. At a

physiological level, the importance of the cellular sources is difficult to assess in a general fashion, although they might provide a large share in maintaining the cellular steady state concentration of the superoxide anion radical. Certainly, also autoxidation reactions such as redox cycling are growing in importance for explaining the oxidative stress caused by several xenobiotics; these include also therapeutic agents of quinone nature, used in cancer chemotherapy (Kappus and Sies, 1981).

It is of interest to note that reactive oxygen intermediates seem often to be metabolized by making use of the principle of dismutation. Not only is the one-electron reduction state eliminated in a disproportionation reaction, but also two-electron reduction products. Whereas the dismutation of the superoxide anion radical and of hydrogen peroxide by the respective enzymes, superoxide dismutase and catalase, yield ground-state triplet oxygen, the dismutation of hydroperoxides as products of lipid peroxidation or prostaglandin G_2 can produce singlet molecular oxygen.

Singlet oxygen is formed in biological systems (a) via photosensitization reactions, an appropriate sensitizer being electronically excited and subsequently transfering energy to oxygen, and (b) via chemiexcitation reactions. These latter pathways of singlet formation occur without activation by light, and therefore were also called "photo chemistry in the dark" (Adam and Cilento, 1982;1983). Pathways of chemiexcitation of oxygen are beginning to be elucidated, and basically there may be two routes. One is through radical-radical interaction (Russell's mechanism) (Russell, 1957; Howard and Ingold, 1968) and the other is through oxene transfer (Cadenas et al., 1983c).

Singlet oxygen may be of particular interest in biological systems, because it is capable of diffusing an appreciable distance in membranes. In stearate monolayers, the diffusion path for singlet oxygen for half-deactivation was measured to be 115 Å (Schnuriger and Bourdon, 1968). The occurence of singlet oxygen in cellular systems has been supported so far mainly by the detection of photoemission via the dimol reaction:

$$^1O_2 + {}^1O_2 \longrightarrow 2\,{}^3O_2 + h\nu\ (634nm,\ 703nm).$$

The use of this "low-level" chemiluminescence as an indicator of $^1O_2$ in intact cells and organs is possible by employing sensitive photon-counting equipment (Boveris et al., 1979; Cadenas and Sies, 1984). Spectral evidence and the enhancement by diazabicyclo-octane (DABCO) and the decrease of photoemission by azide indicate the occurence of singlet oxygen in intact liver during the redox cycling of 2-methyl-1,4-naphthoquinone (menadione) (Wefers and Sies, 1983b) or 1,1-dimethylbipyridylium (paraquat) (Cadenas et al., 1983a). Thus, it is possible that singlet oxygen as a damaging species may be responsible for the toxic effects observed with the compounds. Menadione is mutagenic (Chesis et al., 1984), and singlet oxygen generated by microwave discharge was shown to affect biologically active DNA, causing a loss of transforming activity (Wefers et al., 1986).

Regarding isolated enzymatic systems, the spectra of photoemission resemble that of the H_2O_2/NaOCl reaction (Khan and Kasha, 1970). Two peaks near the 634nm and 703nm regions were observed with isolated ram seminal vesicle prostaglandin hydroperoxidase (cyclooxygenase) (Cadenas et al., 1983b), or with cytochrome P-450 and iodobenzene as substrate (Cadenas et al., 1983c). The monomol photoemission of singlet oxygen occurs at 1270nm, in the infrared. Recently, the lactoperoxidase reaction was shown to photoemit at 1270 nm (Kanofsky, 1984).

OXIDATIVE DAMAGE

Nucleic Acids. Oxidative damage to DNA seems to occur more readily at thymine and guanine than at adenine and cytosine. Thymine glycol as one of the oxidation products is excreted in the urine and has been suggested as a noninvasive indicator for DNA damage (Cathcart et al, 1984). Strand scission and repair are normally occuring events. For a recent discussion, see Sies (1986).

Proteins. Oxidation of amino acid side-chains in proteins has recently begun to be understood as an important biological signal. The amino acids most prone to oxidative damage are methionine (Brot and Weissbach, 1983) histidine (Levine, 1983; Fucci et al., 1983) and tryptophan. Proline may constitute a preferential target for hydrolysis of peptide bonds, yielding a new N-terminal glutamate residue in the fragmented protein (Wolff et al., 1986).

Cysteine will be discussed in some more detail here. While the formation of disulphide bonds as such cannot be considered as damage, because it is a reversible process, disulphides in peptides and proteins may alter biological functions. Thus, alteration in the thiol/disulphide statue has been found to lead to biological consequences including changes in enzyme properties (K_m or V_{max} effects). Thus, the thiol redox state seems to serve as a metabolic signal.

Further, the reversible formation of mixed disulphides between proteins and low-molecular weight thiols, in particular glutathione (ProtSSG), is of interest. ProtSSG in the soluble cytoplasm as well as in membranes has been observed. The S-thiolation of proteins in heart cells treated with diamide and t-butyl hydroperoxide showed distinct patterns, notably proteins with molecular masses of 23, 42 and 97 kD (Grimm et al., 1985; Collinson et al., 1986). The levels of protein-glutathione mixed disulphides are low, about 20-30 nmol/g of liver (Brigelius et al., 1983; Higashi et al., 1985). When GSSG levels were increased, the mixed disulphides also increased (Brigelius et al., 1983; Higashi et al., 1985; Keeling et al., 1982), possibly catalyzed by thiol transferases (Askelof et al., 1974). The disulphides between glutathione and coenzyme A, CoASSG, were found to undergo fluctuations which can be metabolically significant; during oxidative challenge with t-butyl hydroperoxide, the cellular free CoASH pool can be decreased so that coenzyme A-dependent processes are blocked (Crane et al., 1982).

$$CoASH + GSSG \rightleftharpoons CoASSG + GSH$$

In isolated mitochrondria, respiration and ATP synthesis with CoA-dependent substrates such as pyruvate or 2-oxoglutarate is abolished, whereas there is little effect, for example, with β-hydroxybutyrate or succinate as substrates (Sies and Moss, 1978).

Sulphydryl groups may be further oxidised to thiyl radicals and after subsequent oxygen addition lead to the peroxysulphenyl radical:

$$RS^{\cdot} + O_2 \longrightarrow RSO_2^{\cdot}$$

Further rearrangements and oxidation steps yield sulphenates and sulphinates and will finally lead to sulphonates, stable enough to be detectable in assays of enzymatic oxidation. For example, glutathione sulphonate was detected in enzymatic oxidation of glutathione by xanthine oxidase (Wefers and Sies, 1983a) or horseradish peroxidase (Wefers et al., 1985). Thiyl radicals have been detected with ESR methods in horseradish peroxidase-catalysed reactions (Ross et al., 1984; Harman et al., 1986) in vitro; there is no information available yet on the metabolic generation of thiyl radicals in cells.

Carbohydrates. Polysaccharides such as hyaluronic acid can be degraded by oxidative attack, and superoxide dismutase was found to be capable of protecting against the depolymerisation of hyaluronate in synovial fluid (McCord, 1974; Greenwald, 1980).

Lipids. Polyunsaturated fatty acids have become a central area of interest in the chemistry and biochemistry of oxidative reactions. The unspecific oxidation of polyunsaturated fatty acids is known as lipid peroxidation, a radical-mediated pathway leading to a number of stable degradation products. This area is not discussed in detail here (see Kappus, 1985).

DEFENCE LINES: BIOCHEMICAL ANTIOXIDANTS

Detoxication of reactive oxygen species is one of the prerequisites of aerobic life, and the multiple lines of defence which have evolved form veritable antioxidant defence systems are listed in Table 2. The repertoire to counteract the potentially hazardous reactions initiated by oxygen metabolites includes all levels of protection: prevention, interception, and repair. It comprises nonenzymatic scavengers and quenchers denoted by the term antioxidants in the more narrow sense, and also enzymatic systems.

The antioxidant enzymes involved are the intensively studied superoxide dismutases, and various hydroperoxidases such as glutathione peroxidase, catalase and other hemoprotein peroxidases. They are characterised, in general, by high specific cellular content, by specific organ and subcellular localisations which often overlap in a complementary way, and by a specific form of metal involvment in the catalysis including copper, manganese, iron(heme) and selenium. These antioxidant systems have a wide distribution in nature, underscoring their essentiality in coping with the damaging effects of reactive oxygen metabolites in biological systems. Their distribution is crucial in target organ toxicity (Ishikawa et al., 1986a)

It should be noted that a number of additional, or ancillary, systems are of crucial importance. For example, many of the radical or nonradical reactions in cells may lead to thiol oxidation to the disulphide, i.e., the oxidation of glutathione to form GSSG. Thus, the regenerative reaction of reduction to GSH as catalysed by GSSG reductase can become pivotal in antioxidant defence. Likewise, the provision of reducing equivalents to this enzyme is essential. Thus, the NADPH regenerating systems are also of interest.

Diminution of the steady-state levels of reactive

Table 2. Antioxidant Defence in Biological Systems (From Sies, 1985)

System	Remarks
Non-enzymatic	
α-Tocopherol (vitamin E)	Membrane-bound; receptors? Regeneration from chromanoxy radical?
Ascorbate (vitamin C)	Water soluble
Flavonoids	Plant antioxidants (rutin, quercetin, etc)
Chemical	Food additives, e.g. BHA (butylated hydroxyanisole) BHT (butylated hydroxytoluene)
β-Carotene, vitamin A	Singlet oxygen quencher
Urate	Singlet oxygen quencher, radical scavenger?
Plasma proteins	e.g., Coeruloplasmin
Enzymatic	
Superoxide dismutases	CuZn enzyme, Mn enzyme
GHS peroxidases	Selenoenzyme; non-Se enzyme: some GSH S-transferases, e.g., isoenzymes B and AA; Cytosol and mitochrondrial matrix
Catalase	Heme enzyme Predominantly in peroxisomal matrix
Ancillary enzymes	
NADPH-quinone oxidoreductase (DT-diaphorase)	Two electron reduction, dicoumarol-sensitive
Epoxide hydrolase	
Conjugation enzymes	UDP-glucuronyltransferase Sulphotransferase GSH S-transferases
GSSG reductase	
NADPH supply	Glucose-6-phosphate dehydrogenase Isocitrate dehydrogenases Malic enzyme Energy-linked transhydrogenase
Transport systems	GSSG export Conjugate export

compounds capable of generating reactive oxygen species also results in a decreased expression of oxidative stress; in this sense, the two-electron reduction of quinones by NADPH:quinone oxidoreductase (DT-diaphorase) and the subsequent conjugation reactions undergone by the hydroquinone are part of the antioxidant defence (Lind et al., 1982).

Obviously, the export of reactive species in free or conjugated form also serves a detoxication function, so that transport of conjugates as well as of GSSG from cells is of interest here. The binding of conjugates of glutathione to GSSG binding sites may have metabolic significance. It has been shown in kinetic and x-ray crystallographic studies that glutathione conjugates bind to the GSSG-binding site in the active centre of GSSG reductase, causing inhibition of enzymatic activity (Bilzer et al., 1984). An increase in GSSG levels causes metabolic perturbations, including an inhibition of protein synthesis (see Kosower and Kosower, 1978).

The transport system for GSSG and glutathione conjugates have been studied in some detail recently (Sies, 1983; Kaplowitz et al., 1985; Bannai and Tateishi, 1986). In liver, there is mutual competition for biliary export between these two types of glutathione derivative (Akerboom et al., 1982;1984), indicating that the canalicular carrier system may accept both these substrates for transport. There appears to be a GSSG activatable ATPase in the hepatic plasma membrane (Nicotera et al., 1985). Mutual competition for export of GSSG and GS-conjugates was also detected in the heart (Ishikawa and Sies, 1984a; 1984b). Using the creatine kinase reaction as an indicator metabolite system, it was found that GSSG transport across the cardiac plasma membrane was half-maximal at $(ATP/ADP)_{free}$ ratios of approximately 10 in the intact perfused rat heart preparation (Ishikawa et al., 1986c).

Interestingly, a prominent GSH transferase activity is isozyme 4-4, accepting 4-hydroxynonenal as a substrate (Mannervik, 1985) and, therefore, capable of removing this biologically active product of lipid peroxidation (Ishikawa et al., 1986b). Recently, another high-activity isozyme (8-8) was described (Jensson et al., 1986).

Control of the antioxidant capacity. While control of the patterns of antioxidant enzymes is not well-characterised in mammalian cells, it appears that adaptation phenomena may be important in eukaryotes. In this regard, the changes in the biochemical pattern exhibited in cells in hepatic nodules may be considered as adaptive. These nodules contain clones of hepatocytes in which a new state of liver differentiation is acquired, and this is considered as a physiological response to environmental perturbations (Farber, 1984), like the oxyR response in S.typhimurium (Christman et al., 1985). The changes observed in the nodules refer to some of the ancillary antioxidant enzymes mentioned in Table 2; these consist of increases in the cellular activities of some isozymes of glucuronyl transferases, glutathione transferases, gamma-glutamyl transferase, epoxide hydrolase, and NADPH:quinone oxidoreductase. These enzymes are classified as belonging to the Phase II group of enzymes involved in xenobiotic transformation. Interestingly, the enzymes of Phase I, namely cytochromes P-450 and b_5, are drastically decreased in their cellular activities. It appears that these changes in gene expression are related to DNA methylation. In experiments to decrease DNA methylation at the cytosine residues by treatment of the animals with the drug analogue, 5-azacytidine, cytochromes P-450 and b_5 were observed to be decreased (Gooderham and Mannering, 1985), and several isozymes of the glutathione transferases as well as NADPH:quinone oxidoreducatase were increased (Wagner and Sies, 1986) in livers of mice. Recently, NADPH:quinone oxidoreductase was cloned and was described to be hypomethylated in persisting liver noduli (Williams et al., (1986).

Thus, there are interesting relationships between the status of DNA methylation and the expression pattern for some enzymes of importance in defence against oxidative challenge.

Ebselen, a novel selenoorganic compound. This synthetic selenoorganic compound, 2-phenyl-1,2-benzo-isoselenazol-3(2H)-one, has been found to exhibit antioxidant capacity (Muller et al., 1984). In an assay of lipid peroxidation using rat liver microsomes, the lag phase preceding the onset of ascorbate/ADP-Fe-induced lipid peroxidation is increased by the addition of ebselen, whereas the sulphur analogue is inactive; this pertains not only to the low-level chemiluminescence, but also to other parameters of lipid peroxidation like the evolution of ethane and n-pentane or the production of thiobarbiturate-reactive material. In addition to this antioxidant activity, the compound acts catalytically in the GSH peroxidase reaction (Muller et al., 1984; Wendel et al., 1984),

$$2 \text{ GSH} + \text{ROOH} \longrightarrow \text{GSSG} + \text{ROH} + H_2O$$

This activity is thought to be responsible for the protection of isolated hepatocytes against oxidative challenge. Significant protection was afforded against ADP-Fe-induced cell damage in control cells, whereas cells previously made deficient in GSH were not protected by ebselen (Muller et al., 1985). Recently,it was found that ebselen also inhibited the lipoxygenase pathway (Safayhi et al., 1985). Whether this can be explained by the removal of activatory hydroperoxide through the GSH peroxidase reaction, or by yet another site of action, is not clear.

WHERE DOES TOXICITY START

It is evident from the foregoing that damage and repair are continously operative, even under what we might call normal or physiological conditions. In toxicology, one of the major problems may reside in defining, in biochemical terms, a state in which toxicity sets in. The disruption of the delicate pro-oxidant/antioxidant balance in favour of the former has been called oxidative stress (see Sies, 1985). Whether the shape changes associated with formation of blebs (see Orrenius, 1986) and with the damage of the microtubular and microfilamentous system is a major event, or whether the damage to mitochrondrial energy production is decisive, may be a question that should not be asked in a mutally exclusive way. It appears that the general term toxicity, can have a number of underlying biochemical disturbances, so that generalisations should be made with caution.

ACKNOWLEDGMENTS

The work from the author's laboratory was supported by Deutsche Forschungsgemeinschaft, Schwerpunktprogramm "Mechanismen toxischer Wirkungen von Fremdstoffen", and by the National Foundation for Cancer Research, Washington.
Thanks are extended to the coworkers in the laboratory whose contributions are mentioned in the text. The help by Peter Graf in preparing this manuscript is gratefully acknowledged.

REFERENCES

Adam W. and Cilento G., eds. (1982) "Chemical and Biological Generation of Excited States", Academic Press, New York
Adam, W. and Cilento, G. (1983) Angew. Chem. 95,; Int. Ed. 22, 529

Akerboom, T.P.M., Bilzer, M. and Sies, H. (1982) FEBS Lett. 140, 73

Akerboom, T.P.M., Bilzer, M. and Sies, H. (1984) J. Biol. Chem. 259, 5838

Askelof, P., Axelsson, K., Eriksson, S. and Mannervik, B. (1974) FEBS Lett. 38, 263

Bannai, S. and Tateishi, N. (1986) J. Membrane Biol. 89, 1

Bielski, B.H.J., Cabelli, E.E., Arudi, R.L. and Ross, A.B. (1985) J. Phys. Chem. Ref. Data 14, 1041

Bilzer, M., Krauth-Siegel, R.L., Schirmer, R.H., Akerboom, T.P.M., Sies, H. and Schulz, G.E. (1984) Eur. J. Biochem. 138, 373

Boveris, A., Cadenas, E., Reiter, R., Filipkowski, M., Nakase, Y. and Chance, B. (1979) Proc. Natl.Acad. Sci. 77, 347

Brigelius, B., Muckel, C., Akerboom, T.P.M. and Sies, H. (1983) Biochem. Pharmacol. 32, 2529

Brot, N. and Wiessbach, H. (1983) Arch. Biochem. Biophys. 223, 271

Cadenas, E. and Sies, H. (1984) Meth. Enzynol. 105, 221

Cadenas, E., Brigelius, R. and Sies, H. (1983a) Biochem. Pharmacol. 32, 147

Cadenas, E., Sies, H., Graf, P. and Ullrich, V. (1983b) Eur. J. Biochem. 130, 117

Cadenas, E., Sies, H., Nastainczyk, W. and Ullrich, V. (1983c) Hoppe-Seyler's Z. Physiol. Chem., 364, 519

Cathcart, R., Schwiers, E., Saul, R.L. and Ames, B.N (1984) Proc. Natl. Acad. Sci. 81, 5633

Chesis, P.L., Levin, D.E., Smith, M.T., Ernster, L. and Ames, B.N. (1984) Proc. Natl. Acad. Sci. 81, 1696

Collinson, M.W., Beidler, D., Grimm, L.M. and Thomas, J.A (1986) Biochim. Biophys. Acta 885, 58

Christman, M.F., Morgan, R.W., Jacobson, F.S. and Ames, B.N (1985) Cell 41, 753

Crane, D., Haussinger, D. and Sies, H. (1982) Eur. J. Biochem. 127, 575

Farber, E. (1984) Biochim. Biophys. Acta 738, 171

Fucci, L., Oliver, C.N., Coon, M.J. and Stadtman, E.R. (1983) Proc.Natl. Acad. Sci. 80, 1521

Gooderham, N.J. and Mannering, G.J. (1985) Cancer Res. 45, 1569

Greenwald, R.A. (1980) in "Biological and Clinical Aspects of Superoxide and Superoxide Dismutase", (Eds. Bannister, W.H. & Bannister, J.V.) Elsevier, Amsterdam, p 160

Grimm, L.M., Collison, M.W., Fisher, R.A. and Thomas, J.A. (1985) Biochim. Biophys. Acta 844, 50

Harman, L.S., Carver, D.K., Schreiber, J. and Mason, R.P.

(1986) J. Biol. Chem. 261, 1642

Higashi, T., Furukawa, M., Hikita, K., Naruse, A., Tateishi, N. and Sakamoto, Y. (1985) J. Biochem. 98, 1661

Howard, J.A. and Ingold, K.U. (1968) J. Am. Chem. Soc. 90, 1058

Ishikawa, T. and Sies, H. (1984a) FEBS Lett. 169,. 156

Ishikawa, T. and Sies H. (1984b) J. Biol. Chem. 259, 3838

Ishikawa, T., Akerboom, T.P.M. and Sies, H. (1986a) in "Target Organ Toxicity" (Ed. Cohen, G.M.) CRC Press in press

Ishikawa, T., Esterbauer, H. and Sies, H. (1986b) J. Biol. Chem. 261, 1576

Ishikawa, T. Zimmer, M. and Sies, H. (1986c) FEBS Lett. 200, 128

Jensson, H., Guthenberg, C., Alin, P. and Mannervik, B. (1986) FEBS Lett. 201, in press.

Kanofsky, J.R., (1984) J. Photochem. 25, 105

Kaplowitz, N., Yee Aw, T. and Ookhtens, M. (1985) Ann. Rev. Pharmacol. Toxicol. 25, 715

Kappus, H. (1985) in "Oxidative Stress" (Ed. Sies, H.), Academic Press, London, Orlando, 273

Kappus, H. and Sies, H. (1981) Experientia, 37, 1233

Keeling, P.L., Smith, L.L. and Aldridge, W.N. (1982) Biochim. Biophys. Acta 716, 249

Khan, A.U. and Kash, M. (1970) J.Am.Chem.Soc. 92, 3293

Kosower, E. M. and Kosower, N.S. (1978) Int. Rev. Cytol, 54, 109

Levine, R.L. (1983) J. Biol. Chem. 258, 11823

Lind, C., Hochstein, P. and Ernster, L. (1982) Arch. Biochem.Biophys. 216, 178

Mannervik, B. (1985) Adv.Enzymol. 57, 357

McCord, J.M. (1974) Science 185, 529

Muller, A., Cadenas, E., Graf, P. and Sies, H. (1984) Biochem. Pharmacol. 33, 3235

Muller, A., Gabriel, H. and Sies, H (1985) Biochem. Pharmacol. 34, 1185

Nicotera, P., Moore, M., Bellomo, G., Mirabelli, F. and Orrenius, S. (1985) J.Biol.Chem. 260, 1999

Ross, D., Albano, E., Nilsson, U. and Moldeus, P. (1984) Biochem. Biophys.Res.Commun. 125, 109

Russell, G.A. (1957) J.Am.Chem.Soc. 79, 3871

Safayhi, H., Tiegs, G. and Wendel, A. (1985) Biochem. Pharmacol. 34, 2691

Schnuriger, B. and Bourdon, J. (1968) Photochem. Photobiol. 8, 361

Sies, H. (1983) in "Glutathione: Storage, Transport and Turnover in Mammals" (Eds. Sakamoto, Y., Higashi, T. and Tateishi, N.), Scientific Societies Press, Tokyo, 63

Sies, H. (1985) in "Oxidative Stress" (Ed. Sies, H.)
    Academic Press, London, Orlando, p 1
Sies, H. (1986) Angew. Chem. in press
Sies, H. and Moss, K.M. (1978) Eur.J.Biochem. 84, 377
Wagner, G and Sies, H. (1986) to be published
Wasserman, H.H. and Murray, W.A., eds. (1979) "Singlet
    Oxygen", Academic Press, New York
Wefers, H. and Sies, H. (1983a) Eur. J. Biochem. 137, 29
Wefers, H. and Sies, H. (1983b) Arch. Biochem.Biophys. 224,
    568
Wefers, H., Riechmann, E. and Sies, H. (1985)J. Free
    Radicals Biol. Med. 1, 311
Wefers, H., Schulte-Frohlinde, D. and Sies, H. (1986)
    unpublished
Wendel, A., Fausel, M., Safayhi, H., Tiegs, G. and Otter, R.
    (1984) Biochem. Pharmacol. 33, 3241
Williams, J.B., Lu, A.Y.H., Cameron, R.G. and Pickett, C.B
    (1986) J. Biol.Chem. 261, 5524
Wolff, S.P., Garner, A. and Dean, R.T. (1986) TIBS 11, 27

THE RENAL METABOLISM AND TOXICITY OF CYSTEINE CONJUGATES

Imperial Chemical Industries, Plc, Central Toxicology Laboratory, Alderley Park, Macclesfield, Cheshire, UK.

INTRODUCTION

The kidney, containing many of the metabolising enzymes found in the liver, is second only to that organ in its capacity to metabolise foreign chemicals. Although secondary to the liver on an organ to organ basis the anatomy and functional heterogeneity of the kidney can significantly increase the ability of this organ to both concentrate and metabolise foreign chemicals. Several factors combined result in the kidney being exposed to high concentrations of chemicals. Firstly, it is a highly perfused organ receiving about 25% of the cardiac output (Valtin, 1973), 80% of which passes through the renal cortex. Secondly it is the major source of elimination of chemicals and their metabolites and, thirdly, there are several both passive and active mechanisms by which chemicals can be concentrated and accumulated in the kidney.

Within the kidney the more highly perfused, oxygen rich cortex containing the glomeruli and proximal and distal tubules appears to be the principle site of both transport and metabolism of foreign chemicals, rather than the more anaerobic renal medulla. Of the various transport mechanisms within the kidney, organic anion transport will be seen to be the most relevant to the mechanism of action of toxic cysteine conjugates. This type of transport occurs in all three morphologically distinct regions of the proximal tubule, but appears to be located primarily in the S2 and S3 segments in the rat (Tune et al, 1969; Roch-Ramel and Weiner, 1980; Roch-Ramel et al, 1980).

As with the transport mechanisms there is evidence that the metabolising enzymes are located in specific areas of the nephron (Wachsmuth, 1985; Trump et al, 1985) and frequently the intrarenal site of necrosis represents the site of accumulation of the chemical and the location of the activating enzymes. Many of these principles apply to the mechanism of action of toxic cysteine conjugates and provide the explanation of why the kidney is the target organ for these products of glutathione conjugation. This review will discuss the mechanisms whereby a number of cysteine conjugates are concentrated and activated in the kidney to species which are toxic and in some cases also mutagenic. There are basically two mechanisms, one in which the cysteine conjugates are themselves directly reactive, the other in which the conjugates require further metabolic activation to their reactive forms. The normal renal processing of glutathione and cysteine conjugates will also be briefly reviewed since these processes invariably occur alongside those which result in nephrotoxicity.

GLUTATHIONE CONJUGATION AND MERCAPTURIC ACID SYNTHESIS

Glutathione conjugates, the origin of all cysteine conjugates of foreign chemicals, may be formed between glutathione and any chemical possessing an electron-deficient carbon centre. Conjugation is catalysed by cytosolic, microsomal and mitochondrial glutathione-S-transferase enzymes which are found in many tissues including the kidney (Chasseaud, 1979; Jakoby and Habig 1980). Glutathione-S-transferase activity is generally much lower in the kidney than the liver suggesting that most glutathione conjugates are of hepatic origin. However, both the transferase enzymes and glutathione appear to be localised in the cells of the renal proximal tubule (Ross and Guder, 1982). Since this is also the site of necrosis caused by some chemicals which undergo glutathione conjugation, in situ formation of glutathione conjugates in the kidney may be significant.

The activities of the peptidases, γ-glutamyltransferase and cysteinylglycinase, responsible for the degradation of glutathione conjugates to their equivalent cysteine conjugates are significantly higher in the kidney than the liver (Tate 1980; Jakoby et al, 1984). These enzymes are located on the brush border of the proximal tubule where they rapidly degrade glutathione conjugates filtered into the lumen through the glomeruli (Kozak and Tate 1982; McIntyre and Curthoys, 1982; Ross and Guder, 1982). The cysteine conjugates are then readsorbed from the lumen into the proximal cells where they undergo N-acetylation by microsomal N-acetyltransferases prior to excretion in urine as the mercapturic acids (Green and Elce, 1975; Jakoby et al, 1984).

In addition to reabsorption of cysteine conjugates from

the lumen, two distinct mechanisms have been identified for the transport of glutathione conjugates and mercapturates directly into renal cells from the circulating blood. These transport mechanisms are located in the basal-lateral membrane and appear to be responsible for the transport of organic anions and cations (Inoue et al, 1981, 1984; Rankin and Curthoys, 1982; Lash and Jones, 1983, 1984, 1985). Knowledge of these mechanisms of active transport of glutathione and cysteine conjugates has been used extensively in both assessing the toxicity and understanding the mechanisms of action of toxic cysteine conjugates, because it is within renal tubular cells that toxicity is usually expressed and key activating enzymes such as β-lyase appear to be concentrated (Berndt and Mehendale 1979; Hassall et al, 1983; Jaffe et al 1983; Lock and Ishmael 1985; Elfarra et al, 1985; Lock et al, 1986). In conclusion it appears that glutathione conjugates and their cysteine derivatives may enter renal tubular cells either from the lumen after filtration through the glomeruli or by transport through the basal-lateral membrane from the blood.

The relative significance of these two routes will be considered later in this review.

CYSTEINE CONJUGATES THAT ARE DIRECT ACTING TOXINS

1,2-Dichloroethane and 1,2-dibromoethane have been shown to cause damage to several organs including the kidney (Spencer et al, 1951; Rowe et al, 1952). Both dihaloethanes are known to be metabolised by glutathione conjugation to highly reactive S-(2-haloethyl)-glutathione conjugates (Nachtomi et al, 1968; Van Bladeren et al, 1980). Their reactivity is mediated by the formation of episulphonium ions which have been shown to react directly with protein, DNA and glutathione (Figure 1) (Rannug et al, 1978; Guengerich et al, 1980; Van Bladeren et al 1980; Shih and Hill, 1981; Sundheimer et al, 1982; Ozawa and Guengerich, 1983).

Although basically acting through the same mechanism of episulphonium ion formation there appears to be subtle differences in the mechanism of renal toxicity of 1,2-dichloro- and 1,2-dibromoethanes. Exposure to 1,2-dichloroethane lowers hepatic glutathione levels in the rat (Johnson, 1965) while 1,2-dibromoethane exposure lowers both hepatic and renal glutathione levels (Nachtomi et al, 1968; Kluwe, 1981). It is now clear that glutathione conjugation with 1,2-dibromoethane occurs in both liver and kidney and that the conjugate is reactive in situ at its

Figure 1. The formation of episulphonium ions from the glutathione and cysteine conjugates of 1,2-dihaloethanes.

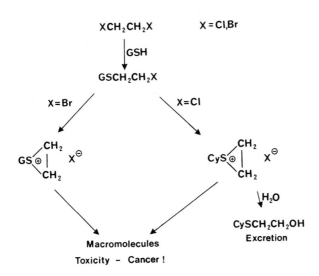

site of formation. Hill et al (1978) have shown renal protein and nucleic acids to have higher concentrations of covalently bound radioactivity than other organs after administration of radioactive 1,2-dibromoethane. The kidney has also been shown to possess high glutathione S-transferase activity with this chemical as substrate providing further evidence that the conjugate is formed and reacts in the kidney. 1,2-Dichloroethane conjugation on the other hand appears to occur only in the liver. The glutathione conjugate which is more stable than either its own cysteine conjugate or the glutathione conjugate of 1,2-dibromoethane is transported via the bile and the gut to the kidney (Elfarra et al, 1985). In the kidney the glutathione conjugate is degraded to the more reactive cysteine conjugate which is toxic through its episulphonium ion (Figure 1). In support of such a mechanism Elfarra et al (1985) have shown that inhibitors of the organic-anion transport system partially protect against the nephrotoxicity of the cysteine conjugate of 1,2-dichloroethane, thus indicating the extra-renal origin of these conjugates.

CYSTEINE CONJUGATES ACTIVATED BY RENAL β-LYASE

The toxicity of cysteine conjugates activated by renal

β-lyase was first recognised in 1959 by McKinney and Biester who identified S-(1,2-dichlorovinyl)-cysteine (DCVC) as a contaminant in cattle feed. DCVC which had been formed during the extraction of soya bean meal with trichloroethylene at high temperatures was subsequently shown to be a potent nephrotoxin in cattle and laboratory animals. Its activation to a toxic metabolite was shown to be catalysed by a renal enzyme known as C-S or β-lyase (Anderson and Shultze, 1965). This enzyme cleaved DCVC at the C-S bond giving ammonia, pyruvate and a reactive species believed to be a thiol (Figure 2). This intermediate was shown to react with glutathione, protein and DNA (Anderson and Schultze, 1965; Bhattacharya and Schultze 1971a and b, 1972; Hassall et al, 1983) and was proposed to inhibit both glutathione reductase and mitochondrial respiration (Stonard and Parker 1971a,b; Stonard 1973). More recent studies (Lash et al, 1986) have confirmed that DCVC and a similar conjugate, S-(2-chloro-1,1,2-trifluoroethyl)-L-cysteine are potent inhibitors of state 3 respiration in rat kidney mitochondria.

Figure 2. The metabolism of haloalkene-cysteine conjugates by renal β-lyase.

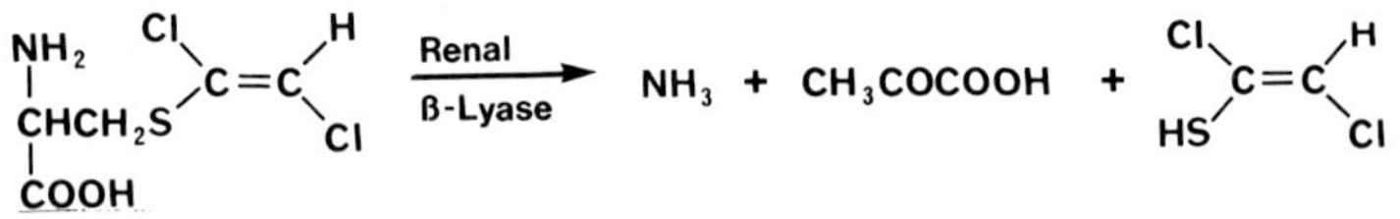

The example shown is the activation of S-(1,2-dichloro-vinyl)-L-cysteine (DCVC).

Following the studies with DCVC a number of haloalkenes and their cysteine conjugates have been shown to damage the pars recta region of the proximal tubule of the kidney. These included chlorotrifluoroethylene, hexafluoropropene (Potter et al, 1981), hexachlorobutadiene (Gradiski et al, 1975; Lock and Ishmael, 1979), tetrafluoroethylene (Dilley et al, 1974) together with their cysteine conjugates and conjugates of several other chloro-fluoroethylenes (Gandolfi et al, 1981; Hassall et al, 1983; Jaffe et al, 1983; Nash et al, 1984; Odum and Green 1984; Dohn et al, 1985; Green and Odum 1985; Elfarra et al, 1986). Several of these studies established that the conjugates were metabolised by kidney slices and isolated tubules to pyruvate and ammonia and to reactive species which had marked effects on organic ion transport mechanisms. Many of these studies were carried out using chemically

synthesised conjugates and there was little or no evidence
for their formation 'in vivo' from the parent haloalkene,
many chemicals in this class being metabolised by
oxidation. Three 'in vitro' studies suggested that
glutathione conjugation could also be a major route of
hepatic metabolism for those haloalkenes which were
nephrotoxic (Bonhaus and Gandolfi, 1981; Dohn and Anders
1982a and b; Wolf et al, 1984). In these studies
glutathione conjugation appeared to be the major metabolic
pathway, chlorinated alkenes forming conjugates by
elimination of a chlorine atom, fluoro-alkenes by addition
of glutathione across a double bond. Both saturated and
unsaturated conjugates were subsequently shown to be
substrates for renal β-lyase (Figure 3) (Green and Odum,
1985).

Figure 3. Proposed mechanism of activation of cysteine
conjugates by β-lyase to toxic (A and B) and mutagenic (A
only) intermediates.

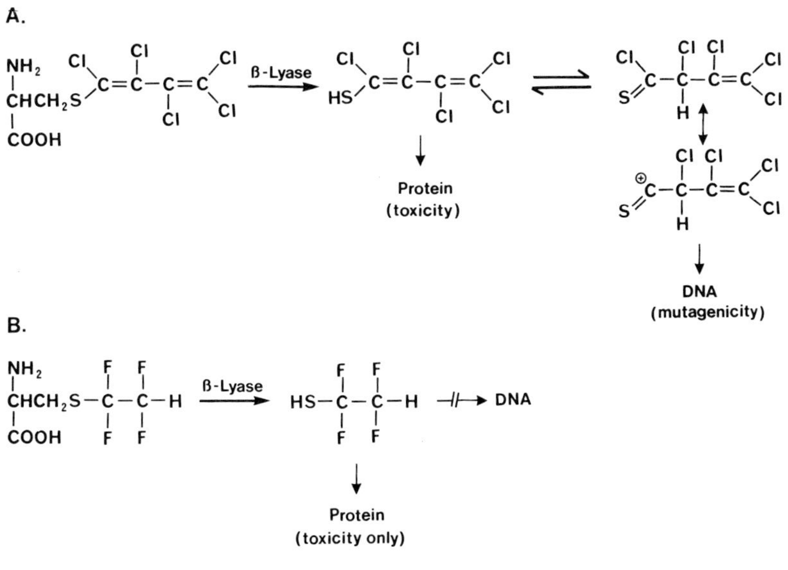

(A) represents the activation of the cysteine conjugate of
hexachloro-1:3-butadiene and (B) the conjugate of
tetrafluoroethylene.

Two 'in vivo' studies finally established glutathione
conjugation and activation by renal β-lyase to be major

metabolic pathways. Both hexachloro-1:3-butadiene (HCBD) and tetrafluoroethylene (TFE) (Nash et al, 1984; Odum and Green, 1984) were shown to be metabolised in rats to glutathione conjugates which were both substrates for β-lyase and also were potent nephrotoxins (Green and Odum, 1985). In one of these studies rats fitted with biliary cannulae were found to be completely protected from the nephrotoxic effects of HCBD suggesting that glutathione conjugation occurred only in the liver, and that the conjugate reached the kidney only after readsorption from the gut (Nash et al, 1984). Uptake into renal tubular cells was shown to occur via the organic anion transport system. Probenecid, a potent inhibitor of organic anion uptake, completely protected against the nephrotoxic effects of HCBD conjugates (Lock et al, 1986).

The earlier studies with DCVC suggested the formation of a reactive intermediate as a result of the action of renal β-lyase. In addition to reacting with various proteins and glutathione this intermediate was also shown to interact with DNA (Bhattacharya and Schultze 1971a and b, 1972; Jaffe et al, 1983). Although the consequence of the interaction of DCVC with DNA are unknown, HCBD, which is known to be metabolised to a similar conjugate, is a renal carcinogen in the rat (Kociba et al, 1977). In this case both the glutathione and cysteine conjugates of HCBD have been shown to be potent mutagens in the Ames bacterial mutation assay when activated by rat kidney fractions. These results indicate that activation by β-lyase can also lead to mutagenicity and presumably cancer in addition to nephrotoxicity (Green and Odum, 1985). The relationshop between structure, β-lyase activity, nephrotoxicity and mutagenicity has been examined for a series of chlorinated and fluorinated cysteine conjugates (Green and Odum, 1985). All of the conjugates studied were substrates for β-lyase and had similar toxicities, but an interesting distinction was found between the conjugates of chloro-alkenes which were mutagenic and those of fluoro-alkenes which were not. It was proposed that the unsaturated thiols generated by the β-lyase cleavage of the chlorinated conjugates reacted with protein sulphydryl groups but in addition they tautomised to thioacyl chlorides which reacted with DNA. The fluorinated conjugates gave a thiol which was similarly reactive with protein, but which was unable to tautomerise to species reactive with DNA because these conjugates are saturated by addition of glutathione across the double-bond during their formation (Figure 3).

For the above haloalkenes glutathione conjugation appears to be the major route of metabolism. Recent studies (Green 1986) with perchloroethylene have identified glutathione conjugation as a minor pathway in addition to the major but saturable oxidative pathway. The product S-(1,1,2 trichlorovinyl)-L-cysteine is a known mutagen (Green and Odum, 1985) and may well account for the low incidence of kidney tumours seen in rats but not mice exposed to perchloroethylene (NTP 1983). Comparisons of the extent of glutathione conjugation in rats and mice indicate that this route is significantly greater in rats in agreement with the observed species differences in carcinogenicity.

It will be apparent from the foregoing that the main class of cysteine conjugates which are substrates for β-lyase are those derived from the halo-alkenes. At the present time there are a few other known examples, the cysteine conjugate of 2-bromohydroquinone (Monks et al, 1984) and S-(2-benzothiazoloyl)-L-cysteine (Dohn and Anders 1982a and b; Lash et al, 1986) being established substrates for renal β-lyase.

β-LYASE

Surprisingly little is known about renal β-lyase. In the kidney β-lyase activity is found in both cytosolic and mitochondrial fractions and appears to be pyridoxal phosphate-dependent (Elfarra et al, 1986), Stonard and Parker 1971a and b; Stevens 1985a and b; Lash et al, 1986). As a pyridoxal phosphate dependent enzyme it is inhibited by aminooxyacetic acid (Elfarra and Anders, 1984). Enzymes also designated β-lyase are present in bovine liver (Anderson and Schultz, 1965), rat liver (Tateishi et al, 1978) and in many species of bacteria (Larsen et al, 1983). The hepatic enzyme appears to be identical to kynureninase (Stevens and Jakoby, 1983; Stevens, 1985a,b) and has a much broader substrate specificity than the renal enzyme. The two enzymes appear to be quite distinct, an antibody to the liver enzyme failing to cross react with the kidney enzyme (Stevens, 1985a).

CONCLUSIONS

Cysteine conjugates derived from the glutathione conjugation of several halo-alkenes and alkanes are potent nephrotoxins either as a result of direct action (haloalkanes) or as a result of activation by renal β-lyase. This enzyme catalyses the conversion of cysteine conjugates to ammonia, pyruvate and a reactive species which is cytotoxic and in some cases mutagenic. At the present time the reactive species have neither been

isolated nor their sites of interactions with
macromolecules identified although the mitochondrion has
been identified as a key target. Direct acting cysteine
conjugates appear to be limited to the 1,2-dihaloethanes
and those activated by β-lyase are mainly from the haloalkene group. However there is already evidence of others,
and it must be expected that amongst the vast range of
chemicals that undergo glutathione conjugation further
examples of toxic cysteine conjugates will be discovered.

REFERENCES

Anderson, P.M. and Schultze, M.O. (1965). Arch. Biochem.
    Biophys, 111, 593.
Berndt, W.O. and Mehendale, H.M. (1979) Toxicology, 14,
    55.
Bhattacharya, R.K. and Schultze, M.O. (1971a). Arch.
    Biochem. Biophys, 145, 565.
Bhattacharya, R.K. and Schultze, M.O. (1971b). Arch.
    Biochem. Biophys, 145. 575.
Bhattacharya, R.K. and Shultze, M.O. (1972). Arch. Biochem.
    Biophys, 153, 105.
Bonhaus, D.W. and Gandolfi, A.J. (1981) Life Sci, 29,
    2399.
Chasseaud, L.F. (1979). Adv. Cancer. Res, 29, 175.
Dilley, J.V., Carter, V.L. and Harris, E.S. (1974).
    Toxicol. Appl. Pharmacol, 27, 582.
Dohn, A.R. and Anders, M.W. (1982a). Biochem. Biophys. Res.
    Commun, 109, 1339.
Dohn, A.R. and Anders, M.W. (1982b). Anal. Biochem. 120,
    379.
Dohn, A.R., Leininger, J.R., Lash, L.H., Quebbemann, A.J.
    and Anders, M.W. (1985) J. Pharmacol. Exp. Ther, 235,
    851.
Elfarra, A.A. and Anders, M.W. (1984). Biochem. Pharmacol,
    33, 3729.
Elfarra, A.A., Baggs, R.B. and Anders, M.W. (1985). J.
    Pharmacol. Exp. Ther, 233, 512.
Elfarra, A.A., Jakobson, I. and Anders, M.W. (1986).
    Biochem. Pharmacol, 35, 283.
Gandolfi, A.J., Nagle, R.B., Soltis, J.J. and Plescia, F.H.
    (1981). Res. Comm. Path. Pharmacol, 33, 249.
Gradiski, D., Duprat, P., Magadur, J-L. and Fayein, E.
    (1975). Eur. J. Toxicol. 8, 180.
Green, R.M. and Elce, J.S. (1975). Biochem. J. 147, 283.
Green, T. (1986). Unpublished data.
Green, T. and Odum, J. (1985) Chem. Biol. Interact, 54,
    15.

Guengerich, F.P., Crawford, W.M., Domoradzki, J.Y., Macdonald, T.L. and Watanabe, P.G. (1980). Toxicol. Appl. Pharmacol, 55, 303.
Hassall, C.D., Gandolfi, A.J. and Brendel, K. (1983). Toxicology, 26, 285.
Hill, D.L., Shih, T.W., Johnson, T.P. and Struck, R.F. (1978). Cancer. Res, 38, 2438.
Inoue, M., Okajima, K. and Morino, Y. (1981). Biochim. Biophys. Acta, 641, 122.
Inoue, M., Okajima, K. and Morino, Y. (1984). J. Biochem. (Tokyo), 95, 247.
Jaffe, D.R., Hassall, C.D., Brendel, K. and Gandolfi, A.J. (1983). J. Toxicol. Environ. Health, 11, 857.
Jakoby, W.B. and Habig, W.H. (1980). in "Enzymatic Basis of Detoxication", Vol II (Ed. Jakoby, W.B). Academic Press, New York, p.63.
Jakoby, W.B., Stevens, J., Duffel, M.W. and Weisiger, R.A. (1984). in "Rev. Biochem. Toxicol" (Ed. Hodgson, E., Bend, J.R. and Philpot, R.M). 6, p.95.
Johnson, M.K. (1965). Biochem. Pharmacol, 14, 1383.
Kluwe, W.M. (1981). in "Toxicology of the Kidney" (Ed. Hook, J.B). Raven Press, New York, p.179.
Kociba, R.J., Keyes, D.G., Jersey, G.C., Ballard, J.J., Dittenber, D.A., Quast, J.F., Wade, C.E., Humiston, C.G. and Schwetz, B.A. (1977). Am. Ind. Hyg. Assoc. J., 38, 589.
Kozak, E.M. and Tate, S.S. (1982) J. Biol. Chem, 257, 6322.
Larsen, G.L., Larson, J.D., Gustafsson, J-A. (1983). Xenobiotica, 13, 689.
Lash, L.H. and Jones, D.P. (1983) Biochem. Biophys. Res. Commun, 112, 55.
Lash, L.H. and Jones, D.P. (1984). J. Biol. Chem, 259, 14508.
Lash, L.H. and Jones, D.P. (1985). Mol. Pharm. 28, 278.
Lash, L.H., Elfarra, A.A. and Anders, M.W. (1986). J. Biol. Chem, 261, 5930.
Lock, E.A. and Ishmael, J. (1979). Arch. Toxicol, 43, 47.
Lock, E.A. and Ishmael, J. (1985). Toxicol. Appl. Pharmacol, 81, 32.
Lock, E.A., Odum, J. and Ormond, P. (1986). Arch. Toxicol, 59, 12.
Monks, T.J., Lau, S.S. and Gillette, J.R. (1984). Abstracts of 6th Int. Symp. on Microsomes and Drug Oxidation, Brighton, Sussex, UK, 5-10th August, 23.
McKinney, L.L., Picken, J.C., Weakley, F.B., Eldridge, A.C., Campbell, R.E., Cowan, J.C. and Biester, H.E. (1959). J. Am. Chem. Soc, 81, 909.

McIntyre, T. and Curthoys, N.P. (1982). J. Biol. Chem, 257, 11915.

Nachtomi, E., Alumot, E. and Bondi, A. (1968). Isr. J. Chem, 6, 803.

Nash, J.A., King, L.J., Lock, E.A. and Green, T. (1984). Toxicol. Appl. Pharmacol, 73, 124.

NTP (1985). NTP technical report on the toxicology and carcinogenesis studies of tetrachloroethylene in F344/N rats and B6C3F1 mice. NIH publication Number 85-2567. Board Draft 8/85.

Odum, J. and Green, T. (1984). Toxicol. Appl. Pharmacol, 76, 306.

Ozawa, N. and Guengerich, F.P. (1983). Proc. Natl. Acad. Sci, 80, 5266.

Potter, C.L., Gandolfi, A.J., Nagle, R. and Clayton, J.W. (1981). Toxicol. Appl. Pharmacol, 59, 431.

Rankin, B.B. and Curthoys, N.P. (1982) FEBS Lett, 147, 193.

Rannug, U., Sundvall, A. and Ramel, C. (1978). Chem. Biol. Interact, 20, 1.

Roch-Ramel, F. and Weiner, I.M. (1980) Kidney Int, 18, 665.

Roch-Ramel, F., White, F., Vowels, L., Simmonds, H.A. and Cameron, J.S. (1980). Amer. J. Physiol, 239, F107.

Ross, B.D. and Guder, W.G. (1982). in "Metabolic Compartmentation", (Ed.Sies, H.) Academic Press, London, p.363.

Rowe, V.K., Spencer, H.C., McCollister, D.D., Hollingsworth, R.L. and Adams, E.M. (1952). Arch. Ind. Hyg. Occup. Med, 6, 158.

Shih, T-W. and Hill, D.L. (1981). Res. Commun. Chem. Path. Pharm, 33, 449.

Spencer, H.C., Rowe, V.K., Adams, E.M., McCollister, D.D. and Irish, D.D. (1951). Arch. Ind. Hyg. Occup. Med, 4, 482.

Stevens, J.L. (1985a). J. Biol. Chem, 260, 7945.

Stevens, J.L. (1985b) Biochem. Biophys. Res. Commun, 129, 499.

Stevens, J. and Jakoby, W.B. (1983). Mol. Pharm, 23, 761.

Stonard, M.D. (1973). Biochem. Pharmacol, 22, 1329.

Stonard, M.D. and Parker, V.H. (1971a). Biochem. Pharmacol, 20, 2429.

Stonard, M.D. and Parker, V.H. (1971b). Biochem. Pharmacol, 20, 2417.

Sundheimer, D.W., White, R.D., Brendel, K. and Sipes, I.G. (1982). Carcinogenesis, 3, 1129.

Tate, S.S. (1980). in "Enzymatic Basis of Detoxification" Vol II, (Ed. Jakoby, W.D.), Academic Press, New York, p.95.

Tateishi, M., Suzuki, S. and Shimizu, H. (1978). J. Biol. Chem, 253, 8854.

Trump, B.F., Berezesky, I.K., Lipsky, M.M. and Jones, T.W. (1985). in "Renal Heterogeneity and Target Cell Toxicity", (Eds. Bach, P.H. and Lock, E.A.) J. Wiley, Chichester, p.31.

Tune, B.M., Burge, M.B. and Patlak, C.S. (1969). Amer. J. Physiol, 217, 1057.

Valtin, H. (1973). Little, Brown, Boston.

Van Bladeren, P.J., Breimer, D.D., Rotteveel-Smijs, G.M.T., De Jong, R.A.W., Buijs, W., Van Der Gen, A. and Mohn, G.R. (1980). Biochem. Pharmacol, 29, 2975.

Wachsmuth, E.D. (1985). in "Renal Heterogeneity and Target Cell Toxicity". (Eds. Bach, P.H. and Lock, E.A.) J. Wiley, Chichester, p.13.

Wolf, C.R., Berry, P.N., Nash, J.A., Green, T. and Lock, E.A. (1984). J. Pharmacol. Exp. Ther, 228, 202.

METABOLIC ACTIVATION BY THE FETUS AND PLACENTA

Olavi Pelkonen, Markku Pasanen and Kirsi Vahakangas

Department of Pharmacology, University of Oulu, SF - 90220
Oulo, Finland.

INTRODUCTION

Metabolism is often called "detoxication", which implies that the products are harmless or inactive. However, in many cases metabolites are more active or toxic than the parent substance and then the process is called "metabolic activation" or "toxification". If an active or toxic metabolite is formed, the outcome, a pharmacological response or a toxic reaction, is determined by the activity of, and the balance between the activating and inactivating enzymes.

FETAL XENOBIOTIC METABOLISM

This topic has been covered extensively in several reviews by us and others (Pelkonen, 1977a; 1980; 1982; 1984a; 1984b; 1985; Juchau, 1980; 1981; Juchau et al, 1980; Nau and Neubert, 1978; Dutton and Leakey, 1981) and here we shall make only short remarks on pertinent aspects of the animal and human fetal xenobiotic metabolism.

When compared with animal fetuses, the human fetus possesses quite an active complex of hepatic xenobiotic-metabolising enzymes (see selected metabolic reactions in Table 1 and comprehensive lists in Pelkonen, 1977a, 1980 and Juchau, 1981). These activities do not seem to be easily inducible in utero by classical inducers. The variability is considerable, as always with human enzymes.

It seems still to be true that mammals other than primates have rather low levels of monooxygenase activities during fetal development. However, with sensitive techniques it has been possible to demonstrate, that rat and mouse embryos possess at least aryl hydrocarbon hydroxylase enzyme very early during development (Galloway et al, 1980; Filler and Lew, 1981). An interesting finding concerning non-mammalian species is that chick embryos seem to be also capable of metabolising benzo(a)pyrene at the adult level or higher very early in ovo (Hamilton et al,

Table 1. Qualitative assessment of xenobiotic-metabolising enzyme systems in human fetal liver and placenta.

	PLACENTA	FETAL LIVER
Oxidations		
Benzo(a)pyrene hydroxylation	inducible	active
7-Ethoxycoumarin O-deethylase	inducible	active
7-Ethoxyresorufin O-deethylase	inducible	active
Aminopyrine N-demethylase	not detected	active
Aniline hydroxylase	not detected	active
Aldrin epoxidase	not detected	active
Biphenyl hydroxylation	not detected	active
Hydrolyses		
Epoxide hydrolase	low	active
Conjugations		
Glucuronidation	very low	very low
Sulphation	very low	active
Glutathione conjugation	low	active
Acetylation	low	active

For original references see Juchau, 1976, 1981; Juchau et al, 1980; Pelkonen, 1977, 1980a.

1983). Also there certainly are large differences between different substrates and metabolic pathways (Lum et al, 1985). Although similar findings will certainly emerge in the future, the primate fetuses seem to stand in their own category with respect to xenobiotic metabolism (Dvorchik and Hartman, 1982; Christ et al, 1983).

The emerging trend has been investigations into the presence or absence of different isozymes of cytochrome P-450. Attempts to purify human fetal hepatic enzymes have been published (Cresteil et al, 1982; Kitada et al, 1985), but still it is difficult to tell, how many isozymes there are in the fetal liver, what are the functions of the purified proteins and how the properties of purified proteins and biotransformation reactions in the microsomes or in vivo can be fitted together. Indirect approaches to study the multiplicity of cytochrome P-450 in different fetal tissues have been employed, including the use of

"isoenzyme-specific" substrates, metabolites or inhibitors
(Kremers et al, 1983) and antibodies developed against
human or animal cytochromes (Cresteil et al, 1982b; Morgan
et al, 1985).

Epoxide hydrolysis (see Pacifici, 1983) and most
conjugation reactions (Cresteil et al, 1982; Steiner et al,
1982; Pacifici et al, 1983; 1986) are rather well developed
in the human fetal liver. The only exception seems to be
glucuronic acid conjugation, which is very low (Pacifici
and Rane, 1982; Steiner et al, 1982). However, Leakey et
al (1983) have demonstrated that UDP-glucuronyltransferase
activity exhibits two developmental groups in liver of
fetal rhesus monkey, the late-fetal activities being from
46 to 114% of adult values. The human situation is not
known.

It is still uncertain whether human fetal xenobiotic
metabolism can be induced in vivo by the exposure to
foreign chemicals (see Pelkonen, 1980). In experimental
animals, it seems fairly well established, that fetal
xenobiotic metabolism is inducible by polycyclic aromatic
hydrocarbons and other compounds capable of inducing
P_1-450-associated activities, whereas óther inducers are
much less efficient. However, there is some evidence that
phenobarbital might have a small inducing effect on fetal
rat or mouse liver enzymes even before birth (Nau and
Gansau, 1981; Cresteil et al, 1982). Experiments with rat
and human fetal cells in cultures indicate that some
monooxygenase activities are inducible even by
phenobarbital (Peng et al, 1984), provided that cells have
been treated by a glucocorticoid (Kremers et al, 1983).
The interrelationship between glucocorticoids and
polycyclic hydrocarbons in perinatal induction of enzymes
in experimental animals seem also to exist (Leakey et al,
1982).

A comprehensive review of different regulatory factors
has appeared recently (Dutton and Leakey, 1981). In spite
of a large body of experimental work we do not know yet
what are the molecular mechanisms controlling the level and
inducibility of xenobiotic metabolism during development
and what triggers the increase during the perinatal
period. However, molecular biological techniques show some
promise, that in the near future we will know much more
about the developmental regulation of different xenobiotic
metabolising enzymes.

METABOLIC ACTIVATION IN THE FETUS

Animal Studies. The formation of reactive metabolites

catalysed by animal fetal tissues has been demonstrated or implicated in several studies (for a review see Pelkonen, 1985). In some studies it has been possible to show that active intermediates produced in in vitro experimental systems by fetal tissues cause effects that are thought to be indicative or analogous to effects in vivo. Some examples are listed in Table 2.

However, the formation of reactive intermediates in in vitro experimental systems does not, in itself, prove that they can reach critical targets and cause harmful effects. It is widely thought that the balance between activating and detoxicating enzymes is of importance in determining the final outcome or at least the possibility of interaction with critical targets. In this context, it is interesting to speculate on the differing ontogenic patterns of activating and detoxicating enzymes and their possible role in fetotoxicity. for example, aryl hydrocarbon hydroxylase activity (an enzyme associated with the initiation of carcinogenesis and toxicity by polycyclic aromatic hydrocarbons) and possibly the formation of reactive epoxide intermediates, is inducible by 3-methylcholanthrene in fetal rat liver, but epoxide hydrolase activity (which converts epoxides to dihydrodiols) is not inducible (Oesch, 1975). Although this finding cannot be interpreted to represent an enhancement of toxicity (because of complex metabolic pathways thought to be operating in the metabolic activation of polycyclic aromatic hydrocarbons), it nevertheless demonstrates that different pathways can be affected differently. The change in the balance of enzymes may lead either to an enhancement or a decrease in fetotoxicity. This area is still largely unexplored.

Human Studies. The ability of the human fetus to oxidise xenobiotics implies that potentially toxic intermediates can be formed and, indeed, some possible candidates have been tentatively identified or postulated in the metabolism of several compounds (Table 3). These examples on the formation of reactive intermediates by fetal tissues in vitro do not constitute proof that toxic reactions actually occur in the fetus. Nevertheless, the existence of these metabolic pathways is a necessary (although not sufficient) prerequisite for toxic manifestations associated with the listed compounds.

Another important factor is that the activity of human fetal enzymes is lower than that of adult enzymes and thus active intermediates are probably formed in smaller quantities. In this respect, however, the sensitivity of

Table 2. Examples of immediate biochemical or biological effects produced by reactive intermediates as catalysed by fetal tissues *in vitro* or after administration *in vivo*.

COMPOUND	FETAL TISSUES IN VITRO OR TARGET IN VIVO	BIOCHEMICAL OR BIOLOGICAL EFFECT OBSERVED
2-Aminoanthracene	Rat liver, lung, intestine, skin	mutagenesis in Salmonella
Benzo(a)pyrene	Rat liver, lung, brain (intestine & skin negative)	mutagenesis in Salmonella
	Mouse liver, lung	mutagenesis in Salmonella
	Mouse fetus in utero	binding to protein & DNA
	Mouse embryos in culture	sister-chromatid exchange
Cigarette-smoke condensate	Rat lung, intestine (liver & skin negative)	mutagenesis in Salmonella
7,12-Dimethyl-benz(a)anthracene	Rat liver, brain, lung	mutagenesis in Salmonella
	Mouse liver, lung	
2-Acetylamino-fluorene	Rat liver, lung	mutagenesis in Salmonella
	Mouse liver, lung, brain	
	Rat embryos in culture	
Nitrofurazone	Mouse fetal liver in vivo	gross malformations
Phenytoin	Mouse fetus in vivo	binding to protein
Cyclophosphamide	Rat embryos in culture	binding to protein, gross malformations

Most original references can be found in Pelkonen, 1985; additional references are Faustman-Watts et al, 1985 and 1986; Greenaway et al, 1982.

Table 3. Potential metabolic activations catalysed by the human fetal tissues *in vitro* and cells in culture.

COMPOUND	METABOLIC PATHWAY DETECTED	HARMFUL EFFECTS IMPLICATED
Benzo(a)pyrene	epoxidation, epoxide hydration, DNA-adducts	mutagenesis, carcinogenesis
7,12-Dimethyl-benz(a)-anthracene	epoxidation, epoxide hydration, DNA-adducts	mutagenesis, carcinogenesis
2-Acetylaminofluorene	N-hydroxylation and ester-ification	mutagenesis, carcinogenesis
Dimethylnitrosamine and other nitrosamines	N-dealkylation, DNA-adducts	mutagenesis, carcinogenesis
Aflatoxin B1	DNA-adducts	mutagenesis, carcinogenesis
Aldrin	epoxidation	increased fetotoxicity
Phenytoin	epoxidation	teratogenesis, fetotoxicity
Aniline	N-oxidation	methaemoglobinemia
Carbon tetrachloride	(free radicals?)	lipid peroxidation, tissue injuries
Paracetamol	GSH conjugate of active metabolite	liver injury

For original references see Pelkonen, 1982 and 1985; additional references Autrup et al, 1984; Oravec et al, 1985.

fetal tissues to exogenous influences is important. It is
likely that fetal tissues and their functions differ from
their adult counterparts with respect to sensitivity to
exogenous influences, such as xenobiotics and their
activated metabolites. The low activities of fetal enzymes
do not necessarily mean that there is less likelihood of
harmful effects being mediated by their metabolites.

Concerning the model toxicant, benzo(a)pyrene, several
studies have demonstrated the presence of AHH activity in
different fetal tissues and the production of different
benzo(a)pyrene metabolites, although at a relatively low
level (see Pelkonen, 1977b, 1982; also Pacifici et al,
1984, 1985; Peng et al, 1984). Also the presence of other
enzymes participating in the metabolism of benzo(a)pyrene,
for example epoxide hydrolase and glutathione S-
transferase, have been detected in human fetal liver (see
Pacifici, 1983). However, the balance between activating
and inactivating enzymes seems to favour inactivation, a
situation resembling that in the adult liver. At least, in
in vitro incubations with human fetal liver microsomes, it
has not been possible to detect the specific binding of
reactive benzo(a)pyrene metabolites to exogenous DNA
(Pelkonen, 1981), a finding quite in contrast with that in
placental studies. The benzo(a)pyrene diol-epoxide-DNA-
adduct can be detected in cultured fetal cells and explants
(Autrup et al, 1984).

Association between metabolic activation and fetotoxicity.
The observation that fetal tissues catalyse the formation
of reactive metabolites is very suggestive with respect to
developmental toxicology, but does not directly prove the
linkage of these two phenomena. However, in some cases
there are strong indications of an association between
reactive intermediates and fetotoxicity. For example,
experimental studies on transplacental carcinogenesis
suggest that agents requiring metabolic activation are
effective only just before birth, when xenobiotic-
metabolising enzymes appear in fetal tissues (Druckrey,
1973).

A promising approach has been the use of the genetic
model developed by Nebert and co-workers (1975). In this
model, the inducibility of aryl hydrocarbon hydroxylase
activity in the liver and other tissues is controlled by
alleles at the so called Ah locus in a manner that obeys
simple Mendelian rules in many genetic crosses. Thus, the
genetic crosses between mice from C57BL/6 and DBA/2
strains, the responsiveness segregates as an autosomal
dominant trait, and in appropriate backcrosses an
association between the Ah locus and the fetotoxicity of a

xenobiotic can be studied without interference from
numerous nonspecific effects of the compound. Because it
has been shown that the induced enzyme produces more
proximal carcinogens, mutagenic metabolites and DNA-bound
metabolites than the control enzyme, both in vitro and in
vivo, it seems very probable that the association between
this genetic trait and the biological effect caused by a
foreign chemical, if demonstrated, is due to reactive
metabolites (Pelkonen and Nebert, 1982).

Studies from Nebert's laboratory demonstrate that there
is indeed a correlation between genetic responsiveness and
the incidence of fetotoxicity. Lambert and Nebert (1977)
demonstrated that responsiveness at the Ah locus was
associated with an increased incidence of stillbirths,
resorptions, and malformations induced by 3-
methylcholanthrene or 7,12-dimethylbenzanthracene. A more
definitive study by Shum et al (1979) showed that
benzo(a)pyrene given at day 7 or 10 of gestation causes in
utero toxicity and tetarogenicity more so in genetically
responsive than in nonresponsive mice. With the use of
backcrosses, they showed that allelic differences at the Ah
locus in the fetus can be correlated with dysmorphogenesis.
Furthermore, they were able to show that the phenotypes of
the mother and the father are of importance in certain
situations, too.

PLACENTAL XENOBIOTIC METABOLISM

On the basis of a number of studies (See Juchau, 1976;
Pelkonen et al, 1979) on the substrate specificity,
relative activity and inducibility of placental xenobiotic-
metabolising enzymes (Table 1), placental xenobiotic
metabolism exhibits a very restricted substrate specificity
in an uninduced state. Only some oxidations induced by
maternal cigarette smoking and conjugations are present to
a significant extent and the placenta in early pregnancy
seems to be devoid of xenobiotic biotransformations and
unresponsive to cigarette smoke induction. It seems likely
that this cigarette smoke-induced enzyme system is not of
importance in pharmacokinetics, but it may be of
toxicological significance.

METABOLIC ACTIVATION IN THE HUMAN PLACENTA

Because the substrate specificity of placental enzyme
systems is very narrow, the possibility for metabolic
activation of foreign chemicals is also very restricted.
Increased human placental microsomal monooxygenases are

able to produce active metabolites from benzo(a)pyrene, 7,12-dimethylbenz(a)anthracene and 2-acetylaminofluorene, which bind covalently to DNA (Pelkonen and Saarni, 1980; Gurtoo et al, 1983) and are mutagenic when tested with Salmonella typhimurium (Jones et al, 1977; Juchau et al, 1978; Vaught et al, 1979). Immunological properties of the placental monooxygenase clearly show it to be of the 3-methylcholanthrene-induced type (Fujino et al, 1982).

We have been attempting to construct the whole sequence of events from the in vitro formation of reactive intermediates by placental microsomes to in vivo fetotoxicity, for example decreased birth weight (Pelkonen et al, 1979; Vahakangas et al, 1982). In in vitro incubations, placental microsomes with induced aryl hydrocarbon hydroxylase activity are able to catalyse the formation of reactive intermediates capable of causing mutations in the Ames test and binding covalently to exogenous DNA (see above). In the latter experimental system it has been possible to demonstrate that the 7,8-diol-9,10-epoxide metabolite is produced as a predominant reactive species (Pelkonen and Saarni, 1980). The production of the diol-epoxide metabolite is dependent on the aryl hydrocarbon hydroxylase activity, as measured by the fluorescent phenol metabolites. When compared with rat liver or human fetal liver, the placental enzyme seems to be more efficient in producing the diol-epoxide metabolite per unit of enzyme activity. The possible reason is that the balance between activating and inactivating enzymes in the placenta in vitro favours the production and survival of the reactive intermediate. With sensitive methods for detecting carcinogen-DNA adducts, such as immunochemical, adduct post-labelling and linear synchronous fluorescence methods, it has been possible to demonstrate that benzo(a)pyrene metabolite-nucleoside adducts are also formed in vivo in human placental DNA, after the exposure to polycyclic aromatic hydrocarbons through cigarette smoking or at work (Vahakangas et al, 1985; Everson et al, 1986). In the next phase it would be desirable to measure the extent of carcinogen binding to placental DNA and correlate it with the biological outcome, be it newborn well-being and characteristics, placental status and hormone production, child development and so on. If the inducibility of placental AHH activity by maternal cigarette smoking is under genetic control, as it seems to be (Pelkonen et al, 1981; Gurtoo et al, 1983), it should be possible to detect "risk pregnancies" with respect to polycyclic aromatic hydrocarbon exposure.

CONCLUSIONS

Although the importance of xenobiotic metabolism in detoxication and metabolic activation of chemicals in the adult organism is firmly established, its overall significance and the relation to toxic reactions during the embryonic and fetal periods is largely a matter of speculation. Many studies have demonstrated the production of reactive metabolites by animal and human fetal and placental tissues and in some cases this production has been shown to be associated with toxic consequences. Indirect evidence suggest that fetotoxic, teratogenic and transplacental carcinogenic effects of some polycyclic hydrocarbons and nitrosamines may be due to the formation of reactive intermediates.

An interesting example is the maternal cigarette smoking-inducible enzyme in the placenta, which metabolises benzo(a)pyrene. The induced enzyme produces both in vitro and probably also in vivo, metabolites, which are able to bind to DNA. Human fetal liver and adrenal gland are also able to metabolise benzo(a)pyrene, but the balance between activating and detoxicating processes seem to favour the latter. Furthermore, fetal hepatic and adrenal enzymes seem not to be inducible by exogenous inducers, at least during the first trimester.

REFERENCES

Autrup, H., Harris, C.C., Wu, S.-M., Bao, L.-Y., Pei, X.-F., Lu, S., Sun, T.-T. and Hsia, C.-C. (1984). Chem. Biol. Interactions, 50, 15.

Christ, W., Hecker, W., Gindler, K. and Stille, G. (1983). Biochem. Pharmacol. 32, 1961.

Cresteil, T., Beaune, P., Kremers, P., Flinois, J.-P. and Leroux, J.-P. (1982a). Pediatr. Pharmacol, 2, 199.

Cresteil, T., Le Provost, E., Flinois, J.-P. and Leroux, J.-P (1982b). Biochem. Biophys. Res. Commun, 106, 823.

Druckrey, H. (1973). Xenobiotica, 3, 271.

Dutton, G.J. and Leakey, J.E.A. (1981). Progr. Drug Res, 25, 189.

Dvorchik, B.H. and Hartman, R.D. (1982). Biochem. Pharmacol, 31, 1150.

Everson et al (1986). Science, 231, 54.

Faustman-Watts, E.M., Namkung, M.J., Greenaway, J.C. and Juchau, M.R. (1985). Biochem. Pharmacol, 34, 2953.

Faustman-Watts, E.M., Giachelli, C.M. and Juchau, M.R. (1986). Toxicol. Appl. Pharmacol, 83, 590.

Filler, R. and Lew, K.J. (1981). Proc. Natl. Acad. Sci,

USA, 78, 6991.
Fujino, T., Park, S.S., West, D. and Gelboin, H.V. (1982).
    Proc. Natl. Acad. Sci, USA, 79, 3682.
Galloway, S.M., Perry, P.E., Meneses, J., Nebert, D.W.,
    Pedersen, R.A. (1980). Proc. Natl. Acad. Sci. USA, 77,
    3524.
Greenaway, J.C., Fantel, A.G., Shephard, T.H. and Juchau,
    M.R. (1982). Teratology, 25, 335.
Gurtoo, H.L., Williams, C.J., Gottlieb, K., Mulhern, A.I.,
    Caballes, L., Vaught, J.B., Marinello, A.J. and Bansal,
    N.K. (1983). Int. J. Cancer 31, 29.
Hamilton, J.W., Densoin, M.S. and Bloom, S.E. (1983). Proc.
    Natl. Acad. Sci. USA, 80, 3372.
Juchau, M.R., Chao, S.T. and Omiecinski, C.J. (1980). Clin.
    Pharmacokin, 5, 320.
Juchau, M.R. (1976). In "Perinatal Pharmacology and
    Therapeutics" (Ed. B. Mirkin). Academic Press, New
    York, p.71.
Juchau, M.R. (1980). Pharmac. Ther, 8, 501.
Juchau, M.R. (1981). In "The biochemical basis of chemical
    teratogenesis" (Ed. M.R. Juchau). Elsevier/North-
    Holland, New York/Amsterdam, p.63.
Juchau, M.R., DiGiovanni, J., Namkung, M.J. and Jones, A.H.
    (1979). Toxicol. Appl. Pharmacol, 9, 171.
Juchau, M.R., Namkung, M.J., Jones, A.H. and DiGiovanni, J.
    (1978). Drug Metab. Disp, 6, 273.
Kitada, M., Kamataki, T., Itahashi, K., Rikihisa, T., Kato,
    R. and Kanakubo, Y. (1985). Arch. Biochem. Biophys,
    241, 275.
Kremers, P., Letawe-Goujon, F., De Graeve, J., Duvivier,
    J., Gielen, J.E., Bastin, M., Frankinet-Collingnon, C.
    and Wolff, D. (1983). Eur. J. Biochem, 137, 603.
Lambert, G.H. and Nebert, D.W. (1977). Teratology, 16, 147.
Leakey, J.E.A., Althaus, Z.R., Bailey, J.R. and Slikker,
    Jr. W. (1983). Biochem. J. 214, 1007.
Leakey, J.E.A., Wishart, G.J. and Dutton, G.J. (1982).
    Biol. Res. Preg, 3, 108.
Lum, P.Y., Walker, S. and Ioannides, C. (1985). Toxicology,
    35, 307.
Jones, A.H., Fantel, A.G, Kocan, R.A., Juchau, M.R.
    (1977). Life Sci, 21, 1831.
Morgan, E.T., Macgeoch, C. and Gustafsson, J.-A (1985). J.
    Biol. Chem, 260, 11895.
Nau, H. and Gansau, C. (1981). In "Culture Techniques"
    (Neubert, D. and Merker, H.-J. eds). Walter de Gruyter
    and Co, Berlin, p.495.
Nau, H. and Neubert, D. (1978). In "Role of
    Pharmacokinetics in prenatal and perinatal toxicology"

(Ed. D. Neubert, H.J., Merker, H., Nau and J. Langman). Georg Thieme, Stuttgart, p.13.

Nebert, D.W., Robinson, J.R., Niwa, A., Kumaki, K. and Poland, A.P. (1975). J. Cell. Physiol, 85, 393.

Newbert, D.W., Levitt, R.C. and Pelkonen, O. (1979). In "Carcinogens : Identification and mechanisms of action" (ed. A.C. Griffin and C.R. Shaw). Raven Press, New York, p.157.

Oesch, F. (1975). FEBS Lett, 53, 205.

Oravec, C.T., Samuel, M.J. and D'ambrosio, S.M. (1985). Drug Metab. Disp, 13, 76.

Pacifici, G.M. (1983). Epoxide detoxication pathways in human fetus. Academic Thesis. Karolinska institutet, Stockholm.

Pacifici, G.M., Bencini, C. and Rane, A. (1986). Pharmacology, 32, 283.

Pacifici, G.M., Colizzi, C., Giuliani, L. and Rane, A. (1983). Arch. Toxicol, 54, 331.

Pacifici, G.M., Colizzi, C., Giuliani, L. and Rane, A. (1984). Pharmacology, 28, 321.

Pacifici, G.M., Glaumann, H. and Rane, A. (1985). Pharmacology, 30, 188.

Pacifici, G.M. and Rane, A. (1982). Br. J. Clin. Pharmacol, 13, 732.

Pelkonen, O. (1977a). In "Progress in Drug Metabolism", vol 2. (Ed. J.W. Bridges and L.. Chasseaud). Wiley, London, p.119.

Pelkonen, O. (1977b). In "Biological reactive intermediates" (Jollow, D.J., Kocsis, J.J., Synder, R. and Vainio, H. eds). Plenum Press, New York, p.148.

Pelkonen, O. (1980a). Pharmac. Ther, 10, 261.

Pelkonen, O. (1980b). Eur. J. Clin. Pharmacol, 18, 17.

Pelkonen, O. (1981). In "Drug metabolism in the immature human" (ed. L.F. Soyka and G.P. Redmond). Raven Press, New York, p.19.

Pelkonen, O. (1982). In "Developmental Toxicology" (Ed. K. Snell). Croom Helm, London, p.167.

Pelkonen, O. (1984a). Dev. Pharmacol. Ther. 7, suppl 1, 11.

Pelkonen, O. (1984b). In "Drugs and Pregnancy : Maternal drug handling-fetal drug Exposure" (Krauer, F., Hytten, F.E. and Del Pozo, E. eds). Academic Press, London. p.63.

Pelkonen, O. (1985). In "Occupational hazards and reproduction"(Ed. K. Hemminki., M. Sorsa and H. Vainio). Hemisphere, Washington, p.113.

Pelkonen, O., Karki, N.T., Koivisto, M., Tuimala, R. and Kauppila, A. (1979). Toxicol. Lett, 3, 331.

Pelkonen, O., Karki, N.T., Korhonen, P., Koivisto, M.,

Tuimala, R. and Kauppila, A. (1979). In "Polynuclear aromatic hydrocarbons" (Ed. P.W. Jones and P. Leber). Ann Arbor Science Publishers, Ann Arbor, p. 765.

Pelkonen, O., Karki, N.T. and Sotaniemi, E.A. (1980). In "Human Cancer. Its Characteristics and Treatment" (Ed. W. Davis., R.K. Harrap and G. Stathopoulos), Excerpta Medica, Amsterdam, p.48.

Pelkonen, O., Karki, N.T. and Tuimala, R. (1981). Cancer Lett, 13, 103.

Pelkonen, O. and Nebert, D.W. (1982). Pharmacol. Rev. 34, 189.

Pelkonen, O. and Saarni, H. (1980). Chem. Biol. Interact, 30, 287.

Peng, D.-R., Pacifici, G.M. and Rane, A. (1984). Biochem. Pharmacol, 33, 71.

Poland, A. and Glover, E. (1980). Mol. Pharmacol, 17, 86.

Shum, S., Jensen, M.N., Nebert, D.W. (1979). Teratology, 20, 365.

Steiner, E., von Bahr, C. and Rane, A. (1982). Dev. Pharmacol. Ther, 5, 14.

Vaught, J.B., Gurtoo, H.L., Parker, N.D., LeBoeuf, R. and Doctor, G. (1979). Cancer Res, 39, 3177.

Vahakangas, K., Hirn, M. and Pelkonen, O. (1982). Toxicol, 10, 81.

Vahakangas, K., Pasanen, M., Trivers, G., Harris, C.C. and Pelkonen, O. (1985). In "26th Congress of the European Society of Toxicology, Abstracts", University of Kuopio, Kuopia, p. C.1.14.

CYTOCHROME P-450 OF THE OLFACTORY EPITHELIUM AND ITS DEGRADATION BY SUICIDE SUBSTRATES IN VIVO

[1]Celia J.Reed, [1]Francesco De Matteis and [2]Edward A. Lock

[1]MRC Toxicology Unit, Carshalton, Surrey, UK and
[2]ICI, Central Toxicology Laboratory, Macclesfield, Cheshire,UK

INTRODUCTION

The olfactory epithelium of several species has been found to contain cytochrome P-450 and to be competent in the metabolism of a variety of substrates (Hadley and Dahl, 1983). In hamsters we have found that, although microsomes prepared from olfactory epithelium contain only 50% of the cytochrome P-450 of those from liver, they are more active in the metabolism of 7-ethoxycourmarin, 7-ethoxyresorufin, hexobarbitone and aniline. Unusually high rates of electron transport were also found in olfactory microsomes, and the ratio of NADPH cytochrome P-450 reductase to cytochrome P-450 shown to be greater in this tissue as compared to the liver. We suggest that facilitated electron flow may contribute to the active drug metabolism of the olfactory cytochrome P-450. Additional evidence for this conclusion may be found in the work of Reed et al (1986); the main purpose of this short paper is to describe the peroxidase activity of olfactory cytochrome P-450, and to compare the effects of three suicide substrates on cytochrome P-450-dependent reactions in the liver and olfactory tissue.

Organic hydroperoxides can interact with cytochrome P-450 and support a number of drug metabolising reactions in the absence of NADPH (Nordblom et al, 1976). They can also be utilised by cytochrome P-450 (acting as a peroxidase) to oxidise dyes such as N,N,N',N'-tetramethylphenylenediamine (TMPD) (Hrycay and O'Brien, 1971) or, in the absence of such acceptor molecules, result in self-catalysed haem destruction. Using cumene hydroperoxide (CuOOH) and TMPD to measure the peroxidase activity of isolated microsomes, we found the olfactory membranes to be 5-fold more active than those from liver (Table 1). However, when the CuOOH-supported deethylation of 7-ethoxycoumarin was studied (in

Table 1. Cumene hydroperoxide-dependent peroxidase and 7-ethoxycoumarin deethylase activities and cytochrome P-450 destruction in hamster hepatic and olfactory microsomes.

TISSUE	PEROXIDASE ACTIVITY	7-ETHOXYCOUMARIN DEETHYLASE ACTIVITY (% CONTROL)	
	nmol TMPD oxidised/ min/mg protein	CuOOH*	CuOOH followed by NADPH[+]
Liver	18.04 $\pm$ 0.98	53	39
Olfactory epithelium	89.58 $\pm$ 5.14	1	16

* samples incubated with CuOOH + 7-ethoxycoumarin for 30 sec.

+ samples incubated with CuOOH for 30 sec. and then with 7-ethoxycoumarin + NADPH for a further 30 sec.

the absence of NADPH) significant activity was found in
hepatic microsomes,   virtually none in olfactory. A
likely interpretation for this finding is that, under these
conditions, the olfactory cytochrome P-450 was much more
active than the hepatic in catalysing its own CuOOH-
dependent degradation. This conclusion is supported by the
finding (Table 1) that when microsomes were preincubated
with the hydroperoxide for 30 sec. and then the drug
substrate and NADPH were added, residual deethylation
activity was considerably less in the olfactory tissue as
compared with the liver. Under these conditions not
significant loss of NADPH cytochrome c reductase activity
was found with either tissue.

     Evidence that the peroxidase activity involves a
cytochrome P-450 pool was obtained by showing that a
suicide substrate of cytochrome P-450 (the 4-ethyl analogue
of 3,5-diethoxycarbonyl-1,4-dihydrocollidine, i.e. 4-ethyl
DDC) caused, in vivo, similar losses of spectrally
determined cytochrome P-450 and peroxidase activity in both
tissues (Figure 1).

**Figure 1. The effect of suicide substrates on cytochrome P-
450 and cytochrome P-450-dependent reactions in (a) hepatic
and (b) olfactory microsomes of male hamsters.**

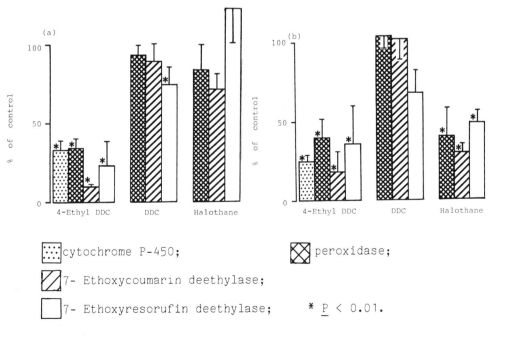

Cytochrome P-450-dependent reactions were affected to similar extents in hepatic and olfactory microsomes following treatment with DDC or 4-ethyl DDC. DDC caused little or no loss of peroxidase, 7-ethoxycoumarin or 7-ethoxyresorufin deethylase activity, while 4-ethyl DDC decreased all three significantly. In contrast, halothane caused loss of the above activities in the olfactory epithelium while having no effect on those of the liver. Halothane can be metabolised by reductive as well as oxidative pathways, but it is the reductive mode that results in destruction of cytochrome P-450 (Krieter and Van Dyke, 1983), and this pathway is favoured in the liver following phenobarbital treatment. The loss of olfactory cytochrome P-450 suggests that reductive metabolism occurs in this tissue, and that the olfactory cytochrome P-450 contains significant amounts of isozyme(s) resembling the phenobarbital inducible forms of the liver. This is substantiated by the particularly high rates of olfactory hexobarbitone and 7-ethoxycouramin metabolism (Reed et al, 1986).

REFERENCES

Hadley, W.M and Dahl, A.R. (1983)Drug Metab. Disp. 11, 275.
Hrycay, E.G. and O'Brien, P.J. (1971)Arch. Biochem. Biophys. 147, 14.
Krieter, P.A. and Van Dyke, R.A. (1983) Chem.-Biol. Interactions 44, 219.
Nordblom, G.D., White, R.E. & Coon, M.J. (1976) Arch. Biochem. Biophys. 175, 524.
Reed, C.J., De Matteis, F. & Lock, E.A. (1986) Biochem. J. (in press).

SUBCELLULAR EFFECTS OF HALOALKENES IN THE KIDNEY

Alf Wallin, Thomas W. Jones, Anibal E. Vercesi,
and Kari Ormstad

Department of Forensic Medicine, Karolinska Institutet,
S-104 01 Stockholm, Sweden.

INTRODUCTION

Several haloalkenes act as selective nephrotoxins in vivo (Lock, 1982). Recently, in vitro toxicity has been demonstrated to occur during incubations of isolated rat renal epithelial cells with the cysteinyl conjugate of trichloroethylene (Elfarra et al, 1986) as well as the glutathione conjugate of hexachlorobutadiene (PCBG) (Jones et al, 1986). Renal bioactivation of PCBG comprises a stepwise degradation in the proximal tubular lumen, exerted by brush-border-associated enzymes, which yields the cysteinyl conjugate (PCBC). After absorption into the tubular epithelial cells PCBC becomes an available substrate to the renal cysteine conjugate β-lyase, which catalyzes the formation of a reactive metabolite (Elfarra and Anders, 1984). The structure of this intermediate is still incompletely known, but it is ascribed the toxic effects on tubular epithelia (Stevens et al, 1986). The exact mechanism beyond PCBC-induced cell toxicity remains to be mapped out, but available knowledge strongly suggests mitochrondria as the major subcellular target (Lash et al, 1986).

The present study focusses on the effects of PCBC on Ca^{2+}-homeostasis and membrane potential in isolated mitochondria from rat kidney cortex.

RESULTS AND DISCUSSION

During exposure to PCBG, isolated renal epithelial cells exhibit a dose-dependent loss of viability preceeded by an increase of cytosolic Ca^{2+}-levels (Jones et al, 1986).

In order to investigate the mechanisms beyond this phenomenon, isolated renal cortical mitochrondria were incubated in the presence of PCBC. Figure 1 demonstrates a dose-dependent release of Ca^{2+} from mitochondria incubated

in a high-Ca^{2+} medium, compared to a control incubation in
the absence of PCBC, where Ca^{2+} is taken up and retained in
the mitrochrondria during respiration.

Figure 1. PCBC-induced mitochondrial Ca^{2+} release

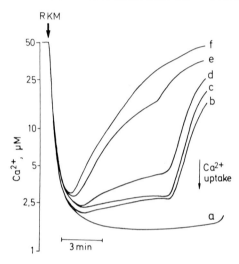

Rat kidney mitochrondria (RKM) were incubated for 15 min at
32°C in a HEPES-buffered medium (5mM) containing 125mM
sucrose, 65 mMKCl, 0.4mM KH$_2$PO$_4$/K$_2$HPO$_4$, 3 μM rotenone,
0.3mM TPP$^+$, and 50 μM CaCl$_2$ (pH7.2). The Ca^{2+}-
concentration in the incubates was recorded by a Ca^{2+}-
selective electrode from Radiometer (Denmark). PCBC was
synthesized according to McKinney (1959) and added to the
incubates at concentrations indicated as follows: 0 M (a),
25 μM (b), 50 μM (c), 100 μM (d), 150 μM (e) , and 250 μM
(f).

Mitochrondrial Ca^{2+} uptake occurs via an uniport
mechanism, and the driving force is the transmembranal
electrochemical potential, i.e. the inside is negatively
charged to ca. 200mV (Akerman and Nicholls, 1983).
Consequently, if the membrane is depolarized, the ability
to retain Ca^{2+} is impaired and calcium is released into the
extramitochondrial space, and then the incubation medium.
    In Figure 2 mitochondria were preincubated with or
without PCBC in a Ca^{2+}-free medium, i.e. all Ca^{2+} present
orginates from the mitochrondrial pool. After 10 minutes
succinate was added to energize the mitochrondria. This
addition results in a rapid uptake of Ca^{2+} from the medium

Figure 2. Comparison of the effect of PCBC on (upper panel) the Ca^{2+} retention and (lower panel) maintenance of the membrane potential in mitochrondria

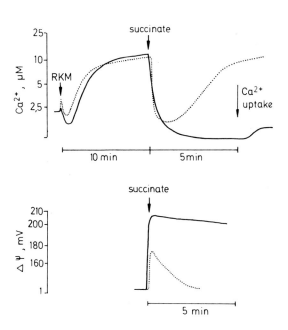

RKM were preincubated in a deenergized state for 10 min in the absence (_____) or presence (.......) of 400 µM PCBC in a Ca^{2+}-deficient medium. Succinate was added after preincubation. The membrane potential was measured by a TPP^+ ion-selective electrode according to Kamo (1979). Tetraphenylphosphonium bromide (TPP^+) was obtained from Aldrich-Chemie (Steinheim, F.R.G.).

in parallel to the build-up of a membrane potential. However, in the presence of PCBC mitochrondria become incapable of maintaining the potential and accordingly Ca2+ is released. Hence, not until succinate induces the electron transport chain and the mitrochondria become energized are these features lost and impairment of mitochondrial functions ensues. This observation demonstrates that ongoing electron transport is necessary to initiate the toxic effects exerted by the reactive metabolite of PCBC against mitochrondria. Our results also indicate that the mitochrondrial inner membrane probably is

the target for the toxic metabolite which may be provoking
an increased proton permeability. Thus, it seems
reasonable to suggest that Ca^{2+} release is an indirect
effect of a collapsed membrane potential.

REFERENCES

Akerman, K.E.O., and Nicholls, D.G. (1983) Rev. Physiol.
   Biochem. Pharmacol. 95, 149.
Elfarra, A.A. and Anders, M.W. (1984) Biochem. Pharmacol.
   33, 3729.
Elfarra, A.A., Lash, L.H. and Anders, M.W.(1986) Proc. Natl.
   Acad. Sci., in press.
Jones, T.W., Wallin, A., Thor, H., Gerdes, R.G., Ormstad, K.
   and Orrenius, S. (1986) Arch. Biochem. Biophys.,
   submitted
Kamo, N., Muratsuga, M., Hangho, R. and Kobatake, Y. (1979)
   J. Memb. Biol. 49, 105.
Lash, L.H., Elfarra, A.A. and Anders, M.W. (1986) J. Biol.
   Chem. 261, 5930.
Lock, E.A.(1982) in "Nephrotoxicity: Assesment and
   Pathogenesis" (Eds Bach, Bonner, Bridges, Lock) John
   Wiley & Sons, p396.
McKinney, L.L., Picken, J.C., Weakley, A.C., Eldridge, A.C.,
   Campbell, R.E., Cowan, J.C. and Biester, H.E. (1959) J.
   Am. Soc. 81, 909.
Stevens, J., Hayden, P. and Taylor G. (1986) J. Biol. Chem.
   261, 3325.

STRONG INHIBITION OF LIPID PEROXIDATION IN VITRO AND IN VIVO BY DITHIOLTHIONE DERIVATIVES

Patrick Dansette, Amor Sassi, Michel Plat, Marie-Odile
Christen and Daniel Mansuy.

Laboratoire de Chimie et Biochimie Pharmacologiques et
Toxicologiques, 45 rue des Saints Peres, 75270 Paris Cedex
06. France. Laboratoire de Chimie Therapeutique, Faculte
de Pharmacie, Rue Jean-Baptiste Clement, 92290 Chatenay-
Malabry, France. Laboratoire de Therapeutique Moderne, 42
rue Rouget de Lisle, 92159 Suresnes, France.

INTRODUCTION

It is now well recognised that during several
pathological situations, an oxidative stress characterised
by an unusual and intense production of species derived
from O_2 reduction occurs in many kinds of cells (Sies,
1985; Reckenagel, 1977). A general consequence of this
oxidative stress is the peroxidation of cell lipids
resulting in a more or less slow degradation of the cell
organisation. Such processes play a key role in the
toxicity induced by acetaminophen (Wendel et al, 1979;
Wendel and Feuerstein, 1979). It thus seems interesting to
find non-toxic compounds that are able to strongly inhibit
lipid peroxidation in vivo, in order to prevent the
deleterious effects of this peroxidation.

Anisyldithiolthione (ADT), 5-(p-methoxyphenyl)-3H-1, 2-
dithiol-3-thione, a drug which has been used for many years
as a choleretic agent was recently described to protect
mice against the acute toxic effects of acetaminophen and
CCl_4 (Ansher et al, 1983). This paper reports results
showing that ADT is a strong inhibitor of lipid
peroxidation both in vitro and in vivo and that low doses
of ADT inhibit ethane exhalation by mice intoxicated by
500mg/kg acetaminophen in addition to the prevention of
mortality caused by acetaminophen overdose. We also
compare ADT to several analogues in order to study the
structural features necessary for these effects.

                                                    Ar   X

	1a	5-anisyl dithiol-thione (ADT)	5 anisyl	S
	1b	5-anisyl dithiolthione-one(ADO)	5 anisyl	O
	2a	5-phenyl dithiol-thione (5PDT)	5-phenyl	S
	3a	4-phenyl dithiol-thione (4PDT)	4-phenyl	S
	4a	5-eugenyl dithiol-thione (EDT)	5-eugenyl	S

RESULTS

Inhibitory Effects of ADT on Lipid Peroxidation In Vitro

ADT inhibits lipid peroxidation induced in rat liver microsomes by classical chemical systems consisting of a ferrous salt associated with a reducing agent such as cysteine or ascorbate (Mansuy et al, 1986; Malvy et al, 1980; Searle and Wilson, 1983). The concentrations (IC_{50}) leading to 50% inhibition of malondialdehyde (MDA) formation were around 3 μM. Analogous IC_{50} values, in the μM range, were found for ADT inhibition of lipid peroxidation induced in rat liver microsomes by enzymatic reduction of CCl_4 in the presence of NADPH (Table 1).

Table 1. Inhibition by ADT derivatives or by antioxidants of lipid peroxidation (malondialdehyde formation) induced chemically or enzymatically in rat liver microsomes.

	Lipid peroxidation in microsomes induced by		
	$FeSO_4$ + Cysteine	$FeSO_4$ + Ascorbate	CCl_4 + NADPH
INHIBITORS	IC_{50} $(10^{-6}M)$[a]		
Promethazine	8.5+0.2	12.5 +0.5	0.4+0.05
Vitamin E	50+25	35 +16	100
ADT (1a)	3.0+0.1	3.01+0.1	2.0+0.1
ADO (1b)	>100	>100	>100
5PDT (2a)	2.3+0.1	2.8 +0.3	5.0+1.0
4PDT (3a)	3.0+0.2	2.8+0.5	3.4+0.2
EDT (4a)	2.5+0.2	2.3+0.3	3.4+0.2

a Mean values $\pm$ SEM (4 experiments)

Under identical conditions, classical inhibitors of lipid peroxidation lead to similar IC_{50} values (promethazine) or to considerably higher values (vitamin E, around 50µM depending upon the chemical or enzymatic nature of induction of lipid peroxidation).

Interestingly, ADO the compound derived from ADT by replacement of its C=S function by a C=O function, showed almost no inhibitory effect toward lipid peroxidation induced either chemically or enzymatically, at concentrations between 10^{-6}M and 10^{-4}M (Table 1).

Effects of ADT on Lipid Peroxidation and Toxicity Induced In Vivo in Mice by Acetaminophen.

As already described (Wendel et al, 1979; Wendel and Feverstein, 1981), untreated NMRI Swiss mice and also mice treated with up to 500mg/kg acetaminophen exhaled only very low amounts of ethane within 3h. If these mice had been starved for 72h in order to deplete hepatic glutathione, they became much more sensitive to acetaminophen toxicity and exhaled large amounts of ethane which could be easily detected (Wendel et al, 1979).

Administration of ADT 3h before acetaminophen reduced ethane exhalation in mice. With ADT doses as low as 5mg/kg ethane decreased to a level identical to that of mice not treated with acetaminophen and the half-maximum effect was obtained with 0.7mg/kg. Whereas i.p. administration of 20 µmoles/kg of ADT to mice 3h before acetaminophen led to a complete inhibition of ethane exhalation, administration of identical amounts of vitamin E, propylgallate of levamisole led only to a partial inhibition of ethane formation (Table 2).

This inhibition of ethane exhalation was accompanied by a protective effect against acetaminophen hepatotoxicity. Whereas all mice treated with 500 mg/kg acetaminophen died within 10 to 24h, all mice pretreated by 50µmoles (12mg) per kg ADT before acetaminophen were alive after 24h. As shown in Table 2, at 20µmoles per kg, ADT is a far better protecting agent than vitamin E.

Effects of Analogues of ADT on Lipid Peroxidation and Hepatoprotection In Vivo in Mice Intoxicated by Acetaminophen.

Several analogues of ADT, with different substituent groups on the dithiolthione ring, were tested at a dose of 20µmole/kg for inhibition of ethane exhalation and their hepatoprotective effect in mice intoxicated by 500 mg/kg acetaminophen. As shown in Table 2, two analogues substituted in the 5 position were excellent inhibitors of

Table 2. Inhibitory effects of ADT and several antioxidants on <u>in vivo</u> lipid peroxidation and hepatotoxicity induced by acetaminophen in mice [a].

COMPOUNDS (20 µmoles/kg)	INHIBITION OF ETHANE EXHALATION	% SURVIVAL AFTER 24h[c]
None	0% [b]	0% (8)
ADT (1a)	100%	70% (10)
ADT (50 µmoles/kg)	100%	100% (5)
Vitamin E	50%	25% (4)
5 PDT (2a)	100%	100%
4 PDT (3a)	0%	0%
EDT (4a)	100%	60%

[a] Mice starved for 72h received 20µmoles/kg of the compound (i.p) and then 500 mg/kg acetaminophen (i.p).
[b] 600 ± 45 nmoles of ethane per kg 3h after acetaminophen administration.
[c] Number of mice used in the experiment.

ethane production and good hepatoprotectors. In fact 5PDT was efficient at even lower doses (10 µmoles/kg, 100% protection). In contrast the compound with a phenyl substitutent in position 4 (4PDT) was a good inhibitor <u>in vitro</u> of lipid peroxidation (Table 1) but did not inhibit ethane production <u>in vivo</u> or protect against mortality.

DISCUSSION

The results of Table 2 confirm previous data (Ansher <u>et al</u>, 1983) on the remarkable ability of ADT to protect animals against the hepatotoxic effects of CCl_4 or acetaminophen. ADT exerts its protective effect at doses as low as 20µmoles/kg. Upon administration of ADT, either i.p. (12 mg/kg) or orally (24 mg/kg, data not shown) at doses considerably lower than those used previously (500 mg/kg (Ansher <u>et al</u>, 1983), 3h before doses of acetaminophen at which all mice die within 24h, a complete protection was observed, all pretreated mice being alive even one week later. Our results also show that ADT exerts a strong inhibitory effect on ethane exhalation by animals treated by acetaminophen. ADT is a better inhibitor of <u>in vivo</u> lipid peroxidation induced in mice by acetaminophen than previously described antioxidants or hepatoprotective agents such as vitamin E, propylgallate or levamisole (Table 2). When compared to these compounds, ADT exhibits an even more pronounced ability to protect mice against the hepatotoxic effects of acetaminophen overdoses. Several other dithiolthiones substituted in the 5 position are equal or better hepatoprotective agents than ADT.

These results suggest that the "antioxidant" effect of ADT and its analogues could play a key role in their protective effect against hepatotoxic manifestations of acetaminophen, by reducing lipid hydroperoxide levels. However, additional experiments are still required to know whether other effects of ADT could be involved. ADT is an interesting new lipid peroxidation inhibitor because : (i) the dithiolthione function seems important for inhibition (ADO is not an inhibitor), (ii) inhibition also occurs in vivo at very low doses and (iii) this drug has been used in man for at least 40 years without significant toxic or adverse effects.

ACKNOWLEDGEMENTS

We thank Laboratoires LATEMA (France) for their scientific and financial support. We also thank Dr. Marcel Delaforge for his scientific assistance.

REFERENCES

Ansher, S.S., Dolon, P. and Bueding, E. (1983). Hepatology, 3, 932-935.
Bottcher, B. (1948). Chem. Ber, 81, 376.
Koster, U., Albrecht, D., Kappus, H. (1977). Toxicol. Appl. Pharmacol, 41, 639-648.
Malvy, C., Paoletti, C., Searle, A.J.F., Willson, R.L. (1980). Biochem. Biophys. Res. Comm, 95, 734-737.
Mansuy, D., Sassi, A., Dansette, P., Plat, M. (1986). Biochem. Biophys. Res. Comm, 135, 1015-1021.
Reckenagel, R.O., Glende, E.D.Jr. and Hruszkewycz, A.M. (1977). in "Free radicals in biology" (W.A. Pryor, ed). vol III, 97-132, Academic Press, New York.
Searle, A.J.F. and Willson, R.L. (1983). Biochem, J. 212, 549-554.
Sies, H. (1985). Oxidative stress, 1-8 and 311-330, Academic Press, London.
Wendel, A. and Feuerstein, S. (1981). Biochem. Pharmacol, 18, p.2531-2520.
Wendel, A., Feuerstein, S. and Konz, K.H. (1979). Biochem. Pharmacol, 13, 2051-205.

METHODS IN DRUG METABOLISM - FUTURE PROSPECTS

James W. Bridges

The Robens Institute, University of Surrey, Guildford GU2 5XH, Surrey, U.K.

INTRODUCTION

The past thirty years have witnessed the introduction of many new techniques which have had a major impact on the practice of drug metabolism. These include: site specific radiolabelling, scintillation counting, gas chromatography, high performance liquid chromatography, mass spectrometry, immunoassay and techniques for preparation of isolated cells, cell fractions and purified enzymes. Moreover a number of older techniques have re-emerged in new forms or for new purposes eg. fluorescence, electrophoresis.

In speculating on future prospects I have drawn on four types of information:
- new techniques where preliminary findings are already showing some promise;
- techniques already in use in other areas of life sciences, but not yet applied to drug metabolism;
- methods which are already in regular use in drug metabolism but whose application might be considerably broadened;
- areas in which there is an undoubted need but no clear indication as to how it will be met.

There are sufficient pressures to improve or change our present methods to ensure that progress in the development of better techniques at least matches and probably surpasses that of the recent past. Major forces in this respect are the growing demands by legislative authorities and others for more and more sophisticated information, increasing cost and efficiency consciousness of managers of research and heightening ethical considerations which are likely to further restrict the use of animals and man for experimental purposes. Consequencies of this strong 'ethical' lobby will probably be a major growth in the use of in vitro and computer modelling techniques, increased replacement of radioisotopes by other labels such as stable isotopes and development of non-invasive sampling techniques eg. analysis of breath, saliva, and sweat and a major extension of the application of whole body NMR and ESR methods.

The purpose of this article is to indicate briefly areas where particular technical progress is likely to be made. It is not intended to be a fully comprehensive assessment and the author apologies to readers if their favourite technique is not mentioned.

CHEMICAL ASPECTS

(i)Fuller Development of Existing Methods (see Table1)

There is a great need to make drug metabolism and toxicology studies more relevant to the actual human exposure situation. This requires that where some preliminary information can be obtained in man the dose regimen administered to animals in toxicity tests is made relevant to the human pharmacokinetics. In this context a greatly extended role for devices, such as implanted minipumps, is envisaged. It will also place even greater demands on the analyst to work with microsamples of animal tissue fluids as well as devising less stressful procedures for obtaining them. In turn good evidence of proper method validation and effective quality control procedures will be required increasingly. If analytical aspects of drug metabolism are to develop optimally means will need to be found of building up a widely available validated data bank which relates physicochemical properties of xenobiotics to their metabolism, pharmacokinetics and method of analysis (see below).

A further major area in which modification of existing methods is likely to play an important part is the adaptation of present methods eg. immunoassays, photometric methods to provide rapid, robust analytical techniques which can be used to identify patient compliance/drug blood levels, pesticide levels in foodstuffs, levels of particular chemicals in the workplace etc. However a significant role is also likely here for biosensor devices

(ii) New Developments

There are a number of general areas where improvements in methods are clearly needed. These include:
- identification of individual enantiomers
- methods for following the distribution of drugs in tissues of live animals;
- availability of simple approaches for characterisation of drug conjugates (other than glucuronides and sulphates and identification of individual binding sites;
- New approaches to sample work up.

Table 1. Some existing chemical techniques in drug metabolism and possible areas for their particular further development

TECHNIQUE	POSSIBLE FURTHER APPLICATION
Derivatisation of chemicals and their metabolites	- additional reagents for post column derivatisation for improving hplc sensitivity and/or specificity
NMR	- Direct identification of drug metabolites in biological fluids
Chemical spot tests	- Development of additional reagents to identify promptly particular functional groups in metabolites
Immunoassays	- Use for rapid field/bedside analysis of environmental/body fluid samples for levels of a chemical
Sampling	- Drug and metabolite analysis by non invasive means eg sampling of saliva, sweat, expired air
Spectrophotrometry	- Improved sensitivity of various spectrophotometric techniques. Use of computerised data banks of spectra for rapid matching

Enantiomers

Many drugs and other chemicals exist as enantiomers eg. propanalol, atenolol, verapimil, amphetamine, buprofen, quinine, phenytoin, promethazine, S-carboxymethylcysteine. Others undergo stereoselective metabolism to form a particular isomeric form. Because in a number of instances

one isomer is found to have quite different pharmacological
or toxicological properties from the other there is likely
to be an increasing requirement to measure separately each
enantiomeric form appearing in tissue fluids. Most of the
available methods have been devised for rather polar
natural products such as amino acids. Progress in this
area depends on development of either more specific chiral
columns/plates for hplc, glc and tlc and/or on the
introduction of enantiomeric derivatisation agents
(Stevenson and Bridges 1986).

In Vivo Distribution of Drugs

To date studies of the in vivo distribution of drugs
have relied almost entirely on noncontinuous invasive
methods such as blood and tissue sampling and whole body
autoradiography. Newly emerging techniques such as whole
body NMR offer the prospect of being able to monitor
continuously the distribution of some drugs directly (eg.
those either bearing a fluorine or phosphorus label or into
which such a label can be inserted). For some others it
may be possible to determine drug distribution through
their effects on cellular biochemistry (eg. in ATP or
creatine phosphate levels) (Gordon 1985). An illustration
of the very considerable potential of whole body NMR both
for animal and human subjects is provided by a study by
Stevens et al (1984) on the uptake of 5-fluorouracil into
the livers of mice. By monitoring the F signal they were
able to not only follow the loss of 5-fluorouracil but also
the rise in the levels of various metabolites and
incorporation of 5-fluorouracil into deoxynucleotides. The
profile with time of changes in metabolites indicated that
degradation of 5 fluorouracil proceeds by reduction of the
pyrimidine ring then hydrolysis to fluoro-β-ureidopropionic
acid which is subsequently hydrolysed to fluoro-β-alanine.

Drug Conjugates

Techniques for identifying drug conjugates with one or
two notable exceptions have lagged well behind those for
phase 1 metabolities. In part this can be ascribed to the
fact that conjugates are commonly poorly, if at all,
extracted by most organic solvents. Many conjugates are
almost certainly simply not recognised because of this.
The problem may be tackled in a number of ways including
direct structural determination without sample work up (eg.
NMR analysis of urine), use of affinity columns
incorporating antibodies to particular types of conjugate
and increasing availability of specific hydrolytic enzymes
for particular conjugates (a consequence of the continuing

success in isolating individual drug metabolising enzymes). The increasing availability of purified drug metabolising enzymes is also of course of great assistance in the production of compounds as references for putative metabolites. It is likely that in many cases improved stability can be achieved by binding the enzymes to a solid support perhaps in combination with the appropriate cofactor regenerating system.

Xenobiotic Residues on Macromolecules

Toxicity often arises through the covalent binding of reactive metabolites of xenobiotics to cellular nucleic acids or proteins. Identification of the nature of the xenobiotic residue and its site of binding may be of considerable value in understanding the mechanisms involved and predicting hazard to man. In addition monitoring of residues in biological fluids may be used as a means of assessing exposure to reactive substances or the ability of an animal to form reactive metabolites. For example exposure to methylating agents can be monitored either by the formation of S-methylcysteine in haemoglobin or by the appearance of N-7-methylguanine in urine (Farmer et al 1986a). Haemoglobin adducts of various kinds have been studied extensively and their formation has been shown to be proportional to exposure for a wide variety of chemical carcinogens (Neumann 1984). Adducts of this kind have the additional advantage that they are fairly easy to isolate and are stable with a lifetime as long as haemoglobin itself. In animals, monitoring adducts in biological fluids has the advantage that appearance of residues with time can be determined without sacrifice of the animals. However perhaps the most important value of monitoring such adducts is in assessing exposure of man to certain chemicals (eg. ethylene oxide, vinylchloride) in the workplace (see Table 2). It is notable that some residues occur in apparently non-exposed individuals. This implies that alkylating arises from a number of environmental sources and/or as a consequence of normal intermediary metabolism. Monitoring is presently conducted using glc-mass spectrometry; although this is likely to continue to be of major value as a primary standardisation method, for routine monitoring purposes it will be replaced by assays based on the use of adduct specific antibodies.

BIOLOGICAL ASPECTS

To date the advances in the chemical aspects of drug metabolism have greatly outstripped the more biological

Table 2. Degree of alkylation of haemoglobin from ethylene
oxide exposed workers and controls

Exposed level	Hydroxyethyl valine (n mol/g Hb)	Hydroxethyl histidine (n mol/g Hb)
High	1.5, 7.7	2.0, 8.0
Low	0.3, 0.4	0.55, 1.0
Controls	0.03, 0.14	0.53, 0.69

From Farmer et al. 1986b

ones. Fundamental questions on the physiological functions
in different organs and regulation mechanisms for
individual drug metabolising enzymes are far from being
resolved. Nonetheless considerable advances have been
made. Techniques for preparing isolated hepatocytes, cell
fractions and purified enzymes are widely used in
laboratories working in drug metabolism and a number are
now introducing the tools of classical molecular biology
with considerable success. The growing pressures to reduce
the use of animals in laboratory experiments will hopefully
encourage further sophistication of the in vitro biological
models which are used (Bridges et al 1983). Despite the
interest in the isolation and primary culture of cells
progress in a number of rather basic areas is still needed,
for example reliable storage techniques have still not been
devised for liver cells; techniques for the isolation of
particular cell types from non-rodent species and from
extrahepatic tissues are as yet not readily transferable
between laboratories and systems for stabilizing drug
metabolising enzyme activity in cells at levels typical of
the in vivo situation remain unsuitable for many
experimental purposes.
    Other needs which hopefully will be fulfilled in the
near future are the availability of more specific subtrates
and inhibitors for individual isoforms of the principal
drug metabolising enzymes and the development of methods
for determining the levels and activities of individual
drug metabolising enzymes in intact cells. In the longer
term the development of in vivo and in vitro preparations
which have been adapted by genetic manipulation to express
or omit a particular drug metabolising activity is a most

exciting prospect.

Specific substrates and inhibitors

More specific substrates and inhibitors of the drug metabolising enzymes are needed for a number of purposes, for example to screen and compare biological preparations for their content of individual isoforms of particular drug metabolising enzymes, to identify the role of a particular isoform in forming a metabolite or in causing toxicity and to investigate mechanisms for the regulation of enzyme activity. Ideally such specific substrates and inhibitors should be utilisable in both in vitro and in vivo investigations. Use of chemically related series of substrates (eg. alkoxyresorufins - M.D. Burke, this volume) has shown considerable promise in studies on individual isoforms of P450 but progress on development of specific substrates and inhibitors for other enzymes is disappointing. Selective inhibitors for oxidative and reductive enzymes likely to be involved in reactive metabolite formation would be particular valuable.

Cellular location and activity of drug metabolising enzymes

The very considerable success in purifying individual drug metabolising enzyme isoforms opens the prospect of widely available specific antibodies to each isoform. The use of labelled antibodies has already proved of considerable value in identifying the distribution of individual drug metabolising enzymes in different cell types and different tissues. However this technique is often misused either through failure to use suitable controls or through inappropriate extension of applications to different species. Development of methods for the quantitation of the extent of immunostaining would considerably enhance the usefulness of the technique. Immunostaining determines total enzyme rather than enzyme activity in fixed tissue. Methods are also needed to measure the activity of individual enzymes in intact cells. Microdensitometry (or microfluorimetry) using colorogenic (or fluorogenic) reagents (Pattison et al 1979) and/or following the spectral changes when substrates interact with P450 are promising approaches. For example the conversion of isosafrole to a carbene metabolite which binds covalently to P450 can be followed by microdensitometry. (Connelly, 1983). Also the capacity of different inducing agents to induce P450 in different regions of a tissue can be followed. Figure 1 illustrates the effect of pretreatment of rats with isosafrole on the distribution of P450 in the liver lobule. It emphasised

Figure 1. Distribution of amplitude of absorbance due to
an isosafrole metabolite: cytochrome P-450 complex across a
lobule of the hepatic median lobe of a male rat pretreated
with isosafrole

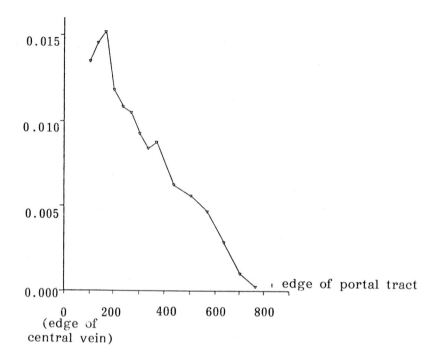

Male rats were pretreated with isosafrole, 0.93mmol/kg in
corn oil daily by i.p injection for 3 days. The
distribution of cytochrome P-450 was measured in a fresh,
frozen section of liver median lobe. The concentration of
cytochrome P-450 was expressed as the absorbance ($A_{455-490}$)
due to an isosafrole metabolite: reduced cytochrome P-450
complex.
(from Connelly, 1983)

the point that morphologically identical cells can differ
markedly in their drug metabolising capability.
Development of colorogenic and fluorogenic agents for the
quantification of individual drug metabolising enzymes
within cells is still in its infancy although several
promising reagents are emerging. This is another area
where the development of more selective inhibitors to
individual enzymes (see above) would be most useful in

order to block alternative or sequential pathways for the metabolism of the substrate.

Genetic manipulation

The techniques of molecular biology have many potentially very important applications to drug metabolism studies. For example at the cellular level it is now feasible to introduce the gene for a particular drug metabolising enzyme in an otherwise non metabolising cell thereby providing a specific model system to assess the relationship between metabolism by that enzyme and toxicity. In a more general application it ought to be possible to develop new cell lines for toxicity testing in which many human derived drug metabolising enzymes are introduced into a particular cell type which manifests a precise endpoint of toxicity. Incorporation into rapidly growing cell lines would be particularly useful. In man such techniques should enable ready typing of individuals for their drug metabolising enzyme profile and allow deficiencies of certain drug metabolising enzymes in at risk groups of the population to be compensated for (eg. Gilberts Syndrome in which there is a deficiency of glucuronyl transferase). Such techniques are likely to prove invaluable too in studying the regulation of individual drug metabolising enzymes. Outside the conventional areas of drug metabolism, cell based, or even cell free systems might be developed to produce particular enzymes on a considerable scale for use in the manufacture of particular chemicals or as a means of removing organic contaminants from important materials.

Other in vitro needs

If in vitro systems are to be used more extensively as a replacement for in vivo methods, means must be found to simulate more effectively in vivo pharmacokinetics in vitro (Bridges et al 1983). This will require for example devises for non continuous exposure to drugs and the resultant metabolites without coexposure of cells to significant levels of organic solvents. The development of computer controlled mimicking of in vivo conditions could also be an important contribution to this goal.

In vivo techniques

For the foreseeable future in vivo models will be necessary for a number of purposes. More effective use of the animals which have to be used is important. This includes selection of conditions for studying metabolism

and pharmacokinetics which are more relevant to the human
exposure situation, improved microsampling techniques for
biological fluids to reduce the need for animal sacrifice
and the more widespread introduction of non invasive
methods (see above). In addition new animal models are
required for certain purposes. For example germ free
rodents have proved very useful in assessing the
contribution of gut microflora to drug metabolism.
However, there are a number of important differences
between the gut microflora of rodents and man. A promising
means of overcoming this difficulty is to establish human
gut microflora in the intestines of germ free rodents
(Chnassia et al 1975). Improved microsurgical technique to
enable direct infusion and/or sampling of the drug
metabolites reaching particular organs would also on
occasion be of great utility.

Computer modelling and data banks

Although there are a very large number of good quality
published papers and unpublished reports in the field of
drug metabolism and pharmacokinetics, over the next few
years the information must be brought together into a
single, properly validated, data bank. If this could be
achieved there would be many great benefits. In scientific
terms it would serve particularly to identify clear cut
structure activity relationships, draw attention to
anomaflies in data and priorities for further
investigation. In toxicity tests, predictive computer
modelling based on such a data bank would enable
optimisation of metabolising systems for each chemical in
short term in vitro tests for toxicity.

CONCLUSIONS

A number of new techniques and important improvements
in existing ones are finding their place in drug metabolism
and pharmacokinetic investigations. There is every reason
to believe that significant progress in this area will
continue steadily.

The tools of molecular biology in particular are
expected to make a dramatic impact on the identification of
the role of individual enzymes in toxicity, in the
development of new cell lines for toxicity testing and in
typing and making good enzyme deficiences in man.

Increasing sophistication of measuring devices is
likely to enhance our knowledge of the interactions of
chemicals and their metabolites with biological components

at the molecular level. It should also greatly assist in the development of non-invasive means for investigating drug metabolism and pharmacokinetics in vivo and in intact tissues and cells.

REFERENCES

Bridges, J.W. Chasseaud, L.F. Cohen, G.M. and Walker,C.H. (1983) in "Animals and alternatives in toxicity testing" (Eds M. Balls, R.J. Riddell and A.N.Worden) Academic Press, London and New York, p31

Chnassia, J.C. Veron, M. Ducluzeau, R. Muller, M.C. and Raibaud, P. (1975) Ann. Microbiol. (Inst. Pasteur) 126B, 367

Connelly, J.C. (1983) PhD Thesis University of Surrey

Farmer, P.B. Schuler, D.E.G and Bird. I (1986a) Carcinogenesis 7, 49

Farmer, P.B. Bailey, E. Gorf, S.M. Tornquist, M. Osterman-Golkar, S. Kautiainen, A. and Lewis-Enright, D.P. (1986b) Carcinogenesis 7, 637

Gordon, R.E. (1985) Physics in medicine and biology 30 (8) 741

Neumann, H.G. (1984)Arch Toxicol 56, 1

Pattison, J.R. Bitensky, L. and Chayen, J. (1979) eds Quantitative Cytochemistry and its Applications Academic Press, London

Stevens, A.N. Morris, P.G. Iles, R.A. Sheldon, P.W. and Griffiths, J.R. (1984) Brit. J. Cancer. 50, 113

Stevenson, D. and Bridges, J.W. (1986) in "Analytical Methods in Human Toxicology" Part 2 (ed Carry, A.S.) MacMillan London, p1

INDEX